**Vascular and
Endovascular Surgery**

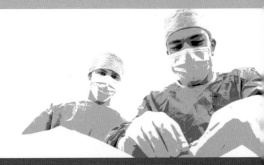

A COMPANION TO SPECIALIST SURGICAL PRACTICE

Series Editors

O. James Garden
Simon Paterson-Brown

Vascular and Endovascular Surgery

FIFTH EDITION

Edited by

Jonathan D. Beard
ChM MEd FRCS

Consultant Vascular Surgeon, The Sheffield Vascular Institute;
Professor of Surgical Education, The University of Sheffield, UK

Peter A. Gaines
FRCP FRCR

Consultant Vascular Radiologist, The Sheffield Vascular Institute;
Professor of Radiology, Sheffield Hallam University, UK

Ian Loftus
MD FRCS

Consultant Vascular Surgeon, St George's Vascular Institute and Reader,
St George's University of London, UK

Edinburgh London New York Oxford Philadelphia St Louis Sydney Toronto 2014

SAUNDERS
ELSEVIER

First edition 1997
Second edition 2001
Third edition 2005
Fourth edition 2009
Fifth edition 2014

ISBN 978-0-7020-4958-3
e-book ISBN 978-0-7020-4966-8

British Library Cataloguing in Publication Data
A catalogue record for this book is available from the British Library

Library of Congress Cataloging in Publication Data
A catalog record for this book is available from the Library of Congress

Notices

ELSEVIER your source for books, journals and multimedia in the health sciences

www.elsevierhealth.com

  Working together to grow libraries in developing countries

www.elsevier.com • www.bookaid.org

The Publisher's policy is to use paper manufactured from sustainable forests

Printed in China

Commissioning Editor: Laurence Hunter
Development Editor: Lynn Watt
Project Manager: Vinod Kumar Iyyappan
Designer/Design Direction: Miles Hitchen
Illustration Manager: Jennifer Rose
Illustrator: Antbits Ltd

Contents

Contents

Contributors

Gillian Atkinson, MCSP
Clinical Specialist Physiotherapist (Amputees),
Mobility and Specialised Rehabilitation Centre,
Northern General Hospital, Sheffield, UK

Jonathan D. Beard, BSc, ChM, MEd, FRCS
Consultant Vascular Surgeon, The Sheffield Vascular
Institute; Professor of Surgical Education, The
University of Sheffield, Sheffield, UK

Jill J.F. Belch, MBChB, MD, FRCP(Glasg),
FRCP(Ed), FRCP
Co-Director, Medical Research Institute; Head, The
Institute of Cardiovascular Research, University of
Dundee, Institute of Cardiovascular Research (TICR),
Division of Cardiovascular & Diabetes Medicine,
Medical Research Institute, Ninewells, Dundee, UK

John R. Bottomley, MBChB, FRANZCR
Endovascular Specialist, Centre for Advanced
Interventional Radiology, North Shore Hospital,
Auckland, New Zealand

Julie Brittenden, MD, FRCS
Professor in Vascular Surgery, Division of Applied
Medicine, University of Aberdeen, Aberdeen, UK

Peter W.G. Brown, BSc, MBChB, FRCS(Ed),
FRCR
Consultant Radiologist, Department of Diagnostic
Imaging, Northern General Hospital, Sheffield, UK

Jan Brunkwall, MD, PhD
Professor and Chairman, Department of Vascular
Surgery, University Clinics, University of Cologne,
Cologne, Germany

Kelly Cheer, MD
Specialty Trainee in Diabetes and Endocrinology,
Tameside Hospital NHS Foundation Trust,
Ashton-under-Lyne, UK

Nicholas J. Cheshire, MD FRCS
Vascular Surgery Research Group, Imperial College,
London, UK

Trevor Cleveland, BMedSci, BMBS, FRCS, FRCR
Consultant Vascular Radiologist, Sheffield Vascular
Institute, Northern General Hospital, Sheffield, UK

Alan G. Dawson, MBChB, BSc (Hons)
Foundation Year Two Doctor, Department of Vascular
Surgery, Aberdeen Royal Infirmary, Aberdeen, UK

Alun H. Davies, MA, DM, FRCS, FHEA, FEBVS,
FACPh
Professor of Vascular Surgery, Honorary Consultant
Surgeon, Head of Academic Section of Vascular
Surgery, Faculty of Medicine Imperial College School
of Medicine; Charing Cross Hospital, London, UK

Richard Donnelly, MBChB(Hons), MD, PhD,
FRCP, FRACP
Professor of Vascular Medicine, University of
Nottingham; Honorary Consultant Physician, Royal
Derby Hospital, Derby, UK

Mark O. Downes, MBBS, DMRD, FRCR
Consultant Vascular/Interventional Radiologist,
Kent and Canterbury Hospital, East Kent Hospitals
University Foundation Trust, Canterbury, UK

Peter A. Gaines, FRCP, FRCR
Consultant Vascular Radiologist, The Sheffield
Vascular Institute; Professor of Radiology, Sheffield
Hallam University, Sheffield, UK

Michael Gawenda, MD, PhD
Professor of Surgery, Vice Chair of the Department
of Vascular Surgery, University of Cologne, Cologne,
Germany

Manjit S. Gohel, MD, FRCS, FEBVS
Cambridge Vascular Unit, Addenbrooke's Hospital &
Imperial College, London, UK

Edward B. Jude, MBBS, MD, MRCP
Consultant Physician and Honorary Reader in
Medicine, Tameside Hospital NHS Foundation
Trust and University of Manchester,
Ashton-under-Lyne, UK

Contributors

Robert Kaikini, BMBCh, MRCP, FRCR
East Kent Hospitals University NHS Foundation Trust,
Canterbury, UK

Robert J. Hinchliffe, MD, FRCS
Senior Lecturer and Honorary Consultant Vascular
Surgeon, St George's Vascular Institute,
London, UK

James E. Jackson, FRCP, FRCR
Consultant Radiologist, Department of Imaging,
Imperial College Healthcare NHS Trust,
Hammersmith Hospital, London, UK

Matthew A. Lambert, MBChB, MRCP
Clinical Lecturer, University of Dundee,
Institute of Cardiovascular Research (TICR),
Division of Cardiovascular & Diabetes Medicine,
Medical Research Institute, Ninewells, Dundee, UK

Johannes Lammer, MD
Professor of Radiology; Director of
the Division of Cardiovascular and Interventional
Radiology; Vice Chairman of the Department of
Radiology, Medical University of Vienna,
Vienna, Austria

Timothy A. Lees, MBChB, FRCS, MD
Consultant Vascular Surgeon, Northern Vascular
Centre, Freeman Hospital, Newcastle upon
Tyne, UK

**Sumaira Macdonald, MBChB, FRCP, FRCR,
PhD, EBIR**
Consultant Vascular Radiologist, Department
of Interventional Radiology, Freeman Hospital,
Newcastle upon Tyne, UK

**Jacobus van Marle, MBChB, MMed (Surg),
FCS(SA)**
Professor of Vascular Surgery, Department of
Surgery, University of Pretoria, Pretoria,
South Africa

David C. Mitchell, MA, MBBS, MS, FRCS
Department of Surgery, Southmead Hospital
North Bristol NHS Trust, Bristol, UK

Robert Morgan, MBChB, MRCP, FRCR, EBIR
Consultant Vascular and Interventional Radiologist,
Radiology Department, St George's NHS Trust,
London

Jonathan G. Moss, MB ChB, FRCS, FRCR, EBIR
Interventional Radiology Unit, Gartnavel General
Hospital, Glasgow, UK

Ramesh Munjal, MS, FRCS
Consultant and Clinical Lead Neurological and Amputee
Rehabilitation, Mobility and Specialised Rehabilitation
Centre, Sheffield Teaching Hospitals, Sheffield, UK

A. Ross Naylor, MD, FRCS
Professor of Vascular Surgery, Vascular Surgery
Group, Division of Cardiovascular Sciences,
Leicester Royal Infirmary, Leicester, UK

**Anthony Nicholson, MSc, FRCR, FFRRCSI(Hon),
EBIR**
Consultant Interventional Radiologist, Department
of Radiology, Leeds Teaching Hospital NHS Trust,
Leeds, UK

Ian Nordon, MSc, MD, FRCS
Consultant Vascular Surgeon, Southampton General
Hospital, Southampton, UK

Janet T. Powell, MD, PhD, FRCPath
Professor of Vascular Biology, Department of
Vascular Surgery, Imperial College, London, UK

Jean-Baptiste Ricco, MD, PhD
Professor of Vascular Surgery, University Hospital
Jean Bernard, University of Poitiers, Poitiers, France

John D. Rose, FRCR
Consultant Interventional Radiologist, Department
of Clinical Radiology, Freeman Hospital, Newcastle
upon Tyne, UK

Dirk A. le Roux, MBChB, FCS(SA), CVS(SA)
Consultant Vascular Surgeon, Department of
Surgery, University of Witwatersrand, Johannesburg,
South Africa

Fabrice Schneider, MD, PhD
Consultant in Vascular Surgery,
University Hospital Jean Bernard, University of
Poitiers, Poitiers, France

**Julian Scott, MD, MBChB, FRCS, FRCSEd,
FEBVS**
Professor of Vascular Surgery, University of Leeds;
Consultant Vascular Surgeon, Leeds Vascular
Institute, Leeds General Infirmary, Leeds, UK

Cliff Shearman, BSc, MBBS, FRCS, MS
Professor of Vascular Surgery, Department of
Vascular Surgery, University Hospital Southampton
Foundation Trust, Southampton, UK

Henrik Sillesen, MD, DMSc
Chairman, Vascular Surgery, Rigshospitalet,
Copenhagen, Denmark

Rob H.W. Strijkers, MD
PhD-candidate, Venous Surgery, Maastricht University
Medical Center, Maastricht, The Netherlands

Matthew Thompson, MA, MBBS, MD, FRCS
Professor of Vascular Surgery, University of London;
Consultant Vascular Surgeon, St George's Vascular
Institute, St George's Healthcare NHS Trust,
London, UK

Hazel Trender, RGN, RM
Vascular Nurse Specialist, Sheffield Vascular Institute,
Sheffield Teaching Hospitals NHS Foundation Trust,
Northern General Hospital,
Sheffield, UK

Cees H.A. Wittens, MD, PhD
Professor of Venous Surgery, Head of Venous
Surgery, Maastricht University Medical Center,
Maastricht, The Netherlands

Michael G. Wyatt, MBBS, MSc (Med. Sci.) MD,
FRCS, FRCSEd (ad hom), FEBVS
Consultant Vascular Surgeon and Honorary Reader,
Northern Vascular Centre, Freeman Hospital,
Newcastle upon Tyne, UK

Series Editors' preface

It is now some 17 years since the first edition of the *Companion to Specialist Surgical Practice* series was published. We set ourselves the task of meeting the educational needs of surgeons in the later years of specialist surgical training and of consultant surgeons in independent practice who wished for contemporary, evidence-based information on the subspecialist areas relevant to their general surgical practice. The series was never intended to replace the larger reference surgical textbooks which, although valuable in their own way, struggle to keep pace with changing surgical practice. This Fifth Edition has also had to contend with increasing specialisation in 'general' surgery. The rise of minimal access surgery and therapy, and the desire of some subspecialties such as breast and vascular surgery to separate away from 'general surgery', may have proved challenging in some countries but has also served to emphasise the importance of all surgeons being aware of current developments in their surgical field. As in previous editions, there has been increasing emphasis on evidence-based practice and contributors have endeavoured to provide key recommendations within each chapter. The eBook versions of the textbook have also allowed the technophile improved access to key data and content within each chapter.

We remain indebted to the volume editors and all the contributors of this Fifth Edition. We have endeavoured where possible to bring in new blood to freshen content. We are impressed by the enthusiasm, commitment and hard work that our contributors and editorial team have shown and this has ensured a short turnover between editions while maintaining as accurate and up-to-date content as is possible. We remain grateful for the support and encouragement of Laurence Hunter and Lynn Watt at Elsevier Ltd. We trust that our original vision of delivering an up-to-date affordable text has been met and that readers, whether in training or independent practice, will find this Fifth Edition an invaluable resource.

O. James Garden, BSc, MBChB, MD, FRCS(Glas), FRCS(Ed), FRCP(Ed), FRACS(Hon), FRCSC(Hon), FRSE
Regius Professor of Clinical Surgery, Clinical Surgery School of Clinical Sciences, The University of Edinburgh and Honorary Consultant Surgeon, Royal Infirmary of Edinburgh

Simon Paterson-Brown, MBBS, MPhil, MS, FRCS(Ed), FRCS(Engl), FCS(HK)
Honorary Senior Lecturer, Clinical Surgery School of Clinical Sciences, The University of Edinburgh and Consultant General and Upper Gastrointestinal Surgeon, Royal Infirmary of Edinburgh

Editors' preface

Vascular and Endovascular Surgery is designed to be a comprehensive and affordable textbook for all those involved with the management of patients with vascular disease, whether they be trainees, vascular or non-vascular specialists, or other healthcare professionals. A modern Vascular Service encompasses many disciplines, and success depends upon a team approach. Whilst the vascular surgeon often remains in overall charge of the patient, management frequently involves vascular nurse specialists, angiologists and interventional radiologists. Other clinicians who may be involved with the management of these patients include diabetologists, neurologists, rheumatologists and haematologists. Physiotherapists and other rehabilitation specialists are also vital for successful patient outcomes. Our choice of authors for this Fifth Edition reflects this multidisciplinary diversity.

Since the structure of the Fourth Edition proved popular, many of the chapters from the Fourth Edition have been retained and extensively revised in line with recently published evidence. The continued move towards non-invasive imaging, medical therapy and endovascular techniques is reflected in the content of this book. For this reason, we have also introduced a new chapter on Future Developments.

To reflect the collaborative nature of a modern vascular service, many of the chapters are co-authored by a vascular surgeon and a vascular radiologist. We have continued to expand our authorship to include more European and World experts with an emphasis on global practice. We are grateful to all our authors for the hard work that they have put into their respective chapters.

This is the last edition of the book that will be edited by ourselves before we retire from clinical practice. We are delighted to welcome Ian Loftus, Consultant Vascular Surgeon at St George's Hospital London, to the editorial team for this volume. Ian will take over as Editor for the 6th Edition in collaboration with a new Vascular Radiologist. We wish them well for future editions of this successful textbook.

Jonathan D. Beard
Peter A. Gaines
Sheffield

Evidence-based practice in surgery

Critical appraisal for developing evidence-based practice can be obtained from a number of sources, the most reliable being randomised controlled clinical trials, systematic literature reviews, meta-analyses and observational studies. For practical purposes three grades of evidence can be used, analogous to the levels of 'proof' required in a court of law:

1. **Beyond all reasonable doubt.** Such evidence is likely to have arisen from high-quality randomised controlled trials, systematic reviews or high-quality synthesised evidence such as decision analysis, cost-effectiveness analysis or large observational datasets. The studies need to be directly applicable to the population of concern and have clear results. The grade is analogous to burden of proof within a criminal court and may be thought of as corresponding to the usual standard of 'proof' within the medical literature (i.e. $P<0.05$).

2. **On the balance of probabilities.** In many cases a high-quality review of literature may fail to reach firm conclusions due to conflicting or inconclusive results, trials of poor methodological quality or the lack of evidence in the population to which the guidelines apply. In such cases it may still be possible to make a statement as to the best treatment on the 'balance of probabilities'. This is analogous to the decision in a civil court where all the available evidence will be weighed up and the verdict will depend upon the balance of probabilities.

3. **Not proven.** Insufficient evidence upon which to base a decision, or contradictory evidence.

Depending on the information available, three grades of recommendation can be used:

a. Strong recommendation, which should be followed unless there are compelling reasons to act otherwise.

b. A recommendation based on evidence of effectiveness, but where there may be other factors to take into account in decision-making, for example the user of the guidelines may be expected to take into account patient preferences, local facilities, local audit results or available resources.

c. A recommendation made where there is no adequate evidence as to the most effective practice, although there may be reasons for making a recommendation in order to minimise cost or reduce the chance of error through a locally agreed protocol.

> ✓ Evidence where a conclusion might be reached **'on the balance of probabilities'** and where there may be other factors involved which influence the recommendation given. This will normally be based on less conclusive evidence than that represented by the double tick icons:
> • III. Evidence from non-experimental descriptive studies, such as comparative studies and case–control studies
> • IV. Evidence from expert committee reports or opinions or clinical experience of respected authorities, or both.

> ✓✓ Evidence where a conclusion can be reached **'beyond all reasonable doubt'** and therefore where a **strong recommendation** can be given.
> This will normally be based on evidence levels:
> • Ia. Meta-analysis of randomised controlled trials
> • Ib. Evidence from at least one randomised controlled trial
> • IIa. Evidence from at least one controlled study without randomisation
> • IIb. Evidence from at least one other type of quasi-experimental study.

Evidence which is associated with either a **strong recommendation** or **expert opinion** is highlighted in the text in panels such as those shown above, and is distinguished by either a double or single tick icon, respectively. The references associated with double-tick evidence are highlighted in the reference lists at the end of each chapter along with a short summary of the paper's conclusions where applicable.

The reader is referred to Chapter 1, 'Evidence-based practice in surgery' in the volume, *Core Topics in General and Emergency Surgery* of this series, for a more detailed description of this topic.

Further reading

The compact format of this book means that it cannot cover every detail of vascular and endovascular surgery, diagnostic imaging and vascular medicine. The books listed below will provide more detail when required.

General vascular

Vascular surgery, 7th edn
Cronenwett JL, Johnson W (eds).
WB Saunders, 2010.
The 'bible' of Vascular Surgery. Encyclopaedic (2 volumes), but expensive, with a strong North American influence.

Comprehensive vascular and endovascular surgery, 2nd edn
Hallet JW, Mills JL, Earnshaw JJ, Reekers JA, Rooke T (eds). Mosby, 2009.
A comprehensive textbook with a transatlantic flavour. Excellent colour illustrations and diagrams.

Atlas of vascular surgery, 2nd edn
Zarins CK, Gewertz BL (eds). Elsevier Churchill Livingstone, 2009.
Clear line diagrams of vascular and endovascular techniques and exposures. A good companion to *Vascular and endovascular surgery.*

Complications in vascular and endovascular surgery
Earnshaw JJ, Wyatt MG (eds). tfm Publishing, 2011.
A useful and affordable guide on avoiding complications and getting out of trouble.

Rare vascular disorders

Eanshaw J, Parvin SD (eds). tfm Publishing, 2005.
A well-illustrated and practical guide for all vascular specialists, covering a host of unusual conditions.

Imaging

Introduction to vascular sonography, 5th edn
Zweibel W (ed.). WB Saunders, 2005.

CT and MR angiography: comprehensive vascular assessment
Rubin GD, Rofsky NM (eds). Lippincott Williams & Wilkins, 2008.

Abrams' angiography: interventional radiology, 2nd edn
Baum S, Pentecost MJ (eds). Lippincott Williams & Wilkins, 2006.

Specialist

Mechanisms of vascular disease: a textbook for vascular surgeons
Fitridge R, Thompson M (eds). Cambridge University Press, 2007.
A good reference book on vascular science and medicine.

Recent advances in thrombosis and haemostasis
Tanaka K, Davie EW (eds). Springer, 2008.

The foot in diabetes, 4th edn
Boulton AJM, Cavanagh PR, Rayman G (eds). Wiley, 2006.

Atlas of amputations and limb deficiencies
Smith DG, Michael JW, Bowker JH (eds). American Academy of Orthopaedic Surgeons, 2004.

The vein book
Bergan JJ (ed.). Elsevier, 2007.

Websites

Books can become outdated, which is why *Vascular and endovascular surgery* is published frequently in an affordable format. Websites and Journals provide up-to-the-minute information on recent trials and technological developments, as well as news of meetings and courses. A few of the more useful websites are listed below.

American Board of Surgery: http://home.absurgery.org/default.jsp?index
American Venous Forum: http://www.venous-info.com
British Society of Interventional Radiology: http://www.bsir.org
Cardiovascular and Interventional Radiological Society of Europe: http://www.cirse.org
European Board of Vascular Surgery: http://www.uemsvascular.com
European Journal of Vascular and Endovascular Surgery: http://www.sciencedirect.com/esvs

Further reading

European Society for Vascular Surgery:
http://www.esvs.org
Vascular Education online learning:
vasculareducation.com
European Venous Forum:
http://www.europeanvenousforum.org

Society for Vascular Surgery (North America):
http://www.vascularweb.org
Vascular Society of Great Britain and Ireland:
http://www.vascularsociety.org.uk

1

Epidemiology and risk factor management of peripheral arterial disease

Richard Donnelly
Janet T. Powell

Introduction

Atherosclerotic peripheral arterial disease (PAD) involving one or more major vessels of the lower limb is common, especially in older patients, due to complex genetic and environmental interactions that result in structural and functional vascular abnormalities and reduced blood flow. PAD may be asymptomatic in the early stages, but is always associated with shortened survival due to the invariable association with atherosclerosis in other arterial territories, especially the coronary, carotid and cerebral circulation. This is highlighted by observational studies showing that reduced ankle–brachial pressure index (ABPI, a marker of disease severity in PAD) is associated with an increased risk of cardiovascular mortality (Table 1.1).[1] However, calcification and sclerosis lead to incompressible arteries, with false elevation of ABPI even in the presence of major distal atherosclerosis. The Strong Heart Study has identified associations between low (<0.90) and high (>1.40) ABPI and increased risk of all-cause and cardiovascular (CV) disease mortality, reporting a U-shaped relationship between a non-invasive measure of PAD and reduced life expectancy (**Fig. 1.1**).[2] For example, adjusted risk estimates for all-cause mortality were 1.69 for low and 1.77 for high ABPI, while the corresponding estimates for CV disease mortality were 2.52 and 2.09.[2]

This chapter considers the epidemiology of PAD, the observational studies identifying reversible and irreversible risk factors for disease progression, and

Table 1.1 • Adjusted relative risk for mortality for levels of ankle–brachial pressure index (ABPI)

ABPI	Relative risk	95% CI	P value
<0.4	3.35	2.16–5.20	<0.001
0.4–0.85	2.02	1.34–3.02	<0.001
>0.85	1.00	Reference	

From McKenna M, Wolfson S, Kuller L. The ratio of ankle and arm arterial pressure as an independent predictor of mortality. Atherosclerosis 1991; 87:119–28. With permission from Elsevier.

the evidence from randomised controlled trials that underpins clinical use of disease-modifying therapies as part of multiple risk factor intervention.

Epidemiology of PAD

Obtaining accurate figures for the prevalence and incidence of PAD has not been straightforward. For example, several epidemiological studies have focused on specific groups, e.g. in the workplace setting or referrals to hospital, which may not be truly representative of the wider population. Thus, workplace screening studies for PAD have excluded those who have retired and those who may be unfit for work. Similarly, epidemiological studies based on inpatient or outpatient referrals tend to underestimate the prevalence of PAD in the community. One of the largest and most reliable sources of information about the overall prevalence of symptomatic and asymptomatic PAD is the Edinburgh Artery Study, which screened large random samples of the general population using age/sex registers from general practices.[3,4]

1

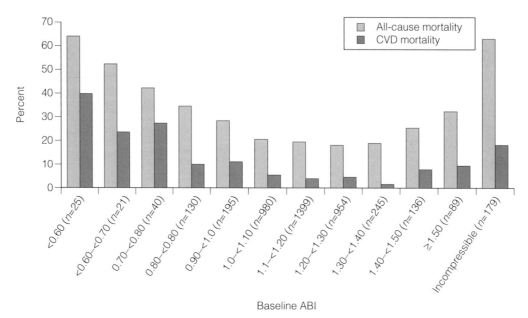

Figure 1.1 • Relationship between ABPI (ankle–brachial pressure index) and survival in patients in the Strong Heart Study.[2] There is a U-shaped relationship such that both low (<0.9) and high (>1.4) ABPI is associated with increased risk of CV and all-cause mortality.

Investigative techniques for epidemiological screening

Clearly, the technique used to establish the presence or absence of PAD will also affect the results of epidemiological surveys. Questionnaires have often been used to establish the nature and severity of symptomatic PAD, e.g. the WHO/Rose questionnaire designed in 1962. The original questionnaire developed by Rose was shown to be highly sensitive but only moderately specific, and therefore in 1985 the tool was modified in a way that increased the specificity, albeit at the expense of a small decrease in sensitivity.[5] The Edinburgh Artery Questionnaire is designed to be self-administered and has a sensitivity of 91% and a specificity of 99% for symptoms of PAD.[6] In general, all questionnaires appear to underestimate the true prevalence of intermittent claudication and the Transatlantic Inter-Society Consensus (TASC) group recommend great caution in interpreting epidemiological studies of symptomatic PAD based solely on questionnaires.

Physical examination to establish the presence or absence of peripheral pulses has also been used in epidemiological surveys to confirm a history of intermittent claudication. However, the absence of a peripheral pulse is not necessarily due to PAD, and at least one pulse may be undetectable in up to 10% of the adult population even though only 3% have symptomatic arterial disease.[7]

Establishing the prevalence of asymptomatic PAD in the general population is equally important. The most useful non-invasive test for this purpose is the ABPI, which is quick and painless and has excellent sensitivity and specificity. An ABPI <0.9 is 95% sensitive and 100% specific for detecting angiogram-positive disease.[8] At the more severe end of the spectrum, most of the data on the prevalence of critical limb ischaemia has been obtained from inpatient records, and only rarely from population-based studies or using ABPI criteria.

Prevalence and incidence of PAD

Evidence from epidemiological studies using ABPI suggests that the prevalence of asymptomatic PAD in the middle-aged and elderly population is around 7–15%.[3,9] However, in the British Regional Heart Study, direct assessment of the femoral artery with ultrasound found that 64% of people aged 56–77 years had significant femoral atherosclerosis and only 10% of these were symptomatic.[10] Autopsy studies have found similar results, suggesting that the true incidence of asymptomatic PAD may be much higher than previously recognised.

Population studies have varied widely in reporting the incidence of intermittent claudication. Most of these are based on questionnaire surveys and therefore prone to some degree of over-reporting.

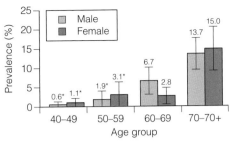

Figure 1.2 • Recent information about the prevalence of PAD from the US National Health and Nutrition Survey, confirming a steep age-related prevalence.[13]

Nevertheless, it is clear that the incidence of intermittent claudication increases steeply with age. The Scottish Heart Study, for example, found a prevalence of 1.1% in subjects aged 40–59 years;[11] in the Limburg study (subjects aged 40–79 years) the reported prevalence varied between 1.4% and 6.1%[12] depending on the criteria used, and the Edinburgh Artery Study indicated a higher prevalence of 4.5%, but in a group (55–74 years) with older mean age.[3]

Information about the prevalence of PAD in the USA has emerged from the National Health and Nutrition Examination Survey (NHANES, 1999–2000).[13] By analysing data from 2174 participants, Selvin and Erlinger found that, among adults aged 40 years and over, the prevalence of PAD was 4.3% (PAD was defined as ABPI <0.90 in either leg). This equates to approximately 5 million people in the USA with PAD. Among those over 70 years old, the prevalence was 14.5%[13] (**Fig. 1.2**).

The incidence of critical limb ischaemia has been estimated to be around 400 cases per million population per year, which equates to a prevalence of 1 in 2500 of the population annually.[14] For every 100 patients with intermittent claudication, approximately one new patient per year will develop critical ischaemia.[8]

Natural history of PAD: cardiovascular and lower limb outcomes

It is important in discussing the natural history of PAD to consider both the progression of the disease in the legs and the fate of the patient as a whole in terms of systemic cardiovascular complications.

Asymptomatic disease

The Edinburgh Artery Study is one of the few studies to have examined the pattern of progression among asymptomatic patients with abnormal ABPIs and the rate of development of symptoms; 7–15% of subjects with asymptomatic PAD developed intermittent claudication over a 5-year period, depending on the initial severity of the disease.[4] A more recent study from the Netherlands reported similar conversion rates, with 27 of 177 asymptomatic patients (15%) developing lower limb symptoms during a 7-year follow-up period.[15]

Information about longitudinal changes in ABPI, and risk factors for declining ABPI, has emerged from the Cardiovascular Health Study.[16] Among 5000 patients with normal ABPI at baseline, 9.5% had a significant decrease in ABPI during a 6-year follow-up. Independent predictors of ABPI decline included age (odds ratio (OR) 1.96 for the 75–84 age group and 3.79 for those >85 years), current cigarette use (OR 1.74), hypertension (OR 1.64), diabetes (OR 1.77) and raised low-density lipoprotein (LDL) cholesterol.[16] Reduced ABPI has also been associated with rising serum creatinine,[17] indicating that even asymptomatic PAD may affect renal outcomes.

There is good evidence that subjects with asymptomatic PAD have a much higher risk of systemic CV complications. The risk of death or disability from cardiac or cerebral events may be much higher than the risk of lower limb symptoms (claudication or acute limb ischaemia). The Edinburgh Artery Study showed that asymptomatic PAD patients have an increased risk of acute myocardial infarction and stroke; in fact, they have almost the same increased risk of CV events and death as that reported among patients with claudication.[3] The reverse also applies, e.g. in men with asymptomatic carotid stenosis ABPI was the strongest predictor of stroke risk.[18]

Intermittent claudication

Large population follow-up studies suggest that up to 50% of patients with intermittent claudication will remain relatively stable (i.e. no deterioration in walking distance) or experience some spontaneous improvement in symptoms during a 5-year period; only 25% of claudicants will develop significant deterioration in walking distance.[19,20] The Basle study[20] is typical of several observational follow-ups in showing that, although two-thirds of patients surviving at 5 years reported no limiting intermittent claudication (i.e. their symptoms had resolved), 63% actually had angiographic progression of the disease. This suggests that although PAD is pathologically progressive, other factors contribute to symptomatology, e.g. collateral vessel formation or physiological and psychological adaptation. Although one-quarter of patients with intermittent claudication have symptoms that worsen over time, only 5% deteriorate sufficiently to merit revascularisation and only 1–2% will require a major amputation.[8]

Although lower limb outcomes are mostly very good for patients with uncomplicated intermittent claudication, the major concern for these patients relates to a heightened risk of CV complications due to silent or symptomatic atherosclerosis in other vascular territories. Patients with intermittent claudication have a 2–4% risk of undergoing a non-fatal CV event within the first year of diagnosis and a 1–3% yearly incidence thereafter.[8] For most patients, however, absolute coronary heart disease (CHD) risk is greater than 30% over 10 years, and all-cause mortality rates are similar to those associated with many forms of cancer. In the CASS study, patients with PAD had a 25% greater likelihood of mortality than patients without PAD.[21]

Critical limb ischaemia

A national survey conducted in 1993 by the Vascular Surgical Society of Great Britain and Ireland found that around 70% of patients with critical ischaemia were offered some form of revascularisation procedure, with a 75% chance of limb salvage. The overall amputation rate, however, was still 21.5% and the mortality rate was 13.5%.[14] Thus, the overall long-term prognosis for these patients is very poor.

The Reduction of Atherothrombosis for Continued Health (REACH) registry

This large multinational registry is providing useful observational data about the spectrum of disease progression, CV outcomes and patterns of treatment in the 21st century. A total of 67 888 patients, aged 45 years or more, from 44 countries were registered in the database if they had either established CV disease or if they were asymptomatic with more than three risk factors (n = 12 389). Among the symptomatic group, patients were enrolled on the basis of coronary artery disease (CAD; n = 40 248), cerebrovascular disease (CVD; n = 18 843) or PAD (n = 8273);[22] 16% of this group had polyvascular disease.

Three-year outcome data for the REACH cohort have been published.[23] Among patients with established CV disease, CV death, myocardial infarction (MI) or stroke rates were 23.0% for patients with CAD, 18.7% for patients with CVD and 33.6% for patients with PAD. Patients with PAD were most likely to have subsequent vascular death (2.9 events per 100 person-years).

The number of vascular territories affected by atherosclerosis was an important determinant of outcome, so those patients with polyvascular disease had the highest rates of major CV events after 3 years.

Epidemiological risk factors for PAD and randomised trials of disease-modifying therapy for secondary prevention

CV risk factors in general

There are numerous CV risk factors associated with atherosclerotic disease progression (**Fig. 1.3**). However, it is important to emphasise the distinction between a CV risk factor and the evidence that intervention to modify that risk factor improves clinical outcomes (i.e. symptoms or survival). Factors such as high serum homocysteine[24] or fibrinogen concentrations may be weak risk factors for PAD, but for clinicians in practice this is largely meaningless without evidence from randomised prospective trials that lowering of homocysteine or fibrinogen affects disease outcome. Indeed, the point is well illustrated by a recent placebo-controlled trial of folic acid and vitamin B (B_6 and B_{12}) supplements, which achieved the aim of producing a sustained reduction in plasma homocysteine levels in patients with established CV disease, but the intervention had no effect on clinical end-points such as mortality or non-fatal CV events.[25]

Risk factors for PAD

In the study, using age- and gender-adjusted logistic regression analyses, the following risk factors (and

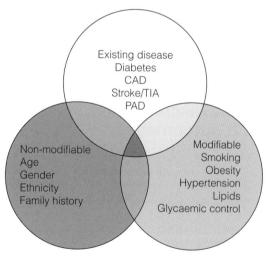

Figure 1.3 • Major CV risk factors can be grouped into: existing disease; non-modifiable risk factors; and modifiable risk factors, where placebo-controlled trials have shown the benefits of intervention.

odds ratios) were significantly associated with PAD: black race/ethnicity (OR 2.83), current smoking (OR 4.46), diabetes (OR 2.71), hypertension (OR 1.75), hypercholesterolaemia (OR 1.68) and poor kidney function (OR 2.00). Elevated fibrinogen and C-reactive protein levels also were associated with PAD.[13] A similar profile of risk factors for PAD has been defined for patients with diabetes using the Atherosclerosis Risk in Communities (ARIC) study database.[26] A recent study indicated that high serum adiponectin is a protective for the development of PAD in women.[27]

Age and gender

There is clear evidence from several studies that increasing age is associated with an increased risk of PAD in both men and women[3,28] (Fig. 1.2). The evidence for a gender difference is slightly less clear. Several studies, including the Framingham Heart Study, have suggested that men have nearly double the risk of developing intermittent claudication compared with women,[28] but the Edinburgh Artery Study failed to show any significant difference between the sexes,[3] and a follow-up to the Limburg study suggested that the incidence of both symptomatic and asymptomatic PAD was greater in women.[15] Family history is an independent risk factor for premature CHD, but studies have failed to show the same (presumably genetic) association for PAD.

Cigarette smoking

Cigarette smoking is associated with excess premature deaths from CV, respiratory and cancer-related diseases. Smoking is undoubtedly the most important modifiable risk factor for PAD. The relationship between smoking and lower limb arterial disease was first identified in 1911 by clinicians who reported a threefold increase in the incidence of claudication among smokers. Smoking not only affects the development of PAD but also affects the clinical outcome in those patients with PAD who continue to smoke. Smokers with PAD are much more likely to progress to critical ischaemia, and more likely to require an amputation or vascular intervention.[29] Furthermore, smoking increases the overall mortality rate among claudicants by a factor of 1.5–3.0.[6]

> ✔✔ In men, smoking cessation reduces overall CV risk to the level of non-smokers within 5–7 years.[30] In women, smoking cessation reduces overall CV risk to the level of non-smokers within 2–4 years.[31]

However, the excess cancer risk associated with smoking often takes 10 years to subside after smoking cessation. In men, the benefits take longer, about 5 years, to take effect. Nevertheless, smoking cessation for CV prevention is highly cost-effective; the benefits appear relatively quickly.

Nicotine is addictive and spontaneous smoking cessation rates are very low (<10%), even among genuinely motivated patients. In terms of helping motivated patients to quit smoking, several approaches are available.

> ✔✔ The antidepressant bupropion, nicotine replacement therapy (NRT) and the newer agent varenicline are all considered to be first-line options; nortriptyline is occasionally used but only as second-line treatment.[32]
> A meta-analysis of more than 100 randomised trials shows that all forms of NRT are equally effective in aiding long-term smoking cessation[33] (Table 1.2). In randomised trials, quit rates after 1 year, on average, are nearly double those following placebo (OR 1.77).[33] Combination NRT (e.g. patch + gum) can also be effective in those patients who have found a single form of NRT insufficient to control nicotine withdrawal symptoms.

Table 1.2 • A summary of more than 100 randomised trials of NRT for smoking cessation

Comparison	Trials (n)	Participants (n)	Pooled OR	95% CI
Gum	52	17 783	1.66	1.52–1.81
Patch	37	16 691	1.81	1.63–2.02
Nasal spray	4	887	2.35	1.63–3.38
Inhaler	4	976	2.14	1.44–3.18
Tablets/lozenges	4	2739	2.05	1.62–2.59
Combination vs. single type	7	3202	1.42	1.14–1.76
Any NRT vs. control	103	39503	1.77	1.66–1.88

The pooled odds ratios show that overall, for different forms of therapy, NRT has a quit rate 1.77-fold higher than placebo at 1 year.[33]

Varenicline, a partial agonist at the $\alpha_4\beta_2$ acetylcholine nicotinic receptor, is licensed for smoking cessation.

✅✅ Varenicline appears to be more effective than NRT,[34] and a meta-analysis of randomised trials showed that quit rates are threefold higher than with placebo and superior to those after use of bupropion (OR 3.22).[35]

Diabetes

Diabetes mellitus is well recognised as an important risk factor for cardiovascular disease and, apart from smoking, is probably the single most important risk factor in the development of PAD. Lower limb arterial disease tends to be more diffuse and distal in diabetics, with both ischaemic and neuropathic ulceration being common. The Edinburgh Artery Study and the Health Professionals Follow-up Study showed that people with diabetes have a 1.5- to 2.5-fold increased risk of symptomatic and asymptomatic PAD compared with non-diabetics, and the lifetime risk of a lower limb amputation is increased 10–16 fold.[36,37] Duration of diabetes is also important, e.g. in the Health Professionals Follow-up Study patients were grouped according to diabetes duration and the relative risks of PAD were 3.63 (diabetes duration 6–10 years), 2.55 (11–25 years) and 4.53 (duration >25 years) compared with patients diagnosed less than 5 years.[37]

✅ Diabetics with critical ischaemia fare less well than their non-diabetic counterparts, e.g. higher amputation rates and less success following revascularisation procedures.[38]

The risks of lower limb ulceration are exacerbated by coexistent microvascular disease and peripheral neuropathy.

Several studies in both type 1 and type 2 diabetes have identified the glucose level as an independent risk factor for PAD.[39,40]

✅ The UK Prospective Diabetes Study (UKPDS) identified a strong association between HbA1c and risk of PAD: each 1% increase in HbA1c was associated with a 28% increased risk of PAD.[40]

However, other important features of the 'metabolic syndrome' of type 2 diabetes include insulin resistance, hypertension, obesity and dyslipidaemia (typically low high-density lipoprotein (HDL) cholesterol and high triglycerides). Epidemiological data have suggested that both insulin resistance and hyperinsulinaemia are independent risk factors for PAD in diabetic and non-diabetic individuals.[41]

Hypertension plays a significant role in the development of PAD in diabetic subjects.

✅✅ In the UKPDS, for every 10 mmHg reduction in systolic blood pressure there was a 12% reduction in overall CV risk, but more specifically a 16% reduction in risk of lower limb amputation or peripheral vascular disease-related mortality.[42]

The Hypertension Optimal Treatment (HOT) trial showed that vigorous blood pressure control had a greater effect in reducing CV events in those patients with diabetes than those without,[43] and effective control of hypertension may limit vascular events even more effectively than tight glycaemic control.[44] The major benefits of glycaemic control appear to be in microvascular protection and prevention of neuropathy and secondary foot complications such as ulceration and infection.

The association of traditional and non-traditional risk factors with PAD incidence in a population of patients with diabetes has been investigated in the ARIC study.[26] This analysis showed that patients with diabetes were more likely to develop PAD if they were smokers (relative risk (RR) 1.87), had CHD at baseline (RR 2.27) and high triglycerides (RR 1.75). Patients taking insulin therapy were also at higher risk.[26]

Blood pressure (BP)

The Framingham and other studies have provided good evidence that hypertension is a powerful predisposing risk factor in the development of intermittent claudication. A BP >160/95 mmHg increased the risk by 2.5-fold in men and fourfold in women during 26 years of follow-up.[28] Hypertension is a major associated CV risk factor, present in up to 55% of patients with PAD.[45] Hypertension also increases the risk of CV complications and mortality in patients with established PAD. Up to 5% of hypertensive patients have been reported to have clinical evidence of PAD at presentation, with a marked age-related increase in hypertension-associated PAD.[46] Isolated or predominantly systolic hypertension is common in PAD patients.

✅ In the Rotterdam Study investigating determinants of PAD, after multivariate analysis each 10 mmHg increase in systolic BP conferred an increased risk of PAD (OR 1.3, 95% CI 1.2–1.5).[47]

Effective antihypertensive therapy is likely to ameliorate the progression of PAD as well as reducing the mortality from stroke and CHD.[48,49] However, there are few randomised trials that have addressed the efficacy of different types of antihypertensive drugs specifically in patients with PAD; rather, patients with PAD have represented small subgroups of much larger studies. Furthermore, BP management in patients with PAD tends to be poor. Systolic hypertension is especially difficult to treat in patients with calcified arteries that have lost their elasticity. In PARTNERS,[50] for example, hypertension was less often treated in new (84%) and previous (88%) patients with PAD as compared to patients with CHD. So what treatments and what guidelines for treatment of hypertension in PAD patients should be recommended?

The treatment of hypertension in patients with PAD has been reviewed recently.[51] There are to date no specific national guidelines for choice of antihypertensive therapy in PAD patients.

> ✅✅ The latest joint British Hypertension Society/National Institute for Health and Clinical Excellence (NICE) guideline[52] states that persistent raised BP with existing cardiovascular disease should be treated if, after measurement on two separate visits, systolic BP, diastolic BP or both are 140/90 mmHg or above.[53]

The aim should be to reduce BP to an optimum target of below 140/85 mmHg among treated hypertensives. It has become clear that small differences in BP translate into relatively large differences in clinical outcome, and that patients achieve worthwhile benefits from antihypertensive therapy even if BP control does not meet the stringent target of <140/85 mmHg.

NICE has reissued guidance in 2011 about the choice of antihypertensive drug, with primacy given to angiotensin-modifying drugs (particularly for those <55 years) and calcium channel blockers to older patients (**Fig. 1.4**). Beta-blockers are no longer a first-line treatment recommendation since they appear less effective in preventing stroke. In practice many hypertensive patients require two or three drugs (angiotensin-converting enzyme (ACE) inhibitor, calcium channel blocker and diuretic) to achieve BP targets.[54]

Renin–angiotensin–aldosterone system blockade

The importance of the renin–angiotensin–aldosterone system (RAAS) in cardiovascular pathophysiology is a continued focus of intense research. There has been considerable interest in whether drugs that block the RAAS confer useful therapeutic and disease-modifying effects, over and above those attributable to BP reduction, in the secondary prevention of CV

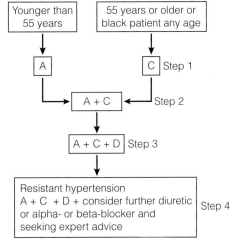

Figure 1.4 • Drug selection and drug sequencing for patients with hypertension. Algorithm published by the British Heart Foundation and endorsed by NICE. Beta-blockers are no longer recommended in step 1, but may be added at step 4. A, ACE inhibitor (consider angiotensin II receptor antagonist if ACE intolerant); C, calcium-channel blocker; D, thiazide-type diuretic. Black patients are those of African or Caribbean descent and not mixed-race, Asian or Chinese patients.

disease.[55] It is well established that ACE inhibitors and angiotensin receptor blockers (ARBs) improve left ventricular (LV) function in heart failure patients and retard the decline in glomerular filtration rate in patients with chronic renal disease. These drugs also improve CV outcomes in patients with atherosclerotic disease (in the absence of LV or renal dysfunction) but whether this is mediated solely via BP lowering, or whether RAAS blockade confers additional (BP-independent) benefits on the blood vessel wall, has been hotly debated.

Serum lipids

The epidemiological evidence relating serum cholesterol levels to CV mortality is well established (**Fig. 1.5**). In terms of PAD, the Framingham Study showed that a fasting cholesterol >7 mmol/L doubled the risk of intermittent claudication,[56] but not all observational studies have reached the same conclusion. Low HDL cholesterol, or an increased LDL:HDL ratio, appear to be independent risk factors for PAD,[3] and there are further independent associations between PAD and circulating levels of apolipoproteins A and B (proteins contained within LDL particles).[57,58]

Circulating cholesterol is derived from two sources (**Fig. 1.6**): (1) endogenous synthesis in the liver, cholesterol is then transported in the blood stream

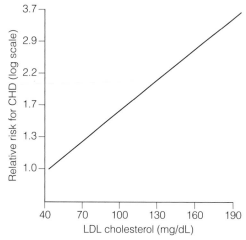

Figure 1.5 • A log-linear relationship between LDL cholesterol levels and the relative risk of CHD. The relationship is steep. For every 30 mg/dL (0.8 mmol/L) change in LDL cholesterol the relative risk of CHD changes in proportion by 30% (divide by 38.46 to convert mg/dL to mmol/L).

via lipoprotein particles and some is secreted into bile; and (2) gastrointestinal absorption of dietary cholesterol and (reabsorption of) bile acids. Statins (drugs that inhibit the rate-limiting enzyme in cholesterol biosynthesis in the liver, hydroxymethylglutaryl (HMG)-CoA reductase) have become the mainstay of clinical practice for lowering cholesterol levels, but a cholesterol absorption inhibitor, ezetimibe, is now available for adjunctive use with statins. Ezetimibe is not systemically absorbed, but

effectively blocks cholesterol transport in the gut, which in turn increases faecal loss of cholesterol and lowers serum cholesterol levels.

The large intervention trials using statins (mostly in CHD and stroke patients) have included only small numbers of patients with coexistent PAD. For instance, patients with PAD contributed only ≈20% of the total patients in the Heart Protection Study; nevertheless, in this subgroup treatment with simvastatin was associated with a substantial reduction in major cardiovascular events (27.6% vs. 34.3% in the placebo group; **Fig. 1.7**).[59]

PAD is now considered a CHD risk equivalent,[60] and unless contraindicated statins should be recommended for all patients with symptomatic PAD.

✓✓ A target LDL cholesterol concentration of <2.6 mmol/L is included in most international guidelines,[61] mainly because of two observations: (1) a retrospective pooled analysis of the achieved LDL cholesterol levels in the placebo and active therapy arms of the major statin trials has shown that the lower the achieved cholesterol level, the lower the risk of major CV events (**Fig. 1.8**); and (2) prospective trials comparing low-dose versus high-dose statin therapy in patients with established CV disease have shown that more intensive cholesterol-lowering (e.g. atorvastatin 80 mg) confers a mortality advantage compared with less intensive cholesterol lowering (e.g. atorvastatin 10 mg) (**Fig. 1.9**).

Achieving a target LDL cholesterol level <2.6 mmol/L is very difficult using standard doses of first-generation

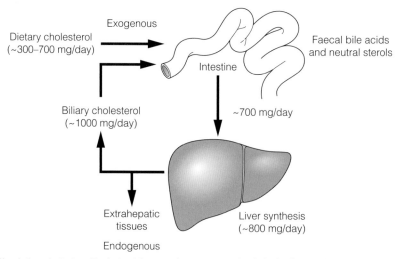

Figure 1.6 • Circulating cholesterol is derived from endogenous synthesis in the liver and exogenous sources (dietary intake and bile acids) absorbed through the gut. Statins block synthesis, ezetimibe blocks gut absorption. The drugs have additive effects on serum cholesterol.

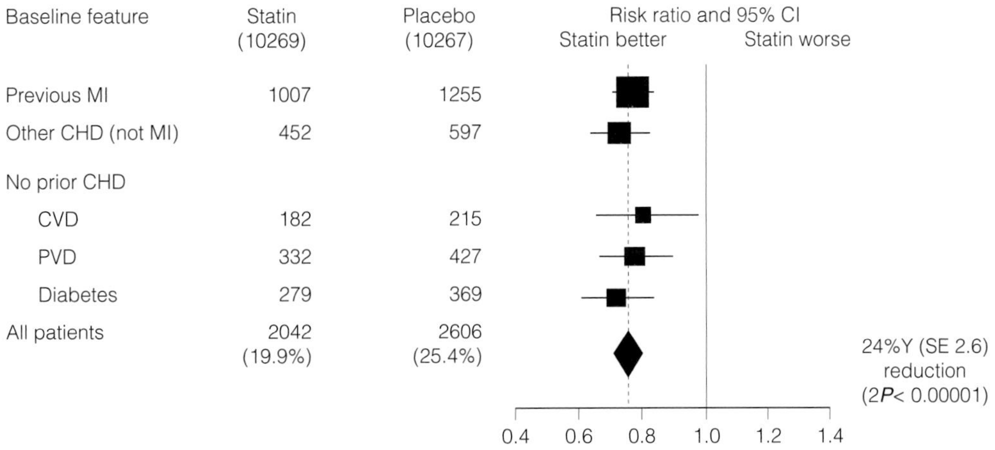

Baseline feature
Statin (10269)
Placebo (10267)
Risk ratio and 95% CI
Statin better
Statin worse
Previous MI 1007 1255
Other CHD (not MI) 452 597
No prior CHD
CVD 182 215
PVD 332 427
Diabetes 279 369
All patients 2042 (19.9%) 2606 (25.4%)
24%Y (SE 2.6) reduction (2P< 0.00001)
0.4 0.6 0.8 1.0 1.2 1.4

Figure 1.7 • In the Heart Protection Study, the benefits of simvastatin 40 mg were evident in those patients with peripheral vascular disease (PVD) at baseline and were independent of age, BP status and baseline cholesterol. Data from the Heart Protection Study Collaborative Group. MRC/BHF Heart Protection Study of cholesterol-lowering with simvastatin in 20,536 high-risk individuals. Lancet 2002; 360:7–22.

Statin
Placebo
4S
4S
LIPID
LIPID
CARE
CARE
HPS
HPS
TNT (10 mg of atorvastatin)
TNT (80 mg of atorvastatin)
Log rank P=0.8
Event (%)
0 5 10 15 20 25 30
0 70 90 110 130 150 170 190 210
LDL cholesterol (mg/dL)

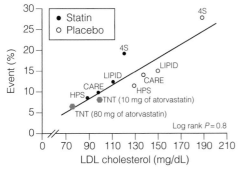

Figure 1.8 • A pooled analysis of achieved LDL cholesterol levels in the placebo group and the active therapy group for each of the major placebo-controlled statin trials. The lower the LDL cholesterol level, the lower the CV event rate (divide by 38.46 to convert mg/dL to mmol/L). Reproduced from LaRosa JC, Grundy SM, Waters DD et al. Intensive lipid lowering with atorvastatin in patients with stable coronary disease. N Engl J Med 2005; 352:1425–35. Copyright © 2005 Massachusetts Medical Society. All rights reserved.

statins. For example, <35% of patients will reach this target using simvastatin 40 mg daily. Thus, clinicians may need to switch to one of the second-generation statins that are more potent, e.g. atorvastatin or rosuvastatin.

A Cochrane review of studies of lipid-lowering therapy in patients with PAD concluded that 'lipid-lowering therapy may be useful in preventing the deterioration of underlying disease and alleviating symptoms' and found a marked, although non-significant, reduction in mortality.[62]

✔✔ There are several trials that have been published since this initial Cochrane review which report that statins are associated with functional improvement in PAD. The largest of these studies showed that atorvastatin (versus placebo) was associated with an increase in pain-free walking distance and quality of life at 12 months.[63] Similar findings were also reported in smaller trials (**Fig. 1.10**).[61]

Patients with PAD benefit from statin therapy, irrespective of the baseline cholesterol concentration. This viewpoint has been confirmed by a recent meta-analysis of trials.[64] Each 1 mmol/L reduction in LDL cholesterol results in about a one-third reduction in mortality from CHD, independent of age, BP and initial cholesterol concentration.

Evidence for dietary control or supplementation

Dietary control is rarely considered for patients with PAD, despite there being at least four important reasons to consider dietary management:

- claudication distance decreases with increasing body weight;[65]
- glucose intolerance increases with increasing body weight;
- increased plasma lipid concentrations are associated with increased atherosclerotic burden;
- reducing salt intake can reduce blood pressure.

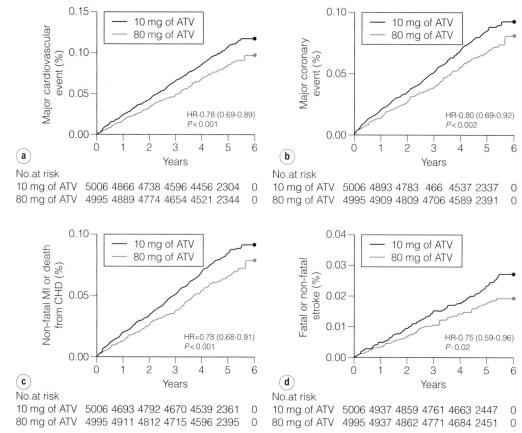

Figure 1.9 • The 'Treating to New Targets' study randomised 10 000 patients with CHD to atorvastatin 80 mg vs. atorvastatin 10 mg once daily. Mean LDL cholesterol levels were 2.0 and 2.6 mmol/L in the two groups, respectively. This difference translated into big differences in CV outcomes. Reproduced from LaRosa JC, Grundy SM, Waters DD et al. Intensive lipid lowering with atorvastatin in patients with stable coronary disease. N Engl J Med 2005; 352:1425–35. Copyright © 2005 Massachusetts Medical Society. All rights reserved.

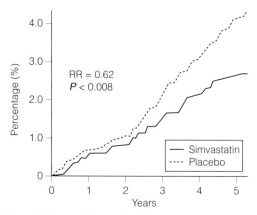

Figure 1.10 • Incidence of new or worsening claudication among 4000 participants in the 4S study of simvastatin vs. placebo in post-MI patients. Reproduced from Pedersen TR, Kjekshus J, Pyörälä K et al. Effect of simvastatin on ischemic signs and symptoms in the Scandinavian Simvastatin Survival Study (4S). Am J Cardiol 1998; 81:333–5. With permission from Elsevier.

Apart from cholesterol and triglycerides, several other dietary components have been associated with effects on atherosclerosis and PAD: these include the polyunsaturated fatty acids, niacin, folate, vitamins B, C and E.

A recent WHO report recommends regular consumption of fish to provide 200–500 mg of eicosapentaenoic acid and docosahexaenoic acid per week, replacement of saturated fat by monounsaturated fat and increased consumption of fruit and vegetables to achieve proper vitamin, antioxidant and fibre status.[66] Increased dietary fish intake is associated with diminished progression of CHD. A Cochrane review has not identified any benefit of omega-3 fatty acid supplementation on clinical outcomes in patients with intermittent claudication.[67]

✓ Meta-analysis of polyunsaturated fatty acid supplementation in patients with PAD has provided no evidence for improved clinical outcomes.[67]

Diets that limit the daily energy intake from fats to 30% or less are effective in reducing plasma lipid and lipoprotein concentrations by 5–20% and can affect weight reduction in those with above average body mass index.

> ✔ A portfolio of dietary changes including reduction of dietary fat, use of soy protein, sterols and almonds may facilitate larger reductions in plasma lipids, similar to those that can be achieved by the first-generation statins, but such diets are very difficult to adhere to.

Therefore, although dietary control is very useful in managing patients with borderline hyperlipidaemia, it cannot replace statins and other drug therapies for the management of hyperlipidaemia.

> ✔ In contrast, moderate intake of alcohol (1–2 units/day) reduces the risk of developing intermittent claudication,[68] and has the beneficial effect of increasing HDL cholesterol concentrations.

There is no consistent evidence for the role of vitamin C or E supplementation on coronary events or other clinical markers of atherosclerosis, although both may have beneficial effects on endothelial function and arterial stiffness in early disease. Similarly, dietary supplementation with folic acid and B vitamins (to lower plasma homocysteine concentrations) has no consistent effect on clinical end-points.[25]

Another diet which merits consideration is the DASH diet (Dietary Approaches to Stop Hypertension).[69] The DASH diet includes increased intake of fruit, vegetables and dietary fibre, together with increased potassium, calcium, magnesium and non-red meat protein, similar to the WHO recommendations. Long-term reduction in dietary salt intake (by 30–40 mmol/day) can also reduce both BP and coronary events in those with marginal hypertension.[70]

Antiplatelet therapy

There is some evidence that PAD is associated with a hypercoagulable state. For example, it has been suggested that patients with intermittent claudication have a higher haematocrit and blood viscosity than the general population, but the Framingham Study found no association between haematocrit and symptomatic PAD. Several studies, however, have confirmed the association of high plasma fibrinogen levels with PAD, and that fibrinogen is a marker of thrombotic risk.

There have been numerous large randomised trials of antiplatelet therapy in patients with cardiovascular disease.

> ✔✔ A Cochrane Review showed that antiplatelet therapy in patients with intermittent claudication reduced the risk of future revascularisation, cardiovascular mortality as well as all-cause mortality.[71] Clopidogrel is estimated to be more cost-effective than aspirin for patients with peripheral arterial disease.[72]

Aspirin has no effect on symptoms of claudication, but some trials have shown that aspirin alone or in combination with dipyridamole delays the angiographic progression of PAD and reduces surgical intervention rates. The standard dose of aspirin for secondary prevention, 75–150 mg daily, is effective in inhibiting platelet function but does not cause the excessive number of gastrointestinal side-effects associated with higher doses.

The CAPRIE trial evaluated the efficacy and safety of clopidogrel compared to aspirin for secondary prevention in 19 185 patients with CV disease.[73] It showed a relative reduction in the risk of MI, ischaemic stroke and vascular death of 8.7% ($P = 0.04$) in favour of clopidogrel after a mean follow-up of 1.9 years, and an absolute risk reduction of 0.51% (number needed to treat = 196 to avoid one ischaemic event during 1.9 years), although a subgroup analysis in PAD patients suggested that the clinical benefit of clopidogrel was greater than 8.7%. Indeed, a recent cost-effectiveness analysis has reported that clopidogrel is more cost-effective than aspirin in patients with peripheral arterial disease.[72]

The combination of clopidogrel and aspirin is superior to aspirin alone in patients with acute coronary syndromes (unstable angina or acute MI), i.e. when there is evidence of unstable plaque, and these benefits are especially evident in patients who require percutaneous coronary intervention or bypass surgery. The CHARISMA trial was performed to assess the effects of dual antiplatelet therapy (clopidogrel + aspirin) in patients with more stable atherosclerotic disease.[74] Overall, there were some safety concerns with dual therapy and no convincing benefit compared with aspirin alone.

> ✔✔ Guidelines for the use of antiplatelet therapy in PAD have been published.[75]

Exercise therapy

The second half of the old adage of treating claudication in five words, 'stop smoking and keep walking' has been put to the test in randomised trials both of exercise versus either no exercise or revascularisation.[76–79] Supervised exercise programmes now have proven benefit in walking ability both before and after revascularisation. One recent trial has shown that supervised exercise can increase walking distance by over 300 m at 12 months.[80]

☑☑ Supervised exercise programmes should be included as first-line therapy for patients with intermittent claudication.[78]

Conclusions

Occlusive arterial disease of the lower limbs is common and disabling; the prevalence increases steeply with age. Although lower limb symptoms and outcomes are variable and generally benign, the associated excess risks of cardiovascular disease (i.e. MI, stroke or sudden death) among patients with PAD are considerable and merit aggressive secondary prevention with atherosclerotic disease-modifying medical therapies. PAD is a CHD risk equivalent, and indeed recent results from the REACH registry indicate that the CV risks associated with PAD have been underestimated.

Epidemiological studies have identified numerous risk factors that, in longitudinal follow-up studies in large populations, are associated with a higher incidence and more rapid progression of PAD. Identifying a risk factor in a population, however, does not necessarily imply that intervention in individuals to lower that risk factor will necessarily improve clinical outcomes. Such evidence only comes from randomised placebo-controlled trials and there are very few that have focused only on patients with PAD. Most of the recommendations derive from studies of patients with other forms of cardiovascular disease.

The major modifiable risk factors are smoking, hyperlipidaemia, hypertension and diabetes. All patients with PAD merit secondary prevention with disease-modifying therapies to lower BP and cholesterol levels, assist with smoking cessation, reduce platelet function and improve glycaemic control.

Key points

- Among adults aged 40 years and over, the prevalence of PAD is 4.3% (PAD defined as ABPI <0.90 in either leg). This equates to approximately 5 million people in the USA with PAD. Among those over 70 years old, the prevalence was 14.5%.
- There is a U-shaped relationship between ABPI and reduced life expectancy. Adjusted risk estimates for all-cause mortality were 1.69 for low ABPI (<0.9) and 1.77 for high ABPI (>1.4), while the corresponding estimates for CV mortality were 2.52 and 2.09.
- The incidence of PAD increases steeply with increasing age and may be slightly more common in men.
- Although lower limb outcomes are relatively good in most patients with PAD, these patients are at very high risk of premature death from other CV events, as illustrated recently by the REACH registry.
- Risk factors for the development of PAD are similar to those for atherosclerotic disease in general, but smoking and diabetes may have a more significant impact in the lower limbs.
- Smoking cessation reduces the excess CV risk within a relatively short period, and treatments to alleviate nicotine withdrawal symptoms include NRT, varenicline or bupropion. NRT doubles quit rates at 1 year, relative to placebo, but the newer agent, varenicline, appears to be superior to NRT and bupropion.
- Other lifestyle modifications, particularly exercise, have been underused and supervised exercise that can increase walking distance and quality of life for claudicants is indicated in nearly all patients.
- Glycaemic control for those with diabetes is important in the prevention of microvascular complications, but other factors in the diabetes syndrome, such as hypertension and dyslipidaemia, may be more important in the development of PAD.
- Lipid-lowering (statin) therapy increases walking distance and survival among patients with CV disease, and all PAD patients should be treated.
- Antiplatelet therapy with low-dose aspirin (or clopidogrel if aspirin is not tolerated) is indicated in all patients with PAD.

References

1. McKenna M, Wolfson S, Kuller L. The ratio of ankle and arm arterial pressure as an independent predictor of mortality. Atherosclerosis 1991;87:119–28.

2. Resnick HE, Lindsay RS, McGrae M, et al. Relationship of high and low ankle brachial index to all-cause and cardiovascular disease mortality: the Strong Heart Study. Circulation 2004;109:733–9.

3. Fowkes F. Edinburgh Artery Study: prevalence of asymptomatic and symptomatic peripheral arterial disease in the general population. Int J Epidemiol 1991;20:384–92.

4. Leng GC. Incidence, natural history and cardiovascular events in symptomatic and asymptomatic peripheral arterial disease in the general population. Int J Epidemiol 1996;25:1172–81.

5. Criqui MH. The sensitivity, specificity, and predictive value of traditional clinical evaluation of peripheral arterial disease: results from noninvasive testing in a defined population. Circulation 1985;71:516–22.

6. Leng GC, Fowkes FG. The Edinburgh Claudication Questionnaire: an improved version of the WHO/Rose Questionnaire for use in epidemiological surveys. J Clin Epidemiol 1992;45:1101–9.

7. Schroll M, Munck O. Estimation of peripheral arteriosclerotic disease by ankle blood pressure measurements in a population study of 60-year-old men and women. J Chronic Dis 1981;34:261–9.

8. Transatlantic Inter-Society Consensus (TASC) Document. Management of peripheral arterial disease. J Vasc Surg 2000;31:S5–35.

9. Newman AB. Ankle–arm index as a marker of atherosclerosis in the Cardiovascular Health Study. Cardiovascular Heart Study (CHS) Collaborative Research Group. Circulation 1993;88:837–45.

10. Leng GC. Femoral atherosclerosis in an older British population: prevalence and risk factors. Atherosclerosis 2000;152:167–74.

11. Smith W, Woodward M, Tunstall-Pedoe H. Intermittent claudication in Scotland. In: Fowkes FGR, editor. Epidemiology of peripheral vascular disease. London: Springer-Verlag; 1991. p. 109–15.

12. Stoffers HE. The prevalence of asymptomatic and unrecognized peripheral arterial occlusive disease. Int J Epidemiol 1996;25:282–90.

13. Selvin E, Erlinger TP. Prevalence of and risk factors for peripheral arterial disease in the United States: results from the National Health and Nutrition Examination Survey (1999–2000). Circulation 2004;110:738–43.
Recent information about the prevalence of PAD in the USA.

14. Critical limb ischaemia: management and outcome. A report of a national survey by The Vascular Surgical Society of Great Britain and Ireland. Eur J Vasc Endovasc Surg 1995;10:108–13.

15. Hooi JD. Incidence of and risk factors for asymptomatic peripheral arterial occlusive disease: a longitudinal study. Am J Epidemiol 2001;153:666–72.

16. Kennedy M, Solomon C, Manolio TA, et al. Risk factors for declining ankle–brachial index in men and women 65 years or older. Arch Intern Med 2005;165:1896–902.

17. O'Hare AM, Rodriguez RA, Bacchetti P. Low ankle–brachial index associated with rise in creatinine level over time. Arch Intern Med 2005;165:1481–5.

18. Ogren M. Ten year cerebrovascular morbidity and mortality in 68 year old men with asymptomatic carotid stenosis. Br Med J 1995;310:1294–8.

19. Bloor K. Natural history of arteriosclerosis of the lower extremities. Ann R Coll Surg Engl 1961;28:36–51.

20. Da Silva A. The Basle longitudinal study: report on the relation of initial glucose level to baseline ECG abnormalities, peripheral artery disease, and subsequent mortality. J Chronic Dis 1979;32:797–803.

21. Eagle KA. Long-term survival in patients with coronary artery disease: importance of peripheral vascular disease. The Coronary Artery Surgery Study (CASS) Investigators. J Am Coll Cardiol 1994;23:1091–5.

22. Bhatt DL, Steg PG, Ohman EM, et al. International prevalence, recognition and treatment of cardiovascular risk factors in outpatients with atherothrombosis. JAMA 2006;295:180–9.
The REACH registry is a large multinational observational study of >67 000 patients with CV disease, including those with PAD. The registry documents clinical outcomes, patterns of disease and treatment in a 21st century setting.

23. Alberts MJ, Bhatt DL, Mas J-L, et al. Three-year follow-up and event rates in the international REduction of Atherothrombosis for Continued Health Registry. Eur Heart J 2009;30:2318–26.
The first outcome data showing what has happened to the 67 000 patients in the registry highlights that PAD confers a substantial risk of MI and stroke.

24. Boers G. Moderate hyperhomocysteinaemia and vascular disease: evidence, relevance and the effect of treatment. Eur J Pediatr 1998;157(Suppl. 2): S127–30.

25. Bonaa KH, Njolstad I, Ueland PM, et al. Homocysteine lowering and cardiovascular events after acute myocardial infarction. N Engl J Med 2006;354:1578–88.
Although serum homocysteine is a risk factor for CV disease in population studies, this intervention trial shows no clinical benefit of homocysteine-lowering therapy (folic A + B vitamins).

26. Wattanakit K, Folsom AR, Selvin E, et al. Risk factors for peripheral arterial disease incidence in

persons with diabetes: the Atherosclerosis Risk in Communities (ARIC) study. Atherosclerosis 2005; 180:389–97.

27. Ho DY, Cook NR, Britton KA, et al. High molecular weight and total adiponectin levels and incident symptomatic peripheral arterial disease in women. Circulation 2011;124:2303–11.

28. Murabito JM, D'Agostino RB, Silbershatz H, et al. Intermittent claudication: a risk profile from The Framingham Heart Study. Circulation 1997;96:44–9.

29. Jonason T, Ringqvist I. Factors of prognostic importance for subsequent rest pain in patients with intermittent claudication. Acta Med Scand 1985;218:27–33.

30. Godtfredsen NS, Holst C, Prescott E, et al. Smoking reduction, smoking cessation, and mortality: a 16-year follow-up of 19,732 men and women from the Copenhagen Centre for Prospective Population Studies. Am J Epidemiol 2002;156(11):994–1001.

31. Rosenberg L, Palmer JR, Shapiro S. Decline in the risk of myocardial infarction among women who stop smoking. N Engl J Med 1990;322:213–7.
Data illustrating the health outcomes following smoking cessation.

32. Aveyard P, West R. Managing smoking cessation. Br Med J 2007;335:37–41.
Modern clinical services to aid smoking cessation using NRT, varenicline and bupropion. Summarises the evidence for smoking cessation and the clinical practicalities.

33. Silagy C, Lancaster T, Stead L, et al. Nicotine replacement therapy for smoking cessation. Cochrane Database Syst Rev 2004;3:CD000146.
Systematic review of NRT.

34. Wu P, Wilson K, Dimoulas P, et al. Effectiveness of smoking cessation therapies: a systematic review and meta-analysis. BMC Public Health 2006;6:300.

35. Cahill K, Stead LF, Lancaster T. Nicotine receptor partial agonists for smoking cessation. Cochrane Database Syst Rev 2007;i:CD006103.
The evidence for smoking cessation treatments.

36. MacGregor AS, Price JF, Hau CM, et al. Role of systolic blood pressure and plasma triglycerides in diabetic peripheral arterial disease. The Edinburgh Artery Study. Diabetes Care 1999;22:453–8.

37. Al-Delaimy WK, Merchant AT, Rimm EB, et al. Effect of type 2 diabetes and its duration on the risk of peripheral arterial disease among men. Am J Med 2004;116:236–40.

38. Da Silva A. The management and outcome of critical limb ischaemia in diabetic patients: results of a national survey. Audit Committee of the Vascular Surgical Society of Great Britain and Ireland. Diabet Med 1996;13:726–8.

39. Beks P. Peripheral arterial disease in relation to glycaemic level in an elderly Caucasian population: the Hoorn study. Diabetologia 1995;38:86–96.

40. Adler A. UKPDS 59: hyperglycaemia and other potentially modifiable risk factors for peripheral arterial disease in type 2 diabetes. Diabetes Care 2002;25:894–9.
A large study conducted in the UK that showed a strong association between glycaemic control and PAD.

41. Price J, Lee A, Fowkes F. Hyperinsulinaemia: a risk factor for peripheral arterial disease in the non-diabetic population. J Cardiovasc Risk 1996; 3:501–5.

42. Adler A. Association of systolic blood pressure with macrovascular and microvascular complications of type 2 diabetes (UKPDS 36): prospective observational study. Br Med J 2000;321:412–9.
Pooled analysis of UKPDS data with respect to achieved BP and outcomes, including lower limb events.

43. Hansson L. Effects of intensive blood-pressure lowering and low-dose aspirin in patients with hypertension: principal results of the Hypertension Optimal Treatment (HOT) randomised trial. HOT Study Group. Lancet 1998;351:1755–62.

44. Beckman J, Creager M, Libby P. Diabetes and atherosclerosis: epidemiology, pathophysiology and management. JAMA 2002;287:2570–81.

45. Lip GY, Makin AJ. Treatment of hypertension in peripheral arterial disease. Cochrane Database Syst Rev 2003;4:CD003075.

46. The sixth report of the Joint National Committee on prevention, detection, evaluation, and treatment of high blood pressure. Arch Intern Med 1997;157:2413–46.

47. Meijer WT, Grobbee DE, Hunink MG, et al. Determinants of peripheral arterial disease in the elderly: the Rotterdam study. Arch Intern Med 2000;160:2934–8.

48. Feringa HH, van Waning VH, Bax JJ, et al. Cardioprotective medication is associated with improved survival in patients with peripheral arterial disease. J Am Coll Cardiol 2006;47:1182–7.

49. Ostergren J, Sleight P, Dagenais G, et al., HOPE study investigators. Impact of ramipril in patients with evidence of clinical or subclinical peripheral arterial disease. Eur Heart J 2004;25:17–24.

50. Hirsch AT, Criqui MH, Treat-Jacobson D, et al. Peripheral arterial disease detection, awareness, and treatment in primary care. JAMA 2001;286: 1317–24.

51. Singer DJ, Kite A. Management of hypertension in peripheral arterial disease: does the choice of drugs matter. Eur J Vasc Endovasc Surg 2008;35:701–8.

52. British Hypertension Society and National Institute for Healthcare Excellence. Hypertension: Management in adults in primary care: pharmacological update, www.nice.org.uk; July 2007. Joint NICE and BHS guidance for BP management.

53. NICE. Hypertension: clinical management of primary hypertension in adults. Clinical Guidelines. CG127, http//guidance./nice/org/uk/CG127; 2011.

54. Williams B, Poulter NR, Brown MJ, et al., British Hypertension Society. Guidelines for management of hypertension: report of the fourth working party of the British Hypertension Society, 2004-BHS IV. J Hum Hypertens 2004;18:139–85.

55. Donnelly R, Manning G. Angiotensin converting enzyme inhibitors and coronary heart disease prevention. J Renin Angiotensin Aldosterone Syst 2007;8:13–22.

56. Kannel WB. Intermittent claudication. Incidence in the Framingham Study. Circulation 1970;41:875–83.

57. Cheng SW, Ting AC, Wong J. Lipoprotein (a) and its relationship to risk factors and severity of atherosclerotic peripheral vascular disease. Eur J Vasc Endovasc Surg 1997;14:17–23.

58. Pilger E. Risk factors for peripheral atherosclerosis. Retrospective evaluation by stepwise discriminant analysis. Arteriosclerosis 1983;3:57–63.

59. Heart Protection Study Collaborative Group. MRC/BHF Heart Protection Study of cholesterol-lowering with simvastatin in 20,536 high-risk individuals. Lancet 2002;360:7–22.

60. Hirsch AT, Haskal ZJ, Hertzer NR, et al. ACC/AHA guidelines for the management of patients with peripheral arterial disease. Circulation 2006;113:463–5.
Updated US guidelines for management of PAD.

61. Erez G, Leitersdorf E. The rationale for using HMG-CoA reductase inhibitors (Statins) in peripheral arterial disease. Eur J Vasc Endovasc Surg 2007;33:192–201.
Effects of statins on PAD.

62. Leng GC, Price JF, Jepson RG. Lipid-lowering for lower limb atherosclerosis. Cochrane Database Syst Rev 2000;2:CD000123.
Analysis of currently available data suggests that lipid-lowering therapy is of benefit for PAD patients to reduce morbidity and possibly mortality.

63. Mohler ER, Hiatt WR, Creager MA. Cholesterol reduction with atorvastatin improves walking distance in patients with peripheral arterial disease. Circulation 2003;108:1481–6.
Effects of statin therapy on functional status in PAD.

64. Prospective studies collaboration. Blood cholesterol and vascular mortality by age, sex and blood pressure: a meta-analysis of individual data from 61 prospective studies with 55 000 vascular deaths. Lancet 2007;370:1829–39.
Overview of the large statin trials, quantifies the benefits of cholesterol reduction.

65. Wyatt MG, Scott PM, Poskitt K, et al. Effect of weight on claudication distance. Br J Surg 1991;78:1386–8.

66. WHO Study Group. Diet, nutrition and prevention of chronic diseases. Technical Report Series No. 916. Geneva: World Health Organisation; 2003.

67. Sommerfield T, Price J, Hiatt WR. Omega-3 fatty acids for intermittent claudication. Cochrane Database Syst Rev 2007;17:CD003833.

68. Djousse L, Levy D, Murabito JM, et al. Alcohol consumption and risk of intermittent claudication in the Framingham Heart Study. Circulation 2000;102:3092–7.
Relationship between alcohol intake and PAD in observational follow-up studies.

69. Sacks FM, Svetkey LP, Vollmer WM, et al. Effects on blood pressure of reduced dietary sodium and the Dietary Approaches to Stop Hypertension (DASH) diet. N Engl J Med 2001;344:3–10.

70. Cook NR, Cutler JA, Obarzanek E, et al. Long term effects of dietary sodium reduction on cardiovascular disease outcomes: observational follow-up of the trials of hypertension prevention (TOHP). Br Med J 2007;334:885.

71. Greenhalgh J, Bagust A, Boland A, et al. Clopidogrel and modified-release dipyridamole for the prevention of occlusive vascular events (review of Technology Appraisal No. 90): a systematic review and economic analysis. Health Technol Assess 2011;15:1–178.

72. Wong PF, Chong LY, Mikhailidis DP, et al. Antiplatelet agents for intermittent claudication. Cochrane Database Syst Rev 2011;11:CD001272.
Meta-analysis of the effects of antiplatelet therapy in intermittent claudication.

73. CAPRIE Steering Committee. A randomised, blinded trial of clopidogrel versus aspirin in patients at risk of ischaemic events (CAPRIE). Lancet 1996;348:1329–39.

74. Bhatt DL, Fox KAA, Hacke W, et al. Clopidogrel and aspirin versus aspirin alone for the prevention of atherothrombotic events (CHARISMA). N Engl J Med 2006;354:1706–17.

75. Peripheral Arterial Disease Antiplatelet Consensus Group. Antiplatelet therapy in peripheral arterial disease: Consensus statement. Eur J Vasc Endovasc Surg 2003;26:1–16.
Recent, evidence-based consensus guidelines for use of antiplatelet therapy in different clinical scenarios related to PAD.

76. Housley E. Treating claudication in five words. Br Med J 1988;296:1483–4.

77. Watson L, Ellis B, Leng GC. Exercise for intermittent claudication. Cochrane Database Syst Rev 2008; CD000990.

78. Frans FA, Bipat S, Reekers JA, et al. Systematic review of exercise training or percutaneous transluminal angioplasty for intermittent claudication. Br J Surg 2012;99:16–28.

79. Murphy TP, Regensteiner JG, Mohler FR, et al. Supervised exercise versus primary stenting for claudication resultion from aorto-iliac peripheral artery disease: 6-month outcomes from the CLEVER study. Circulation 2011;Nov 16 (Epub).

80. Nicolaï SP, Teijink JA, Prins MH. Exercise therapy in Peripheral Arterial Disease Study Group multicenter randomised clinical trial of supervised exercise therapy with and without feedback versus walking advice for intermittent claudication. J Vasc Surg 2010;52:348–55.

2

Assessment of chronic lower limb ischaemia

Henrik Sillesen
John R. Bottomley

Introduction

Atherosclerosis is a systemic disease involving the arterial tree throughout the body. The most commonly affected sites are the coronary, carotid, iliac and femoral arteries. When atherosclerosis affects the peripheral circulation it is referred to as peripheral arterial disease (PAD). The pattern of disease is often thought of as affecting three levels – the aorto-iliac, the femoropopliteal and the tibial segments. Intermittent claudication is typically the first symptom of PAD, most commonly located to the calf muscles, and usually occurs when PAD affects one level – most often iliac or femoropopliteal. More severe disease affecting two or three levels may result in critical limb ischaemia with rest pain, ulceration or gangrene involving the toes or forefoot. The tibial arteries are commonly affected by calcification in patients with diabetes, end-stage renal disease and those of advanced age. This chapter deals with the assessment of patients with chronic lower limb ischaemia and the principles of vascular imaging.

✔ There are several classifications based on the severity of PAD. The simplest is the Fontaine classification (Table 2.1). The Rutherford classification (Table 2.2) is more detailed, useful for reporting standards, but rarely used in clinical practice.

Intermittent claudication (IC)

✔✔ IC is a frequent symptom in the elderly, occurring in 14% of men over the age of 65 years, increasing to 21% in those over the age of 85 years (see Chapter 1).

The classic feature of IC is that pain develops on walking in the muscle groups distal to the arterial obstruction, most commonly in the calf, but also in the thigh or buttock, depending on the location of the atherosclerotic lesion. The pain is not felt at rest or when the first few steps are taken, but typically develops progressively on walking and is described as an ache, cramp or tightening in the muscle that usually forces the patient to stop. Occasionally, mild claudication may be felt only while walking uphill or quickly. Pain develops due to ischaemia of muscles and is therefore located to these and not to joints, which is helpful when considering differential diagnoses. Pain from claudication is rapidly relieved by rest and reappears after walking a similar distance.

The differential diagnosis includes osteoarthritis of the hip or knee and lumbar nerve route irritation. Patients with spinal stenosis may have symptoms of IC that are very similar to intermittent claudication due to vascular disease.[1] Whereas patients with vascular claudication get pain relief by just standing still, patients with spinal stenosis need to relieve the pressure in the spinal canal, which they do by sitting or lying down. A history of pain on standing as well as walking therefore suggests neurogenic claudication due to spinal stenosis. Patients with osteoarthritis of the hip with referred pain down the leg and a history similar to claudication usually experience some pain in the buttock or groin when turning their body, even in a sitting or supine position. The pain is not relieved by standing still as the patient needs to lessen the burden on the joint. In addition, pain from osteoarthritis typically begins when walking and gets better after

Table 2.1 • Fontaine classification of the severity of PAD

Fontaine stage		Description
I	Asymptomatic	PAD present but no symptoms
II	Intermittent claudication	Cramping pain in leg muscles precipitated by walking and rapidly relieved by rest
III	Rest pain	Constant pain in feet (often worse at night)
IV	Tissue loss	Ischaemic ulceration or gangrene

Table 2.2 • Rutherford classification of the severity of PAD

Grade	Category	Description
0	0	Asymptomatic
I	1	Mild claudication
I	2	Moderate claudication
I	3	Severe claudication
II	4	Ischaemic rest pain
II	5	Minor tissue loss
III	6	Major tissue loss

some exercise. Although the diagnosis can usually be established by history and examination alone, minimally invasive investigations, including an exercise test to exclude arterial disease, may be reassuring.

Lumbar nerve route irritation may also cause aching in the calf or down the back of the leg from buttock to ankle. The sensation appears to be very similar to that of claudication, particularly when confined to the calf. Direct enquiry for these symptoms is helpful, but the key feature is again the need to sit or lie to obtain relief. Spinal flexion may release the involved nerve roots, whereas a straight leg raise will often precipitate the pain. When both sciatic nerve irritation or spinal stenosis and PAD coexist in the same patient, it can be extremely difficult to identify which is contributing most to the patient's symptoms.

The cornerstones in the assessment of chronic lower limb ischaemia are a careful history, palpation of pulses and ankle–brachial pressure index (ABPI) measurement. The important point is to verify that the clinical findings correlate well with the patient's symptoms. As the patients get older so does the arterial tree. The mere presence of PAD (i.e. reduced ABPI, atherosclerosis visible on ultrasound examination) does not mean that it is the cause of the symptoms. The history should include the duration of symptoms and the mode of onset. Most patients gradually become aware of pain on

walking, which is typical in progressive PAD. The patient experiences pain when the arterial supply to the leg muscles is insufficient to meet the metabolic needs during exercise.

✓✓ The blood supply required by resting muscles is relatively small (130–150 mL/min) and may be increased five- to tenfold during exercise.[2]

Arterial occlusions can be well tolerated when collaterals can develop, which may provide the same volume flow at rest as in normal individuals.[3] Examples include the thigh muscles around the superficial femoral artery at the adductor canal, which is well collateralised by the profundafemoris artery and occlusions of the iliac arteries, where collaterals through the pelvis and buttock may result in normal resting pressures and even a palpable foot pulse (**Fig. 2.1**). Significant PAD is usually associated with an ABPI of <0.9 (see later), but in such cases an exercise challenge will result in a fall in ankle pressures and disappearance of the distal pulses. If such patients have only limited physical activity they may be asymptomatic.

Critical ischaemia

Ischaemic rest pain, ischaemic ulceration or gangrene of the feet requires urgent investigation and revascularisation in order to avoid limb loss due

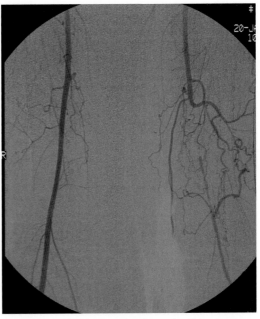

Figure 2.1 • Arteriogram showing well-collateralised occlusion of left superficial femoral artery. The patient had palpable foot pulses and almost normal resting ABPIs. These fell on the left side after exercise.

to progressive tissue necrosis and/or infection. Untreated, the prognosis is poor both for the patient and the leg, and recognition of critical ischaemia is therefore vitally important. There have been several attempts at a consensus for the definition of critical limb ischaemia (CLI).

> ✔ The European Consensus defines CLI as rest pain for more than 2 weeks, or ulceration/gangrene, and an ankle pressure of <50 mmHg or a toe pressure of <30 mmHg.[4]

However, this definition has been criticised because the pressures required for healing in the presence of ulceration or gangrene may be higher and ankle pressures are often falsely elevated in patients with diabetes (see later).[5] The Trans-Atlantic Inter-Society Consensus (TASC) II suggests that an ankle pressure of <70 mmHg or a toe pressure of <50 mmHg is more realistic in the presence of ulceration or gangrene.

> ✔ The precise definition is more relevant for reporting standards than for clinical use and the consensus document recommends that the term critical limb ischaemia should be used for all patients with chronic ischaemic rest pain, ulcers or gangrene attributable to objectively proven arterial occlusive disease.[6]

CLI in its very mild form may start with pain in the forefoot at night sufficient to disturb the patient's sleep when the patient is in supine position, thereby cancelling the effect of gravity on blood flow to the lower limbs.[7] When the patient hangs the leg out of the bed or if they stand up and walk, thereby increasing the blood flow to the foot, the pain is relieved. If the patient constantly hangs their feet out of bed at night, or even sleeps sitting in a chair, the limb swells due to dependency oedema. This can lead to a vicious circle with more tissue damage and the key is to use strong painkillers (usually opiates) so that the limb can be kept in the supine position overnight to relieve the oedema prior to arterial reconstruction.

To the experienced eye the diagnosis of CLI seems obvious, but it is easy to miss a small ischaemic lesion on the heel or between the toes. When established necrosis or gangrene is present with absent limb pulses there is no doubt about the diagnosis. The stage when critical ischaemia without necrosis or gangrene is present (Rutherford II 4) is characterised by pallor when the leg is elevated above the heart and by redness when hanging down (Buerger's or Ratshow's test positive). The dark red colour is caused by the dilated capillaries of the foot (**Fig. 2.2**). Normally, only one-third are open at any time but in the state of critical ischaemia autoregulation is

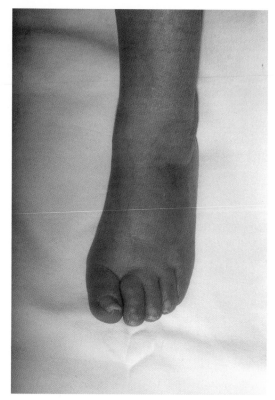

Figure 2.2 • Sunset red foot due to dilated capillaries caused by critical (limb-threatening) ischaemia. Elevation of the foot will result in pallor (Buerger's or Ratshow's test positive).

paralysed and, as a consequence, all capillaries are open.[8] It may take a while for pallor on elevation to occur but capillary refill will be abolished immediately.

Rare causes of ischaemia

The vast majority of cases of chronic lower limb ischaemia are caused by atherosclerotic PAD, but some rare conditions exist that tend to affect a younger age group. A good history of IC in a young patient should be taken seriously, as some of these conditions may progress rapidly to CLI. Resting ABPIs should be measured in all patients with leg pain on exercise, especially if foot pulses are absent. Those with a good history of IC and palpable foot pulses or normal ABPI should also undergo an exercise test and post-exercise ABPIs. Persistent sciatic artery is so rare that in my 30 years I may have seen one case.

Persistent sciatic artery

In this congenital anomaly, the embryonic axial limb artery, the sciatic artery, does not obliterate and remains continuous with the popliteal artery,

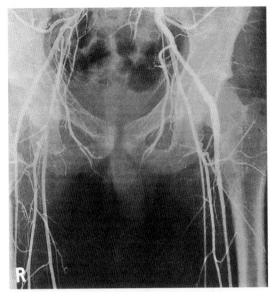

Figure 2.3 • Persistent bilateral sciatic arteries arising from the common iliac arteries with dilatation and intimal irregularity of the left sciatic artery at the level of the acetabulum.

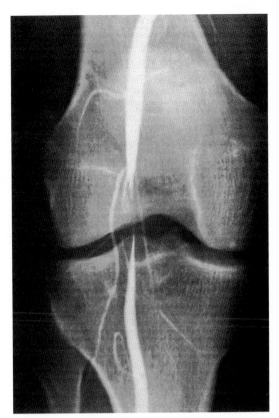

Figure 2.4 • Smooth 'hourglass' stenosis of popliteal artery due to cystic adventitial disease. A similar appearance may be seen in popliteal entrapment, especially during active plantar flexion.

providing the major blood supply to the lower limb. The anomaly is bilateral in 22% of cases and is commonly associated with failure of the iliofemoral vessels to develop properly. The presenting symptoms include pain and a pulsatile mass in the buttock due to aneurysmal degeneration of the artery as it emerges from the sciatic foramen. Thrombosis or distal embolism may lead to acute ischaemia.[9] Although pedal pulses may be present, the femoral pulse will be reduced or absent if the iliofemoral vessels are hypoplastic (Cowie's sign) and IC will result if neither system has developed properly (**Fig. 2.3**). Symptomatic patients can be treated by combined bypass grafting and endovascular exclusion of the aneurysm.[9] Asymptomatic patients should be monitored for aneurysm development.

Cystic adventitial disease (CAD)

CAD, caused by a cystic abnormality of the adventitia of the artery, most commonly affects the popliteal artery and may present with IC. The contents resemble that of a ganglion and the cysts may be connected to the synovium of the knee joint. IC may be severe and of rapid onset. The condition should be particularly suspected in young patients without significant risk factors for PAD. Pedal pulses sometimes disappear on knee flexion. Arteriography may show an unusually smooth 'hourglass' or eccentric stenosis (**Fig. 2.4**). Ultrasound scanning will demonstrate the cystic

abnormality, as will computed tomography (CT) or magnetic resonance (MR) scanning. Angioplasty is ineffective. The affected segment of artery requires resection and repair with an interposition vein graft via a posterior approach.[10]

Popliteal artery entrapment

The condition is not common but should be suspected when a young patient, particularly an athlete, complains of classic critical ischaemia. It can be anatomical or functional; in the anatomical variant, the artery courses around the medial head of the gastrocnemius muscle rather than between the two heads or, more rarely, passes deep to the popliteus muscle. Compression of the artery occurs during flexion, resulting in IC. Aneurysmal degeneration and/or thrombosis may develop. Two-thirds of cases are bilateral and the popliteal vein is involved in 10%.[11] Examination may reveal reduction or obliteration of pedal pulses during active plantar flexion. Duplex scanning or arteriography using this manoeuvre may also demonstrate kinking or compression of the popliteal artery. CT or MR scanning can also demonstrate the anatomical abnormality. Symptomatic patients should be treated by the division of the medial head of gastrocnemius and/or reconstruction of the popliteal artery. Surgery may be indicated for an asymptomatic contralateral limb whenever anatomical entrapment is detected.[12] In the functional variant of the condition, an anatomically normally positioned artery is compressed against a hypertrophied gastrocnemius or the soleal muscle ring. Unlike the anatomical variant, functional entrapment should only be treated when symptomatic.

Fibromuscular dysplasia (FMD)

Although FMD usually affects the renal and carotid arteries, it can affect the proximal upper and lower limb arteries in young people, causing IC. The external iliac artery appears the commonest site of involvement and arteriography may demonstrate a classic beaded appearance (**Fig. 2.5**). Patients with iliac FMD should be screened for renal involvement. Symptomatic stenoses usually respond well to angioplasty.[13]

Buerger's disease

Buerger's disease (thromboangiitis obliterans) is a systemic vasculitis that affects medium-sized arteries and veins. It should be considered in any heavy smoking young male claudicant, especially if they are of Middle or Far Eastern origin.[14] Vasospastic symptoms and superficial thrombophlebitis commonly occur and patients may progress rapidly to, or present with, CLI.

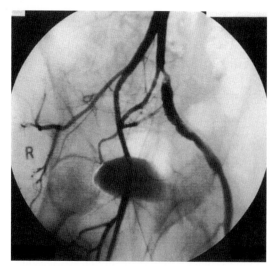

Figure 2.5 • Fibromuscular dysplasia affecting the left external iliac artery of a 12-year-old boy.

> ✔✔ The crural vessels are usually severely affected, with patent arteries to the knee joint and typical 'corkscrew' collaterals in the calf.[15]

The pathophysiology and management of this condition and other causes of vasculitis such as Takayasu's are covered in Chapter 12.

History and examination

History

> ✔✔ As all patients with PAD are at risk of myocardial infarction or stroke, a full history for other cardiovascular diseases and risk factors is essential (see Chapter 1).

In addition to previous myocardial infarction, stroke, coronary artery bypass grafting and arterial surgery, direct enquiry should include symptoms suggestive of angina or transient cerebral ischaemia. Although approximately 30% of patients with symptoms of limb ischaemia will have a history of myocardial infarction, it is not uncommon that angina or transient ischaemic attacks are diagnosed for the first time. The investigation and treatment of these symptoms usually have a higher priority than PAD (see Chapter 3). The enquiry for cardiovascular risk factors is equally important and obviously covers smoking, diabetes mellitus, hypertension, dyslipidaemia, and a detailed drug and family history. Upper extremity exertional pain, postprandial abdominal pain and erectile dysfunction in men are other important potential clues to the presence of significant occlusive atherosclerotic disease in other vascular territories.

Smoking may also cause chronic obstructive pulmonary disease. This and any cardiac disease will limit exercise capacity, limiting the benefit of any revascularisation, and may render the patient unfit for any open vascular reconstruction. Enquiry should be made, therefore, of any symptoms that may suggest that the patient may be unfit for intervention.

Examination

Signs of atherosclerosis and its risk factors in any part of the cardiovascular system should be elicited as well as examination findings to establish the site and severity of PAD. Examination should be systematic and include the following: measurement of blood pressure in both arms and the inter-arm difference; palpation of all peripheral and central pulses; pulse rate, rhythm and heart sounds; examination of the hands and abdominal aorta; careful inspection of the feet, particularly of skin integrity, colour and temperature. In addition, skin changes and calf hair loss may also be suggestive of chronic lower limb ischaemia.[16]

The body mass index (BMI) should be calculated by measuring height and weight.[17] This is a good estimate of obesity, a predictor of life expectancy and anaesthetic risk, but also adds to the patient's walking incapacity. In some cases, weight loss will reduce the patient's symptoms substantially.

Palpation of pulses is subjective, and is influenced by the sensitivity of the fingers, the experience of the examiner, the obesity of the patient and the warmth of the room. Any patient with symptoms from the lower limb that could be of ischaemic origin should have ABPI assessed. The femoral artery should always be palpable, whether it is pulsatile or occluded, if it is examined properly, unless the patient is very obese (**Fig. 2.6**). If it is occluded it can often be palpated as a hard cord due to atherosclerosis. If the pulse feels weak it is often because of proximal obstruction causing reduced femoral artery blood pressure. The popliteal pulse is more difficult to palpate, particularly in a well-muscled or obese subject, but should always be felt to exclude an aneurysm (**Fig. 2.7**). Palpation of the foot pulses should always be described. It may be difficult when the foot is swollen or the room is cold. Presence or absence of foot pulses on physical examination is a 'weak' and subjective sign of PAD and should always be supplemented by objective measurements (ABPI). The absence of a single foot pulse may have little clinical significance and, although it should be recorded, it is not an indication for more detailed investigation.

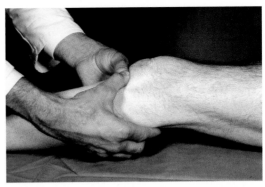

Figure 2.7 • A popliteal pulse is best felt using both hands with the leg relaxed in slight flexion.

Exercise challenge

Patients present occasionally with a classic history of IC, but with palpable foot pulses. These patients may have been investigated previously for joint disease or lumbar nerve root irritation even though their history may be 'typical' of claudication. Most often, there is proximal aorto-iliac disease with collaterals through the pelvis, sufficient to produce adequate or even normal pulses at rest. In patients who complain of symptoms only on exercise, it is rewarding to examine the leg following an exercise challenge. This can be done quite simply in the consulting room or by asking the patient to walk up and down the corridor (or on a treadmill if available). Even elderly patients find it easy to exercise the calf muscle by a repeated 'tiptoe' while leaning on the couch (**Fig. 2.8**). The patient returns to the couch so that the pulses can be examined immediately after exercising for 1 minute. More important, the post-exercise ABPI is measured.

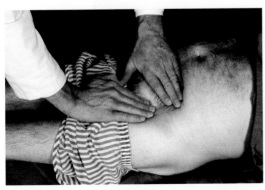

Figure 2.6 • Palpation of the femoral pulse may require both hands except in the thin patient. One hand pushes the lower abdomen out of the way and the other palpates the femoral artery/pulse.

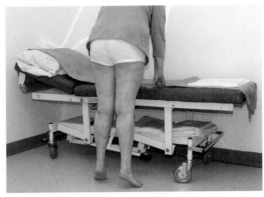

Figure 2.8 • Simple 'tiptoe' exercise of the calf muscle causes vasodilatation with disappearance of pulses and the emergence of bruits on examination immediately after the exercise.

ABPI measurement using a hand-held Doppler device

> ✔ ABPI assessment should be a routine part of a vascular examination.[6]

The perfusion pressure at the ankle can be measured using a tourniquet and insonating the pedal arteries with Doppler ultrasound. The patient should be rested for more than 5 minutes, lying supine, and a standard blood pressure tourniquet applied just above the ankle, with the tourniquet being 50% wider than the limb diameter. The tourniquet cuff is inflated above the systolic pressure, when the pedal Doppler signal should disappear. On gradually lowering the cuff pressure, the Doppler signal reappears at the ankle systolic pressure (**Fig. 2.9**). The probe should be held at a 30–60° angle to the vessel in order to achieve the optimal signal. The systolic blood pressure is then taken from the brachial artery in the same way and the ABPI calculated as the ratio of the ankle to the brachial systolic pressures. Blood pressures should be assessed on both arms at the patient's first visit since 3–5% of PAD patients may have supra-aortic obstructive disease as well. The higher of the two brachial blood pressures should be used as the reference for calculating ABPI.

> ✔ The systolic pressure at the ankle is normally higher, due to superimposed pulse waves down the arterial tree with an ABPI of 1.0–1.2. An ABPI of <0.9 suggests arterial disease and serves as the lower limit of normal. An ABPI of <0.5 is often associated with critical ischaemia.[6]

As falsely high ankle arterial pressures may be measured if the calf arteries are rigid due to calcification, as is often seen in diabetics and patients with chronic kidney insufficiency (dialysis patients), the finding of very high ankle pressures or incompressible ankle arteries should always raise suspicion of a false result. In such cases, measurement of toe pressures (see below) will reveal a true pressure as the small digital arteries very rarely become affected with media calcification. Alternatively, if toe pressure measurement is not possible, the pedal Doppler signal should also be assessed for normal triphasic or biphasic waveforms (see later). When the Doppler signal in the foot is monophasic due to proximal disease, pressures above the brachial pressure suggest falsely high readings due to vascular calcification.

Assessment of ABPI is clearly indicated for all patients with leg ulceration and foot ulcers. The technique is particularly important in diabetic 'neuropathic' ulcers or infection involving the toes or feet, where missed proximal arterial disease may lead to amputation due to rapidly progressing infection. The ABPI is also useful in elderly patients referred with foot symptoms that do not appear to be vascular when a normal measurement is reassuring.

Toe pressures

Toe pressure measurements may be useful when the calf arteries are incompressible or when severe distal arterial disease in the foot is suspected, i.e. in cases with high ABPI but non-healing ulcers at toe or forefoot level.

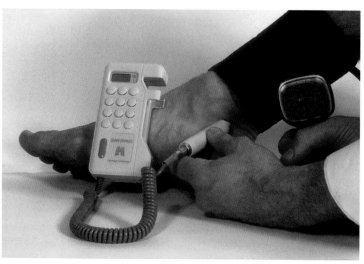

Figure 2.9 • A hand-held Doppler can be used to detect the presence of an arterial signal at the ankle. Assess the waveform – abnormal (monophasic/damped) or normal (biphasic/triphasic) – and measure the ABPI.

✓✓ A small toe cuff should be used and placed around the proximal phalanx of the great, second or third toe with a photoelectric cell on the toe distally.[18]

The toe pressure can be measured using the strain-gauge technique, photo-plethysmography or laser Doppler to detect the disappearance and reappearance of the pulse as the cuff is inflated and deflated.[19] A warm room is essential to avoid vasospasm and most often the feet need a 15- to 20-minute warm-up period. Expressed as a ratio to brachial artery pressure, toe pressures are normally lower than ABPI at 0.8–0.9.

✓ Critical ischaemia is unusual with toe–brachial pressure ratios >0.3 or absolute toe pressures >40 mmHg and two or more serial measurements are of greater value in predicting outcome than an initial single assessment.[20]

The ischaemic angle

As a refinement to Buerger's test, the level at which a pedal Doppler signal disappears on elevation of the foot may be taken as a crude measure of ankle arterial pressure when the calf arteries are incompressible.[21] This technique has been called the 'pole test' as the foot is raised alongside a calibrated pole marked in mmHg (0.73 mmHg=1 cmH$_2$O). This technique is only useful in severe ischaemia as it is not possible to raise the foot high enough to measure normal pressures.

Risk factors

All patients should be investigated for risk factors for atherosclerosis as modification reduces both the risk of fatal cardiovascular events and the need for arterial reconstruction. The risk factors associated with PAD are essentially the same as those for ischaemic heart disease, and include smoking, lack of exercise, unhealthy dietary habits (too much fat from meat, dairy fat, too little fish and vegetables), dyslipidaemia, diabetes mellitus and hypertension (see Chapter 1).

All patients with PAD require a full blood count, erythrocyte sedimentation rate (ESR), urea and electrolytes, plus random blood glucose, and lipids. Anaemia can present with symptoms of leg ischaemia, as can polycythaemia. An elevated ESR (or viscosity) may indicate raised fibrinogen, which seems an important factor in the development of PAD and vascular thrombosis. Renal impairment is often associated with PAD and requires

Box 2.1 • Blood tests in patients suffering PAD

All patients
Full blood count and ESR (or plasma viscosity)
Anaemia
Polycythaemia
Thrombocythaemia
Biochemical profile
Diabetes
Renal impairment
Dyslipidaemia
Hypertriglyceridaemia
Selected patients
(Age <50 years or acute unusual thrombosis)
Thrombophilia screen
Hyperhomocysteinaemia
'Ex' smokers
Thiocyanate, carboxyhaemoglobin or urinary cotinine

ESR, erythrocyte sedimentation rate

detection before contemplating both imaging and intervention. Arterial thromboembolism is relatively infrequent in patients under the age of 50. Young patients with PAD should have a thrombophilia screen as antiphospholipid antibodies or antithrombin III deficiency may lead to repeated rethrombosis following either angioplasty or reconstruction. Hyperhomocysteinaemia can cause accelerated atherosclerosis and should be excluded in young patients with PAD. Acute peripheral ischaemia in a younger patient with no history of PAD should warrant cardiac work-up, including at least electrocardiogram (ECG) and echocardiography. The investigation of cardiovascular risk factors is summarised in Box 2.1. As 25% of patients who claim to have stopped smoking may be lying, measuring a smoking marker may be required, although the effect of such 'proof' on smoking cessation is questionable.[22]

Vascular laboratory

Waveform assessment and segmental pressures

The use of Doppler waveforms, originally implemented using hand-held continuous-wave Doppler devices, still has an important role in the investigation of PAD. The elasticity in normal arteries gives a characteristic triphasic waveform (see Fig. 2.11c). The blood pressure may be reduced distal to a stenosis and, consequently, the resistance in the peripheral vascular bed is reduced, changing the shape of this waveform. Distal to a moderate stenosis (50% diameter reduction) the waveform is biphasic, and with a >70% stenosis the waveform becomes monophasic (see Fig. 2.11d).[23,26] Waveform shape can be affected by distal disease, dilatation of arteries, multisegment disease, complete occlusion of an artery and also ambient temperature. Waveform shape can only give an indication of disease and should be used in conjunction with segmental pressures to determine which segments in the leg are diseased, i.e. since percutaneous transluminal angioplasty (PTA) is minimally invasive and generally provides good results in the iliac arteries, knowing that a pressure-reducing lesion is located in this anatomical region may strengthen the indication for invasive treatment in a patient with severe IC.

Clinicians frequently see patients with multisegment disease. Segmental arterial pressures have some additional value in both determining the level of disease and predicting whether proximal arterial reconstruction will be adequate to treat critical ischaemia (**Fig. 2.10**). However, duplex ultrasound or arteriography are more useful in this respect.

Laser Doppler and transcutaneous oximetry

These are both techniques used to assess the viability of skin perfusion. Laser Doppler measures the Doppler shift in light emitted by a diode and measures overall skin perfusion to a depth of approximately 1.5 mm.

✔✔ It is most appropriately used as a trend instrument and has failed to gain any useful clinical applications in PAD even though the newer probes, with several measuring points, are more reliable.

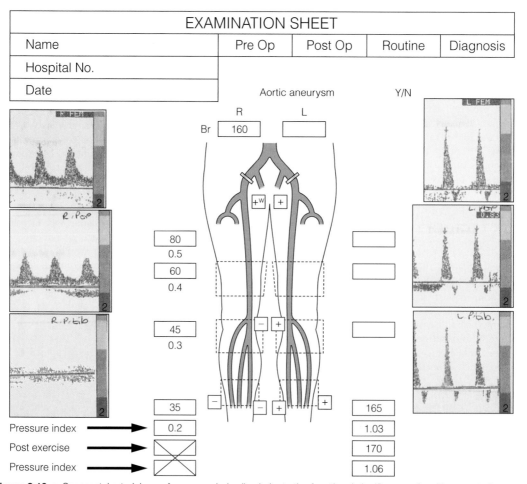

Figure 2.10 • Segmental arterial waveforms may help discriminate the functional significance of multisegment disease, such as the right iliac and superficial femoral occlusions in this patient. Theoretically, normalising the low thigh pressure will approximately double the ankle arterial pressure to a level that should relieve ischaemic rest pain.

Transcutaneous oximetry can be used to measure the partial pressure of oxygen diffusing through the surface of the skin as an indirect measure for oxygen tension in the underlying tissue. It was hoped that $tcPO_2$ measurements of calf skin might be used to determine whether healing would occur following below-knee amputation.[24] Unfortunately, neither $tcPO_2$ nor ABPI is reliable for this as the changes in skin perfusion after the distal limb has been removed cannot be predicted. Where there is severe proximal disease, removing the distal limb is unlikely to heal.

Duplex ultrasound (DUS)

DUS allows the visualisation and haemodynamic assessment of arteries using grey-scale, also known as B-mode imaging, colour-flow Doppler mapping, power Doppler and pulsed-wave Doppler interrogation of blood flow. It is an operator-dependent examination; however, in the hands of an experienced sonographer, it can be used to map the length of an artery and identify the severity and location of disease. As with all tests being used to assess patients, the accuracy in the local setting must be evaluated.

> ✅✅ DUS of the extremities has been given a class 1 recommendation (supported by multiple randomised controlled trials or meta-analyses) for the diagnosis, the anatomical location and degree of stenosis of PAD, as well as for routine surveillance after femoral–popliteal or femoral–tibial pedal bypass with a venous conduit.[25]

The value of duplex is that the diseased artery may be imaged clearly using grey-scale ultrasound, which visualises echogenic plaques and the anatomy of the artery/disease. Real-time colour-flow Doppler is used to identify blood flow through the colour box positioned in the grey-scale image. Colour filling will only occur where blood is moving and can therefore be used to enhance the grey-scale image by identifying 'soft' echolucent atheroma or thrombus as an area of absent colour filling. Colour flow also allows identification of increased blood velocity by a change in colour within the lumen of the artery. Combining grey-scale and colour-flow mapping, a severe stenosis can be seen as grey echoes reducing the diameter of the colour filling and a 'mosaic' of colours indicating increased velocity and turbulence. Grey-scale and colour flow do not provide a quantitative means of determining the severity of a stenosis other than by direct luminal diameter or area loss measurement (**Fig. 2.11a,b**).

Accurate quantification of the severity of the stenosis requires the use of pulsed-wave Doppler. With this technique the ultrasound signal is pin-pointed to a specific depth by the sampling box, which is kept small within the central lumen. The change of frequency (Doppler shift) in this reflected signal is determined by the transmitted frequency, angle of insonation and the velocity of blood. Modern DUS machines allow automated calculation of blood velocity but the accuracy of this relies heavily on the correct determination of the position of the pulsed-wave Doppler box and angling of the central cursor to the axis of blood flow. The peak systolic velocity is measured in the normal artery proximal to a stenosis and then in the stenosis identified by colour flow. The shape of the Doppler waveform (triphasic, biphasic or monophasic), degree of spectral broadening (range of velocity profiles within the wave spectra secondary to turbulence) and change in peak systolic velocity relative to the upstream normal artery all help to determine the severity of a given stenosis (Table 2.3).[26] A twofold increase in the peak systolic velocity generally indicates a 50% narrowing of the artery, while a 2.5-fold increase indicates a narrowing of greater than 50%. Distal to a stenosis, the Doppler waveform changes shape due to damping with reduction in peak systolic velocity and a slower acceleration time (time from end diastole to peak systole; **Fig. 2.11c**).

Certainty of the diagnosis of a complete occlusion as opposed to high-grade stenosis with trickle flow within an artery may be difficult and depends heavily on the experience of the sonographer. The shape of the Doppler waveform proximally and distally, colour-flow images and the presence of collaterals all contribute to differentiating these lesions. Difficulties can arise with deep or tortuous arteries, where signal return is reduced and optimum angles of insonation are difficult to obtain. Multiple stenoses along the length of an artery reduce the accuracy of flow velocity measurements in the assessment of more distal stenoses. The sonographer must thus use valuable years of experience and knowledge of more subtle changes in blood velocity to determine the severity of a given stenosis when there are tandem or multiple stenoses.

Assessment of suprainguinal arteries

This can be difficult due to respiratory movements, the depth of arteries, arterial tortuosity, overlying bowel gas and if arterial wall calcification obscures the vessel lumen, particularly in the presence of slow flow. Varying the plane of insonation may occasionally help by 'throwing off' obscuring and distracting anatomy and pathology.

> ✅ Aorto-iliac DUS arterial assessment has been shown to match catheter angiography, with a sensitivity of 0.89 and specificity of 0.90.[27]

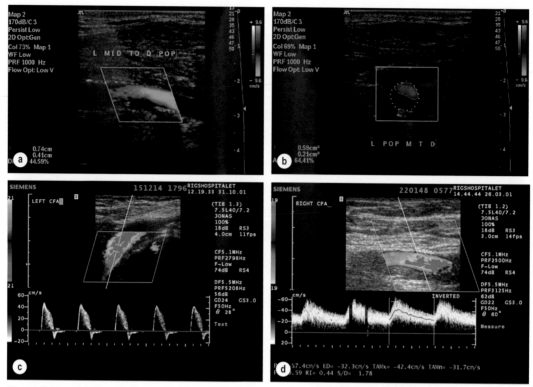

Figure 2.11 • (a) A longitudinal colour Doppler image of a mid to distal left popliteal artery stenosis with a diameter reduction of 45%. **(b)** The area reduction of the same lesion on transaxial imaging is 64%. **(c,d)** Doppler waveforms from common femoral artery, just proximal to stenosis **(c)** and distal to stenosis **(d)**. Notice how the waveform is triphasic with steep acceleration phase signalling high resistance **(c)**, and monophasic, and dampened distal to the stenosis, where the stenosis has caused a pressure drop with reduction in resistance as a result **(d)**.

Table 2.3 • Diagnostic criteria for peripheral arterial diameter reduction

	Diameter reduction (%)	Waveform	Spectral broadening	PSV distal/ PSV proximal
Normal	0	Triphasic	Absent	No change
Mild	1–19	Triphasic	Present	<2:1
Moderate	20–49	Biphasic	Present	<2:1
Severe	50–99	Monophasic	Present	>2:1*

PSV, peak systolic velocity.
*>4:1 suggests >75% stenosis, >7:1 suggests >90% stenosis.

An experienced vascular sonographer will report any study limitations. Changes in the Doppler waveform before and after an inadequately viewed segment give an indication of disease and the need for further investigation. A simple test is to evaluate the Doppler waveform in the common femoral artery. If it is triphasic, the likelihood of a severe obstructive lesion in the aorto-iliac segment is very small.[28]

Assessment of infrainguinal arteries

✅ In experienced hands, DUS is accurate at identifying disease from the common femoral to the distal popliteal artery, with a sensitivity of 84–87% and specificity of 92–98% compared to catheter angiography.[29,30]

The crural arteries can be more difficult, especially when there is severe proximal disease.[31,32] In large calves, the depth of insonation attenuates the signal return, making it difficult to visualise the proximal crural arteries.[32] Accuracy can be improved by using a 4.2-MHz curved-array abdominal probe, which allows deeper penetration. Alternatively, power Doppler, which is more sensitive to slow flow, can help to detect the optimum tibial artery for revascularisation.[33,34]

Radiological investigations

The choice of imaging modality for the investigation of chronic lower limb ischaemia was reviewed as part of the recently published, August 2012, UK National Institute of Clinical Evidence (NICE) 'Lower limb peripheral arterial disease: diagnosis and management', Clinical Guideline 147. The question as to the most clinical and cost-effective method for assessment of PAD revealed eight relevant publications from which the following broad recommendations were made.

✔✔ 1. Offer duplex ultrasound as first-line imaging to all people with peripheral arterial disease for whom revascularisation is being considered.
2. Offer contrast-enhanced magnetic resonance angiography (CE-MRA) to people with peripheral arterial disease who need further imaging (after duplex ultrasound) before considering revascularisation.
3. Offer computed tomography angiography to people with peripheral arterial disease who need further imaging (after duplex ultrasound) if CE-MRA is contraindicated or not tolerated.[35]

Many vascular centres use DUS as the first-line imaging modality to investigate PAD due to its greater availability, lower cost and limited access to MR scanner time. Relying solely on DUS, however, prior to lower limb revascularisation, risks underestimation of the severity and number of sites of vascular disease, particularly at challenging-to-reach anatomical areas such as the iliac and proximal infragenicular crural arteries. CE-MRA, on the other hand, provides better overall diagnostic accuracy and may also serve as a first-line imaging modality.[36,37] CE-MRA provides an excellent overview when maximum intensity projection (MIP) presents 'angiographic' type images and is increasingly being extended to image the foot arteries. DUS can then be utilised in a complementary role, focused on problem solving, to address specific equivocal haemodynamic questions that may affect the treatment strategy. This optimises the sonographer's time and eliminates redundant duplication of imaging normal arterial segments twice.

Contrast media

Iodinated intravascular contrast media, whether for use in catheter angiographic procedures or for vascular or tissue enhancement in CT examinations, continues to pose risks for the development of contrast-induced nephrotoxicity (CIN). This is most commonly defined as an acute decline in renal function with an increase in serum creatinine (SCr) by more than 25% of the baseline value or a 44 μmol/L (0.5 mg/dL) absolute increase of SCr occurring within 48–72 hours, following the intravascular administration of a contrast medium in the absence of an alternative aetiology.[38]

In a multivariate analysis several risk factors have been identified (Box 2.2).[39] Methods to reduce the incidence of CIN have been highly contentious and have included usuing alternative imaging techniques, varying the choice of contrast, minimising contrast volume, pharmacological manipulation by stopping nephrotoxic drugs and metformin, and intravenous volume expansion.[40]

A CIN Consensus Working Panel composed of experts in the contrast field undertook an extensive review of the literature and produced ten consensus statements (Box 2.3).[41]

✔✔ The CIN Consensus Working Panel agreed that for an estimated glomerular filtration rate (eGFR) of 30–59 mL/min, intravenous volume expansion reduces the risk for CIN and that patients should receive adequate intravenous volume expansion with isotonic crystalloid (1.0–1.5 mL/kg per hour) for 3–12 hours before the procedure and for 6–24 hours afterwards. If the eGFR is <30 mL/min a nephrology consultation is recommended with dialysis planning should CIN occur.

Box 2.2 • Risk factors for contrast-induced nephropathy (CIN) identified in multivariate analysis

Chronic kidney disease (stage 3 or greater: eGFR <60 mL/min/1.73 m²)
Diabetes mellitus (type 1 or 2)
Volume depletion
Nephrotoxic drug use (NSAIDs, ciclosporin, aminoglycosides)
Preprocedural haemodynamic instability
Other comorbidities:
• Anaemia
• Congestive heart failure
• Hypoalbuminaemia

eGFR, estimated glomerular filtration rate;
NSAIDs, non-steroidal anti-inflammatory drugs.

Box 2.3 • Consensus statements agreed upon by the CIN Consensus Working Panel

1. CIN is a common and potentially serious complication following the administration of contrast media in patients at risk for acute renal injury.
2. The risk of CIN is elevated and of clinical importance in patients with chronic kidney disease (particularly when diabetes is also present), recognised by an eGFR <60 mL/min/1.73 m².
3. When serum creatinine or eGFR is unavailable, then a survey may be used to identify patients at higher risk for CIN than the general population.
4. In the setting of emergency procedures, where the benefit of very early imaging outweighs the risk of waiting, the procedure can be performed without knowledge of serum creatinine or eGFR.
5. The presence of multiple CIN risk factors in the same patient or high-risk clinical scenarios can create a very high risk for CIN (50%) and ARF (15%) requiring dialysis after contrast exposure.
6. In patients at increased risk for CIN undergoing intra-arterial administration of contrast, ionic high-osmolality agents pose a greater risk for CIN than low-osmolality agents. Current evidence suggests that for intra-arterial administration in high-risk patients with chronic kidney disease, particularly those with diabetes mellitus, non-ionic, iso-osmolar contrast is associated with the lowest risk of CIN.
7. Higher contrast volumes (100 mL) are associated with higher rates of CIN in patients at risk. However, even small (30 mL) volumes of iodinated contrast in very-high-risk patients can cause CIN and ARF requiring dialysis, suggesting the absence of a threshold effect.
8. Intra-arterial administration of iodinated contrast media appears to pose a greater risk of CIN above that which occurs with intravenous administration.
9. Adequate intravenous volume expansion with isotonic crystalloid (1.0–1.5 mL/kg per hour) for 3–12 hours before the procedure and continued for 6–24 hours afterwards can lessen the probability of CIN in patients at risk. The data on oral fluids as opposed to intravenous volume expansion as a CIN prevention measure are insufficient.
10. No adjunctive medical or mechanical treatment has been proved to be efficacious in reducing the risk of CIN. Prophylactic haemodialysis or haemofiltration have not been validated as effective strategies.

ARF, acute renal failure; CIN, contrast-induced nephropathy; CKD, chronic kidney disease; eGFR, estimated glomerular filtration rate.

Much debate has surrounded which contrast agent might have an advantage in reducing the incidence of CIN, with much support for the use of iso-osmolar, non-ionic contrast media over low-osmolar, non-ionic agents. A recent meta-analysis of randomised controlled trials showed that the route of administration may affect the renal safety of contrast agents. Specifically, iodixanol may be a better choice for patients receiving intra-arterial contrast.[42]

✔✔ In the PREDICT study, a randomised double-blind comparison of CIN after low- or iso-osmolar contrast agent exposure, 248 patients with moderate to severe chronic kidney disease and diabetes mellitus were randomised to receive at least 65 mL of iopamidol 370 (low-osmolar) or iodixanol 320 (iso-osmolar) for a CT procedure. There was no significant difference in the incidence of CIN at 48–72 hours after contrast administration.[43]

Metformin is excreted unchanged in the urine. In the presence of renal failure, either pre-existing or induced by iodinated contrast medium, metformin may accumulate in sufficient amounts to cause the serious complication of lactic acidosis. Metformin does not cause renal failure.[38] Contrast agents should therefore be administered with caution, particularly those with known renal impairment, and it is essential that the renal function (serum creatinine) is checked in these patients prior to the examination.

If >100 mL of intravenous iodinated contrast is to be administered for intra-arterial contrast, metformin should be withheld for 48 hours after the procedure.

✔ If there is biochemical evidence of renal impairment, i.e. serum creatinine >120 μmol/L, metformin should also be withheld for 2 days before and after contrast administration. Serum creatinine should be rechecked 48 hours post procedure and the metformin reinstituted only if renal function remains stable (less than 25% increase compared to baseline).

Patients with a baseline serum creatinine of >150 μmol/L should not be taking metformin. If patients are referred on metformin despite this level of chronic kidney disease, the metformin should be discontinued indefinitely and the patient referred back for alternative hypoglycaemic therapy prior to the procedure.

Nephrogenic systemic fibrosis (NSF) is a newly described phenomenon of skin, muscle and organ fibrosis that may produce severe disability or even death. Its incidence may vary from negligible up to 2–5% in selected high-risk clinical situations. As of May 2007 the total number of worldwide cases was 215. The cause of NSF is rapidly emerging and has been largely attributed to gadolinium-based contrast agents (GBCAs) used in contrast-enhanced MR imaging and occurs particularly in the setting of moderate to severe renal impairment. Specific subtypes of gadolinium MR contrast agents given to patients with chronic kidney disease (CKD 4 and 5; **Box 2.3**) have been implicated in the majority of cases and it is believed that macrocyclic gadolinium chelates are more stable and less likely to release free gadolinium ions,[44] thought to be central to the underlying pathophysiology.

Blood pool contrast agents (BPCAs), which are also GBCAs, have recently emerged and have provided a number of new imaging opportunities in the assessment of vascular disease. Gadofosveset Trisodium or Ablavar® (Lantheus Medical Imaging) is an albumin-bound gadolinium chelate that stays within the vascular compartment, allowing vascular imaging up to 30–40 minutes after a single injection. It is 90% renally excreted and has the highest T1 relaxivity of any gadolinium agent, thus providing good signal strength for first-pass arterial imaging. High-resolution images can subsequently be obtained to interrogate equivocal stenoses or the vessel wall. To date, there have been no cases of NSF attributed to Gadofosveset®, thought to be due possibly to the lower concentration of gadolinium required.

Magnetic resonance angiography (MRA)

There are many MR techniques for the assessment of vessels and vessel patency, all of which continue to evolve at a rapid pace. In recent years, phase-contrast and time-of-flight MRA have largely given way to three-dimensional contrast-enhanced MRA (CE-MRA), which employs subtraction, bolus chase and stepping table movements. CE-MRA provides a non-invasive, three-dimensional luminal assessment of vessels without the risk of iodine-based contrast agents and without the use of ionising radiation. It has now become the preferred first-line imaging technique for the investigation of PAD. This is advocated in international guidelines, as well as by the TASC II document and recently published NICE Clinical Guideline 147 on the diagnosis and management of PAD.[6,36] Analyses of the accuracy of MRA and comparisons of the merits of differing MR techniques have been performed.

> ✅✅ In a meta-analysis of 32 studies including 1022 patients, CE-MRA was concluded to have high accuracy for identifying or excluding clinically relevant arterial steno-occlusions in adults with PAD symptoms.[45]

Technique
There are a wide variety of techniques for performing peripheral lower limb MRA that depend on the MR hardware, software sequences, moving or continuous-table capability, peripheral and surface coils, preferred contrast agent and injection protocol. As crural (tibial) vessel venous contamination has been the Achilles heel of consistently high-quality peripheral MRA, techniques have been developed to overcome this by obtaining this imaging station either faster using parallel imaging (acceleration techniques) or, first, using dynamic time-resolved MRA, followed by the more usual three- or four-station stepping-table 'bolus chase' technique (**Fig. 2.12a**). More recent developments have included greater efforts at imaging the foot vessels as distal intervention has become of increasing importance (**Fig. 2.12b**).

Contraindications
Contraindications to MRA include the presence of a pacemaker or certain types of metallic prosthetic cardiac valve implants, intracranial aneurysm clips, cochlear implants or metallic intraocular foreign bodies. Up to 5% of patients may be claustrophobic in the MR bore, which may be overcome using open bore systems or by using psychotherapy relaxation techniques. Occasionally, sedation or rarely a general anaesthetic may be required.[6]

Computed tomographic angiography (CTA)

Over the last 15 years, CT scanners have developed from single-slice to ever increasing numbers of simultaneously acquired helical multislice systems, progressing through four, eight, 16, 32, 64 dual-energy source systems to 256 slices. CTA today is invaluable in the acute setting for the diagnosis of acute bleeding and vessel injuries, and relies heavily on excellent contrast timing techniques.[46] Calcification within the lower limb arterial tree has greatly limited its use as the preferred imaging modality for the assessment of chronic lower limb ischaemia.

> ✅✅ The UK National Clinical Guideline Centre, 'Lower limb peripheral arterial disease: diagnosis and management', NICE Clinical Guideline 147, August 2012, recommends computed tomography angiography to people with peripheral arterial disease who need further imaging prior to revascularisation (after duplex ultrasound) if CE-MRA is contraindicated or not tolerated.[35]

Technique
With each of the multislice systems, the tube continuously rotates and acquires information as the patient is fed through the scanner. The volume scanned is then divided into many volume elements (voxels) and the central processor reconstructs slices

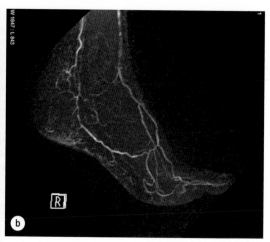

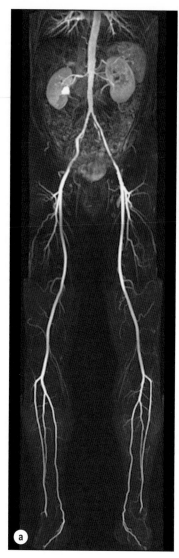

Figure 2.12 • **(a)** Coronal MIP of contrast-enhanced aorta and lower limb MRA at 3 T using a stepping, bolus chase technique and image fusion. **(b)** Sagittal MIP of optimal arterial filling during dynamic contrast enhanced MRA of the foot. Images provided by Dr A. Holden, Auckland City Hospital.

from this dataset. Because a *volume* of tissue has been scanned, these slices can be reconstructed in any plane (multiplanar and curved planar reconstructions). Complex reconstructions can also be performed, with the subtraction of bone or other detail that may obscure the arteries. As arterial wall calcification is close to the Hounsfield unit of arterially opacified blood, care must be taken to ensure that no normal part of the vessel has been subtracted when using automated subtraction algorithms. This also applies to vessels that lie in close proximity to bone, for example the tibial arteries, which may be subtracted if the bones are automatically removed. The radiologist must therefore review the source data in the plane of greatest spatial resolution (with 0.6-mm slice thickness in modern multislice

systems, this now includes any plane, including oblique planes) as well as the reconstructions.

MIP images can be constructed, selecting the highest density voxel along a given plane or planes (**Fig. 2.13a**). This produces a two-dimensional angiographic-like image that can be rotated to allow multiple viewing angles. A variety of three-dimensional volume rendered reconstructions can also be displayed in colour, with preset colour maps determined to best display the anatomy required (**Fig. 2.13b**). With the exception of complex vascular anatomy, such as arteriovenous malformations or intracranial aneurysms, little additional purely diagnostic information is gained. These images are, however, useful for surgical and endovascular planning, producing accurate vessel diameters,

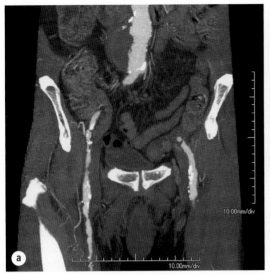
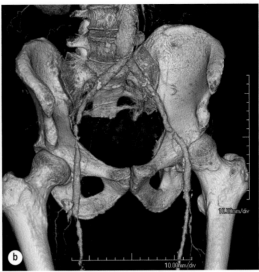

Figure 2.13 • (a) An oblique coronal thin MIP reconstruction created for an elderly male patient with chronic bilateral limb ischaemia. **(b)** A volume-rendered CT angiogram of the lower abdominal aorta, iliac and proximal femoral arteries, demonstrating extensive peripheral vascular disease. High-grade stenoses are present in both external iliac arteries and the proximal right superficial femoral artery.

permitting consideration of catheter selection to take place ahead of interventions, or allowing planning of optimal angulation of fluoroscopic and digital subtraction angiographic tube positions.

Catheter angiography

Digital subtraction angiography (DSA) was, for a long time, considered the 'gold standard' in the investigation of peripheral vascular disease; however, as an invasive procedure placing patients at risk of harm, albeit at low incidence levels (Table 2.4), this has now given way to non-invasive imaging modalities and is no longer recommended in guidelines. Diagnostic angiography is also expensive, requires informed consent, a day-case bed, ties up numerous members of angiography suite staff and negatively impacts on time available for planned therapeutic interventions.[47,48]

Table 2.4 • Royal College of Radiologists recommendations for upper limit of complications arising from diagnostic angiography

Haematoma (requiring transfusion, surgery or delayed discharge)	3.0%
Occlusion of the artery	0.5%
Pseudo-aneurysm	0.5%
Arteriovenous fistula	0.1%
Distal embolisation	0.5%
Occlusion of distal arteries	2.0%

Technique

DSA takes the output from an image intensifier and digitises the image. A single image is taken before the injection of contrast (the mask image); following contrast injection, further images are taken that can be subtracted from the mask. This removes bony detail, leaving a clear image of the arterial tree. In CLI, good-quality images of the crural (tibial) arteries and plantar arch are important in planning distal bypass operations. These distal images are prone to movement artefacts in the critical limb and adequate analgesia is therefore essential.

Basic angiographic access is by the modified Seldinger technique[49] using a hollow puncture needle and a floppy guidewire, usually with a J-tip placed down the central lumen of the needle into the artery lumen. A catheter is then passed over the wire once the puncture needle has first been removed. Most angiograms for lower limb ischaemia require the injection of contrast by mechanical pumps using catheters with multiple side holes. This ensures that the contrast is distributed evenly within the circulating blood and that the catheter remains stable in position. Usually, diagnostic angiograms involve placing a pigtail catheter in the abdominal aorta with images from the infrarenal aorta to the foot. Intra-arterial pressure gradients can also be measured across stenoses of uncertain significance. With care, diagnostic angiography is safe with 3- or 4-Fr catheters in patients with international normalised ratios of prothrombin time up to 3.0, provided the blood pressure is well controlled.

Risks and limitations

The risks of conventional catheter angiography may be related to contrast media or technique.

Contrast related

- Allergic: these are not dose related and probably result from mast cell degranulation. The incidence of severe anaphylactic reactions due to ionic contrast media is 0.01–0.02%, but non-ionic low-osmolar iodinated contrast agents are 5–10 times safer than their predecessors. Patients with severe asthma or hay fever are at increased risk of an allergic reaction, which may be severe. Steroid prophylaxis should be considered. Patients with known contrast allergy should be imaged using alternative techniques.
- Toxic: these are dose related and manifest themselves as a metallic taste in the mouth, feelings of warmth, nausea or vomiting, cardiac arrhythmias and pulmonary oedema. They are more likely to occur in patients with severe vascular disease.
- Renal (CIN – see above).

Technique related

- Pseudo-aneurysm/haematoma: haematoma around the puncture site is common. This can be reduced by using smaller catheters and a good manual haemostasis arterial compression technique for at least 10 minutes. Arterial closure devices are rarely indicated for diagnostic angiography using 3- and 4-Fr catheters, although this may allow faster ambulation of patients and be useful with uncorrected clotting profiles.
- Dissection: a dissection flap is usually caused by poor technique using undue force or hydrophilic guidewires. Although small flaps are rarely a problem, larger or antegrade flaps may significantly slow blood flow or occlude the artery.
- Infection is rare with good aseptic technique.
- Arteriovenous fistula: as the femoral artery and vein are contained within the femoral sheath they may both be punctured during arterial access when a blind puncture is performed. Where ultrasound is available, this should be used to avoid anterior wall plaques and accurately identify the common femoral artery.
- Embolisation: if atheromatous material lining the artery is inadvertently dislodged, it will embolise distally. This may be retrieved using suction aspiration but may need surgical embolectomy or bypass surgery.

Key points

- The Fontaine classification for the severity of PAD has the benefit of simplicity and is clinically useful.
- Risk factors must be identified and treated in all patients with PAD.
- A careful history is essential, especially in patients with coexisting spinal problems.
- Patients with a good history of claudication and palpable pulses should be examined after exercise and/or an exercise test performed.
- Rare causes of ischaemia should not be forgotten, especially in younger patients.
- Documentation of the severity of ischaemia by Doppler pressures/waveforms is mandatory in all patients with absent or weak pulses who are complaining of leg pain, weakness or numbness.
- Further investigation is not warranted unless revascularisation is being considered.
- Critical ischaemia requires urgent investigation and revascularisation in order to avoid limb loss due to progressive tissue necrosis and/or infection.
- Offer duplex ultrasound as first-line imaging to all people with peripheral arterial disease for whom revascularisation is being considered. Offer CE-MRA to people with peripheral arterial disease who need further imaging (after duplex ultrasound) before considering revascularisation.
- Contrast-induced nephrotoxiciy remains a serious concern for all procedures requiring iodinated contrast medium. Serum creatinine or eGFRs must be known and provided on all patients at risk for developing this complication and must also be checked at 48 hours post-contrast injection.

- Nephrogenic systemic fibrosis is a rare but potentially serious condition occurring in chronic kidney disease patients receiving gadolinium-based contrast agents. Serum creatinine levels or eGFR must be known and provided on all patients referred for CE-MRA who are at risk of developing this condition (stage 3, 4 and 5 chronic kidney disease).
- CTA provides detailed angiographic imaging in peripheral arterial disease but is limited in severely calcified disease and those with known severe PAD. It is particularly useful in the acute assessment of limb ischaemia where potentially embolising sources may be identified.
- Catheter angiography is invasive and is no longer recommended as a first-line imaging modality in the diagnosis of PAD. It should be limited to patients in whom therapeutic intervention is planned at the same time.

References

1. Porter RW. Spinal stenosis and neurogenic claudication. Spine 1996;21:2046–52.

2. Leyk D, Baum K. Cardiac output, leg blood flow and oxygen uptake during foot plantar flexions. Int J Sports Med 1999;20:510–5.
   Parallel determinations of cardiac output, leg blood flow (LBF) and pulmonary oxygen uptake were performed in nine healthy male subjects at the onset and cessation of dynamic foot plantar flexions. Within the first 10 seconds of exercise LBF increased from 400 to about 1000 mL/min at all exercise intensities. During the subsequent 5 minutes of exercise, LBF decreased to about 800 mL/min at the lowest intensity. By contrast, it increased to about 1900 mL/min at the highest intensity.

3. Pena CS, McCauley TR. Quantitative blood flow measurements with cine phase-contrast MR imaging of subjects at rest and after exercise to assess peripheral vascular disease. AJR Am J Roentgenol 1996;167:153–7.

4. Second European Consensus Document on Chronic Critical Leg Ischemia. Eur J Vasc Surg 1992;6:1–4.

5. Thompson MM, Sayers RD, Varty K, et al. Chronic critical leg ischemia must be redefined. Eur J Vasc Surg 1993;7:420–6.

6. Norgren L, Hiatt WR, Dormandy JA, et al., on behalf of the TASC II Working Group. Inter-Society Consensus for the Management of Peripheral Arterial Disease (TASC II). Eur J Vasc Endovasc Surg 2007;33:S1–75.

7. Jelnes R, Tonnesen KH. Nocturnal foot blood flow in patients with arterial insufficiency. Clin Sci (Lond) 1984;67:89–95.
   Twenty-four-hour continuous recording of xenon (^{133}Xe) washout from the forefoot was performed on patients with normal circulations ($n=10$) and on patients with different degrees of arterial insufficiency ($n=36$). During day hours the calculated subcutaneous blood flow in the forefoot was the same in patients with normal circulation and in patients with different degrees of arterial insufficiency (2.0 ± 0.8 mL/min per 100 g). During sleep the blood flow nearly doubled in patients with normal circulation, no systematic change was seen in patients with IC, and in patients with severe ischaemia the blood flow decreased by approximately 50%.

8. Eickhoff JH. Local regulation of subcutaneous blood flow and capillary filtration in limbs with occlusive arterial disease. Studies before and after arterial reconstruction. Dan Med Bull 1986;33:111–26.

9. Maldini G, Teruya TH. Combined percutaneous endovascular and open surgical approach in the treatment of a persistent sciatic artery aneurysm presenting with acute limb-threatening ischemia – a case report and review of the literature. Vasc Endovasc Surg 2002;36:403–8.

10. Macfarlane R, Livesey SA. Cystic adventitial arterial disease. Br J Surg 1987;74:89–90.

11. Levien LJ, Veller MG. Popliteal artery entrapment syndrome: more common than previously recognized. J Vasc Surg 1999;30:587–98.

12. Turnipseed WD. Popliteal entrapment syndrome. J Vasc Surg 2002;35:910–5.

13. Hui C, Baker D, Platts A. The role of percutaneous transluminal angioplasty in the treatment of carotid fibromuscular dysplasia. Eur J Vasc Endovasc Surg Extra 2003;5:102–5.

14. Mills JL. Buerger's disease in the 21st century: diagnosis, clinical features, and therapy. Semin Vasc Surg 2003;16:179–89.

15. Suzuki S, Yamada I. Angiographic findings in Buerger disease. Int J Cardiol 1996;54(Suppl.):S189–95.
    One hundred and forty-four angiographic images of the lower extremities of 119 patients with Buerger's disease were studied. The collateral vessels had a 'corkscrew' appearance in 39 (27%) of 144 limbs affected by Buerger's disease, whereas this appearance was seen in only 2 (3%) of 63 limbs of patients with atherosclerosis ($P < 0.001$). The appearance of corkscrew-shaped vessels is the most characteristic feature of Buerger's disease and represents a dilated vasa vasorum of the occluded main arteries.

16. Adam AJ, Beard JD, Cleveland T, et al. BASIL trial participants. Bypass versus angioplasty in severe ischaemia of the leg (BASIL): multicentre, randomised controlled trial. Lancet 2005;366:1925–34.
A prospective randomised controlled trial of surgery versus angioplasty in patients with severe lower limb ischaemia. At entry into the trial, only one-third were on a statin, over one-third were not on an antiplatelet agent and over one-third were still smoking.

17. NHS Direct. What is the body mass index?, www.nhsdirect.nhs.uk/articles/article.aspx?ArticleId=850; 2008.

18. Pahlsson HI, Laskar C. The optimal cuff width for measuring toe blood pressure. Angiology 2007;58:472–6.
To determine the optimal cuff width for measuring toe blood pressure in patients with lower limb ischaemia, this study examined 20 patients with symptoms of PAD referred for vascular examination or vascular surgery. Toe blood pressure was measured hydrostatically by the pole test using cuffs of different widths. The pole test reflects the true physiological blood pressure value and was the reference method. The 2.5-cm cuff most accurately reflected the pole test.

19. Ubbink DT. Toe blood pressure measurements in patients suspected of leg ischemia: a new laser Doppler device compared with photo-plethysmography. Eur J Vasc Endovasc Surg 2004;27:629–34.

20. Varatharajan N, Pillay S. Implications of low great toe pressures in clinical practice. Aust N Z J Surg 2006;76:218–21.

21. Smith FCT, Shearman CP, Simms MH, et al. Falsely elevated ankle pressures in severe leg ischemia. The pole test: an alternative approach. Eur J Vasc Surg 1994;8:408–12.

22. Silagy C, Mant D, Fowler G, et al. Meta analysis on efficacy of nicotine replacement therapies in smoking cessation. Lancet 1994;343:139–42.

23. Cole SEA, Walker RA, Norris R. Vascular laboratory practice, IPEM Part III. York: Institute of Physics and Engineering in Medicine; 2001.

24. De Graaff JC, Ubbink DT, Legemate DA, et al. Evaluation of toe pressure and transcutaneous oxygen measurements in management of chronic critical leg ischemia: a diagnostic randomised clinical trial. J Vasc Surg 2003;38:528–34.

25. ACC/AHA Guidelines for the Management of Patients with Peripheral Arterial Disease (Lower Extremity, Renal, Mesenteric, and Abdominal Aortic): a collaborative report from the American Association for Vascular Surgery/Society for Vascular Surgery, Society for Cardiovascular Angiography and Interventions, Society for Vascular Medicine and Biology, Society of Interventional Radiology, and the ACC/AHA Task Force on Practice Guidelines (Writing Committee to Develop Guidelines for the Management of Patients with Peripheral Arterial Disease). J Am Coll Cardiol 2006;47(6):1239–312.

26. Gerhard-Hermana M, Gardin JM, Jaff M, et al. Guidelines for noninvasive vascular laboratory testing: a report from the American Society of Echocardiography and the Society for Vascular Medicine and Biology. Vasc Med 2006;11:183–200.

27. Kohler TR, Nance DR, Cramer MM, et al. Duplex scanning for the diagnosis of aortoiliac and femoropopliteal disease: a prospective study. Circulation 1987;76:1074–80.

28. Eiberg JP, Jensen F, Grønvall Rasmussen JB, et al. Screening for aortoiliac lesions by visual interpretation of the common femoral Doppler waveform. Eur J Vasc Endovasc Surg 2001;22(4):331–6.

29. Cossman DV, Ellison JE, Wagner WH, et al. Comparison of contrast arteriography to arterial mapping with color-flow duplex imaging in the lower extremities. J Vasc Surg 1989;10:522–9.

30. Moneta GL, Yeager RA, Antonovic R, et al. Accuracy of lower extremity arterial duplex mapping. J Vasc Surg 1992;15:275–84.

31. Larch E, Minar E, Ahmadi R, et al. Value of colour duplex sonography for evaluation of tibioperoneal arteries in patients with femoropopliteal obstruction: a prospective comparison with anterograde intraarterial digital subtraction angiography. J Vasc Surg 1997;25:629–36.

32. Grassbaugh JA, Nelson PR, Rzucidlo EM, et al. Blinded comparison of preoperative duplex ultrasound scanning and contrast arteriography for planning revascularization at the level of the tibia. J Vasc Surg 2003;37:1186–90.

33. Wain RA, Berdejo GL, Delvalle WN, et al. Can duplex scan arterial mapping replace contrast arteriography as the test of choice before infrainguinal revascularization? J Vasc Surg 1999;29:100–9.

34. Ligush Jr. J, Reavis SW, Preisser JS, et al. Duplex ultrasound scanning defines operative strategies for patients with limb-threatening ischemia. J Vasc Surg 1998;28:482–91.

35. National Clinical Guideline Centre. Lower limb peripheral arterial disease: diagnosis and management. NICE Clinical Guideline 147, August 2012
1. Offer duplex ultrasound as first-line imaging to all people with peripheral arterial disease for whom revascularisation is being considered.

2. Offer CE-MRA to people with peripheral arterial disease who need further imaging (after duplex ultrasound) before considering revascularisation.

3. Offer computed tomography angiography to people with peripheral arterial disease who need father imaging (after duplex ultrasound) if CE-MRA is contraindicated or not tolerated.

36. Collins R, Burch J, Cranny G, et al. Duplex ultrasonography, magnetic resonance angiography, and computed tomography angiography for diagnosis and assessment of symptomatic, lower limb peripheral arterial disease: systematic review. Br Med J 2007;334(7606):1257.

37. Visser K, Hunink MG. Peripheral arterial disease: gadolinium enhanced MR angiography versus color-guided duplex US – a meta-analysis. Radiology 2000;216:67–77.

38. European Society of Urogenital Radiology (ESUR). Guidelines on Contrast Media, version 6.0. February 2007.

39. McCullough PA, Adam A, Becker CR, et al. Risk prediction of contrast-induced nephropathy. Am J Cardiol 2006;98(Suppl. 6A):27K–36K.

40. Thomsen HS, Morcos SK, Barrett BJ. Contrast-induced nephropathy: the wheel has turned 360 degrees. Acta Radiol 2008;49(6):646–57.

41. Stacul F, Adam A, Becker CR, et al. Strategies to reduce the risk of contrast-induced nephropathy. Am J Cardiol 2006;98(Suppl. 6A):1K–4K.

42. Dong M, Jiao Z, Liu T, et al. Effects of administration route on the renal safety of contrast agents: a meta-analysis of randomized controlled trials. J Nephrol 2012;25(3):290–301.
Administration route may affect the renal safety of contrast agents. Specifically, iodixanol may be a better choice for patients receiving intra-arterial contrast.

43. Kuhn MJ, Chen N, Sahani DV, et al. The PREDICT study: a randomized double-blind comparison of contrast-induced nephropathy after low- or isoosmolar contrast agent exposure. AJR Am J Roentgenol 2008;191(1):151–7.
Two hundred and forty-eight patients with moderate to severe chronic kidney disease and diabetes mellitus were randomised to receive at least 65 mL of iopamidol 370 (low osmolar) or iodixanol 320 (iso-osmolar) for a CT procedure. There was no significant difference in the incidence of CIN at 48–72 hours after contrast administration.

44. European Society of Urogenital Radiology (ESUR) Guideline. Gadolinium based contrast media and nephrogenic systemic fibrosis (17 July 2007) opinion of only the Academic members of the ESUR Contrast Media Safety Committee.

45. Menke J, Larsen J. Meta-analysis: accuracy of contrast-enhanced magnetic resonance angiography for assessing steno-occlusions in peripheral arterial disease. Ann Intern Med 2010;153(5):325–34.
A total of 32 studies met the inclusion criteria. The pooled sensitivity of MRA was 94.7% (95% confidence interval (CI): 92.1–96.4%) and the specificity was 95.6% (CI: 94–96.8%) for diagnosing segmental steno-occlusions. The pooled positive and negative likelihood ratios were 21.56 (CI: 15.7–29.69) and 0.056 (CI: 0.037–0.083), respectively. MRA correctly classified 95.3%, overstaged 3.1% and understaged 1.6% of arterial segments.

46. Heijenbrok-Kal MH, Kock MCJM, MyriamHunink MG. Lower extremity arterial disease: multidetector CT angiography-meta-analysis. Radiology 2007;245(2):433–9.
A total of 12 studies met the inclusion criteria. Multidetector CT angiography was used to evaluate 9541 arterial segments in 436 patients. The pooled sensitivity and specificity for detecting a stenosis of at least 50% per segment were 92% (95% CI: 89–95%) and 93% (95% CI: 91–95%), respectively. There was no significant difference in the diagnostic performance in the infrapopliteal segments from that in the aorto-iliac and femoro-popliteal segments.

47. Kock MR, Adriaensen ME, Pattynama PM, et al. DSA versus multi-detector row CT angiography in peripheral arterial disease: randomized controlled trial. Radiology 2005;237(2):727–37.

48. Edwards M-B. 25 years of heart valve replacements in the United Kingdom. A guide to types, models and MRI safety. United Kingdom Heart Valve Registry. London: Hammersmith Hospital; 2000.

49. Seldinger S. Catheter replacement of the needle in percutaneous angiography. Acta Radiol 1953;39:368–76.

3

Medical treatment of chronic lower limb ischaemia

Cliff Shearman

Introduction

Peripheral arterial disease (PAD) is an extremely common condition.

> ✓✓ In the Edinburgh Artery Study of men and women aged 55–74 years of age, 4.5% had symptomatic PAD, in other words intermittent claudication. However, a further 8% had evidence of major asymptomatic disease and 16.6% had abnormal haemodynamic parameters suggesting minor PAD.[1] Five years later all new cases of intermittent claudication in the study group were in subjects previously found to have asymptomatic disease.[2]

This is encouraging as it suggests that there may be a window of opportunity in which to identify and try to slow or reverse the progression of PAD. In this study the prevalence of both symptomatic and asymptomatic PAD increased with age and was more common in lower socio-economic groups. Both of these are important issues to consider when comparing the treatment of PAD with other cardio-vascular diseases.

Patients with symptomatic PAD have reduced mobility and quality of life, which equates to some cancers, but PAD is also a powerful marker of cardiovascular risk, equating to a previous myocardial infarction.[3] In a survey of 1886 patients with PAD, 58% had coronary artery disease and 34% had suffered a cerebrovascular event.[4]

> ✓✓ Overall, individuals with PAD are six times more likely to die from cardiovascular disease than those with no PAD.[5] Although the risk of a cardiovascular event increases in symptomatic patients, the risk is also present for asymptomatic individuals.

Five years after diagnosis of PAD the mortality risk of the patient is twice that of a patient with breast cancer.

> ✓✓ In the Reduction of Atherothrombosis for Continued Health (REACH) registry of patients with either known cardiovascular disease or who are at increased cardiovascular risk, the highest cardiovascular event rate was in the 5986 patients with PAD. At 1-year follow-up 18.2% of PAD patients had suffered a cardiovascular death, myocardial infarction (MI), a stroke or had been hospitalised for a cardiovascular event compared with 13.3% of the coronary artery disease group and 10% of the cerebrovascular disease group.[6] The group that had the highest cardiovascular event rates were those with evidence of polyvascular arterial disease, i.e. disease in three arterial beds (e.g. cerebral, cardiac and peripheral).

In summary, PAD is present in over 29% of the adult population and in the majority is asymptomatic. Apart from the impact on the patient in those with symptoms, PAD also identifies patients at extremely high risk of cardiovascular events, particularly if they

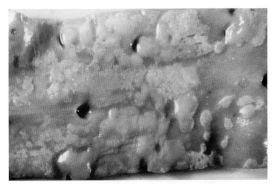

Figure 3.1 • Early atheromatous changes in aorta of asymptomatic patient. Courtesy of Dr P. Gallagher.

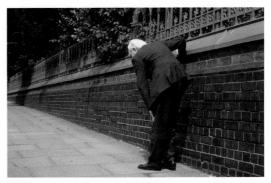

Figure 3.2 • Patient handicapped by intermittent claudication.

have arterial disease elsewhere (**Fig. 3.1**). The key aims of treatment of PAD should be reduction of cardiovascular risk and improvement of the symptoms. Despite these stark figures, evidence suggests that many patients with PAD remain undiagnosed and even those who have been identified get suboptimal treatment, especially when compared to patients with coronary artery disease.[7] This chapter will address the diagnosis and detection of PAD, factors affecting cardiovascular risk and medical treatments that may improve the symptoms of PAD.

PAD diagnosis and screening

Identification of PAD may be relevant to three patient groups. Firstly, in patients who present with primary symptoms affecting the legs who are at increased cardiovascular risk and may also be suitable for treatment of their claudication. Secondly, patients already at increased cardiovascular risk (e.g. after MI or stroke) when the diagnosis of PAD identifies a subgroup (polyvascular disease) who are at extremely high risk of cardiovascular events. The final group is asymptomatic patients in whom the identification of PAD may allow attempts to reduce cardiovascular risk and prevent disease progression. The evidence of identifying arterial disease in each of these groups is examined.

In symptomatic patients the diagnosis of PAD can be made on structured questioning, examination and measurement of ankle–brachial pressure index (ABPI). Typical muscular pain in the calf or thigh and buttocks on walking, combined with absent lower limb pulses, is strongly suggestive of PAD (**Fig. 3.2**). However, many patients have comorbidities, such as arthritis, which can confuse the history and pulse palpation may be difficult. Based on the above clinical criteria alone PAD will be missed in many individuals, and objective methods of assessment are needed, especially in asymptomatic people.[8] Measurement of ABPI has

been shown to be a reproducible method of confirming the diagnosis and is widely applicable in primary and secondary care[9] (**Fig. 3.3**).

In a few patients in whom there remains uncertainty about the diagnosis, duplex ultrasound scanning should be undertaken to identify PAD. Treadmill exercise testing may be helpful to determine the dominant pathology in patients with other comorbidities that limit walking, such as arthritis.

> ✅ PAD can usually be diagnosed on clinical history, examination and measurement of ABPI. Despite the ease of diagnosis many symptomatic patients go unrecognised and remain at increased cardiovascular risk. Ironically it is often not until the patient with PAD develops coronary heart disease (CHD) or stroke that they begin to receive correct treatment. Even those with identified PAD often go untreated, identifying a lack of awareness amongst physicians and patients.

This lack of awareness of the significance of PAD has been partly addressed at a national level. In the UK reduction of cardiovascular deaths is a stated aim of the Government and there are financial incentives through the General Medical Services (GMS) contract in primary care to identify and treat risk factors in patients with CHD and stroke. In April 2012 diagnosis of PAD will be included in the GMS contract and the National Institute of Health and Clinical Excellence (NICE) will publish guidelines on the mangement of PAD in mid 2012.

> ✅✅ The Inter-Society Consensus for the Management of Peripheral Arterial Disease (TASC II) and a number of international expert bodies have recognised that PAD is a major health issue and should be identified and treated.[10–14]

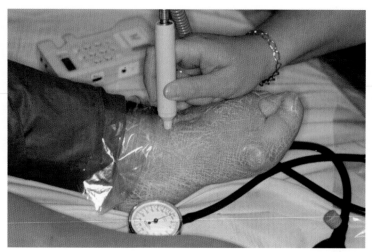

Figure 3.3 • Measurement of ankle–brachial pressure index in a patient with PAD. The technique should be standardised. The patient should be supine and rested. The cuff size should be appropriate for the patients limbs and placed just above the malleoli. Using an 8-MHz Doppler ultrasound probe the systolic pressures in the anterior tibial (illustrated) post-tibial and peroneal arteries should be recorded. The pressures in both arms should be recorded. The ankle–brachial pressure index (ABPI) is the highest ankle pressure divided by the highest arm pressure.

✔ In patients with established CHD or stroke the identification of PAD places them in the highest risk group for further cardiovascular events. At present few patients with stroke or CHD are routinely screened for PAD but this is likely to improve with the introduction of new national guidelines.

The diagnosis of PAD in these groups would place them in an extremely high-risk group for further cardiovascular events and appropriate attention could be given to modifying their risk factors.

The observation that a reduced ABPI, even in asymptomatic patients, correlates with increased cardiovascular risk prompts the concept of screening the adult population.[15]

✔✔ The lower the ABPI, the more likely is the patient to have polyvascular disease and hence the greatest cardiovascular risk.[16]

PAD is common in the adult population and identification using ABPI is a simple, inexpensive test. Perhaps one of the most attractive aspects of using ABPI is that it identifies a high-risk individual before they develop clinical problems such as angina, MI or stroke.

Although appealing, at present there is no evidence that screening the adult population in general for PAD using ABPI would be of benefit or cost-effective and further work is needed to clarify this.

However, the evidence for the measurement of ABPI in all patients with leg pain on walking, or with evidence of coronary or cerebrovascular disease, and patients with risk factors known to increase cardiovascular risk (e.g. diabetes, hypertension and raised cholesterol) is very strong.

Modifying cardiovascular risk

There is overwhelming evidence for the benefits of identifying and correcting risk factors such as hypertension, dyslipidaemias, diabetes and obesity in patients with PAD. Active intervention to aid smoking cessation, increased exercise as well as the use of antiplatelet agents will result in a marked reduction in cardiovascular morbidity and mortality (see Chapter 1). Despite such evidence the delivery of this aspect of medical treatment remains poor. In the ongoing REACH registry of patients at increased cardiovascular risk principally being managed in primary care, only a minority of patients with PAD receive adequate medical treatment.[17] Even in patients referred to secondary care only 70% were on antiplatelet therapy and 44% taking a statin.[18] Perhaps most disappointing of all, even after secondary care involvement there still remains a number of patients receiving inadequate treatment. In a retrospective review of 109 patients who had undergone amputation due to PAD at the time of referral for prosthesis fitting only 41% had been prescribed a statin and only 60% were taking an antiplatelet agent; 39% of patients were on both a statin and antiplatelet agent, but 32% had been prescribed neither.[19]

Lay knowledge of PAD too is poor compared to CHD and stroke. In a group of 2501 adult Americans only 26% had ever heard of PAD. Of those with awareness of PAD 56% were aware it was associated with smoking and approximately 25% were aware it was linked to MI, stroke and amputation.[20] Secondary prevention clinics for CHD have been demonstrated to save lives and it seems reasonable to extrapolate this benefit to patients with PAD.[21]

Medical treatments for symptomatic PAD

It is important that all patients receive clear and appropriate advice about their condition and how they can improve their prognosis.

Exercise

Exercise is widely held to be of benefit to patients with PAD and not only improves walking distance but may also help reduce cardiovascular mortality. Unfortunately only 27% of vascular surgeons in the UK have access to such programmes.[22]

Although most studies comparing exercise with other therapies have been small and used different exercise regimens there is good evidence for the improvement in muscle function, vascular endothelial cell function and metabolic adaptations with exercise.[23]

✔✔ A meta-analysis of 21 studies of the effect of exercise on patients with intermittent claudication suggested an improvement in walking distance of 122%.[24] Supervised programmes in which the patient exercised for 30 minutes at least three times per week for 6 months had the most benefit. Programmes not directly supervised have less, if any, benefit.[25]

Numerous mechanisms have been proposed for this apparent benefit, including metabolic adaptation of the muscle, transformation of the muscle fibre type, increased muscle capillary blood flow and haemorheological factors such as a reduction in fibrinogen, but the optimum programme or method of exercise remains to be determined.

In a randomised controlled trial of three treatments for intermittent claudication due to femoropopliteal disease, angioplasty, supervised exercise or a combination of angioplasty and supervised exercise, all treatments improved walking distance

and quality of life (QOL) at 12 months. The combination of exercise and angioplasty tended to gain more improvement in the short term than either treatment alone but the QOL gain was equal in all groups.[26] The MIMIC Trial also showed a benefit of combining supervised exercise, best medical therapy and angioplasty over best medical therapy and angioplasty for patients with either superficial femoral artery disease or aortoiliac disease.[27]

✔✔ Supervised exercise programmes should be available for all patients with intermittent claudication and offered before interventional treatments are considered.

Angioplasty may offer some short-term benefit,[28] but exercise appears more effective at improving walking distance over the longer term. If angioplasty is undertaken it should be combined with best medical therapy and supervised exercise.

In a randomised controlled study of surgical revascularisation compared to surgery and exercise or exercise alone, the surgery and exercise group had the biggest improvement in walking distance. However, patients undergoing surgery had a 20% excess risk of adverse events.[29]

A sedentary lifestyle is a major risk factor for cardiovascular disease and individuals who undertake exercise on a regular basis have half the cardiovascular mortality risk of those who are inactive.[30] Although intensive exercise such as long-distance running reduces cardiovascular risk markedly, moderate increases in activity also confer a significant benefit.[31] The National Institutes of Health conference on physical activity and health concluded that all children and adults should build up to a total of 30 minutes of moderate intense activity such as brisk walking each day.[32] Interestingly, there is a direct correlation between levels of activity and ABPI, suggesting that a physically active lifestyle may help prevent PAD.[33] For adults who increase their activity there is evidence of a significant reduction in cardiovascular mortality compared to subjects who maintain a sedentary lifestyle.[34] This benefit is lost if the subject becomes unfit again and so exercise programmes need to ensure that the patients maintain their exercise regimen.

Exercise in patients with claudication is associated with increases in some inflammatory mediators, a type of ischaemia–reperfusion injury. On this basis it has been postulated that exercise may cause endothelial damage and even contribute to the high risk of cardiovascular events suffered by this group. However, regular supervised exercise has been shown not only to improve walking distance, but is associated with a significant reduction in serum markers of the periexercise inflammatory response, suggesting exercise has a positive effect.[35]

✅ Exercise appears to be of established value in improving walking distance in patients with claudication and should be offered to all patients with intermittent claudication. Although few patients currently have access to this therapy and compliance in patient groups remains low, when serious concerted attempts are made to address cardiovascular risk, compliance improves.[36]

Drug treatment

Vasoactive drugs

NICE have recently evaluated four drugs currently used in ther treatment of intermittent claudication: cilostazol (Pletal), naftidrofuryl oxalate (Praxilene), pentoxyfylline (Trental) and inositol nicotinate (Hexopal). A large number of randomised controlled trials were conducted and it was concluded that pentoxyfylline improved absolute walking distance by 60% compared to placebo and cilostazol by 25%. In three head-to-head trials there was no conclusive evidence of an advantage of one agent over the other and so taking into account the cost-effectiveness of treament it was recommended that if vasoactive drugs were indicated then naftidrofuryl should be used.[37]

✅✅ In a review of the evidence available from all randomised controlled studies of vasoactive drugs for the treatment of claudication, naftidrofuryl was the most cost-effective. The benefits are relatively small, with an estimated 60% improvement in absolute walking distance compared to placebo and have not been compared to other therapies. Naftidrofuryl should be the only agent used.

Although side-effects are relatively uncommon it is questionable whether this treatment is cost-effective and also what clinical utility these relatively small improvements have from the patient's perspective.

✅ The use of agents such as cilostazol and naftidrofuryl varies across countries and is relatively low in the UK compared to other European countries. The reason for this is not entirely clear, but probably reflects doubt about the clinical value of the small increases in walking distance, together with cost. It is unlikely that these therapies will be cost-effective compared to supervised exercise.
   Patients started on naftidrofuryl should be reassessed at 3 months and treatment continued only if they have gained benefit.

A range of other drugs and agents have been explored, including vitamin E, buflomedil and carnitine, without any firm evidence of benefit. Omega-3 fish oils have been found to reduce re-infarct rates after MI and reduce inflammation in atherosclerotic plaques. They have been explored in patients with PAD in uncontrolled studies, but there is no evidence to support their widespread use at present.[38]

Although primarily given for their lipid-lowering properties, plaque regression has been reported in studies when statins are given in high doses. Atorvastatin 80 mg/day was shown to improve walking distance in patients with intermittent claudication.[39] Although interesting, it is unclear whether this is likely to be of clinical relevance. In studies of plaque regression in the coronary circulation very high doses of statins have to be administered to see an effect that is likely to be associated with increased side-effects.

Prostanoids

Prostaglandin E_1 (PGE_1) and stable prostacyclin (PGI_2) have a number of properties that make them theoretically useful in the treatment of PAD. They are powerful vasodilators, have an anti- and disaggregatory effect on platelets, and seem to optimise vascular endothelial function. PGE_1 is metabolised in the lung on first pass and so is usually administered bound to a carrier. PGI_2 has a half-life of 1–2 minutes and itself is of limited value. Iloprost is a stable prostacyclin analogue with a half-life of approximately 30 minutes. Both PGE_1 and iloprost are given intravenously and commonly cause side-effects of headaches, nausea, facial flushing and hypotension. Their use, therefore, is effectively confined to patients in a hospital setting and is labour intensive.

✅✅ There have been several studies of prostanoids in intermittent claudication without any evidence of benefit. In patients with critical limb ischaemia pain reduction, rate of ulcer healing, amputation and survival were advantaged by iloprost.[40] In 133 patients diagnosed with Buerger's disease (thromboangitis obliterans) there were significant improvements in terms of ulcer healing and pain relief compared to aspirin and placebo.[41]

However, these were low-quality studies and there is no recent evidence to support the use of these agents other than in a small number of individual patients when the clinician feels there is no alternative, and these should ideally be submitted to a registry.

Angiogenesis

Gene therapy

The development of new blood vessels in ischaemic tissue, therapeutic angiogenesis, has appeal in patients in whom conventional revascularisation procedures are not possible. A number of angiogenic growth factors have been identified and it is thought that by raising levels of these at the site of potential collateral formation it may be possible to improve limb blood flow. It is possible to insert a gene coding for a growth factor into a DNA plasmid. These can either be injected as naked plasmids into the muscle of the ischaemic limb or via a viral vector such as human adenovirus. In early human trials using growth factors including vascular endothelial growth factor, fibroblast growth factor and platelet-derived growth factor there has been evidence of increased vascularity and limb blood flow. However, the trials are very small, uncontrolled and there are potential risks of new vessel growth at other sites such as the eye, and malignancy.[42]

Cell therapy

Endothelial progenitor cells are attracted to sites of endothelial injury and ischaemia. They are involved with endothelial repair and new vessel growth. The origin of these cells is unclear but they can be identified from monocyte or endothelial origins. There is evidence to show that bone marrow-derived mononuclear cells, which include endothelial progenitor cells, are attracted to areas of ischaemia. Early reports suggest some benefit from intramuscular injection of these cells into ischaemic muscle. Studies are in the very early stage at present and it is too soon to say whether this approach will have any clinical relevance.

Spinal cord stimulation

Spinal cord stimulation is a technique that can be used for chronic pain relief. An epidural electrode is inserted and connected to a stimulator box implanted beneath the skin. Based on the gate theory, stimulation of the spinal cord at the level of L3–4 is thought to reduce pain sensation and produces a sensation of warmth and paraesthesia in the limb. Implantation is relatively straightforward, but positioning the electrode to get pain relief can be difficult and getting the correct impulse frequency and strength may be problematic. Spinal cord stimulation is used primarily for intractable pain in patients with unreconstructable PAD. A single, large randomised controlled study of 120 patients failed to identify any benefit in terms of reduction of amputation or survival between the treatment and control groups.[43]

✔✔ NICE recommends that spinal cord stimulation should not be used for chronic pain of ischaemic origin outside a clinical trial.[44]

Lumbar sympathectomy

✔ Sympathetic denervation of the lower limbs has been advocated as a treatment for patients unsuitable for reconstruction with critical limb ischaemia for many years. It is suggested that destruction of the L2 and L3 lumbar sympathetic ganglia improves skin blood flow and modifies pain. There is no evidence for the role of sympathectomy and older studies found variable results in terms of pain relief. The procedure is offered to relatively few patients with critical limb ischaemia and there is wide variation in its use geographically.

Intermittent pneumatic compression

Intermittent pneumatic compression of the calf and foot has been shown to increase popliteal artery blood flow. The mechanism for this is unclear but it is thought that the sustained reduction in venous pressure during treatment may be a factor. In one small study sustained benefits in terms of walking ability were found up to 12 months. Since the devices can be used by the patients in their own homes they may prove to be a useful therapy.[45]

Conclusions

PAD remains underdiagnosed and undertreated. Considering how prevalent it is in the population this seems surprising, but there remains considerable lack of awareness of the significance of the condition amongst both clinicians and the public. The finding of PAD is an indication that the individual is at excess cardiovascular risk and there is overwhelming evidence for the role of risk factor management in this group. Exercise will improve walking distance in patients with claudication, appears as good as any other current therapy, and should certainly be offered to patients prior to other treatments. Other medical therapies may help but generally the benefit is either very modest or unproven. Prostanoids may be of help in some patients, such as those with Buerger's disease. The key to improving the treatment of PAD seems to be in raising awareness of the condition and organising risk factor and lifestyle advice clinics.

Key points

- 29% of the adult population over 55 years have PAD but only 4.5% are symptomatic.
- PAD can be easily diagnosed on history, examination and a reduced ABPI.
- A low ABPI is a marker of cardiovascular risk.
- Patients with leg pain on walking should have ABPI measured.
- Patients with established cardiovascular disease should have ABPI measured.
- Further evidence is needed to recommend screening of the adult population for reduced ABPI.
- Although all patients with PAD should receive aggressive management of their risk factors, currently less than 50% receive correct medical treatment.
- Supervised exercise should be available and offered to patients with intermittent claudication.
- Naftidrofuryl may be of value in patients who cannot undertake exercise programmes and do not wish interventional treatment.
- Prostanoids have a limited role and may be of help in patients with Buerger's disease but the evidence is very weak.
- Angiogenesis is an exciting concept but at present needs considerable further evaluation.

References

1. Fowkes FGR, Housley E, Cawood EHH, et al. Edinburgh Artery Study: prevalence of symptomatic and asymptomatic peripheral arterial disease in the general population. Int J Epidemiol 1991;20:384–91.

2. Leng GC, Lee AJ, Fowkes FGR, et al. Incidence, natural history and cardiovascular events in symptomatic and asymptomatic peripheral arterial disease in the general population. Int J Epidemiol 1996;25:1172–81.

   These two reports from the Edinburgh Artery Study are important as they reveal the true prevalence of PAD in the community. The 5-year follow-up data also reinforce the high risk of cardiovascular events that these patients experience.

3. St Pierre AC, Cantin B, Lamarche B, et al. Intermittent claudication: from its risk factors to long term prognosis in men. The Quebec cardiovascular study. Can J Cardiol 2010;26(1):17–21.

4. Aronow WS, Ahn C. Prevalence of coexistent coronary artery disease, peripheral artery disease and atherothrombotic brain infarction in men and women ≥62 years of age. Am J Cardiol 1994;74:64–5.

5. Criqui MH, Langer RD, Fronek A, et al. Mortality over a period of 10 years in patients with peripheral arterial disease. N Engl J Med 1992;326:381–6.

   This is an important study of 565 men and women over a 10-year period. All subjects with evidence of PAD had a significantly increased risk of cardiovascular death. Those with the most severe disease had a 15-fold increased risk of cardiovascular death.

6. Steg PhG, Bhatt DL, Wilson PWF, et al. One-year cardiovascular event rates in outpatients with atherothrombosis. JAMA 2007;297:1197–206.

   The REACH registry is important as it is a contemporaneous registry of the outcome and treatment of over 68 000 patients worldwide at increased risk of cardiovascular events. Interestingly, the group with PAD appears to have the highest morbidity and mortality compared to coronary heart disease and cerebrovascular disease.

7. Hirsch AT, Criqui MH, Treat-Jacobsen D, et al. Peripheral arterial disease detection and awareness and treatment in primary care. JAMA 2001;286:1317–24.

8. Criqui MH, Fronek A, Klauber MR, et al. The sensitivity, specificity, and predictive value of traditional clinical evaluation of peripheral arterial disease: results from noninvasive testing in a defined population. Circulation 1985;71:516–22.

9. Caruana MF, Bradbury AW, Adam DJ. The validity, reliability, reproducibility and extended utility of ankle to brachial pressure index in current vascular surgical practice. Eur J Vasc Endovasc Surg 2005;29:443–51.

10. Hirsch AT, Haskal ZJ, Hertzer NR, et al. ACC/AHA 2005 guidelines for the management of patients with peripheral arterial disease (lower extremity, renal mesenteric and abdominal aortic): executive summary. JACC 2006;47:1239–312.

11. Abramson BL, Huckell V, Anand S, et al. Canadian Cardiovascular Society Consensus Conference: peripheral arterial disease – executive summary. Can J Cardiol 2005;21:997–1006.

12. Scottish Intercollegiate Guideline Network (SIGN 89). Diagnosis and management of peripheral arterial disease. A national clinical guideline. 2006.

13. Norgren L, Hiatt WR, Dormandy JA, et al. Inter-Society consensus for the management of peripheral arterial disease (TASC II). J Vasc Surg 2007;45(Suppl. S): S5–67.

14. JBS 2. Joint British Societies Guidelines on prevention of cardiovascular disease in clinical practice. Heart 2005;91(Suppl. V).
    The guidelines outlined in Refs 10–14 all identify PAD as a major cardiovascular risk that should be treated the same way as other risk factors.

15. Heald CL, Fowkes FG, Murray GD, et al. Ankle brachial index collaboration. Atherosclerosis 2006;189:61–9.

16. Fowkes FGR, Low L-O, Tuta S, et al., on behalf of AGATHA Investigators. Ankle brachial index and the extent of atherothrombosis in 8891 patients with or at risk of vascular disease: results of the international AGATHA study. Eur Heart J 2006;27: 1861–7.
    This large international study recruited 8891 patients. They found that the ABPI was related to the risk profile of the patient and a low ABPI was associated with arterial disease in more than one bed.

17. Bhatt DL, Steg PG, Ohman E, et al. International prevalence, recognition, and treatment of cardiovascular risk factors in outpatients with atherothrombosis. JAMA 2005;295:180–9.

18. Khan S, Flather M, Mister R, et al. Characteristics and treatments of patients with peripheral arterial disease referred to UK vascular clinics: results of a prospective registry. Eur J Vasc Endovasc Surg 2006;33:442–50.

19. Bradley L, Kirker SGB. Secondary prevention of arteriosclerosis in lower limb vascular amputees: a missed opportunity. Eur J Vasc Endovasc Surg 2006;32:491–3.

20. Hirsch AT, Murphy TP, Lovell MB, et al. Gaps in public knowledge of peripheral arterial disease. The first national PAD public awareness survey. Circulation 2007;116:2086–94.

21. Murchie P, Campbell NC, Ritchie LD, et al. Secondary prevention clinics for coronary heart disease: four year follow up of a randomised controlled trial in primary care. Br Med J 2003;326:84.
    Patients with a history of coronary heart disease (n=1343) were randomised to receive an invitation to attend a secondary prevention clinic or continue usual care. The mean follow-up was 4.7 years. A reduction in deaths and coronary events was found in the intervention group (proportional hazards ratio 0.76 for coronary events).

22. Stewart AHR, Lamont PM. Exercise for intermittent claudication. Br Med J 2001;323:703–4.

23. Stewart K, Hiatt W, Regensteiner J. Exercise training for claudication. N Engl J Med 2002;347: 1941–51.

24. Gardner AW, Peohlman ET. Exercise rehabilitation programs for the treatment of claudication pain. JAMA 1995;274:975–80.
    This meta-analysis still remains the best evidence for advising exercise in patients with claudication. Based on this, TASC II (recommendation 14) states: 'supervised exercise should be made available as part of the initial treatment for all patients with peripheral arterial disease'. Attempts at larger studies of the role of exercise failed due to lack of recruitment of patients.

25. Bendermacher BLW, Willigendael EM, Teijink JAW, et al. Supervised exercise therapy versus nonsupervised exercise therapy for intermittent claudication. Cochrane Database Syst Rev 2006;(2), Art. No.:CD005263. doi:10.1002/14651858.CD005263. pub2.

26. Mazari F, Khan JA, Carradice D, et al. Randomized clinical trial of percutaneous transluminal angioplasty, supervised exercise and combined treatment for intermittent claudication. Br J Surg 2012; 99:39–48.
    178 patients with intermittent claudication due to superficial femoral artery disease were randomised to supervised exercise, angioplasty or supervised exercise and angioplasty. Their clinical outcomes were recorded and quality of life assessed up to 12 months. Although all treatment groups gained improvement there was an advantage in terms of walking distance in the group that received both angioplasty and exercise.

27. The Mimic Trial Participants. The adjuvant benefit of angioplasty in patients with mild to moderate intermittent claudication (MIMIC) managed by supervised exercise, smoking cessation advice and best medical therapy: results from two randomised trials in stenotic fenoropopliteal and aortoiliac disease. Eur J Vasc Endovasc Surg 2008;36:680–86.
    144 patients with intermittent claudication were randomised to best medical treatment, supervised exercise and angioplasty or best medical treatment, supervised exercise. Patients were stratified according to the level of the arterial disease: 93 femoropopliteal and 34 aortoiliac. Follow-up was for 24 months. Patients gained greater benefit from angioplasty and exercise combined but the subgroups were very small, limiting the value of the results.

28. Fowkes FGR, Gillespie IN. Angioplasty (versus nonsurgical management) for intermittent claudication. Cochrane Database Syst Rev 1998;(2), Art: CD000017. doi:10.1002/14651858.CD000017
    There have been two trials involving 98 patients randomised to angioplasty versus exercise or angioplasty compared with medical treatment. At 6 months the angioplasty group had higher ABPIs than the non-angioplasty group. However, despite a long-term follow-up over a year there was no identifiable benefit in terms of walking distance.

29. Lundgren F, Dahllof A-G, Lundholm K, et al. Intermittent claudication – surgical reconstruction or physical training? A prospective randomized trial of treatment efficiency. Ann Surg 1989;209:346–55.

Seventy-five patients were randomised in this study and follow-up was 1 year. Patients who were operated on generally did better and more were likely to lose their symptoms completely. However, there was morbidity associated with the surgery and a number of patients did not complete exercise training. The added effects of exercise and surgery are interesting, but need further evaluation. This is an old study and all of the therapies have changed significantly, making it difficult to compare with current practices.

30. Powell KE, Pratt M. Physical activity and health. Br Med J 1996;313:126–7.

31. Winslow E, Bohannon N, Brunton SA, et al. Lifestyle modification: weight control, exercise and smoking cessation. Am J Med 1996;101(Suppl. 4A):25S–33.

32. NIH Consensus Development Panel on Physical Activity and Cardiovascular Health. NIH Consensus Conference: physical activity and health. JAMA 1996;267:241–6.

33. Gardner AW. Physical activity is related to ankle/brachial index in subjects without peripheral arterial disease. Angiology 1997;48:883–9.

34. Blair SN, Kohl HW, Barlow CE, et al. Changes in physical fitness and all cause mortality: a prospective study of healthy and unhealthy men. JAMA 1995;273:1093–8.

35. Tisi PV, Husle M, Chulakadabba A, et al. Exercise training for intermittent claudication: does it adversely affect biochemical markers of the exercise induced inflammatory response. Eur J Vasc Endovasc Surg 1997;14:344–50.

36. Noble J, Modest GA. Managing multiple risk factors: a call to action. Am J Med 1996;101(Suppl. 4A): 79S–81.

37. NICE Technology Appraisal Guidance 223. Cilostazol, naftidrofuryl oxalate, pentoxifylline and inositol nicotinate for the treatment of intermittent claudication in people with peripheral arterial disease, www.nice.org.uk/guidance/TA223.

All published trials of the use of these agents were reviewed and the quality of the data assessed by a panel of experts and patients. The evidence for improvements in absolute walking distance seems strong but it is not clear how these compare to other treatments such as supervised exercise. It was concluded that on cost-effectiveness grounds naftidrofuryl should be the only agent used.

38. Sommerfield T, Price J, Hiatt WR. Omega-3 fatty acids for intermittent claudication. Cochrane Database Syst Rev 2004;(3), Art. No.:CD0038333. doi:10.1002/14651858.CD003833.pub3.

39. Mohler ER, Hiatt WR, Creager MA. Cholesterol reduction with atorvastatin improves walking distances in patients with peripheral arterial disease. Circulation 2003;108:1481–6.

40. Loosemore TM, Chalmers TC, Dormandy JA. A meta-analysis of randomized placebo control trials in Fontaine stages III and IV peripheral occlusive disease. Int Angiol 1994;13:133–42.

41. Fiessinger JN, Schafer M. Trial of iloprost versus aspirin treatment for critical limb ischaemia of thromboangiitis obliterans. Lancet 1990;335:555–7.

In this study 87% of the treated group was thought to respond to treatment. Complete pain relief was obtained in 63% and 35% of the treatment group compared to 28% and 13% of the control group at 6 months.

42. Mughal NA, Russell DA, Ponnambalam S, et al. Gene therapy in the treatment of peripheral arterial disease. Br J Surg 2012;99:6–15.

43. Klomp HM, Spincemaille GH, Steyerberg EW, et al. Spinal cord stimulation in critical limb ischaemia: a randomised trial. Lancet 1999;353:1040–4.

44. NICE Technology Appraisal Guidance 159. Spinal cord stimulation for chronic pain of neuropathic or ischaemic origin, www.nice.org.uk/TA159.

Four randomised controlled trials failed to show any sustained benefit of spinal cord stimulation compared to other treatments for pain reduction, avoidance of amputation or quality of life in patients with ischaemic pain due to PAD.

45. Ramaswami G, D'Ayala M, Hollier LH, et al. Rapid foot and calf compression increases walking distance in patients with intermittent claudication: results of a randomized study. J Vasc Surg 2005;41:794–801.

4

Intervention for chronic lower limb ischaemia

Anthony Nicholson
Julian Scott

Introduction

This chapter will focus upon intervention for chronic lower limb ischaemia. Exercise therapy is considered in Chapter 3. The decision to treat patients with chronic lower limb ischaemia by endovascular or open surgery will depend upon the severity of symptoms, associated comorbidity, technical considerations and evidence-based outcomes. Open surgery is usually reserved for patients in whom conservative or endovascular treatments are not an option or where they have failed to produce significant relief of symptoms. The basic principles of open vascular surgery include the identification of an adequate inflow, a suitable conduit and adequate run-off. Patients must be made aware that any intervention runs the risk of failure or other complications, which may result in limb loss and/or death.

Patient selection

The symptoms of patients with chronic lower limb ischaemia can range from mild claudication to limb-threatening ischaemia. The decision to intervene in claudication will depend on walking distance, the patient's current lifestyle and their desire to regain their loss in quality of life. This has to be reviewed against the potential risk of any intervention, the long-term durability of the procedure and the need for further intervention. For instance, younger patients who claudicate at 400 metres might be severely handicapped if they can no longer work effectively

or take part in leisure activities. Conversely, elderly patients with a claudication distance of 50–100 metres might not be particularly handicapped if they have good access to local amenities and a supportive family. These two scenarios highlight the importance of considering quality of life in the treatment equation. Box 4.1 summarises the factors influencing the decision to intervene in claudication.

The decision regarding conservative management or intervention in patients with intermittent claudication was recently informed by two randomised trials (the MIMIC and CLEVER trials).

The CLEVER trial[1] randomised 111 patients to best medical care (BMC) alone, BMC plus supervised exercise or BMC plus iliac stenting. At 6 months those patients who received BMC plus supervised exercise had a significantly better treadmill walking distance than those who had received BMC and stenting, and both did significantly better than the group receiving BMC alone. However, the patients who had stents inserted reported significantly better quality of life than those who received supervised exercise. This difference in end-points was not explained but is likely to be a placebo effect of perceived treatment over non-treatment if the patients fail to see supervised exercise as an intervention.

The MIMIC trial assigned patients with the relevant level of claudication to angioplasty plus best medical therapy plus supervised exercise or supervised exercise plus best medical therapy alone. Thirty-four patients with aorto-iliac disease and 93 with femoropopliteal disease were randomised. Both the absolute walking distance and the claudication distance improved by 30% more in the

Box 4.1 • Factors affecting the decision to intervene in claudication

For
Short walking distance
Employment/ lifestyle affected
No improvement with exercise
Stenosis/short occlusion
Unilateral symptoms
Against
Short history
Not significantly lifestyle limiting
Still smoking
Other limiting conditions, e.g. chronic airways disease, arthritis
Long occlusion/diffuse disease
Bilateral symptoms

femoropopliteal groups and by 78% more in the aorto-iliac group in the angioplasty arm of the study.[2] Though criticised as a small trial it is significantly larger than the often quoted other randomised controlled trials (RCTs) from Oxford and Edinburgh,[3,4] which randomised patients to angioplasty or exercise and found that exercise was more effective. Also, the degree of improvement in the angioplasty arm would have made it difficult ethically to continue the MIMIC study.

The results of these two trials confirm that, for the majority of claudicants, whether they have aorto-iliac or femoropopliteal disease, risk factor modification, BMC and exercise are the front-line treatments that should be offered. Intervention should be reserved for those who fail to improve on such a regime, for those with severe symptoms and for those who cannot participate in – or do not have available – a supervised exercise programme.

Unlike patients with intermittent claudication, most patients with critical limb ischaemia (CLI) require some form of intervention. There are some situations

when this would be inappropriate and these patients should not undergo unnecessary investigation or treatment. If the general condition of the patient is poor, and the chances of survival limited due to coexistent pathology, the involvement of a palliative care team is recommended (**Fig. 4.1**). However, if the patient has a reasonable quality of life and is likely to survive for more than a few months, it is probably better to attempt revascularisation whenever possible. No one wishes to see a patient spend the remaining few months of life struggling with an amputation as well as their primary disease. Some patients present with such advanced ischaemia that there is little viable tissue left on the weight-bearing area of the foot. It is sometimes possible, with revascularisation to the relevant angiosome and a customised forefoot amputation, to achieve a functional foot, but if this is not possible a primary amputation is the better option (see Chapter 5). The chair- or bed-bound patient can provide a challenge when deciding on whether to intervene. Fixed flexion deformities may also make amputation the best option. However, the rehabilitation team should be involved in this decision, as the patient's ability to transfer from a chair to the bed or toilet may depend on preservation of that limb.

Preoperative independence and mobility have been shown to be good predictors of postoperative independence and mobility after infrainguinal bypass for CLI.[5] Only one of 25 survivors who were not living independently before surgery achieved independent living 6 months postoperatively. Therefore, there seems little point in undertaking extensive revascularisation in the hope of achieving independence for a patient already requiring community care.

Cost-effectiveness

The cost-effectiveness of any intervention requires careful evaluation. A retrospective analysis of CLI in elderly patients found that the hospital cost of reconstruction was nearly twice the cost of primary amputation.[6] However, if the community costs were added,

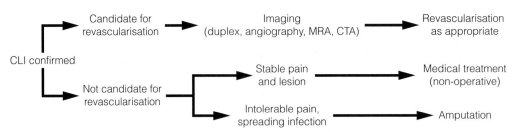

Figure 4.1 • Algorithm for treatment of patients with critical limb ischaemia. CTA, computed tomography angiography; MRA, magnetic resonance angiography. Adapted from Norgren L, Hiatt WR, Dormandy JA et al. TASC II Working Group. Inter-Society Consensus for the Management of Peripheral Arterial Disease (TASC II). J Vasc Surg 2007; 45(Suppl S):S5–67. With permission from the Society for Vascular Surgery.

amputation was more than twice as expensive, partly because 66% of reconstructed patients were able to return home compared to only 33% of amputees. A more recent prospective study also found that amputation was more expensive than revascularisation at 1 year.[7] There was little difference between the cost of successful endovascular treatment compared with surgical reconstruction, because the length of inpatient stay was related more to the state of the foot than the treatment received.

A prospective study of 150 patients with CLI found that activities of daily living and pain scores improved significantly after successful reconstruction and primary amputation, but mobility was only improved by successful reconstruction.[8] Thus, the improvement in the overall quality of life of those undergoing successful reconstruction seems largely due to better mobility. Patients whose reconstruction fails, leading to secondary amputation fare badly, both in terms of quality of life and cost, emphasising the need for a high success rate if undertaking this type of reconstruction. This is especially true for infrainguinal bypass procedures. In one study, the surgical ideal of an uncomplicated infrainguinal bypass operation, with rapid relief of pain, swift wound healing, a rapid return to premorbid function and no further intervention, was only achieved in 16 of 112 patients.[9]

TASC recommendations

✅ The Trans-Atlantic Inter-Society Consensus (TASC) Working Group and the Society of Interventional Radiology (SIR) have made recommendations for the type of lesion that is suitable or unsuitable for endovascular or open surgical treatment.[10,11]

There are differences between these recommendations but these are not particularly significant and they are summarised in Table 4.1. The recommendations have been updated to account for advances in endovascular techniques. Both classify peripheral arterial disease according to the level of the disease (e.g. aortic, iliac, femoropopliteal or crural) and by the severity of the disease (e.g. types A–D). As the disease becomes more severe and/or more diffuse, the recommendations move from endovascular to open intervention:

- type A lesions should usually be treated by endovascular means;
- type B lesions should preferentially be treated by endovascular means;

Table 4.1 • Endovascular therapy or open surgery: summary of recommendations of the TASC II Working Group

Segment/ recommendation	Usually PTA (type A)	PTA preferred (type B)	Surgery preferred (type C)	Usually surgery (type D)
Infrarenal aorta		Stenosis ≤3 cm		Aortic occlusion
Iliac (CIA/EIA)	Stenosis ≤3 cm	Stenosis 3–10 cm	Bilat. CIA occlusions Unilat.	Bilat. EIA occlusions
		Unilat. CIA or EIA occlusion	CIA+EIA occlusion	Disease extending into aorta and/or CFAs
Femoral	SFA stenosis ≤10 cm	SFA stenosis or occlusion ≤15 cm	SFA stenosis or occlusion >15 cm	Complete SFA or popliteal occlusions
Popliteal	Occlusion ≤5 cm	Popliteal stenosis	Recurrent disease	
Crural	Crural interventions have severe outcomes if they go wrong. Therefore there is no category A or B		Stenoses ≤4 cm or occlusions ≤2 cm	Diffuse disease or occlusions >2 cm
Outcomes	Excellent results can be expected from an endovascular approach in all segments		PTA/stent only has modest results and is indicated when surgery is contraindicated for technical or patient reasons	Endovascular approach is not advised unless symptoms are limb threatening and surgery is not possible

The presence of calcification or multiple lesions generally moves a recommendation towards open surgery, e.g. type B to type C. CFA, common femoral artery; CIA, common iliac artery; EIA, external iliac artery; PTA, percutaneous transluminal angioplasty; SFA, superficial femoral artery.

- type C lesions should preferentially be treated by open revascularisation;
- type D lesions should usually be treated by open surgery.

When diagnostic imaging is based on magnetic resonance angiography, which cannot image arterial calcification, the distinction between a type B and C lesion can be difficult and may lead to incorrect management decisions.

Suprainguinal endovascular intervention

Abdominal aorta

Haemodynamically significant stenoses of the infrarenal aorta are rare and usually seen in short, obese female smokers with a small-calibre aorta. Prior to the advent of endovascular therapies these patients would have undergone a localised aortic endarterectomy but primary stenting is now the first-line treatment (**Fig. 4.2**), with 5-year patency rates of 50%.[12] Complications are rare and usually relate to embolisation, pseudoaneurysm formation and recurrent disease.[13] Complete aortic occlusions

are best treated by an aorto-bifemoral bypass (see later). In an unfit patient aorto-uni-iliac stenting, combined with a femorofemoral crossover, may be a better alternative to an axillo-bifemoral bypass.[14] Kissing stents can be used but there is a risk of one stent compressing the other.

Iliac arteries

Though the European guidelines on the management of CLI and the diabetic foot[18] state that there are no randomised studies of percutaneous transluminal angioplasty (PTA) to open surgery in the iliac arteries, this is incorrect.

There is one RCT that compares open surgery to angioplasty in symptomatic iliac disease.[19] In this study, 263 men with iliac disease that was a major component to either rest pain or lifestyle-limiting claudication underwent either bypass surgery (n=123) or angioplasty (n=129). There were three deaths in the surgery group and none in the angioplasty group. There was no difference in patency and limb salvage rates, at a median follow-up of 4 years. The authors concluded that the lower morbidity and mortality rate in the angioplasty group supported the concept of angioplasty first strategy as outcomes between the

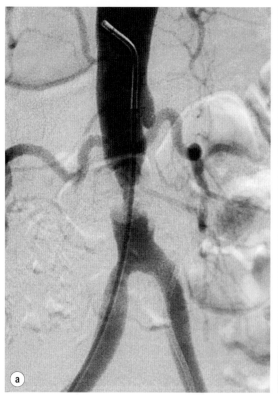 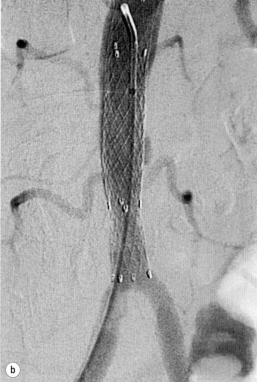

Figure 4.2 • Localised infrarenal aortic stenosis **(a)** successfully treated with self-expanding nitinol stents **(b)**.

two treatments were no different. The study was, however, limited by (i) the absence of women, who have smaller arteries and (ii) the relatively small numbers, which precluded subgroup analysis.

In a second, non-randomised comparative study the complication rate, primary patency and cost of stent deployment were compared with direct surgical reconstruction for the treatment of severe aorto-iliac occlusive disease.[20] Sixty-five patients underwent stent deployment and 54 patients had surgical reconstruction. No significant difference was observed between the groups in terms of clinical presentation, demographics and late complications. The cumulative primary patency rate for bypass grafts was, however, significantly better than for iliac stents at 18 months (93% vs. 73%), 30 months (93% vs. 68%) and 42 months (93% vs. 68%). Multivariate analysis suggested that females, anyone with ipsilateral superficial femoral artery (SFA) occlusion, and patients who had procedure-related vascular complications and hypercholesterolaemia were more likely to thrombose their bypass graft or stent. Costs did not differ significantly.

So here we have two studies with very different conclusions. The first is an RCT and the second an observational study. It is difficult to determine which of the many variables in the observational study affected which group, and it is of course possible that patients who were less fit for open surgery were treated by endovascular means. The fact is that the literature remains controversial.

✅✅ The TASC Working Group has looked at all the available evidence and concluded that endovascular treatment is the treatment of choice for type A aorto-iliac lesions and open surgical treatment for type D lesions.[11] The TASC considers that the evidence for the efficacy of one treatment instead of another was inadequate for type B and C lesions.

When is an iliac lesion significant?

The arteriographic grading of stenoses is hampered by wide intra- and inter-observer variability.[21] Intravascular ultrasound provides better measurements of cross-sectional area but it is expensive and not widely available. In theory, pressure gradient measurements at the time of angiography should be a relatively simple procedure. However, there is no consensus in the literature regarding what constitutes a significant pressure gradient[22] and there is little or no information on the role of vasodilators (doses), systolic versus mean pressures and peripheral resistance in assessing stenotic vessels. Tetteroo et al. reported that they would have stented between 4% and 87% of their patients, emphasising the overall lack of consensus.[23]

They suggested that a mean gradient of 10 mmHg at rest or after vasodilation should be used as a marker of significance and this is generally accepted, though there is no evidence at all for this.

Who should have an angioplasty or a stent?

Early aorto-iliac angioplasty had a high rate of embolic complications, particularly when dealing with occlusive rather than stenotic disease.[24] As a result stenting became the first-line treatment of iliac occlusive disease based on this observation. RCTs have been performed, but these have been compounded by flawed design and study methodology. Such a study demonstrated 4-year patency rates of 91.6% for stents and 74.3% for PTA alone, but the results have never been fully published.[25]

There is only one peer-reviewed, published RCT that compares primary stent placement with PTA followed by stent placement if needed in the iliac arteries. The Dutch Iliac Stent Trial (DIST)[26] randomised patients to either a primary Palmaz stent or PTA alone. In the latter group stents were reserved for patients with suboptimal PTA results. The authors reported that 43% of patients randomised to PTA received iliac stents and that 2-year cumulative patency rates for the two groups were similar at 71% versus 70%. They concluded that because angioplasty followed by selective stent placement is less expensive than primary stent placement, the former should be the treatment of choice for lifestyle-limiting intermittent claudication caused by iliac artery occlusive disease. However, only 29 iliac artery occlusions were treated among 279 patients and, by study design, patients with occlusions more than 5 cm in length were ineligible for enrolment. PTA alone failed in 10 out of 12 subjects (83%). Although stents seem to offer special benefits in the treatment of longer segment lesions, little guidance about such patients is provided by this trial. Furthermore, most patients in the DIST study had mild clinical symptoms, and only 22% of patients in each group were classified as having Society for Vascular Surgery/International Society for Cardiovascular Surgery (SVS/ISCVS) grade 3–5 ischaemia. As a consequence, the milder pattern of atherosclerotic disease observed in the DIST study differed from that encountered in many interventional practices. In addition, the study was designed to have a 90% likelihood of detecting a 10% difference in post-treatment arterial patency after 12 months between the two groups (power=90%). Unfortunately, the trial was terminated after less than 80% of the intended sample had been enrolled. Outcome information after as little as 1 year is available in the published report for about 60% of subjects who ultimately enrolled, a fraction that actually represents less than 45% of the intended patient sample. Thus, even though the authors did not observe 'substantial differences' in clinical outcomes between their experimental groups, the DIST study was more likely to miss than to detect the same potential 10% improvement in 12-month patency rates that was used to configure the trial, as the actual power was less than 50%. Because of under-recruitment, the authors attempted to amplify their sample by reporting the number of lesions treated, rather than the number of subjects actually involved. For example, a patient with simultaneous common and external iliac stenoses or occlusions was classified as two treated lesions, rather than as a single person. As a result, little information about crucial patient subgroups (e.g. occlusions vs. stenoses, common iliac vs. external iliac lesions) can be gleaned from this report. Despite these problems the authors continued to publish from the original dataset, reporting patency rates and patient survival at 5 years.[27]

There is a second RCT of stent versus angioplasty in complete iliac occlusions (the STAG trial). This is not yet published in the peer-reviewed literature but has been presented.[28] The results suggest that there are significantly fewer major complications, particularly embolisation, following stent compared to PTA, but that stents confer no benefit in terms of patency (P. Gaines, personal communication). If so, we are brought full circle to the original premise that stenting infers benefits in terms of reduced complications in iliac occlusions, rather than improved patency. Though the authors are not in a position to comment until the publication of this study, much will depend on the original design and power of the study in terms of its primary and secondary end-points.

✅✅ A meta-analysis of such studies has been performed.[29] This found a better technical success rate for stent (97%) rather than PTA (91%) ($P<0.05$). It also found a better overall 4-year primary patency for iliac stents in CLI (67% vs. 35%), though this was not the case for claudicants (77% vs. 65%). This emphasises the need for significant subgroup analysis in any study. A cost-effectiveness analysis[30] of aorto-iliac stenotic disease suggested that PTA and selective stent insertion for suboptimal results is the most cost-effective option, but did not deal specifically with technically more difficult and potentially complicated occlusive disease.

Iliac stenoses

In iliac stenotic disease, angioplasty alone should be the procedure of choice. The end-point for aorto-iliac revascularisation procedures is determined by intra-arterial haemodynamic measurements, which are readily obtained in this arterial segment. Ideally, simultaneous waveforms obtained above and below the treated segment should overlap, with no mean or systolic gradient (**Fig. 4.3**).

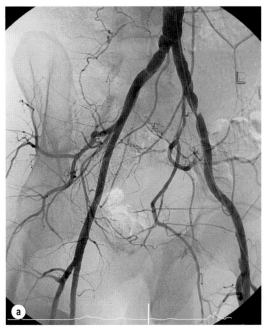
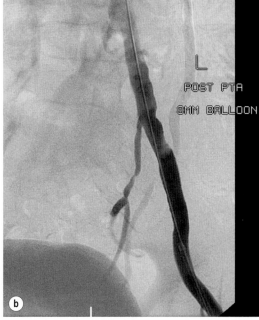

Figure 4.3 • (a) There is a severe focal stenosis of the left external iliac artery. **(b)** After balloon dilatation there is minor residual stenosis. However, there is no pressure gradient across the lesion and stenting is not required.

Often, ideal haemodynamic results are not achieved because of recoil or patient intolerance to balloon inflation to a calibre consistent with elimination of the gradient. This situation may demand a stent of suitable diameter and length. Balloon-mounted stents are normally preferred in this situation, though self-expanding stents may be desirable if the problem is intolerance.

Iliac occlusions

Chronic iliac occlusions can be crossed from the ipsilateral or contralateral side and stented to reduce the risk of embolic complications. This requires the insertion of a stent prior to PTA (**Fig. 4.4**). Self-expanding stents are indicated and in the authors' experience this will always traverse the chronic occlusion over the wire. Heparin is mandatory immediately after arterial access. Once a stent of appropriate diameter and length has been deployed it can then be inflated with a suitable sized balloon. If there is a suitable iliac stump of the ostium, a uni-iliac stent will work well. If, however, the occluded iliac artery does not have a stump and the aortic lumen tapers smoothly to the occlusion, then 'kissing' iliac stents may have to be used, even when the contralateral iliac artery does not have a significant stenosis.[31] This should be avoided if at all possible. Early results are good[32] but, in small arteries, the long-term patency is not as good as uni-iliac stenting. The external iliac artery is slightly more prone to rupture than the common iliac, but responds well to stenting.

Complications

The third British Iliac Angioplasty Study (BIAS)[33] followed 2233 patients for 12 months to 8 years. The complication rate in patients suffering intermittent claudication was 2.6% and in patients with critical leg ischaemia was 11.6%, reflecting the difference in age, comorbidity and disease extent. However, only 2.4% of patients overall required unplanned surgery, unplanned endovascuscular intervention or some other procedure that delayed discharge from hospital. The overall mortality for inpatient intervention was 2.8% and for day-case intervention no deaths were reported. Importantly, arterial perforation remains rare, with an overall mortality of 0.17%.

Potentially serious complications include the following:

Bleeding and pseudoaneurysm development

This can be treated by direct digital pressure but if there is a pseudoaneurysm, ultrasound-guided compression can be used,[34] though thrombin injection, endovascular stent graft or open surgery may be necessary.[35]

Arterial rupture

Often, when rupture occurs during PTA, the patient experiences severe pain. But rupture has occurred without pain or other symptoms; therefore, it is very important to perform an arteriogram immediately after angioplasty. Gross extravasation of contrast is generally seen in cases of frank rupture (**Fig. 4.5**). Once an arterial rupture is recognised, rapid action is required to prevent death. It is always wise to ask for help from a colleague vascular interventionist. Tamponade of the leak with the angioplasty balloon followed by a covered stent graft to seal the rupture is the most appropriate treatment. Resultant hypotension and bradycardia should be treated with resuscitative therapy.[36–38]

Embolisation

Embolisation occurs in 2–7% of patients,[33] and is more common in occlusive disease and in patients with CLI. The nature of the emboli (plaque, thrombus or cholesterol) determines the success of the different therapeutic options. Local thrombolytic infusion works poorly if the embolus is solid material (plaque). Suction thrombectomy is good for either thrombus or plaque. It requires a non-tapered catheter with a large end hole. Occasionally, large emboli have to be surgically removed.

Stent-related complications

Device-related problems such as (i) failure to deploy or misplacement and (ii) infection are rare and beyond the scope of this chapter.[36] Patients with infected stents should, however, be started on intravenous antibiotic therapy and investigated with a view to removal of the stent with revascularisation using autologous vein, preferably via an extra-anatomical route.

Suprainguinal open surgical intervention

The surgical approach to patients with significant aorto-iliac disease is determined by the patient's general fitness and whether or not they have had previous abdominal surgery (**Fig. 4.6**). In general terms all patients should undergo cardiorespiratory assessment, e.g. respiratory function tests, left ventricular ejection fraction (echo or multiple gated acquisition scan, MUGA), and preferably a cardiopulmonary exercise test. If they can exercise to a VO_2 peak that implies an adequate reserve for surgery (>15 mL/kg/min), further investigation may not be required. However, if they cannot exercise due to claudication pain then a dobutamine stress echocardiogram or Myoview scan might be more appropriate.[39]

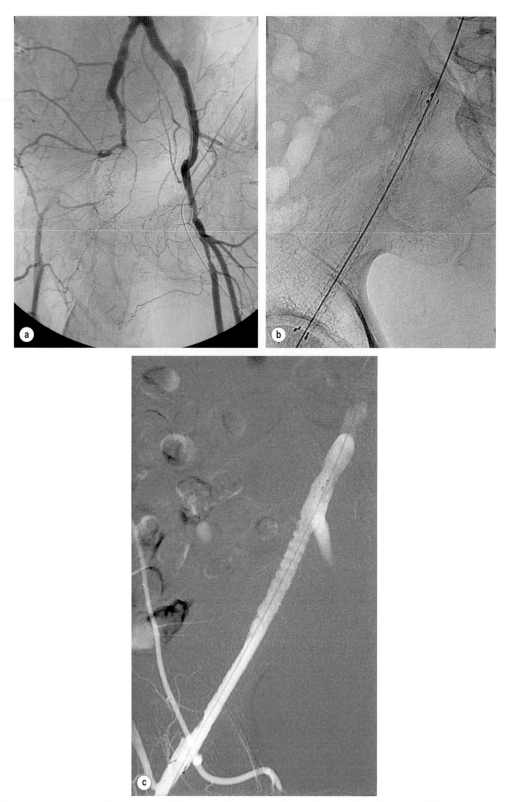

Figure 4.4 • Long right iliac occlusion **(a)** successfully treated with a self-expanding nitinol stent **(b)**, showing appearance after percutaneous transluminal angioplasty of the stent **(c)**.

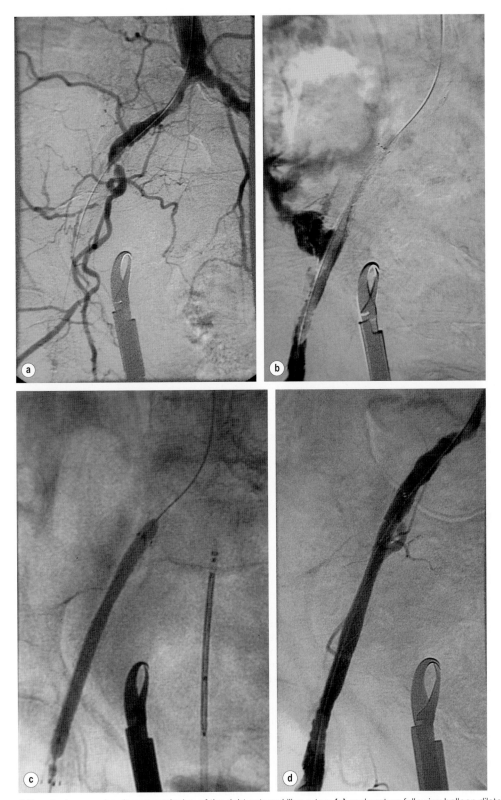

Figure 4.5 • Angiogram showing an occlusion of the right external iliac artery **(a)** and rupture following balloon dilatation **(b)**. Control was achieved with an occlusion balloon **(c)** and the artery repaired with a covered stent **(d)**.

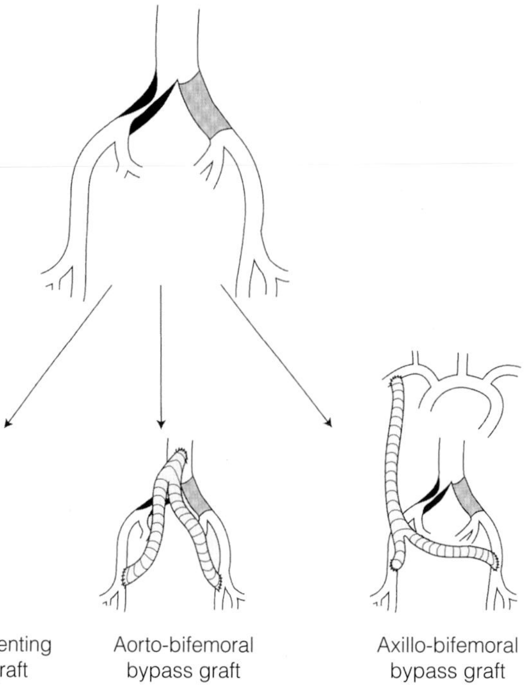

Figure 4.6 • Possible treatment options in a patient with aorto-iliac disease. Axillo-bifemoral bypass should be reserved for patients with critical ischaemia.

Iliac angioplasty/stenting and crossover graft

Aorto-bifemoral bypass graft

Axillo-bifemoral bypass graft

✓✓ To date there is no evidence of efficacy for preoperative methicillin-resistant *Staphylococcus aureus* (MRSA) screening, but in England all patients undergoing prosthetic grafting should either be screened or receive standard MRSA prophylaxis, nasal mupirocin and chlorhexidine bathing. Individual units should consider their admission policy for elective and emergency vascular cases, particulary in terms of transmission rates.[40]

Aorto-bifemoral bypass

The infrarenal abdominal aorta can be approached laparoscopically or by conventional open surgery. Laparoscopic aortic surgery has been introduced in many European countries and advocates claim lower morbidity and mortality rates and shorter hospital stays.[41,42] There remains no convincing evidence to support these claims as there have been no randomised trials. Laparoscopic aortic surgery requires extensive training and the procedure times are longer than for open surgery. With regard to open surgery, there is little or no evidence to favour either a transperitoneal versus a retroperitoneal approach or a vertical versus transverse incision, although transverse incisions are favoured by anaesthetists as the top end of a vertical incision often 'escapes' an epidural. End-to-end anastomoses are used for flush occlusions below the renal arteries (**Fig. 4.7**). If the proximal infrarenal aorta is patent, then an end-to-side anastomosis can preserve flow to a patent inferior mesenteric and/or internal iliac artery, thus reducing the risk of pelvic ischaemia.

✓ The majority of surgeons would favour a Dacron graft over polytetrafluoroethylene (PTFE). There are some theoretical data showing that PTFE grafts are more resistant to infection than Dacron, but this is outweighed by the superior handling and suturing characteristics of Dacron. Rifampicin soaking and/ or silver impregnation have been shown to improve the infection resistance of Dacron in vitro. There is little clinical evidence to support their use but they do no harm.[43] There is some observational evidence that young patients with premature atherosclerosis (<55 years) do better with superficial femoral vein bypass grafts compared to conventional Dacron prostheses.[44] Despite the initial success of these procedures there remains a significant postoperative morbidity and a high rate of buttock and hip claudication (see Table 4.2).[45]

Axillo-bifemoral bypass

Often described as the last resort of the destitute, this has its place in the very unfit patient and those with a 'hostile' abdomen.

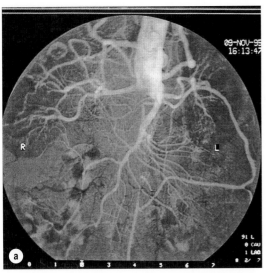
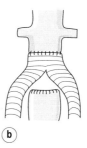
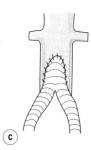

Figure 4.7 • Aortogram showing occlusion of the aorta below the level of the renal arteries **(a)**. In this case the proximal anastomosis of an aorto-bifemoral bypass should be end to end **(b)**. If there is continuity with the inferior mesenteric artery or internal iliac arteries, then an end-to-side anastomosis **(c)** may be preferable.

✔ The procedure is associated with a 5% in-hospital mortality, and 5-year limb salvage and patient survival rates of 74% and 34–39%, respectively.[46,47] A randomised clinical trial has reported improved 3-year graft patency rates in grafts with a flowsplitter (86%) versus a contralateral limb taken off at 90° (38%).[48]

Unilateral iliofemoral bypass

This procedure is indicated where there is extensive disease within the external iliac artery, which has failed to respond to endovascular intervention or where the disease extends into the common femoral artery.

✔✔ A recent study from France has demonstrated a superior outcome at 4 years in those patients who underwent iliofemoral grafting over femorofemoral crossover grafting.[49]

Table 4.2 • Outcome following aorto-bifemoral grafting[36]

Operative mortality	5%
Patient survival	73–88% at 5 years
Primary patency	85% at 5 years
	60% at 10 years
Re-operation	33%
Graft infection	1% for 10 years
False aneurysm	1% for 10 years

The key to success is a good inflow in the form of a disease-free common iliac artery and appropriate run-off into the SFA or profunda femoris artery (PFA). In the majority of cases a common femoral artery (CFA) endarterectomy and patch will have to be performed to gain access to the run-off vessels. In the rare cases where the common iliac is poor, the distal aorta can be used as a source of inflow. The common iliac artery is approached through a classical Rutherford–Morrison incision and an 'Omnitract' or ring retractor is a valuable tool in maintaining exposure of the vessels. Care should be taken to identify and preserve the ureter. Proximal control of the common iliac artery is essential, and some surgeons would avoid dissecting around the back of the vessel, as torrential venous bleeding can ensue, especially if there has been an inflammatory response around the vessels. Some surgeons would therefore advocate not to fully mobilise the vessel, but merely clamp it, without slings. Previous abdominal surgery, e.g. appendicectomy, or inguinal hernia repair may affect access to the retroperitoneal space and should be considered prior to any planned surgery. Externally supported 8-mm Dacron or PTFE are the conduits of choice and are usually sewn end-to-side to the common iliac. A tunnel is then created, from above and below the inguinal ligament, taking care not to injure the vein that overlies the CFA at the level of the inguinal ligament and the distal anastomosis completed to the CFA. In those cases where the SFA is occluded it is essential to extend the anastomosis down to at least the first bifurcation of the PFA.

Iliofemoral crossover

This procedure is indicated where the affected limb has no inflow vessel but the contralateral limb has a relatively disease-free iliac inflow. Use of the contralateral iliac artery avoids exposure of both groins. In addition, if the donor iliac artery develops significant atherosclerosis over time, this can be treated percutaneously via the donor femoral artery, thus avoiding direct puncture of the graft and/or anastomotic site. The donor iliac vessels are approached via a Rutherford–Morrison incision and the graft (Dacron/PTFE externally supported 8 mm) is placed in a lazy' S position. It is essential that the patient is catheterised and great care should be taken tunnelling the graft into the contralateral groin as there is the potential to damage the bladder and the iliofemoral veins.

Femorofemoral crossover

Femorofemoral crossover grafting is considered to be a low-risk procedure with an operative mortality between 0% and 5%. However, these figures are influenced by the presence of critical ischaemia, previous surgery and the need for combined iliac interventions.[51] Pursell et al., in a recent review, reported a 22% complication rate, including a 6% graft infection rate.[52] Like the iliofemoral graft, the procedure can be considered when the affected limb has no inflow and the contralateral iliac and femoral vessels are free of disease. The one contraindication is a large abdominal apron, which can affect the lie of the graft, especially in the seated position. The approach does, however, avoid an abdominal incision, but in theory exposes the patient to a higher rate of wound-related problems in the groin, notably infection. Two types of configuration are described: (1) lazy S and (2) inverted U. There are no convincing data to support either approach and it is often best decided at the time of surgery.

✔✔ One randomised trial has demonstrated no difference between externally supported 8-mm Dacron or PTFE.[53] However, Mingoli et al. reported 5- and 10-year primary patency rates of 80% and 60%, respectively, for supported grafts versus 69% and 21% for unsupported grafts.[54] Combined or delayed iliac angioplasty at the time of femorofemoral crossover bypass grafting should be avoided in those patients with iliac lesions in excess of 5 cm. Aburahma et al. reported 3-year primary patency rates of 85% and 31% in patients with iliac lesions 3–5 cm and >5 cm, respectively.[55]

Femoral endarterectomy and profundaplasty

The CFA and deep femoral artery (profunda femoris) origin is a common site for exophytic calcific atherosclerotic disease (**Fig. 4.8**). It is generally considered that the nature and location of the disease at a bifurcation subject to flexion is not usually suitable for angioplasty or stenting. However, there is no evidence for the superiority of endarterectomy over angioplasty (**Fig. 4.9**). Though there are several small cohort studies claiming safety and efficacy of CFA angioplasty/stent, none represents anything more than level IV evidence. A randomised trial is badly needed in view of the significant complications, especially the complications associated with CFA endarterectomy.

Femoral endarterectomy and repair using a patch that extends into the profunda is the preferred treatment at the moment. The choice of patch includes vein or prosthetic (Dacron or PTFE). If the SFA is occluded, this can be harvested and endarterectomised to form a useful patch, preserving the long saphenous vein and avoiding the risk of infection

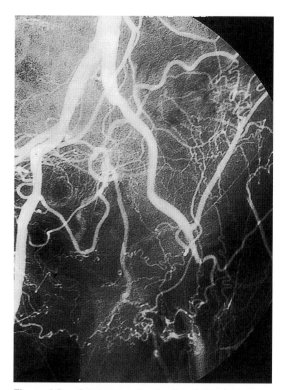

Figure 4.8 • Arteriogram of a claudicant showing a localised occlusion of the left common femoral artery, suitable for endarterectomy and patch repair.

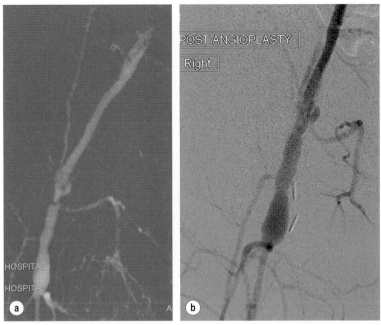

Figure 4.9 • A 65-year-old patient with short distance intermittent claudication and grade 3 chronic renal disease amongst other comorbidities. Carbon dioxide angiography confirmed the magnetic resonance angiography diagnosis of a common femoral stenosis **(a)**, which was angioplastied with a good result **(b)**. The CFA remained patent with minimal re-stenosis at 18 months.

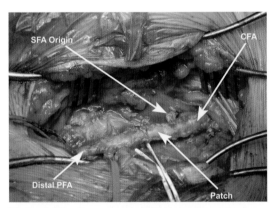

Figure 4.10 • Femoral and profunda endarterectomy and repair using a patch of endarterectomised SFA. This avoids the infection risk associated with prosthetic material and preserves the long saphenous vein.

associated with prosthetic material (**Fig. 4.10**). Femoral endarterectomy can be combined with iliac angioplasty or stenting, if there is proximal disease that would be difficult to access percutaneously. Femoral endarterectomy can also be combined with a femoropopliteal/distal bypass. In this case, the proximal end of the graft is used as the patch.

It is inadvisable to cross-clamp a proximal stent if arterial control is required for distal reconstruction. Clamping may crush the stent or tear the arterial wall. Arterial control can be achieved with an occlusion balloon, passed up the artery over a J-tip guide-wire. This trick is also useful whenever the proximal inflow is heavily calcified. In patients who require endovascular intervention down to or across the inguinal ligament in combination with CFA disease, consideration should be made as to the possibility of an extensive CFA/external iliac artery (EIA) endarterectomy via a vertical incision placed over the CFA extending over the inguinal ligament and curved towards the anterior superior iliac spine. This allows access to the retroperitoneal space and the EIA, and in particular the narrow space beneath the inguinal ligament.

Infrainguinal reconstruction

There are several treatment options for patients with isolated disease of the SFA (**Fig. 4.11**). Multilevel infrainguinal disease often requires more extensive revascularisation, and would normally only be justified in a patient with critical ischaemia (**Fig. 4.12**). Over the last decade there has been a significant reduction in the number of infrainguinal bypass grafts. The reasons for this are unclear, but may well relate to improvements in general medical care and risk factor modification, a renewed realisation of the benefits of exercise therapy, earlier referral, better access to interventional vascular radiology and improved endovascular techniques (see later).

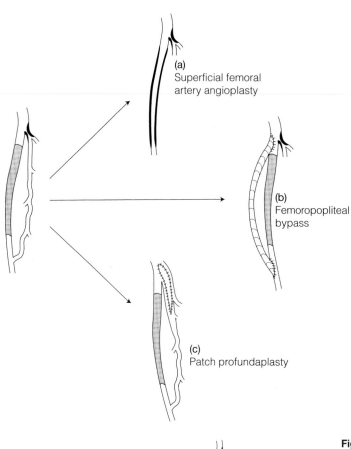

Figure 4.11 • Possible treatment options for a patient with localised SFA disease. Angioplasty **(a)** should be the first line of treatment for stenoses and occlusions less than 15 cm in length. Longer lesions will require a femoropopliteal bypass graft **(b)**. Profundaplasty **(c)** may be sufficient to improve claudication or rest pain, but will not usually heal ulceration or necrosis.

(a) Superficial femoral artery angioplasty

(b) Femoropopliteal bypass

(c) Patch profundaplasty

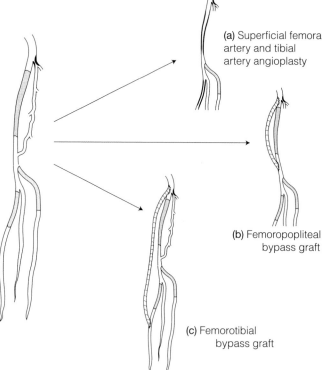

Figure 4.12 • Possible infrainguinal revascularisation options in a patient with critical limb ischaemia due to multilevel disease. Angioplasty **(a)** should be attempted if possible but may need to be extensive, with the risk of early re-occlusion. Femoropopliteal bypass **(b)** may fail to reperfuse the foot unless at least one calf artery is patent into the foot. Extensive tissue loss or sepsis usually requires a femorotibial bypass graft **(c)**, especially in a diabetic.

(a) Superficial femoral artery and tibial artery angioplasty

(b) Femoropopliteal bypass graft

(c) Femorotibial bypass graft

✓✓ Smoking cessation is vital, as continued smoking results in a threefold increased risk of graft failure.[52] Preoperative screening for hypercoagulability is also important as this adversely affects graft patency, limb salvage and survival.[56,57]

Successful infrainguinal bypass is dependent upon a good inflow, a reasonable size conduit and adequate run-off. It is important to have access to a contemporary set of images (usually within 6 months) and to have all inflow issues resolved either before or at the time of surgery. The CFA is the usual site for the proximal anastomosis, but if the vein will not reach, then either the profunda femoris or SFA can be used. If the SFA is diseased, it can be endarterectomised.

In terms of the outflow, grafts to the above-knee popliteal should only be undertaken if there is limited vein available or if there is no evidence of disease in that segment. As such, the below-knee popliteal is the preferred site of the distal anastomosis. By contrast, the tibioperoneal trunk is often diseased and represents a poor alternative to a crural vessel. Restoration of foot pulses is usually required to heal necrosis, especially in the presence of diabetes. If there are concerns about the run-off vessels, antegrade angiography or dedicated calf and foot magnetic resonance angiography may provide additional information. The posterior tibial artery is the easiest crural artery to access as it lies deep to the long saphenous vein (LSV). The mid-peroneal artery is also accessible from the medial side between the posterior tibial and soleus muscles. Access to the lower peroneal artery requires resection of a short length of fibula (**Fig. 4.13**). The anterior tibial artery is reached via an incision 4 cm lateral to the anterior edge of the fibula. The decision as to which vessels are grafted is dependent upon their size and continuity to the pedal arch and the angiosomes of the foot, as there is evidence that directly revascularising the affected angiosome territory improves outcome.[58]

Choice of graft material

The LSV is the conduit of choice in femoropopliteal grafting. Preoperative ultrasound mapping is essential. In general, a single non-varicose LSV is usable as long as it is not too small.

✓✓ A small LSV <3 mm is associated with a twofold risk of early failure and should be discarded or used as a venous patch or cuff.[59]

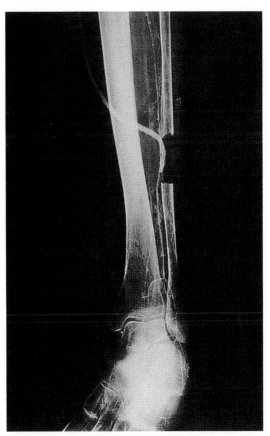

Figure 4.13 • Completion arteriogram of a femoro-peroneal vein bypass graft showing the fibulectomy required to access the peroneal artery from the lateral side of the leg.

By contrast, large veins (>6 mm) are often associated with focal varicosities that may require excision and splicing or alternatively plication of a local blow-out. The use of complex LSV systems (two or more) is associated with increased dissection, local haematoma formation and skin necrosis. If the LSV has been removed or is of poor quality one should consider removing the contralateral LSV. If this is not an option the short saphenous veins (SSVs) or arm veins can be scanned; however, for most femoropopliteal grafts, both will be needed. Bilateral SSV harvesting is best approached with the patient in the prone position (**Fig. 4.14**). If the arm veins are to be harvested, it is important to remind junior doctors and phlebotomists not to use them for blood sampling.

✓ In general, arm veins should only be used for rest pain, ulceration and/or gangrene; however, there are odd exceptions but patients need to be aware of the lower patency rates and the increased technical difficulties in harvesting and anastomosing these veins.[60]

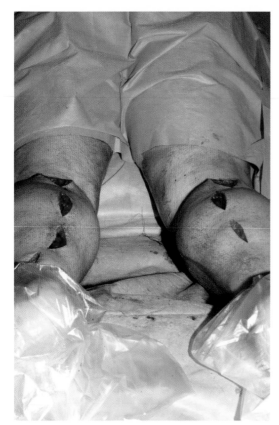

Figure 4.14 • Bilateral short saphenous vein harvesting for a redo left femoro-anterior tibial vein graft.

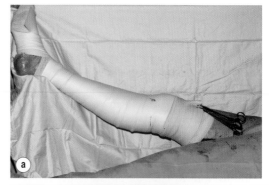

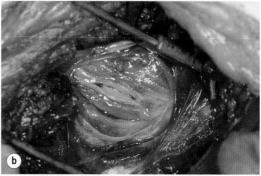

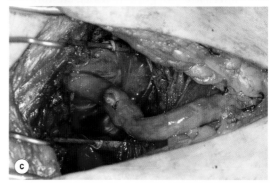

Figure 4.15 • (a) Esmarch tourniquet applied over a crepe bandage. (b) Exposed posterior tibial artery and venae commitantes after the application of the tourniquet. Note no clamps and no bleeding, which facilitates the anastomosis. (c) Completed distal anastomosis to the posterior tibial artery. A Boazul cuff can be used in the same way (see Chapter 17).

In situ versus reversed vein

There is no good clinical evidence to suggest that either technique is better than the other. However, the in situ technique is less forgiving than the conventional reverse graft, especially with uniform good-quality veins. The in situ technique lends itself to femorotibial bypass grafts to the posterior tibial, peroneal and dorsalis pedis arteries. By contrast, grafts to the anterior tibial artery are best tunnelled in the lateral position. Grafts tunnelled via the medial to lateral aspect via the interosseous membrane can be difficult to access if they develop a stenosis within this segment. The key step to success is the correct use of the valvulotome and one should be familiar will all types, including the disposable versions (LeMaitre). If the reversed technique is preferred it is essential to follow a strict tunnelling protocol to avoid twisting or kinking, especially if simultaneous anastomoses are undertaken. The use of a tourniquet is particularly useful in femorodistal bypass surgery as it reduces the need for extensive dissection and facilitates the anastomosis, as no clamps are required because of the bloodless field (Fig. 4.15). Alternatively, fine silastic slings or intraluminal occluders are preferable to clamps, and magnifying loupes are essential.

Prosthetic grafts

The use of prosthetic material for both intermittent claudication and critical ischaemia has fallen dramatically because of poor patency rates and concerns about graft infection.[61]

✓✓ The patency rates for femoropopliteal bypass for CLI from a meta-analysis by Hunink et al. gave primary patencies of 66% for vein (any level), 47% for above-knee PTFE and 33% for below-knee PTFE at 5 years.[62] The pooled weighted data for primary patency rates for femoro-distal (tibial or pedal) bypass are reported in TASC as 85%, 80% and 70% for femorodistal bypass with vein and 70%, 35% and 25% for femorodistal bypass with prosthetic at 1, 3 and 5 years, respectively.[11]

A Cochrane review reported no differences between PTFE and Dacron.[63] However, a subsequent multicentre randomised study of PTFE or Dacron for above-knee femoropopliteal bypass has reported a significant difference in the 2-year secondary patency rates for Dacron over PTFE.[64]

When no vein is available, most surgeons favour a vein cuff at the distal anastomosis. The Joint Vascular Research Group RCT of Miller vein cuff versus non-cuff for femoropopliteal PTFE grafts demonstrated significantly higher patency rates for prosthetic grafts with a vein cuff at the below-knee level at 3 years.[65]

Graft surveillance

This remains a controversial subject. Three randomised clinical trials demonstrated no benefit from a vein graft surveillance programme.[66–68] These studies were, however, criticised on the basis of the duplex criteria for an 'at-risk' graft and the timing of the initial scan (see Table 4.3).[69]

✓ On the basis of these observations, Mofidi et al., in an observational study using rigid duplex criteria, reported that a duplex scan at 6 weeks could predict those patients who require continued vein graft surveillance.[70] In addition, patients undergoing grafting using arm veins should be targeted as they are prone to develop stenoses and aneurysms.[71] Further work is required to define this population in more detail, but at present a 6-week scan should identify those vein grafts that require continued surveillance.

✓ In the case of PTFE grafts the data are limited, but there is observational evidence to support the practice of an early duplex to identify those with low graft flow. These patients can then be considered for long-term anticoagulation.[72]

Table 4.3 • Ultrasound criteria for 'at-risk' femorodistal vein grafts

Authors	Year	Machine	PSV (cm/s)	V2/V1
Lundell et al.[66]	1995	Diasonics CV 400	>200	–
		Acuson XP10	<45	–
Ihlberg et al.[67]	1998	ATL ultramark 9	<45	>2
Davies et al.[68]	2005	–	<45	>2

PSV, peak systolic velocity.

Infrainguinal endovascular intervention

Femoropopliteal angioplasty

The angioplasty literature suggests a 1-year patency rate for femoropopliteal stenosis of 70% and for occlusions of 50%. The literature is, however, generally poor and rarely defines the type of lesion that is being treated. The TASC document[11] is probably more realistic about the type of lesion that should be treated. In order to improve outcomes, many different alternatives to angioplasty have been proposed, including stents, cutting balloons,[73] cryoplasty[74] and drug-eluting stents. Critical analysis of a confusing literature on cryoplasty would suggest it is no better than angioplasty alone.[75]

Subintimal angioplasty

Although often described as a novel technique, subintimal angioplasty has been around for more than 20 years. It is perhaps considered novel because it has only been described in detail in the last 10 years. Using an antegrade catheter and a hydrophilic guidewire the subintimal space above a femoropopliteal occlusion is accessed and the wire pushed down like a surgical ring stripper (**Fig. 4.16**). If the artery is not too calcified the wire will invariably re-enter the true lumen below the obstruction and dilatation with a 5- or 6-mm angioplasty balloon will produce a patent though dissected channel offering a clean surface to blood flow. As a limb salvage procedure this technique works extremely well, with salvage rates of >75% being reported.[75–77]

Femoropopliteal stents

The results of femoropopliteal stents are variable and depend on an adequate inflow, the size of the artery treated and good run-off. Early results

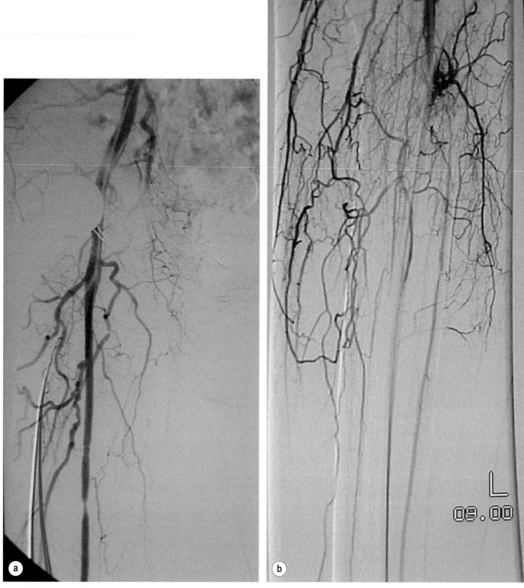

Figure 4.16 • (a,b) Angiograms of a patient with right-sided tissue loss demonstrating an occluded SFA with a stenosed left profunda femoris, an isolated popliteal segment, and patent peroneal and anterior tibial arteries.

from placement of stents did not demonstrate advantage over simple angioplasty, in part probably due to a poor understanding of the biomechanics of the SFA.[78–80] There are now four randomised trials comparing SFA angioplasty to SFA stenting in claudicants.[81–84] None has compared like with like, using different length lesions with non-matched comorbidities, and different risk factors. All have used surrogate end-points. The results from three

have been very positive for the use of stents and the fourth showed no significant difference, perhaps because it tested a very rigid stent prone to fracture against angioplasty.[84] Three meta-analyses of these trials have not supported the use of stents over PTA in the femoropopliteal segments.[85–87] In any event, there is also doubt as to whether data from any one trial can be transferred to all stents since there are data to indicate that design does matter.[88]

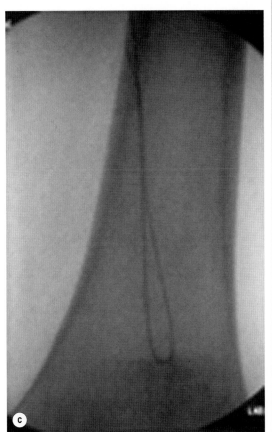

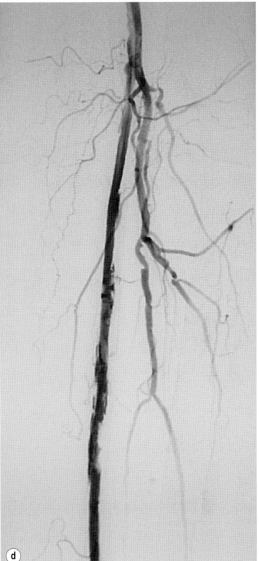

Figure 4.16 • cont'd **(c)** This captured image demonstrates the classic loop of hydrophilic wire used to strip a passage through the subintimal space. **(d,e)** Following 6-mm PTA the femoropopliteal segment is patent with good flow. The irregularities are caused by the deliberately dissected intimal flap. These are rarely (but occasionally) flow limiting.

(Continued)

✓ Patency rates of nearly 90% at 1 year and 78% at 3 years have been reported.[80–84] These good results are mainly in claudicants. Stent fractures also occur more commonly in the femoropopliteal segment due to flexion and overlapping of multiple stents. Stent fractures are associated with a higher risk of re-stenosis and occlusion. At the moment there are no good data to support the routine use of primary stenting in the femoropopliteal segments.[85–88]

Drug-eluting stents/balloons

Sirolimus-eluting stents have been tested and results from animal models demonstrated marked effects on smooth muscle proliferation and cell migration, with reduction in intimal hyperplasia following stent placement.

In a multicentre study from Germany, angioplasty balloons coated in paclitaxel produced significantly better results at 6 and 24 months in terms of

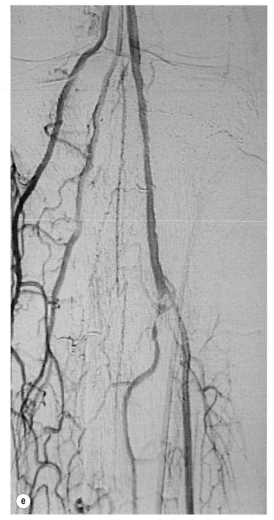

(e)

Figure 4.16 • cont'd

been criticised for significant commercial bias. At present there are no robust data to suggest that DES should be used over bare metal stents as a rescue where angioplasty fails.

late lumen loss and target lesion revascularisation compared to PTA alone or PTA plus paclitaxel-containing contrast media.[93] However, as shown in SIROCCO, it may be that the effect eventually wears off and that late complications may arise as seen in the coronary arteries treated with drug-eluting stents. Therefore, at present further data are required before their routine use as a primary technique could be recommended. In patients with limited revascularisation options and especially if treating recurrent stenoses, drug-eluting balloons may have a role. However, the authors' experience of using drug-eluting balloons in this scenario has been disappointing.

Covered stent grafts

✔ A small single-centre randomised trial of Viabahn expanded PTFE/nitinol stent grafts versus femoral to above-knee popliteal expanded PTFE or Dacron bypass grafts showed no difference in primary and secondary patency rates at 12 months (73.5% and 83.9% vs. 74.2% and 83.7%, respectively).[94]

This trial has been criticised for the large proportion of patients with claudication and the preferential use of prosthetic bypass material, rather than autologous vein. Also, few patients were taking best medical therapy including a statin and antiplatelet agent. Other trials have been similarly criticised but have found no difference in patency rates[95] or better patency rates for surgical bypass.[96] Nevertheless, if a patient does not have a suitable vein, then a stent graft seems a reasonable, but expensive, option. The superiority of stent grafts over open stents has not been demonstrated and there are no trials of stents versus bypass grafts to the below-knee popliteal level, which is more commonly required in patients with CLI.

The Surgical versus Percutaneous Bypass (SuperB)[97] trial is designed to compare the use of heparin-bonded stent grafts for the treatment of long lesions of the SFA to the venous surgical femoropopliteal bypass in a multicentre RCT. It will determine comparative patency rates and also complication rates with a number of secondary endpoints such as quality of life. Many of the criticisms of previous trials have been considered in this trial. It will publish data at 1, 3 and 5 years but as yet has not reported.

✔✔ In the SIROCCO trial of sirolimus-eluting stents (DES) versus bare SMART nitinol stents for TASC C lesions, the re-stenosis rate at 24 months was 22.9% and 21.1%, respectively.[89,90] There is a second randomised trial of the Zilver nitinol stent coated with paclitaxel against PTA in less than 10-cm stenotic or occluded segments. Twelve-month results demonstrated significant superiority of DES,[91] but a finding of superiority at 2 years for DES has recently been published.[92] Most of the patients in this trial had intermittent claudication and there are no data at all about statin use. The trial methodology has been criticised because of potential bias, as more than 50% of patients 'assigned' to DES had already had failed PTA and were therefore almost certain to get an improved result with a secondary stent. The trial has also

Crural artery intervention

Endovascular crural artery recanalisation in patients with tissue loss is associated with limb salvage rates of 81% at 12 months.[98,99] The use of self-expandable stents may have additional benefit at 1 year.[100] The success of the procedure is dependent upon a good inflow, stenotic rather than occlusive disease and focal rather than widespread atherosclerosis. Where crural intervention is done for tissue loss it is desirable to recanalise the appropriate angiosome if at all possible (**Fig. 4.17**). There is no evidence for this but it is a logical approach. A trial is needed to see if the recanalisation of the appropriate angiosome artery is superior to recanalisation of any of the three tibial arteries in terms of ulcer healing.

Infrainguinal bypass versus angioplasty

✓✓ In the BASIL trial (Bypass versus Angioplasty in Severe Ischaemia of the Leg) angioplasty was compared against infrainguinal bypass.[101–103] The primary outcome measure was amputation-free survival. Secondary outcome measures included all-cause mortality, morbidity and reintervention, quality of life and hospital costs. A total of 452 patients were randomised; 30-day mortality was low in both groups (5% for surgery and 3% for angioplasty). Surgery was associated with a significantly higher morbidity (57% vs. 41%), mainly due to myocardial infarction and wound infection. Those having surgery also stayed in hospital longer and this contributed to the cost of

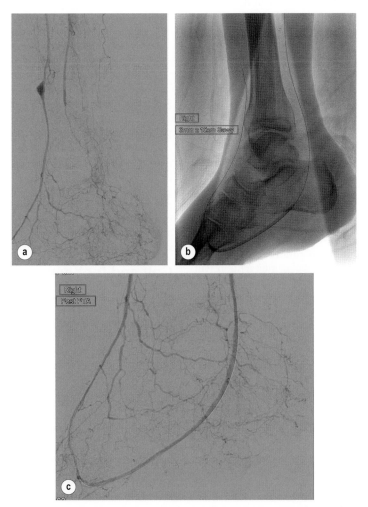

Figure 4.17 • An 80-year-old patient with a very painful left heel ulcer that was not getting any better despite intensive management. A previous distal bypass to the anterior tibial artery had occluded **(a)**. Posterior tibial and peroneal arteries were occluded and there was a very poor foot arch. The posterior tibial artery and foot arch were crossed with wire and catheter and angioplastied to 3 mm **(b)** with a good result, which allowed healing of the ulcer over the next month **(c)**.

surgery being one-third higher than angioplasty at 1 year. However, by 3 years there was no significant difference in costs because those having angioplasty had a significantly higher failure rate (20% vs. 3% within 12 months), resulting in a higher reintervention rate (28% vs. 17%). There was no difference in quality of life, amputation-free survival or all-cause mortality at any time interval out to 2 years, and by 5 years 36% of patients had died. Subgroup analysis suggests that surgery is the best option for fit patients likely to survive a significant period of time with a usable vein, and PTA where they have no suitable vein and where there is no viable bypass option.

The trial has been criticised for the combined endpoint, the high mortality that accounted for 75% of the end-points, the failure to address the secondary risk factors and the absence of data on diabetic control. Despite improvements in drug therapy for secondary prevention since the BASIL trial was recruiting, the arms of the trial were well matched and an analysis of the cases in the trial by one of these authors, who was a member of the data monitoring committee, suggests that it was a trial of very difficult surgery versus very difficult angioplasty, a view contrary to the assumption made by the authors of the European guidelines on critical limb ischaemia.[18] In addition, critics of 'the vein bypass if fit' strategy point out that patients suffering from CLI invariably have serious comorbidities that result in earlier death than might otherwise be the case. They and their relatives should be aware of the higher open surgical mortality and question the ability of even the most skilled doctor to predict within a group of patients with CLI who is likely to survive a significant period of time post-intervention. In addition, the decision regarding surgery or endovascular intervention will depend on whether the patient has rest pain alone or tissue loss (ulceration) alone. A surgical option will probably give better long-term results for patients suffering rest pain, which of course brings the debate back to the prediction of life span.

Non-interventional treatment for CLI

Please see Chapter 21 for a discussion of the future potential of gene therapy.

Iloprost

✓✓ A meta-analysis of six randomised controlled studies of iloprost, involving more than 700 patients with CLI, suggests a significant reduction in death and amputation at 6 months (35% vs. 55%) for those patients receiving the drug.[104]

However, the long-term benefit remains unclear for this expensive drug and its use in the UK has declined over the last few years.

Spinal cord stimulation

✓ Two controlled studies of spinal cord stimulation have demonstrated no improvement in ulcer healing, limb salvage and mortalilty rates.[105,106] More recently, a further study has confirmed the role of spinal cord stimulation in non-reconstructable vascular disease. The authors reported that preoperative transcutaneous PO_2 measurements and preoperative sceening improved the probability of limb salvage.[107]

Sympathectomy

Lumbar sympathectomy is an option in patients with unreconstructable occlusive disease and rest pain. The duration of the benefit remains, however, in question. In those patients with rest pain and tissue loss, sympathectomy is of limited use. Published results are old and variable: some report long-term pain relief in 78% of cases, with 11% requiring amputation;[108] others report pain relief in only 6%, with 70% requiring early amputation.[109]

Calf and foot compression

✓✓ In a small-scale community-based observation study, Kavros et al. reported their experience of intermittent pneumatic compression (IPC) of the foot, calf or both in patients with chronic lower limb ischaemia. IPC was delivered at an inflation pressure of 85–95 mmHg, applied for 2 seconds with rapid rise (0.2 seconds), three cycles per minute; three 2-hourly sessions per day were requested. Significant improvements in wound healing and limb salvage rates were noted over a control group.[110]

Key points

- The TASC offers sensible guidelines for the treatment of both supra- and infrainguinal disease.
- Best medical therapy and supervised exercise in patients with claudication should be the initial treatment of choice but is underutilised because it is under-resourced and often not considered.
- Iliac occlusions should be treated by primary stenting if exercise therapy fails or cannot be undertaken. Complication rates are low.

- Suprainguinal surgery remains a useful treatment option for bilateral/diffuse disease, but great care should be taken in the era of MRSA.
- Infrainguinal surgery is in decline but autologous vein remains the conduit of choice.
- In the absence of leg vein, arm vein should be considered.
- Prosthetic grafts should only be used as a last resort and only with a venous cuff.
- Graft surveillance remains contentious and requires further research.
- Infrainguinal endovascular intervention requires further study.
- The long-term results of the BASIL trial favour surgery for CLI if the anatomy is suitable, there is a good vein, the patient is relatively young, has no other comorbidities likely to cause early death and the patient is fit to undergo open surgery. Otherwise PTA is the treatment of choice.
- There is no role for vasodilators in CLI.
- Sympathectomy continues to be used despite little or no evidence.
- Some patients with CLI are best treated by primary amputation.

References

1. Murphy TP, Cutlip DE, Regensteiner JG, et al. Supervised exercise versus primary stenting for claudication resulting from aortoiliac peripheral artery disease: six-month outcomes from the claudication: exercise versus endoluminal revascularization. Circulation 2012;125:130–9.
   In iliac arteries supervised exercise when adhered to is objectively superior to iliac intervention when walking distance is measured, but quality of life is subjectively better post-intervention.

2. Greenhalgh RM, Belch JJ, Brown LC, et al. The adjuvant benefit of angioplasty in patients with mild to moderate intermittent claudication (MIMIC) managed by supervised exercise, smoking cessation advice and best medical therapy: results from two randomised trials for stenotic femoropopliteal and aortoiliac arterial disease. Eur J Vasc Endovasc Surg 2008;36:680–8.
   Supervised exercise therapy and endovascular intervention work. The two may work well together.

3. Perkins JMT, Collin J, Creasy TS, et al. Exercise training versus angioplasty for stable claudication. Long and medium term results of a prospective, randomised trial. Eur J Vasc Endovasc Surg 1996;11:409–13.

4. Whyman MR, Fowkes FGR, Kerracher EMG, et al. Randomised controlled trial of percutaneous transluminal angioplasty for intermittent claudication. Eur J Vasc Endovasc Surg 1996;12:167–72.

5. Abou-Zamzam Jr. AM, Lee RW, Moneta GL, et al. Functional outcome after infrainguinal bypass for limb salvage. J Vasc Surg 1997;25(2):287–97.

6. Humphreys WV, Evans F, Watkin G, et al. Critical limb ischaemia in patients over 80 years of age: options in a district general hospital. Br J Surg 1995;82(10):1361–3.

7. Singh S, Evans L, Datta D, et al. The costs of managing lower limb-threatening ischaemia. Eur J Vasc Endovasc Surg 1996;12(3):359–62.

8. Johnson BF, Singh S, Evans L, et al. A prospective study of the effect of limb-threatening ischaemia and its surgical treatment on the quality of life. Eur J Vasc Endovasc Surg 1997;13(3):306–14.

9. Nicoloff AD, Taylor Jr. LM, McLafferty RB, et al. Patient recovery after infrainguinal bypass grafting for limb salvage. J Vasc Surg 1998;27(2):256–66.

10. Society of Interventional Radiology Standards of Practice Committee. Guidelines for percutaneous transluminal angioplasty. J Vasc Interv Radiol 2003;14:S209.

11. Norgren L, Hiatt WR, Dormandy JA, et al. TASC II Working Group. Inter-Society Consensus for the Management of Peripheral Arterial Disease (TASC II). J Vasc Surg 2007;45(Suppl. S):S5–67.
    Comprehensive guidelines on the treatment of peripheral arterial disease.

12. Stoeckelhuber BM, Meissner O, Stoeckelhubr M, et al. Primary endovascular stent placements of focal infrarenal aortic stenosis. Initial and mid term results. J Vasc Interv Radiol 2003;14:1443–7.

13. Simons PC, Nawijn AA, Bruijninckx CM, et al. Long-term results of primary stent placement to treat infrarenal aortic stenosis. Eur J Vasc Endovasc Surg 2006;32:627–33.

14. Naylor AR, Ah-See AK, Engeset J. Axillofemoral bypass as a limb salvage procedure in high risk patients with aortoiliac disease. Br J Surg 1990;77(6):659–61.

15. Benson K, Hartz AJ. A comparison of observational studies and randomised control trials. N Engl J Med 2000;342:1878–86.

16. Concato J, Shah N, Howitz RI. Randomised control trials, observational studies in the hierarchy of research design. N Engl J Med 2000;342:1887–92.

17. Ioannidis JPA, Haidich AB, Lau J. Any casualties in the clash of randomised and observational evidence? Br Med J 2001;322:879–90.

18. Setacci C, de Donato G, Tera M, et al. Management of critical limb ischaemia and diabetic foot clinical practice guidelines of the European Society for Vascular Surgery. Eur J Vasc Endovasc Surg 2011;42:S43–60.

19. Wolf GL, Wilson SE, Cross AP, et al. Surgery or balloon angioplasty for peripheral vascular disease; a randomised clinical trial. J Vasc Interv Radiol 1993;4:639–48.

A multicentre prospective trial comparing PTA versus surgery for both supra- and infrainguinal disease. Both treatment arms were successful in terms of improving quality of life and haemodynamics; however, no difference was observed in outcomes at 4 years.

20. Ballard JL, Burgen JJ, Singh P, et al. Aorto iliac stent deployment vs surgical reconstruction; analysis of outcome and cost. J Vasc Surg 1998;28:94–101.

21. Kaufmann SL, Barth KH, Kadir S, et al. Haemodynamic measurements in the evaluation and follow up of transluminal angioplasty of the iliac and femoral arteries. Radiology 1982;142:329–36.

22. Kamphius AG, van Engelen AD, Tetteroo E, et al. Impact of different haemodynamic criteria for stent placement after suboptimal iliac angioplasty. Dutch Iliac Stent Trial Study Group. J Vasc Interv Radiol 1999;10:741–6.

23. Tetteroo E, Haaring C, van der Graaf Y. Randomised comparison of primary stent placement versus primary angioplasty followed by selective stent placement in patients with iliac-artery occlusive disease. Lancet 1998;341:1153–9.

24. Ring EJ. Percutaneous recanalisation of common iliac occlusions; an unacceptable complication rate. AJR Am J Roentgenol 1982;139:587–9.

25. Richter GM, Noeldge G, Roeren T, et al. First long term results of a randomised muticentre trial: iliac balloon expandable stent placement vs PTA. Radiology 1990;177(P):152.

26. Tetteroo E, van der Graaf Y, Bosch JL, et al. Randomised comparison of primary stent placement versus primary angioplasty followed by selective stent placement in patients with iliac-artery occlusive disease. Dutch Iliac Stent Trial Study Group. Lancet 1998;351:1153–9.

A multicentre randomised clinical trial (1993–7) comparing direct stent placement versus primary angioplasty with or without subsequent stent placement in patients with intermittent claudication. No difference was observed in the quality of life, patency and reintervention rates.

27. Klein WM, van der Graaf Y, Seegers J, et al. Dutch Iliac Stent Trial: long-term results in patients randomized for primary or selective stent placement. Radiology 2006;238:734–44.

28. Hersey N, Cleveland T, Gaines P. STAG trial: a multicentre randomised clinical trial comparing angioplasty and stenting for the treatment of iliac occlusion: comparison of clinical outcomes and complications. Abstract. British Society of Interventional Radiology 2010;.

29. Bosch JL, Hunink MG. Stent or PTA in iliac "occlusive" disease meta-analysis of the results of PTA and stent placement in aortoiliac occlusive disease. Radiology 1997;204:87–96.

A meta-analysis of data from 1990 onwards, which included six PTA studies (1300 patients) and eight stent placement studies (816 patients). No differences were observed between the two groups in terms of mortality and complications, but technical success was higher in the stented group.

30. Bosch JL. Iliac arterial disease: cost effectiveness analysis of stent placement vs PTA. Radiology 1998;208:641–81.

31. Dyet JF, Cook AM, Nicholson AA. Self expanding stents in iliac arteries. Clin Radiol 1993;48:117–9.

32. Dyet JF, Gaines PA, Nicholson AA. Treatment of chronic iliac occlusions by means of percutaneous endovascular stent placement. J Vasc Interv Radiol 1997;8:349–53.

33. Third BSIR Iliac Angioplasty and Stenting Report. British Society of Interventional Radiology. Oxfordshire: Dendrite Clinical Systems; 2008. http://www.bsir.org; [accessed 29.11.12].

34. Lewis DR, Davies AH, Irvine CD, et al. Compression ultrasonography for false femoral artery aneurysms: hypocoagulability is a cause of failure. Eur J Vasc Endovasc Surg 1998;16:427–8.

35. Tisi PV, Callam MJ. Surgery versus non-surgical treatment for femoral pseudoaneurysms. Cochrane Database Syst Rev 2006;1:CD004981.

36. Hogg ME, Peterson BG, Pearce WH, et al. Bare metal stent infections: case report and review of the literature. J Vasc Surg 2007;46:813–20.

37. Redman A, Cope L, Uberoi R. Iliac artery injury following placement of the memotherm arterial stent. Cardiovasc Intervent Radiol 2001;24:113–6.

38. Chatziioannou A, Mourikis D, Katsimilis J. Acute iliac artery rupture: endovascular treatment. Cardiovasc Intervent Radiol 2007;30:281–5.

39. Carlisle J, Swart M. Mid-term survival after abdominal aortic aneurysm surgery predicted by cardiopulmonary exercise testing. Br J Surg 2007;94:966–9.

40. Thompson M. An audit demonstrating a reduction in MRSA infection in a specialised vascular unit resulting from a change in infection control protocol. Eur J Vasc Endovasc Surg 2006;31:609–15.

A prospective audit that demonstrated the effectiveness of an isolation policy on MRSA infection rates.

41. Coggia M, Javerliat I, Di Centa I, et al. Total laparoscopic bypass for aortoiliac occlusive lesions: 93-case experience. J Vasc Surg 2004;40:899–906.

42. Štádler P, Šebesta P, Vitásek P, et al. A modified technique of transperitoneal direct approach for totally laparoscopic aortoiliac surgery. Eur J Vasc Endovasc Surg 2006;32:266–9.

43. Schmacht D, Armstrong P, Johnson B, et al. Graft infectivity of rifampin and silver-bonded polyester grafts to MRSA contamination. Vasc Endovasc Surg 2005;39:411–20.

44. Jackson MR, Ali AT, Bell C, et al. Aortofemoral bypass in young patients with premature atherosclerosis: is superficial femoral vein superior to Dacron? J Vasc Surg 2004;40:17–23.

45. Jaquinandi V, Picquet J, Bouyá P, et al. High prevalence of proximal claudication among patients with patent aortobifemoral bypasses. J Vasc Surg 2007;45:312–8.

46. Hertzer NR, Bena JF, Karafa MT. A personal experience with direct reconstruction and extra-anatomic bypass for aortoiliofemoral occlusive disease. J Vasc Surg 2007;45:527–35.

47. Harrington ME, Harrington EB, Haimov M, et al. Axillofemoral bypass: compromised bypass for compromised patients. J Vasc Surg 1994;20:195–201.

48. Wittens CH, van Houtte HJ, van Urk H. European Prospective Randomised Multi-centre Axillo-bifemoral Trial. Eur J Vasc Surg 1992;6:115–23.
   A prospective multicentre RCT comparing two designs: (i) contralateral branch at an angle of 90° and (ii) a flow-splitter. At a median follow-up of 12 months the flow-splitter group had a significantly better patency rate at 2 years. No differences were observed in terms of mortality and graft infection.

49. Ricco JB, Probst H. Long-term results of a multicenter randomized study on direct versus crossover bypass for unilateral iliac artery occlusive disease. J Vasc Surg 2008;47:45–53.
   A prospective multicentre RCT (France and Switzerland) between 1986 and 1991, which demonstrated superior assisted primary and secondary patency rates for iliofemoral grafting over femoro-femoral bypass. The latter should be reserved for high-risk cases not amenable to interventional radiology.

50. Ascer E, Kirwin J, Mohan C, et al. The preferential use of the external iliac artery as an inflow source for redo femoropopliteal and infrapopliteal bypass. J Vasc Surg 1993;18:234–9.

51. Kim YW, Lee JH, Kim HG, et al. Factors affecting the long-term patency of crossover femoro-femoral bypass graft. Eur J Vasc Endovasc Surg 2005;30:376–80.

52. Pursell R, Sideso E, Magee TR, et al. Critical appraisal of femorofemoral crossover grafts. Br J Surg 2005;92:565–9.

53. Eiberg JP, Røder O, Stahl-Madsen M, et al. Fluoropolymer-coated Dacron versus PTFE grafts for femorofemoral crossover bypass: randomised trial. Eur J Vasc Endovasc Surg 2006;32:431–8.
   A randomised multicentre clinical trial comparing Dacron versus PTFE in femoro-femoral reconstruction demonstrated no differences in outcome.

54. Mingoli A, Sapienza P, Feldhaus RJ, et al. Femorofemoral bypass grafts: factors influencing long-term patency rate and outcome. Surgery 2001;129:451–8.

55. Aburahma AF, Robinson PA, Cook CC, et al. Selecting patients for combined femorofemoral bypass grafting and iliac balloon angioplasty and stenting for bilateral iliac disease. J Vasc Surg 2001;33(Suppl. 2):S93–9.

56. Willigendael EM, Teijink JAW, Bartelink M-L, et al. Smoking and the patency of lower extremity bypass grafts: a meta-analysis. J Vasc Surg 2008;42:67–74.
   A meta-analysis of 29 studies that evaluated the influence of smoking on the patency rates of lower limb arterial reconstruction.

57. Curi MA, Skelly CL, Baldwin ZK, et al. Long term outcome of infrainguinal bypass grafting in patients with serologically proven hypercoagulability. J Vasc Surg 2003;37:301–6.
   A retrospective analysis of consecutive patients from January 1994 to January 2001, which demonstrated that patients with evidence of hypercoagulability have a worse outcome in terms of long-term patency, limb salvage and survival rates.

58. Neville RF, Attinger CE, Bulan EJ, et al. Revascularization of a specific angiosome for limb salvage: does the target artery matter? Ann Vasc Surg 2009;23:367–73.

59. Shanser A, Hevelone N, Owens CD, et al. Technical factors affecting autogenous vein graft failure: observations from a large multicentre trial. J Vasc Surg 2007;46:1180–90.
   Analysis of the PREVENT III trial database of 1404 North American patients who underwent lower limb arterial reconstruction with autogolous vein.

60. Faries PL, Arora S, Pomposelli Jr. FB, et al. The use of arm vein in lower-extremity revascularization: results of 520 procedures performed in eight years. J Vasc Surg 2000;31:50–9.

61. Veith FJ, Gupta SK, Ascer E, et al. Six-year prospective multicenter randomized comparison of autologous saphenous vein and expanded polytetrafluoroethylene grafts in infrainguinal arterial reconstructions. J Vasc Surg 1986;3(1):104–14.

62. Hunink MG, Wong JB, Donaldson MC, et al. Patency results of percutaneous and surgical revascularization for femoropopliteal arterial disease. Med Decis Making 1994;14(1):71–81.
   The authors used a method based on the proportional hazards model and the actuarial life-table approach; the results were adjusted for differences in case mix of the study populations. Adjusted 5-year primary patencies after surgery varied from 33% to 80%, the best results being for saphenous vein bypass performed for claudication.

63. Mamode N, Scott RN. Graft type for femoropopliteal bypass surgery. Cochrane Database Syst Rev 1999;2:CD001487.
   A Cochrane review of nine trials that included 1334 patients. No clear evidence was identified as to which type of graft is best. No difference was observed between in situ and reversed. Vein cuffs offer better primary patency rates for below-knee femoro-popliteal PTFE grafts.

64. Jensen LP, Lepäntalo M, Fossdal JE, et al. Dacron or PTFE for above knee femoropopliteal bypass. A multicenter randomised study. Eur J Vasc Endovasc Surg 2007;34:44–9.

A prospective multicentre RCT (1993–8) comparing Dacron versus PTFE. No difference was observed in terms of limb salvage, mortality and major complications. Secondary patency rates were better in the Dacron group.

65. Griffiths GD, Nagy J, Black D, et al. Randomized clinical trial of distal anastomotic interposition vein cuff in infrainguinal polytetrafluoroethylene bypass grafting. Br J Surg 2004;91:560–2.
A prospective RCT of cuff versus no cuff for femoro-popliteal PTFE reconstructions. Three-year patency rates were significantly better in the cuff group in the below-knee setting; however, no differences were observed in limb salvage rates (above and below knee).

66. Lundell A, Lindblad B, Bergqvist D, et al. Femoropopliteal–crural graft patency is improved by an intensive surveillance program: a prospective randomised study. J Vasc Surg 1995;21:26–34.
A prospective RCT of intensive versus routine surveillance. Primary and secondary patency rates were better in the intensive group, but no difference was observed in the PTFE grafts.

67. Ihlberg L, Luther M, Tierala E, et al. The utility of duplex scanning in infrainguinal vein graft surveillance: results from a randomised controlled study. Eur J Vasc Endovasc Surg 1998;16:19–27.
Entry into this trial was based upon a patent graft at 1 month. Patients were prospectively randomised to clinical observation versus duplex. No beneficial effect was noted in the duplex group.

68. Davies AH, Hawdon AJ, Sydes MR, et al on behalf of the VGST participants. Is duplex surveillance of value after leg vein bypass grafting? Circulation 2005;112:1985–91.
A multicentre prospective RCT where patients with a patent graft at 1 month were randomised to clinical versus duplex assessment. No differences were observed between the two groups in mortality, primary and secondary patency rates and limb salvage rates.

69. Bandyk D. Surveillance after lower extremity arterial bypass. Perspect Vasc Surg Endovasc Ther 2007;19:376–83.

70. Mofidi R, Kleman J, Berry O, et al. Significance of early postoperative duplex results in infrainguinal vein bypass surveillance. Eur J Vasc Endovasc Surg 2007;34:327–32.

71. Armstrong PA, Bandyk D, Wilson JS, et al. Optimizing infrainguinal arm vein bypass patency with duplex ultrasound surveillance and endovascular therapy. J Vasc Surg 2004;40:724–31.

72. Brumberg RS, Back MR, Armstrong PA, et al. The relative importance of graft surveillance and warfarin therapy in infrainguinal prosthetic bypass failure. J Vasc Surg 2007;46:1160–6.

73. Rabbi JF, Kiran RP, Gersten G, et al. Early results with infra-inguinal cutting balloon angioplasty limits distal dissection. Ann Vasc Surg 2004;18:640.

74. Laird J, Jaff MR, Biamino G, et al. Cryoplasty for the treatment of femoro-popliteal arterial disease; results of a prospective multi-centre registry. J Vasc Interv Radiol 2005;16:1067–73.

75. Karthik S, Tuite DJ, Nicholson AA, et al. Cryoplasty for arterial restenosis. Eur J Vasc Endovasc Surg 2007;33:40–3.

76. Spinosa DJ, Leung DA, Matsumoto AH, et al. Percutaneous intentional extraluminal recanalization in patients with chronic critical limb ischemia. Radiology 2004;232:499–507.

77. Lazaris AM, Salas C, Tsiamis AC, et al. Factors affecting patency of subintimal infrainguinal angioplasty in patients with critical lower limb ischemia. Eur J Vasc Endovasc Surg 2006;32:668–74.

78. Sabeti S, Schillinger M, Amighi J, et al. Primary patency of femoro-popliteal arteries treated with Nitinol stainless steel self expanding stents: propensity score adjusted analysis. Radiology 2004;232:516–21.

79. Vogel TR, Shindelman LE, Nackman JB, et al. Efficacious use of Nitinol stents in the femoral and popliteal arteries. J Vasc Surg 2003;38:1178–84.

80. Jahnke T, Voshage G, Müller-Hülsbeck S, et al. Endovascular placement of self expanding Nitinol coiled stents for the treatment of femoro-popliteal obstructive disease. J Vasc Interv Radiol 2002;13:257–66.

81. Laird JR, Katzen BT, Scheinert D, et al. Nitinol stent implantation versus balloon angioplasty for lesions in the superficial femoral artery and proximal popliteal artery: twelve-month results from the RESILIENT randomized trial. Circ Cardiovasc Interv 2010;3(3):267–76.

82. Krankenberg H, Schlüter M, Steinkamp HJ. Nitinol stent implantation versus percutaneous transluminal angioplasty in superficial femoral artery lesions up to 10cm in length. The Femoral Artery Stenting Trial (FAST). Circulation 2007;116:285–92.

83. Dick P, Wallner H, Sabeti S, et al. Balloon angioplasty versus stenting with nitinol stents in intermediate length superficial femoral artery lesions. Catheter Cardiovasc Interv 2009;74:1090–5.

84. Schillinger M, Sabeti S, Loewe C, et al. Balloon angioplasty versus implantation of nitinol stents in the superficial femoral artery. N Engl J Med 2006;354(18):1879–88.

85. Mwipatayi BP, Hockings A, Hofmann M, et al. Balloon angioplasty compared with stenting for treatment of femoropopliteal occlusive disease: a meta-analysis. J Vasc Surg 2008;47:461–9.

86. Kasapis C, Henke PK, Chetcuti SJ, et al. Routine stent implantation vs. percutaneous transluminal angioplasty in femoropopliteal artery disease: a meta-analysis of randomized controlled trials. Eur Heart J 2009;30:44–55.

87. Bachoo P, Thorpe PA, Maxwell H, et al. Endovascular stents for intermittent claudication. Cochrane Database Syst Rev 2010;1:CD003228.

88. Rits J, van Herwaarden JA, Jahrome AK, et al. The incidence of arterial stent fractures with exclusion of coronary, aortic and non-arterial settings. Eur J Vasc Endovasc Surg 2008;36:339–45.

89. Duda SH, Bosier SM, Lammer J, et al. Sirolimus eluting vs bare Nitinol stents for obstructive superficial femoral artery disease. The SIROCCO II trial. J Vasc Interv Radiol 2005;16:331–8.
A randomised double-blind trial comparing bare stents against sirolimus-eluting stents. No difference was observed between the groups in terms of the primary endpoint of in-stent lumen diameter at 6 months.

90. Duda SH, Bosiers M, Lammer J, et al. Drug-eluting and bare nitinol stents for the treatment of atherosclerotic lesions in the superficial femoral artery: long-term results from the SIROCCO trial. J Endovasc Ther 2006;13:701–10.
A randomised double-blind trial comparing bare stents against sirolimus-eluting stents. At 24 months no difference was observed between the two groups in terms of mortality, ankle–brachial index and restenosis rates.

91. Dake M, Ansell G, Jaff M, et al. Paclitaxel-eluting stents show superiority to balloon angioplasty and bare metal stents in femoropopliteal disease. Twelve-month Zilver PTX randomized study results. Circ Cardiovasc Interv 2011;4:495–504.

92. Dake M. The Zilver PTX randomized trial of paclitaxel-eluting stents for femoropopliteal disease: 24-month update. Presented at 7th edition of the Leipzig Interventional Course (LINC) 2011 2011 Leipzig, Germany; 19–22 January.

93. Tepe G, Zeller T, Albrecht T, et al. Local delivery of paclitaxel to inhibit restenosis during angioplasty of the leg. N Engl J Med 2008;14:689–99.
A randomised multicentre trial that compared paclitaxel-coated angioplasty balloons and paclitaxel dissolved in the angiographic contrast medium during angioplasty of the leg. At 6 months there was a significant reduction in late lumen loss and requirement for target lesion revascularisation.

94. Kedora J, Hohmann S, Garrett W, et al. Randomised comparison of percutaneous Viabahn stent grafts vs prosthetic femoro-popliteal bypass in the treatment of superficial femoral arterial occlusive disease. J Vasc Surg 2007;45:10–6.

95. McQuade K, Gable D, Pearl G, et al. Four-year randomized prospective comparison of percutaneous ePTFE/nitinol self-expanding stent graft versus prosthetic femoral–popliteal bypass in the treatment of superficial femoral artery occlusive disease. J Vasc Surg 2010;52:584–90.

96. Lepäntalo M, Laurila K, Roth WD, et al. Scandinavian Thrupass Study Group. PTFE bypass or thrupass for superficial femoral artery occlusion? A randomised controlled trial. Eur J Vasc Endovasc Surg 2009;37:578–84.

97. Lensvelt MM, Holewijn S, Fritschy WM, et al. SUrgical versus PERcutaneous Bypass: SUPERB-trial; heparin-bonded endoluminal versus surgical femoro-popliteal bypass: study protocol for a randomized controlled trial. Trials 2011;12:178.

98. Soder HK, Manninen HI, Jaakkola P, et al. Prospective trial of infrapopliteal artery balloon angioplasty for critical limb ischemia: angiographic and clinical results. J Vasc Interv Radiol 2000;11:1021–31.

99. Vraux H, Hammer F, Verhelst R, et al. Subintimal angioplasty of tibial vessel occlusions in the treatment of critical ischaemia: mid-term results. Eur J Vasc Endovasc Surg 2000;20:441–6.

100. Peregrin JH, Smirová S, Koznar B, et al. Self-expandable stent placement in infrapopliteal arteries after unsuccessful angioplasty failure: one year follow up. Cardiovasc Intervent Radiol 2008;31:860–4.

101. Adam AJ, Beard JD, Cleveland T, et al. BASIL trial participants. Bypass versus angioplasty in severe ischaemia of the leg (BASIL): multicentre, randomised controlled trial. Lancet 2005;366:1925–34.
A prospective RCT of surgery versus angioplasty in patients with severe lower limb ischaemia. The primary end-point of the study was amputation. At the end of 6 months there was no difference between the two groups in terms of amputation-free survival rates and quality of life.

102. Bradbury AW, Adam DJ, Bell J, et al. Bypass versus Angioplasty in Severe Ischaemia of the Leg (BASIL) trial: an intention-to-treat analysis of amputation-free and overall survival in patients randomized to a bypass surgery-first or a balloon angioplasty-first revascularization strategy. J Vasc Surg 2010;51:5S–17S.

103. Bradbury AW, Adam DJ, Bell J, et al. Bypass versus Angioplasty in Severe Ischaemia of the Leg (BASIL) trial: analysis of amputation free and overall survival by treatment received. J Vasc Surg 2010;51:18S–31S.

104. Loosemore TM, Chalmers TC, Dormandy JA. A meta-analysis of randomized placebo control trials in Fontaine stages III and IV peripheral occlusive arterial disease. Int Angiol 1994;13:133–42.
A meta-analysis of six RCTs of iloprost in the treatment of patients with Fontaine stage III and IV peripheral arterial occlusive disease unsuitable for arterial reconstruction. Significant ($P < 0.05$) beneficial effects with regards to the probability of being alive with both legs at 6 months follow-up were reported.

105. Jivegard LE, Augustinsson LE, Holm J, et al. Effects of spinal cord stimulation (SCS) in patients with inoperable severe lower limb ischaemia: a prospective randomised controlled study. Eur J Vasc Endovasc Surg 1995;9:421–5.

106. Klomp HM, Spincemaille GH, Steyerberg EW, et al. Spinal-cord stimulation in critical limb ischaemia: a randomised trial. ESES Study Group. Lancet 1999;353:1040–4.

107. Amann W, Berg P, Gersbach P, et al. European Peripheral Vascular Disease Outcome Study SCS-EPOS. Spinal cord stimulation in the treatment of non-reconstructable stable critical leg ischaemia: results of the European Peripheral Vascular

Disease Outcome Study (SCS-EPOS). Eur J Vasc Endovasc Surg 2003;26:280–6.

108. Persson AV, Anderson LA, Padberg Jr. FT. Selection of patients for lumbar sympathectomy. Surg Clin North Am 1985;65:393–403.

109. Fulton RL, Blakeley WR. Lumbar sympathectomy: a procedure of questionable value in the treatment of arteriosclerosis obliterans of the legs. Am J Surg 1968;116:735–44.

110. Kavros SJ, Delis KT, Turner NS, et al. Improving limb salvage in critical ischemia with intermittent pneumatic compression: a controlled study with 18-month follow-up. J Vasc Surg 2008;47:543–9.
A retrospective observational study looking at the efficacy of intermittent pneumatic compression (IPC) in the community in patients with chronic limb ischaemia. Wound healing and limb salvage were significantly better in the IPC group.

5

The diabetic foot

Kelly Cheer
Edward B. Jude

Introduction

Foot problems are one of the most common complications of diabetes, with 15% of patients developing a foot ulcer in their lifetime.[1] Foot complications account for more hospital admissions than other complications of diabetes[2] and are associated with considerable morbidity and mortality.[3] The main aetiological factors in foot ulcer development are peripheral neuropathy and peripheral vascular disease, either alone or in combination with biomechanical abnormalities and susceptibility to infection.

Diabetic foot problems can include a wide range of conditions, including peripheral neuropathy and associated neuropathic pain, peripheral vascular disease, ulceration, osteomyelitis, Charcot neuroarthropathy and, ultimately, lower limb amputation. People with diabetes are eight to 24 times more likely than those without diabetes to have a lower limb amputation,[4] and it is suggested that about 85% of those amputations could be avoided by early detection and involvement of a specialist foot team.[5] Patients with diabetes often exhibit multiple complications of their diabetes, including retinopathy, nephropathy and ischaemic heart disease, and as such their care can be complicated and require a multidisciplinary team of physicians, surgeons and allied health professionals.

Epidemiology

The estimated global prevalence of diabetes in 2010 was 285 million, expected to rise to 438 million by 2030.[6] In the UK, in 2011, there were 2.9 million people diagnosed with diabetes,[7] a figure that will rise to more than 4 million by 2025,[6] and as such the prevalence and incidence of foot ulceration are likely to increase also. There have been a number of population studies looking at incidence of foot ulceration in patients with diabetes, in various community-based populations. In a 2002 study from the north-west of England, the annual incidence of foot ulceration was reported as 2.2% among 10 000 community-based patients with type 2 diabetes.[8] In the Wisconsin study, the 4-year incidence of ulcers in patients with type 1 and type 2 diabetes was 9.5% and 10.5%, respectively.[9] A later study from the USA showed that 5.8% of patients followed up over 3 years developed a foot ulcer, nearly 2% per year.[10]

When considering the aetiology of foot ulcers, 45–60% of ulcers are neuropathic, around 10% purely ischaemic and the remaining 25–45% of ulcers are of mixed neuroischaemic origin. A study of all patients attending a foot clinic over a 7-year period showed a slight reduction in the proportion of neuropathic ulcers, at 36%, with 52.3% neuroischaemic and 11.7% ischaemic.[11] This may represent a changing pattern of presentation of diabetic foot ulcers, as a result of patient education, and the introduction of multidisciplinary foot clinics; further research is needed to establish if this is the case.

In 2005, the International Diabetes Federation wrote a position statement on care of the diabetic foot, which states that, every 30 seconds, a leg is lost to diabetes somewhere in the world.[12] Evidence suggests that 100 patients with diabetes per week

- Peripheral neuropathy 20–40%
- Peripheral vascular disease 20–40%
- Foot ulceration: 5% of patients with diabetes per year
- Foot infection and osteomyelitis: 22–66% of all foot ulcers
- Amputation: 0.5% of patients with diabetes per year
- Charcot's neuroarthropathy: 0.1–0.4% of patients with diabetes per year

lose a toe, foot or lower limb,[13] and up to 70% of patients die within 5 years of having an amputation due to diabetes.[14]

✓✓ The National Institute for Health and Clinical Excellence (NICE) has produced guidelines for management of foot disease in diabetes (Box 5.1).[15]

Aetiology of foot ulceration

Diabetic neuropathy

The numerous manifestations of diabetic neuropathy affect up to 50% of patients, but despite much intensive research, the pathophysiology remains unclear and opinion is divided between microvascular disease leading to nerve hypoxia, and the direct effects of hyperglycaemia on neuronal metabolism.

There are a number of manifestations of diabetic neuropathy, from simple mononeuropathies to complex polyneuropathies with autonomic involvement. In the lower limbs, distal sensory polyneuropathy is the commonest presentation, but motor and autonomic fibres can also be involved. The development of neuropathy is linked to poor glycaemic control over many years, and therefore increases in frequency with both duration of diabetes and advancing age. Estimates of the prevalence of neuropathy vary due to differences in diagnostic criteria and populations. A number of studies have indicated a prevalence of approximately 30% among patients with diabetes in hospital, with lower rates closer to 20% in population-based samples;[16]

these figures are likely to be higher when examining an elderly population, and may be as high as 50%. Regular foot examination is essential to identify when neuropathy is present, so that appropriate education can be instituted and treatment given where appropriate to prevent complications resulting from loss of protective sensation. Unless proper foot examination is carried out, the diagnosis can be missed in a significant number of patients.[17]

Not every patient with diabetic neuropathy will describe symptoms; indeed, they may be completely unaware of their marked sensory loss, which can therefore only be detected by regular screening of the asymptomatic patient with diabetes. Over time, as the neuropathy evolves, patients may experience symptoms. These can be extremely painful, such as burning, altered temperature perception, paraesthesia or allodynia (touch perceived as a painful stimulus), or may be so-called negative symptoms, such as numbness or deadness in the limb. Symptoms of neuropathy can be differentiated from intermittent claudication more easily by the nocturnal exacerbations, lack of relationship to exercise and location of symptoms (Table 5.1).

Coexistent autonomic neuropathy can reduce sweating in the skin and open arteriovenous shunts, leading to increased blood flow to the leg.[18] The neuropathic foot is therefore typically warm with bounding pulses and has dry, sometimes cracked, skin. Motor neuropathy mainly affects the intrinsic muscles of the foot (as they are most distal) and can lead to wasting (guttering between the metatarsals) and altered foot shape, with clawed toes and prominent metatarsal heads. This, in turn, increases the risk from unperceived external trauma (e.g. ill-fitting shoes), repetitive painless injury to high-pressure areas under the metatarsal heads when walking, and easy access for infection through the dry cracked skin. Early neuropathy can be suggested by callus formation on weight-bearing areas. Neuropathy is responsible for a high proportion of foot ulcers; in the Eurodiale study, which looked at 1232 patients across 14 European centres, peripheral neuropathy was present in 86% of patients undergoing treatment for foot ulcers.[19]

Table 5.1 • Comparison of signs and symptoms of neuropathic and ischaemic pain

	Neuropathic pain	Intermittent claudication	Ischaemic rest pain
Site	Foot/shin	Calf/thigh	Foot/calf
Nature	Tingling, burning, shooting	Cramping	Aching
Exacerbating factors	Night time	Exercise	Elevation
Relieving factors	Exercise	Rest	Dependency of foot
Clinical signs in the foot	Warm, bounding pulses	Weak/absent pulses	Cold/pulseless

The diagnosis of peripheral neuropathy is usually simple and can be made by clinical examination, which reveals a 'stocking' distribution of sensory loss to one or more of pain, temperature and vibration modalities. Quantitative sensory testing can be performed for perception of vibration, pressure and temperature thresholds, but the perception of pressure threshold is the simplest and most commonly used in clinical practice. A nylon monofilament is used; by pressing against the skin until it buckles, a load of 10 g of pressure can be accurately applied. Patients unable to feel this on the sole of the foot are at high risk of ulceration. Simple bedside testing is often all that is required to identify the foot at risk for neuropathic ulceration; nerve conduction studies are rarely needed in clinical practice.

> ✅ Using a 128-Hz tuning fork to check vibration sensation on the apex of the great toe and a 10-g monofilament to test light touch sensation at 10 sites on the foot can identify 87% of patients with loss of protective sensation in the foot and therefore risk of ulceration.[20]

> ✅✅ No drugs have been demonstrated to improve the underlying neuropathy, but NICE has produced guidelines on the treatment of painful neuropathy in patients with diabetes.[21]
>
> - First line:
>   - Duloxetine, starting at 60 mg daily and increasing if needed to maximum 120 mg daily.
>   - If contraindicated, start amitriptyline 10 mg daily and increase to maximum 75 mg daily.
> - Second line:
>   - If first-line duloxetine, switch to amitriptyline or pregabalin, or combine with pregabalin.
>   - If first-line amitriptyline, switch to or combine with pregabalin.
> - Third line:
>   - Refer to specialist pain service.
>   - Consider tramadol or topical lidocaine whilst waiting for review.

> ✅✅ Good glycaemic control is fundamental in preventing the development of neuropathy, as shown by the landmark Diabetes Control and Complications Trial (DCCT)[22] and the United Kingdom Prospective Diabetes Study (UKPDS).[23] These showed that intensive glycaemic control reduced clinical neuropathy by 60% and abnormal nerve conduction by 44%. Review of glycaemic control therefore should not be underestimated when dealing with a patient with a foot ulcer.

Peripheral vascular disease

Atherosclerotic vascular disease is probably present (at least in a subclinical form) in all patients with long-duration of diabetes.[24] Patients with diabetes often have risk factors for peripheral arterial disease, including hypertension, hyperlipidaemia or smoking.

> ✅ Vascular disease (in all forms) is a major cause of morbidity and mortality in people with diabetes, and accounts for 44% of deaths in type 1 and 52% in patients with type 2 diabetes.[25] The Eurodiale study showed that peripheral arterial disease was present in 49% of patients with a foot ulcer.[19]

The distribution of vascular disease in the lower limb is thought to be different in diabetes, with more frequent involvement of vessels below the knee. One study of patients referred for angiography showed no difference in proximal disease (iliac, femoropopliteal vessels) but distal disease (calf vessels) was twice as high in patients with diabetes as those without.[26] Disease was also more commonly found in multiple locations within the vasculature, and stenoses may also be present in collateral vessels (**Fig. 5.1**).

The difficulties posed by the distribution may be further complicated by a reduced ability to develop collateral supply, but despite these problems revascularisation procedures are frequently successful, although a more distal anastomosis may be required. Comparative studies have shown similar long-term outcomes of revascularisation for patients with and without diabetes,[27] and diabetes does not have a significant negative impact on distal revascularisation.[28]

Patients with diabetes and peripheral vascular disease may develop intermittent claudication, but often this is absent, due to coexistent diabetes-related peripheral neuropathy. The first clinical presentation may be ischaemic foot ulceration.[24] Typically, the ischaemic ulceration is at the ends of the toes, and in the absence of neuropathy can be painful. The foot is usually cool with absent pulses, but the presence of warmth in a neuroischaemic foot with swelling may suggest underlying deep infection or Charcot neuroarthropathy. The most helpful non-invasive investigation is measurement of the ankle–brachial pressure index (ABPI).[29] A combination of a history of calf pain on walking, absent peripheral pulses and an ABPI of less than 0.9 predicts the presence of peripheral arterial disease with 95% sensitivity and specificity.[30] ABPI may be falsely elevated (>1.3) with calcification of blood vessel wall, a phenomenon frequently seen in patients with diabetic neuropathy (**Fig. 5.2**). In this situation, the Doppler waveform seems useful, as loss of the normal triphasic waveform indicates vascular disease. Transcutaneous

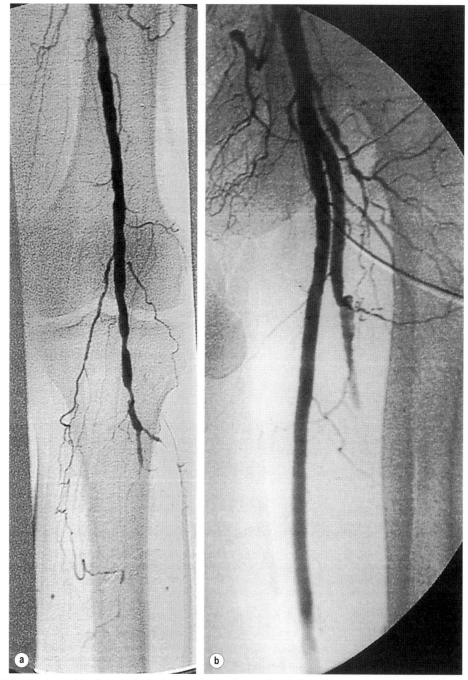

Figure 5.1 • Typical distribution of atherosclerosis affecting the popliteal trifurcation and tibial arteries **(a)**. The distal profunda is also affected **(b)**, which reduces the ability for collaterals to develop around a superficial femoral occlusion.

oxygen tension (measured by an electrode placed on the foot) accurately reflects skin oxygenation and can be used to determine the severity of ischaemia and the likelihood that an ischaemic ulcer will heal.[31] Despite advances in non-invasive investigations, arteriography (which should include the pedal arteries) remains the gold standard for both diagnosis and planning of treatment. Magnetic resonance (MR) is the modality of choice for arteriography in patients with diabetes as it avoids the risk of nephropathy and metabolic acidosis associated with the use of iodinated contrast (see Chapter 3 for medical management).

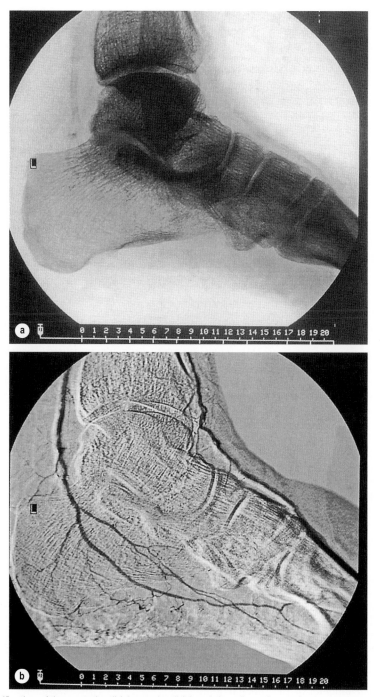

Figure 5.2 • Calcification of the posterior tibial, anterior tibial and dorsalis pedis arteries in a patient with diabetes **(a)**. The calcification is in the media and may falsely elevate Doppler pressures and make pulses difficult to palpate. However, good arterial flow may still be present **(b)**.

Revascularisation will usually be required for isch-aemic or neuroischaemic ulceration. The suitability of an individual for vascular reconstruction needs to be considered carefully, and depends on appropriate anatomy and the presence of other medical condi-tions. For example, a decision to amputate rather than revascularise in a patient with renal failure and ischaemic heart disease may be based on their substantial perioperative risk from a prolonged distal bypass, rather than the availability of a vessel to graft on to. An aggressive approach to revascularisation is known to save limbs, but other conditions may need treating or optimising as far as possible prior to vascular surgery. When severe foot infection is present, this needs treating with incision, drainage and debridement, and only once infection is controlled can revascularisation be performed.

Biomechanical aspects

The most important cause of foot ulceration is loss of protective pain sensation, permitting 'painless' repetitive trauma and tissue injury. Vertical pressure applied to the plantar surfaces of the feet during standing when walking can predispose to ulceration. Plantar pressures can be measured by a number of methods, both dynamic and static. Patients with peripheral neuropathy and particularly patients with foot ulcers have high plantar pressures, although high pressures alone in the absence of insensitivity do not lead to ulceration. Frykberg et al.[32] used an F-scan pressure mat system, and identified patients at risk of ulceration with foot pressures >6kg/cm². Stacpoole-Shea et al.[33] studied a Pedar in-shoe pressure analysis system, and demonstrated its ability to predict potential sites for foot ulceration with a sensitivity of 83% and a specificity of 69%.

Neuropathy and altered proprioception, and small muscle wasting can, in themselves, lead to alteration of the foot architecture and shape, resulting in clawing of the toes, prominent metatarsal heads and a high arch, all of which result in changes in foot pressures.[34] To some extent, this can be reviewed clinically and raises suggestions as to where ulcers are likely to occur on the foot. The more severe deformities associated with Charcot neuroarthropathy, with joint dislocation and bony deformities, can also result in increased foot pressures and subsequent ulceration.

Limited joint mobility is a further contributing factor to elevated plantar pressures. Chronic hyperglycaemia results in glycosylation of proteins and, when collagen is involved, the collagen bundles become thickened and cross-linked. This results in thick, tight, waxy skin and restriction of joint movement. Limited joint mobility of the subtalar joint alters the mechanics of walking and is strongly associated with high plantar pressures.[35]

Neuropathy alone does not lead to spontaneous ulceration, but requires trauma in the context of insensitivity to result in tissue damage. Trauma can be a single event, like standing on a nail, but more frequently involves repeated minor trauma, such as an unperceived shoe rubbing to the toes, or increased pressure beneath the metatarsal heads during walking. As mentioned above, it is possible to measure plantar pressures, and a prospective study showed that 28% of patients with high foot pressures developed a foot ulcer during a 30-month follow-up period, with ulcers occurring in those with neuropathy and high foot pressures.[36] The presence of callus (produced in response to pressure) may exacerbate the problem by acting as a foreign body, thereby increasing pressure further.[37] Removal of callus significantly reduces foot pressures,[38] and should be done regularly by an experienced podiatrist.

The accurate measurement of foot pressures requires sophisticated and often expensive systems, which are currently only available in specialist centres. However, clinical examination that inspects foot shape and identifies the presence of callus provides very valuable information, which can be used to select patients in need of pressure relief (see management section). Footwear should also be inspected as part of this assessment.[15] Indeed, the presence of callus may, in some ways, be superior to pressure measurement, as it results not only from vertical pressure, but also from shear forces, which currently cannot be measured. The presence of haemorrhage into callus should be seen as a pre-ulcerative phenomenon and requires urgent attention.

Other risk factors

Advancing age is frequently accompanied by other risk factors for ulceration, such as impaired vision and immobility, both of which make the recommended regular inspection of the feet more difficult; this in turn can delay the time when help is sought for an ulcer. The prevalence of both neuropathy and peripheral vascular disease is higher among elderly patients.

NICE[15] have suggested guidelines for assessing the risk of ulceration and frequency of foot care in patients with diabetes, as shown in Box 5.2.

Box 5.2 • Summary of NICE guidelines for foot risk screening

Each patient should receive an assessment which places them into one of the following groups:

- Low current risk (normal sensation, palpable pulses): education and annual review
- Increased risk (neuropathy or absent pulses): refer to specialist foot team and review every 3–6 months
- High risk (neuropathy or absent pulses, plus deformity, skin change, or previous ulcer): review by foot protection team every 1–3 months
- Foot ulcer: urgent assessment within 24 hours by multidisciplinary team

The pathway to ulceration

As identified previously, there are a number of risk factors for the occurrence of foot ulcers in patients with diabetes: previous ulceration, neuropathy, peripheral vascular disease, altered foot shape, high plantar pressures, increasing age, visual impairment and living alone. The pathway to ulceration and amputation is often complex, and two or more of the above elements are almost always required. Ulceration of the insensate foot only occurs when it is subjected to trauma; the addition of peripheral vascular disease reduces the external pressure required to cause local ischaemia and tissue breakdown. Conversely, in patients with elevated plantar pressures due to rheumatoid arthritis, ulceration does not occur as sensation is intact and pain protects the feet from repeated injury.

The corollary of this multifactorial aetiology is that pathways can be interrupted at any point. Tight glycaemic control in the early years of treatment for diabetes will help to prevent the development of neuropathy. The provision of good foot care education and well-fitting shoes may be equally successful at preventing ulceration. It therefore follows that each of these individual components must be addressed to enable a foot ulcer to heal.

Management

The management of diabetic foot problems requires input from a number of different healthcare professionals (**Fig. 5.3**), and evidence strongly suggests that specialist diabetic foot clinics can significantly reduce ulceration and amputation rates. One retrospective study showed a 75% reduction in major amputation after introduction of a multidisciplinary foot clinic and improved facilities for revascularisation of ischaemic limbs.[39] Care of patients with diabetes who develop foot ulcers should take place in a specialist clinic. The multidisciplinary team should consist of a doctor with an interest in diabetes and foot disease, podiatrists and orthotists, with access to services of vascular and orthopaedic surgeons.[40]

The 'at-risk' foot

The identification of patients at risk of foot ulceration should be done on an annual basis for all patients with diabetes. Screening does not require expensive equipment and testing can be done in an ordinary clinic setting. Foot examination is frequently overlooked,[41] perhaps because healthcare professionals are reassured by patients not reporting any symptoms. However, as discussed earlier, neuropathy, vascular disease and even ulceration can frequently be asymptomatic but easily diagnosed by simple clinical examination.[42] Peripheral neuropathy can be recognised with standard clinical tools by finding reduced or absent vibration, pinprick or thermal sensation in the foot. Testing with a 128-Hz tuning fork to check vibration sensation on the apex of the great toe and a 10-g monofilament to test light touch sensation at 10 sites of the foot will correctly identify 87% of patients with loss of protective sensation in the feet, who are therefore at risk of ulceration.[43] Quantitative sensory testing can also be a useful adjunct. Dry and cracked skin on the feet usually signifies autonomic neuropathy; neuropathic symptoms (burning, paraesthesiae, etc.) should be sought. Peripheral vascular status is usually assessed by palpation of the peripheral pulses, and it should be remembered that absent foot pulses may be due to arterial wall calcification and not necessarily absent flow. The ABPI should be measured whenever there is any doubt, but further investigation will be dictated by individual clinical requirements.

If a patient is identified as 'at risk', by the presence of one or both of peripheral neuropathy and peripheral vascular disease, then a more detailed assessment of additional risk factors is required. Foot inspection may reveal deformities of foot shape and areas of callus that indicate sites exposed to high pressure or friction. Immobility or social circumstances may influence a patient's ability to understand and carry out appropriate foot care. A history of previous ulceration should be sought, as this is probably the strongest single predictor of future ulceration.

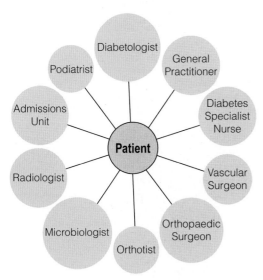

Figure 5.3 • Multidisciplinary team involved in the care of a patient with a foot ulcer.

As most of the risk factors (with the exception of peripheral vascular disease) are not directly modifiable by treatment, the most important element of management of at-risk patients is the provision of good education on foot care.

> ✔ Even a simple approach can have considerable success, as demonstrated by Malone et al.,[44] who reported a two-thirds reduction in amputation and ulceration as a result of a 1-hour educational session. A number of different educational strategies have been tested, and shown to have an outcome on rates of ulceration and amputation.[45]

Areas to be covered by education need to include correction of patient misconceptions, as well as advice on foot care (see Box 5.3). This can be delivered in the form of group sessions, printed material or opportunistic education in clinic. With regard to advice on foot care, it is important to concentrate on positive recommendations rather than prohibitions. Patients also need to know how to gain rapid access to advice and treatment from the foot-care team, and in the event of a new foot ulcer, urgent assessment by a multidisciplinary team should be made within 24 hours.[15]

Extra-depth shoes can provide enough room for clawed toes, and cushioned insoles can reduce plantar pressures. Most patients can be fitted with 'off-the-shelf' extra-depth shoes, with custom-made shoes being reserved for patients with major foot deformity. Further shoe modifications are possible – for example, a rigid rocker-bottom sole can be added.

Box 5.3 • Principles of foot-care education

1. Target the level of information to the needs of the patient. Those not at risk require only general advice about foot hygiene and footwear
2. Make positive rather than negative recommendations:
   a. DO inspect the feet daily
   b. DO report any problems, even if painless
   c. DO buy shoes with a square toe box and laces
   d. DO inspect the inside of the shoes for foreign objects every day before putting on
   e. DO attend a fully trained podiatrist regularly
   f. DO cut your nails straight across and not rounded
   g. DO keep your feet away from heat (fires, radiators, hot-water bottles) and check bath water with your hand or elbow
   h. DO always wear something on your feet to protect them and never walk barefoot
3. Repeat the advice at regular intervals and check for compliance
4. Disseminate advice to other family members or those involved in the patient's care

With the rocker axis posterior to the metatarsal heads, metatarsal head pressure can be reduced by up to 40%.[46] Regular podiatry is needed for most at-risk patients. Callus needs to be debrided regularly; although it develops in response to pressure and friction, its removal can reduce pressure, as stated previously. Callus can sometimes hide ulceration, which will only be revealed when the callus is removed. Without removal, infection and abscess formation are more likely, but it is important to explain to the patient that the podiatrist has not caused the underlying ulcer revealed when the callus is removed. The presence of callus should always prompt a search for its cause, and shoe modification may be necessary.

The surgical correction of specific foot deformities is sometimes necessary to prevent ulceration. This should only be done after confirming that there is good peripheral circulation and it is important to remember that correction of a hallux valgus may leave a rigid hallux with resultant high plantar pressures. Correction of deformity is usually only performed in patients with a history of ulceration, rather than for primary prevention.

Ulcer management

All patients with diabetes presenting with foot ulcers need a full examination of the foot, including peripheral sensation and circulation (supplemented with measurement of ABPI if there is any doubt at all about the circulation) in order to classify an ulcer. They also need assessment of footwear and deformities.

> ✔ Guidelines devised by the International Working Group on the Diabetic Foot in 2007 stress the importance of inspecting footwear, evaluating the type of ulcer, documenting location, size and depth, and checking for infection in patients presenting with a new foot ulcer.[47]

Foot ulcers can be classed as neuropathic, ischaemic or neuroischaemic, and the University of Texas or Wagner classification systems can be used to communicate more information. The Wagner classification[47] grades ulcers on the depth of penetration and the extent of tissue necrosis. It makes no reference to aetiology, which is a feature of the University of Texas wound classification system,[48] which has been validated in clinical practice.[49] The University of Texas system assesses ulcer depth, presence of wound infection and any signs of lower-extremity ischaemia (Table 5.2). For example, an infected neuroischaemic ulcer penetrating to bone would be IIID.

Neuropathic ulcers

Typically, the foot is warm and well perfused with bounding pulses and distended veins. The ulcer is

Table 5.2 • Texas wound classification system

Stage	Grade			
	0	**I**	**II**	**III**
A	Completely epithelialised wound	Superficial wound	Wound penetrates to tendon or capsule	Wound penetrates to bone or joint
B	Plus infection	Plus infection	Plus infection	Plus infection
C	Plus ischaemia	Plus ischaemia	Plus ischaemia	Plus ischaemia
D	Plus infection and ischaemia	Plus infection and ischaemia	Plus infection and ischaemia	Plus infection and ischaemia

usually at the site of repetitive trauma, and most commonly due to a shoe rub on the dorsum of the toes, or a high-pressure area under the metatarsal heads. The ulcer may be hidden under callus. Occasionally, a foreign body causes ulceration, for example a nail penetrates the sole of the shoe, or a stone is found inside the shoe. Patients with neuropathy may walk on a foreign body for hours or even days without realising it.

The key to management is pressure relief and offloading.[50] With shoe-induced ulcers, appropriate footwear must be provided, irrespective of any protestations from the patient that their own shoes (which caused the ulcer) are comfortable. Merely providing the shoes may not be enough; patients often fail to wear the shoes due to appearance, or a belief that they are only to be used outside the home.

To relieve pressure from a plantar ulcer, a more aggressive approach can be required. Bed rest is simple, but expensive in hospital and difficult to enforce in a patient who feels well and is pain free, so ambulatory methods have been designed. The total contact cast was originally used for patients with neuropathic ulcers due to leprosy, and modified by Paul Brand for use in patients with diabetic neuropathic ulcers. The cast extends from below the knee and encases the whole foot. Only minimal padding is used, except in the forefoot.

✓✓ Excellent healing rates have been reported and, in a randomised controlled trial, the total contact cast was associated with faster healing compared with other removable devices.[51]

The total contact cast works by transferring load from the forefoot to the heel, and directly to the leg via the cast wall, as well as reducing oedema and shear forces.[52] The main disadvantages are that it is labour intensive, as it may need frequent changes, and signs of wound infection or new ulceration secondary to the cast may not be seen. A frequently used alternative is the Scotch cast boot. This is a removable fibreglass boot that is moulded to the contours of the plantar surface of the foot (**Fig. 5.4**). A number

of commercially produced pressure-relieving boots are now available, and although their capacity to reduce pressure has been demonstrated, only the total contact cast has been tested in trials of ulcer healing. However, since these alternative devices are removable, patients may take them off whilst at home, and therefore impede further healing. These can be made non-removable by wrapping the removable cast with fibreglass casing material. Evidence suggests that healing with this form of offloading was almost on a par with total contact casting.[53]

The second important element of management of neuropathic ulcers is debridement of callus. Wounds heal from the margins and callus prevents the migration of epidermal cells from the wound margin, and encourages and masks wound infection. Debridement of callus and necrotic tissue is usually required on a weekly basis, and continued presence or rapid reaccumulation of callus should prompt a review of the pressure relief used.

Ischaemic and neuroischaemic ulcers

Purely ischaemic ulcers are relatively rare and most are, in fact, neuroischaemic. Typical sites include the toes, heel and medical aspect of the first metatarsal head. Callus is usually absent and the ulcer is often surrounded by a rim of ischaemia and may have a necrotic centre. The presence of pain depends on the degree of neuropathy. Ulceration is often precipitated by minor trauma; again, the most common culprit is ill-fitting shoes. Prompt vascular assessment is crucial and angiography is often required. Revascularisation should be performed whenever possible, both for ulcer healing (ischaemic and neuroischaemic ulcers only rarely heal without improvements in blood flow) and to prevent future ulceration.

Gangrene and amputation are among the most feared complications of diabetes. Although gangrene may complicate neuropathic ulceration (microorganisms in infected digital ulcers may produce necrotising toxins, which lead to thrombotic occlusion of digital arteries and subsequent gangrene), it usually only occurs when significant vascular disease is present. Gangrenous tissue must be removed, and

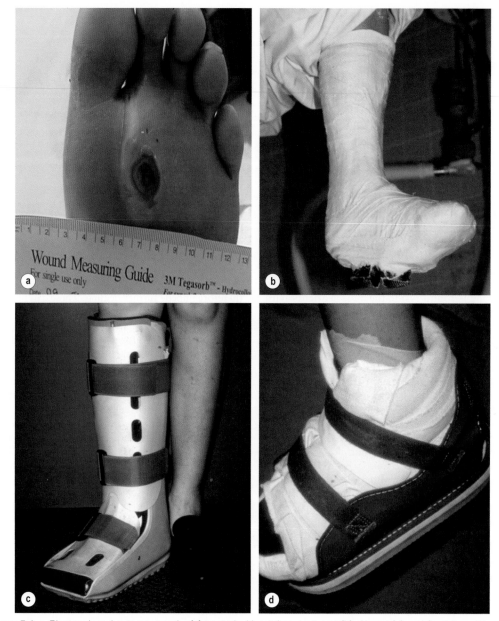

Figure 5.4 • Plantar ulcer due to neuropathy **(a)** treated with total contact cast **(b)**, Aircast **(c)** and Scotch cast boot **(d)**.

when it involves a dry digit with a clear demarcation line, this will usually occur spontaneously, leaving a healed stump (**Fig. 5.5**). However, when these conditions are not met, local amputation is mandatory.

Local amputation includes simple removal of a toe, ray amputation (toe and metatarsal), or transmetatarsal amputation. The general rule is to remove all necrotic and infected tissue, ensuring that no bone is left exposed, while leaving part of the wound open to allow drainage. Bone should

be sent for culture as the organisms responsible for osteomyelitis may be different from those grown from the ulcer. A foot X-ray after local amputation is a useful baseline if progression of osteomyelitis is subsequently suspected. If arterial reconstruction is possible, this can be combined with amputation to enable healing of the amputation site. This is not possible when major sepsis is present, and in such circumstances revascularisation should be done at a second procedure when

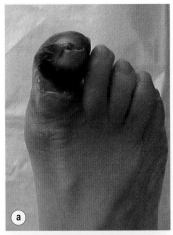

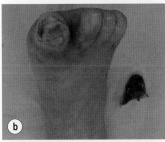

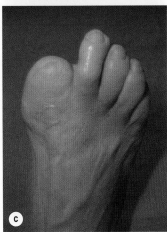

Figure 5.5 • Patient with digital gangrene **(a)**, resulting in autoamputation **(b)** and healing of the wound **(c)**.

infection has been controlled by debridement and antibiotics. The amputation site is determined by both the extent of tissue involvement and the level at which the circulation will support wound healing. Transcutaneous oxygen tension can be helpful to determine the relevant level of circulation; in a large study, values under 40 mmHg were strongly associated with failure of healing at the amputation site.[54]

Infection

Infection in diabetic foot ulcers can vary from superficial cellulitis to deeper infection of the soft tissues and bones. An infected foot ulcer can lead to limb loss in a matter of days, but by no means are all ulcers infected, although bacterial colonisation seems universal. The distinction between colonisation and infection can be difficult and often not aided by microbiological investigations.[55] Clinical signs are the most reliable indicators of infection. Evidence of systemic upset (fever, leucocytosis) is frequently absent, and signs of local inflammation, swelling and presence of pus are usually used to dictate the need for antibiotic therapy. No one clinical sign is a reliable marker for infection. With severe infection, crepitus may be present due to gas formation and fluctuance can indicate the presence of an abscess. Infections are usually polymicrobial, with typically three to six organisms identified per ulcer.[56] The most commonly found organisms include staphylococci, streptococci, Gram-negative species such as *Proteus* and *Pseudomonas*, and anaerobes such as *Bacteroides*; synergy between organisms may increase pathogenicity. More recently, methicillin-resistant *Staphylococcus aureus* (MRSA) has posed an increasing problem, and has been found to be present in up to 30% of ulcers in specialised foot clinics.[57] In non-limb-threatening infections, microbiological investigation is not essential, but when swabs are taken the method is important. Superficial swabs are likely to isolate colonising rather than pathogenic bacteria; the deeper the sample, the more reliable the results. Ideally, curettings from the ulcer base should be transported and cultured aerobically and anaerobically.

> ✔ Osteomyelitis should be suspected in any deep ulcer if a sinus tract is present, or if an ulcer fails to heal despite adequate pressure relief.

Osteomyelitis is an important predisposing factor for amputation, and occurs in 22–66% of patients with diabetes and a foot ulcer.[58] Plain radiography is often used as the first-line test, but the characteristic changes of bone destruction (**Fig. 5.6**) can take 2 weeks or longer to develop and do not occur until 30–50% of the bone has been destroyed.[59]

Other imaging modalities include three-phase bone scans, and indium-labelled white cell scans or Leucoscan, along with magnetic resonance imaging. Guidelines from the Infectious Diseases Society of America recommend magnetic resonance imaging and bone sampling.[60] Magnetic resonance imaging can also prove useful by showing marrow oedema before cortical bone loss occurs, and is potentially valuable in differentiating osteomyelitis from Charcot neuroarthropathy. Interestingly, a simple clinical test (the ability to probe to bone with a blunt instrument at the

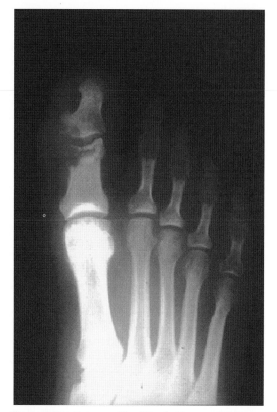

Figure 5.6 • Osteomyelitis of the first toe causing bony destruction.

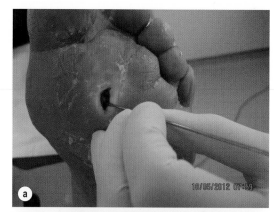

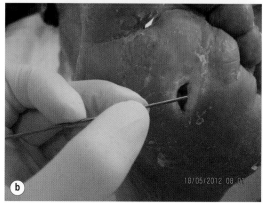

Figure 5.7 • Probing an ulcer with a sterile probe will detect sinus tracts and help diagnose underlying osteomyelitis.

base of the ulcer; see **Fig. 5.7**) has been proven as a useful test for osteomyelitis,[61] with a sensitivity of 66% and a positive predictive value of 89% (i.e. bone can be probed in 66% of cases of osteomyelitis, and in ulcers where bone can be probed 89% have osteomyelitis). Simple laboratory markers, such as erythrocyte sedimentation rate and C-reactive protein, may assist in the diagnosis.

The threshold for initiating antibiotic treatment should be low, and the agents used should have a spectrum of activity to include the known common pathogenic organisms.[62] There is limited evidence on which to base the choice of antibiotic regimen, although it has been demonstrated that antibiotic treatment is not required in neuropathic ulcers that are not clinically infected.[63]

Factors to be considered when choosing antibiotic treatment should include the appropriate route, spectrum of activity, duration of treatment and local policy. If the patient has systemic signs of infection, intravenous antibiotics are needed. Several antibiotics have been proven to be beneficial in clinical trials, but treatment is often empirical.

Mild infections can often be treated with relatively narrow-spectrum antibiotics with coverage against Gram-positive cocci, for example oral amoxicillin–clavulanic acid, flucloxacillin or oral clindamycin. Ciprofloxacin can be added if Gram-negative infection is suspected, although the potential for this particular antibiotic to be implicated in *Clostridium difficile* diarrhoea should be considered. In severe infections, initial empirical treatment includes amoxicillin–clavulanic acid, broad-spectrum cephalosporins, or combinations of clindamycin and ciprofloxacin. As mentioned previously, MRSA is causing increasing problems in foot clinics. Local antibiotic guidelines should be followed when treating MRSA in foot wounds, and often contact with microbiologists for advice is necessary.

There are a number of other factors that must be addressed to ensure healing of an infected foot wound. Attention must be paid to the patient's general medical condition, and it is important to correct hyperglycaemia, renal failure or electrolyte disturbance where possible to aid with wound healing. Regular debridement is important to remove necrotic and devitalised tissue, pus should be drained and the foot offloaded. The principles of dressing a healing wound include keeping it moist, managing exudates and protecting the surrounding intact skin.[64] Limb-threatening infections require urgent hospitalisation, bed rest, surgical debridement and broad-spectrum antibiotics.

> ✓ Various newer topical therapies have been recently researched and shown to be of some benefit in the healing of chronic foot wounds in patients with diabetes. These include platelet-derived growth factor (becaplermin), living dermal equivalent (Dermagraft) and living human skin equivalents (Graftskin). However, they are not appropriate for all patients and should be used in selected circumstances. Their availability should not obscure the fact that most ulcers respond to simple care, comprising pressure relief, debridement and control of infection, and must not be seen as a replacement, but as an addition to good wound care.

Larva debridement therapy

Larval debridement therapy (the use of maggots to cleanse wounds) is hardly new. Indeed, an early reference to larval therapy was made during the Napoleonic wars, when it was observed that wounds which had maggots in them did not become infected and appeared to heal better.

In recent years, the use of sterile larvae (from the greenbottle fly, *Lucilia sericata*) has been investigated with encouraging results, and is becoming increasingly popular as a therapy for infected and necrotic wounds.[65] It is thought that maggots remove necrotic tissue by secreting powerful enzymes that break down dead tissue into a liquid form, which is then ingested.[66] The mechanisms by which larvae prevent or combat infection are also complex, but there is anecdotal evidence that they may also help in combating antibiotic-resistant strains of bacteria. There is a growing body of clinical experience with the use of larval therapy that suggests that it is useful in the management of patients with necrotic, sloughing or often neuroischaemic ulcers. The use of this therapy is now quite widespread for foot care for infected ulcers, with some evidence that it is effective in eradicating MRSA.[67]

Medical problems on the surgical ward

Patients with diabetes on the vascular surgical ward will often have multiple comorbidities and other complications related to their diabetes. Apart from peripheral neuropathy and peripheral vascular disease, they may have evidence of ischaemic heart disease, diabetic nephropathy and autonomic neuropathy, all of which can affect their eventual outcomes. These comorbid conditions need to be considered and addressed – for example, patients with significant renal impairment may need a renal review prior to any procedures.

> ✓✓ Angiography with contrast media carries a risk of worsening renal function.

Metformin must be stopped for 48 hours prior to elective catheter angiography due to a risk of worsening renal failure and lactic acidosis. Coronary artery disease and cardiac autonomic neuropathy increase the risk of intraoperative cardiac events, and should be addressed prior to surgery. The hormonal and metabolic changes associated with surgery create a particular problem in diabetes and intravenous insulin infusions (with dextrose and potassium) are usually needed for the perioperative period, unless the duration of anaesthesia is short (<45 minutes) and the patient is not on insulin.

Patients with neuropathy are at great risk of developing posterior heel ulcers whilst lying immobile in bed for several days. These can be difficult to heal, are entirely preventable and medicolegally indefensible. The simple provision of foam leg troughs is often all that is needed to relieve pressure on the heels whilst the patient is in bed, and should be done routinely in patients at risk. The Ipswich Touch Test[68] has been shown to identify those at risk for ulceration. Light touch with a finger is applied to the tips of the first, third and fifth toes of each foot, with patients who are unable to feel two or more sites deemed to be at risk, and treated with foot protection.

Charcot neuroarthropathy

Charcot neuroarthropathy is characterised by bone and joint destruction, fragmentation and remodelling. It can be one of the most devastating foot complications of diabetes, and was first described as a complication of tabes dorsalis. It can develop in any joint, and has been reported in most sensory neuropathies, but diabetes is now the commonest cause of the Charcot foot. Although once thought to be very rare, it is now known to affect nearly 10% of patients with neuropathy and over 16% of those with a history of neuropathic ulceration.[69] Charcot neuroarthropathy is thought to occur due to trauma of the foot, which may be mild and go unnoticed in the context of neuropathy. In the early stages, the foot becomes swollen, warm (usually > 2 °C compared to the contralateral foot) and erythematous, and may be incorrectly diagnosed as being due to a sprain, gout, cellulitis or deep vein thrombosis. If not treated promptly, osteolysis and osteopenia can occur; ligaments can become lax and gradual remodelling of the foot occurs, with chronic deformity and fusion of the bones in abnormal positions. Periarticular erosions have been noted to be common around affected joints and may precede fractures and fragmentation of bone, suggesting that inflammatory arthropathy (possibly secondary to trauma) is the first stage in the process, and then ongoing weight-bearing prolongs this phase, leading to bone resorption and fractures.

Most textbooks describe this as a painless condition, but there is frequently some discomfort, although usually not enough to prevent walking. The presentation may be several weeks after the onset of symptoms and, because of the lack of significant pain, plain radiographs are not always performed. Plain radiography is usually adequate to make the diagnosis, but isotope scans and magnetic resonance imaging are sometimes needed to exclude osteomyelitis. The natural history is such that, after a number of months, during which bone resorption continues, the swelling and warmth begin to resolve. Treatment is aimed at shortening the time in order to minimise bone and joint destruction. The midfoot is a common site of Charcot neuroarthropathy and, when affected, can result in midfoot collapse, with a plantar bony prominence and 'rocker-bottom deformity', which has a very high risk of ulceration (**Fig. 5.8**). The mainstay of treatment is rest and immobilisation, usually in a total contact cast, which may need to be continued for many months until disease activity has subsided. Disease activity is usually judged by measuring the temperature of the skin with an infrared thermometer; when this is

2 °C warmer than the other foot, an inflammatory response is still present.

✔️✔️ In a randomised trial, a single infusion of pamidronate resulted in a significant reduction in symptoms as well as an additional improvement in disease activity, and a reduction in bone turnover markers compared with standard care.[70] The oral bisphosphonate, alendronate (70 mg weekly), has also been shown to reduce bone turnover markers and symptoms, but no difference in disease activity was demonstrated.[71]

Surgery to the foot is contraindicated in the early stages, due to the gross hyperaemia of the involved bone, and the risk that it (like trauma) will trigger bone resorption. However, corrective surgery may be useful at a later stage in order to remove bony prominences, which may increase risk of ulceration. During the early stages of the condition, appropriate (usually custom-made) footwear is required, and great care should be taken of the other foot as there is a high risk of contralateral Charcot changes. Medical treatment should therefore be instituted immediately a diagnosis of Charcot foot is made. The cornerstone of treatment of acute Charcot neuroarthropathy is immediate effective offloading, typically with total contact casting, and reduction in weight-bearing. The main current targets of pharmacological intervention are the inhibition of excess osteoclastic activation and suppression of an excess proinflammatory cytokine response. Long-term follow-up is necessary as recurrence is common and further foot ulceration can occur.[72]

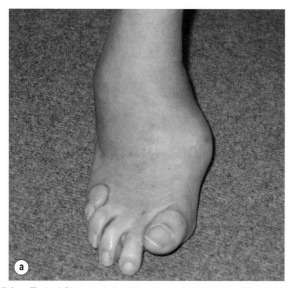
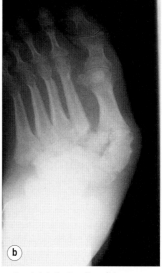

Figure 5.8 • Typical Charcot deformity with midfoot collapse **(a)** and xray showing joint destruction **(b)**.

Key points

- The management of the diabetic foot is challenging and requires a multidisciplinary approach, ideally coordinated by a specialised clinic.
- Identification of high-risk patients requires screening that must be both comprehensive and regular, and patient education should be part of this process.
- Once ulceration has developed, aggressive management can achieve excellent results with a significant reduction of both amputation and re-ulceration rates.
- Future research may ultimately enable the prevention of foot ulcers and predisposing factors that lead to ulceration and may demonstrate superior ways of healing ulcers. However, the dissemination of current 'best practice' is already starting to have a major impact on the outlook for this condition.

References

1. Sanders LJ. Diabetes mellitus: prevention of amputation. J Am Podiatry Assoc 1994;84:322–8.

2. Krentz AJ, Acheson P, Basu A, et al. Morbidity and mortality associated with diabetic foot disease: a 12-month prospective survey of hospital admissions in a single UK centre. Foot 1997;7:144–7.

3. Boyko EJ, Ahroni JH, Smith DG, et al. Increased mortality associated with diabetic foot ulcers. Diabet Med 1996;13:967–72.

4. Fosse S, Hartemann-Heurtier A, Jacqueminet S, et al. Incidence and characteristics of lower limb amputations in people with diabetes. Diabet Med 2009;26:391–6.

5. Holstein P, Ellitsgaard N, Bornefeldt Olsen B, et al. Decreasing incidence of major amputations in people with diabetes. Diabetologia 2000;43:844–7.

6. Diabetes UK. Diabetes in the UK 2010: key statistics on diabetes, http://www.diabetes.org.uk/Documents/Reports/Diabetes_in_the_UK_2010.pdf; 2010.

7. Diabetes UK. Diabetes prevalence 2011. 2011. http://www.diabetes.org.uk/Professionals/Publications-reports-and-resources/Reports-statistics-and-case-studies/Reports/Diabetes-prevalence-2011-Oct-2011/

8. Abbott CA, Carrington AL, Ashe H, et al. The North-West Diabetes Foot Care Study: incidence of, and risk factors, for new diabetic foot ulceration in a community-based patient cohort. Diabet Med 2002;19:377–84.

9. Moss SE, Klein R, Klein B. The prevalence and incidence of lower extremity amputation in a diabetic population. Arch Intern Med 1992;152:610–3.

10. Ramsey SD, Newton K, Blough DK, et al. Incidence, outcomes and cost of foot ulcers in patients with diabetes. Diabetes Care 1999;22(3):3820–7.

11. Oyibo SO, Jude EB, Voyatzoglou D, et al. Clinical characteristics of patients with diabetic foot problems: changing patterns of foot presentation. Pract Diabetes Int 2002;19:10–2.

12. International Diabetes Federation. Position statement – the diabetic foot, http://www.idf.org/position-statement-diabetic-foot; 2005.

13. National Diabetes Support Team. Diabetic foot guide, http://www.diabetes.nhs.uk/document.php?o=219; 2006.

14. Schofield CJ, Libby G, Brennan GM, et al. Mortality and hospitalization in people after amputation: a comparison between patients with and without diabetes. Diabetes Care 2006;29(10):2262–6.

15. National Institute for Health and Clinical Excellence (NICE). Type 2 diabetes: prevention and management of foot problems, www.nice.org.uk/guidance/CG10; 2004.
NICE guidance for management of patients with foot problems and type 2 diabetes.

16. Young MJ, Boulton AJ, MacLeod AF, et al. A multicentre study of the prevalence of diabetic peripheral neuropathy in the UK hospital clinic population. Diabetologia 1993;36:150–4.

17. Herman WH, Kennedy L. Underdiagnosis of peripheral neuropathy in type 2 diabetes. Diabetes Care 2005;28:1480–1.

18. Boulton AJM, Scarpello JS, Ward JD. Venous oxygenation in the neuropathic diabetic foot: evidence of arteriovenous shunting. Diabetologia 1982;22:6–8.

19. Prompers L, Huijberts M, Apelqvist J, et al. High prevalence of ischaemia, infection and serious comorbidity in patients with diabetic foot disease in Europe. Baseline results from the Eurodiale study. Diabetologia 2007;50:18–25.
Large multicentre study across Europe looking at a variety of factors in patients with diabetes-related foot ulceration.

20. Boulton AJM, Vinik AI, Arezzo JC, et al. Diabetic neuropathies: a statement by the American Diabetes Association. Diabetes Care 2005;28:956–62.
Testing with a 10-g monofilament and 128-Hz tuning fork can be used to screen patients for peripheral neuropathy.

21. National Institute for Health and Clinical Excellence (NICE). Neuropathic pain: pharmacological management, www.nice.org.uk/guidance/CG96; 2010.
Recommendations for pharmacological management of neuropathic pain in patients with diabetes.

22. The Diabetes Control Complications Trial Research Group. The effect of intensive treatment of diabetes on the development and progression of long-term complications in insulin-dependent diabetes mellitus. N Engl J Med 1993;329(14):977–86.
Landmark study in diabetes care showing that tight glycaemic control reduced the risk of microvascular complications.

23. Turner RC, Cull CA, Holman RR. The UK Prospective Diabetes Study. Diabetes Care 1996;19:182–3.

24. Jude EB. Intermittent claudication in the patient with diabetes. Br J Diabetes Vasc Dis 2004;4:238–42.

25. Morrish NJ, Wang SL, Stevens LK, et al. Mortality and causes of death in the WHO multinational study of vascular disease in diabetes. Diabetologia 2001;44(Suppl. 2):s14–21.

26. Jude EB, Oyibo SO, Chalmers N, et al. Peripheral arterial disease in diabetic and non-diabetic patients: a comparison of severity and outcome. Diabetes Care 2001;24:1433–7.

27. Karacagil S, Almgren B, Bowald S, et al. Comparative analysis of patency, limb salvage and survival in diabetic and non-diabetic patients undergoing infrainguinal bypass surgery. Diabet Med 1995;12:537–41.

28. Faires PL, LoGerfo FW, Hook SC, et al. The impact of diabetes on arterial reconstructions for multilevel arterial occlusive disease. Surg Gynecol Obstet 2001;181:251–5.

29. Weitz JL, Byrne J, Glaggett GP, et al. Diagnosis and treatment of chronic arterial insufficiency of the lower extremities: a critical review. Circulation 1996;94:3026–49.

30. Jude EB, Boulton AJM. End stage complications of diabetic neuropathy. Diabetes Rev 1999;7:395–410.

31. Ruangsetakit C, Chinsakchai K, Mahawongkajit P, et al. Transcutaneous oxygen tension: a useful predictor of ulcer healing in critical limb ischaemia. J Wound Care 2010;19(5):202–6.

32. Frykberg RG, Lavery LA, Pham H, et al. Role of neuropathy and high foot pressures in diabetic foot ulceration. Diabetes Care 1998;21:1714–9.

33. Stacpoole-Shea S, Shea G, Lavery L. An examination of plantar pressure measurements to identify the location of diabetic forefoot ulceration. J Foot Ankle Surg 1999;38:109–15.

34. Boulton AJM. The pathogenesis of diabetic foot problems: an overview. Diabet Med 1996;13(Suppl. 1):S12–6.

35. Fernando DJ, Masson EA, Veves A, et al. Relationship of limited joint mobility to abnormal foot pressures and diabetic foot ulceration. Diabetes Care 1991;14:8–11.

36. Veves A, Murray HJ, Young MJ, et al. The risk of foot ulceration in diabetic patients with high foot pressures: a prospective study. Diabetologia 1992;35:660–3.

37. Murray HJ, Young MJ, Hollis S, et al. The association between callus formation, high pressures and neuropathy in diabetic foot ulceration. Diabet Med 1996;13:979–82.

38. Abouaesha F, van Schie CH, Griffiths GD, et al. Plantar tissue thickness is related to peak plantar pressure in the high-risk diabetic foot. Diabetes Care 2001;24:1270–4.

39. Holstein P, Ellitsgaard N, Bornefeldt Olsen B, et al. Decreasing incidence of major amputations in people with diabetes. Diabetologia 2000;43:844–7.

40. Cheer K, Shearman C, Jude EB. Managing complications of the diabetic foot. Br Med J 2009;339:1304–7.

41. Herman WH, Kennedy L. Underdiagnosis of peripheral neuropathy in type 2 diabetes. Diabetes Care 2005;28:1480–1.

42. Apelqvist J, Bakker K, van Houtum WH, et al. Practical guidelines on the management and prevention of the diabetic foot: based upon the International Consensus on the Diabetic Foot (2007). Prepared by the International Working Group on the Diabetic Foot. Diabetes Metab Res Rev 2008;24(Suppl. 1):S181–7.

43. Boulton AJM, Vinik AI, Arezzo JC, et al. Diabetic neuropathies: a statement by the American Diabetes Association. Diabetes Care 2005;28:956–62.

44. Malone JM, Snyder M, Anderson G, et al. Prevention of amputation by diabetic education. Am J Surg 1989;158:520–3.

45. Singh M, Armstrong DG, Lipsky BA. Preventing foot ulcers in patients with diabetes. JAMA 2005;293(2):217–28.

46. Schaff PS, Cavanagh PR. Shoes for the insensitive foot: the effect of a 'rocker bottom' shoe modification on plantar pressure distribution. Foot Ankle 1990;11:129–40.

47. Wagner Jr FW. The dysvascular foot: a system for diagnosis and treatment. Foot Ankle 1981;2:64–122.

48. Armstrong DG, Lavery LA, Harkless LB. Validation of a diabetic wound classification system: the contribution of depth, infection and ischaemia to risk of amputation. Diabetes Care 1998;21:855–9.

49. Oyibo S, Jude EB, Tarawaneh I, et al. Comparison of two diabetic foot ulcer classification systems: the Wagner and University of Texas systems. Diabetes Care 2001;24:84–8.

50. Bus SA. Priorities in offloading the diabetic foot. Diabetes Metab Res Rev 2012;28(Suppl. 1):54–9.

51. Armstrong DG, Nguyen HC, Lavery LA, et al. Offloading the diabetic foot: a randomised clinical trial. Diabetes Care 2001;24:1019–21.
Proper offloading of the diabetic foot ulcer was shown to enhance wound healing.

52. Shaw JE, Hsi WL, Ulbrecht JS, et al. The mechanism of plantar unloading in total contact casts: implications for design and clinical use. Foot Ankle Int 1997;18:809–17.

53. Katz IA, Harlan A, Miranda-Palma B, et al. A randomized trial of two irremovable off loading devices in the healing of diabetic wounds: a randomized controlled trial. Diabetes Care 2005;28:551–4.

54. Jacobs MJ, Ubbink DT, Kitslaar PJ, et al. Assessment of the microcirculation provided additional information in critical limb ischaemic. Eur J Vasc Surg 1992;6:135–41.

55. Lavery LA, Armstrong DG, Wunderlich RP, et al. Risk factors for foot infections in individuals with diabetes. Diabetes Care 2006;29:1288–93.

56. Lipsky BA, Pecoraro RE, Wheat LJ. The diabetic foot. Soft tissue and bone infection. Infect Dis Clin North Am 1990;(4)409–32.

57. Dang CN, Prasad YDM, Boulton AJM, et al. Methicillin-resistant Staphylococcus aureus in the diabetic foot clinic: a worsening problem. Diabet Med 2003;20:159–61.

58. Lavery LA, Peters EJ, Armstrong DG, et al. Risk factors for developing osteomyelitis in patients with diabetic foot wounds. Diabetes Res Clin Pract 2009;83:347–52.

59. Tomas MB, Patel M, Marwin SE, et al. The diabetic foot: pictorial review. Br J Radiol 2000;73:443–50.

60. Lipsky BA, Berendt AR, Deery HG, et al. Diagnosis and treatment of diabetic foot infections. Clin Infect Dis 2004;39:885–910.

61. Grayson ML, Gibbons GW, Balogh K, et al. Probing to bone in infected pedal ulcers: a clinical sign of underlying osteomyelitis in diabetic patients. JAMA 1995;273:721–3.

62. Jude EB, Unsworth PF. Optimal treatment of diabetic foot ulcers. Drugs Aging 2004;21:833–50.

63. Chantelau E, Tanudjaja T, Altenhofer F, et al. Antibiotic treatment for uncomplicated neuropathic forefoot ulcers in diabetes: a controlled trial. Diabet Med 1996;13:156–9.

64. Steed DL, Attinger C, Coolaizzi T, et al. Guidelines for treatment of diabetic foot infections. Wound Repair Regen 2006;14:680–92.

65. Thomas S, Jones M, Shutler S, et al. Using larvae in modern wound management. J Wound Care 1996;5:60–9.

66. Casu RE, Eisemann CH, Vuoclo T, et al. The major excretory/secretory protease from Luciliacuprina larvae is also a gut digestive protease. Int J Parasitol 1996;26:623–8.

67. Bowling FL, Salgami EV, Boulton AJ. Larval therapy: a novel treatment in eliminating methicillin-resistant Staphylococcus aureus in diabetic foot ulcers. Diabetes Care 2007;30:370–1.

68. Rayman G, Vas PR, Baker N, et al. The Ipswich Touch Test: a simple and novel way to identify inpatients with diabetes at risk of foot ulceration. Diabetes Care 2011;34(7):1517–8.

69. Cavanagh PR, Young MJ, Adams JE, et al. Radiographic abnormalities in the feet of patients with diabetic neuropathy. Diabetes Care 1994;17:201–9.

70. Jude EB, Selby PL, Mawer B, et al. Pamidronate in diabetic Charcot neuroarthropathy: a randomised placebo controlled trial. Diabetologia 2001;44:2032–7.
This trial showed the efficacy of bisphosphonates in treating acute Charcot arthropathy.

71. Pitocco D, Ruotolo V, Caputo S, et al. Six-month treatment with alendronate in acute Charcot neuroarthropathy: a randomised controlled trial. Diabetes Care 2005;28(5):1214–5.
This trial showed the reduction in symptoms, bone turnover markers and improvement in bone density in the feet of Charcot patients treated with the bisphosphonate, alendronate.

72. Fabrin J, Larsen K, Holstein PE. Long-term follow up in diabetic Charcot feet with spontaneous onset. Diabetes Care 2000;23:796–800.

6

Amputation, rehabilitation and prosthetic developments

Ramesh Munjal
Gillian Atkinson

Introduction

For some patients with lower limb ischaemia, amputation may be the only interventional option because revascularisation is not possible, has failed or the leg is unsalvageable. Amputation may also be a better option than complex revascularisation when patients are bed-bound and/or demented. Amputation should not be regarded as 'failure' of treatment but should be seen by patients as well as clinicians as a positive procedure. Amputation should aim to relieve pain, remove dead, severely ischaemic or infected tissue, and improve quality of life. This is true even for those who may not be able to walk with a prosthesis.

The planning and process of rehabilitation for amputees should start prior to amputation and continue into the community. Expert and holistic assessment of the patient leading to careful selection of the level of amputation, good surgical technique and optimal postoperative management are all vital in the initial stage of amputee rehabilitation. The process then dovetails into postamputation early rehabilitation, e.g. use of early walking aids, wheelchair and home assessments, prosthetic rehabilitation where appropriate, and continuing follow-up and support to patients and their families in the community.

This chapter concentrates on the rehabilitation of patients undergoing amputation because of lower limb ischaemia, although the principles involved are similar for amputations due to other causes, such as trauma.

Epidemiology

Peripheral arterial occlusive disease accounts for the vast majority of lower limb amputations in westernised societies. More than 80% of all amputations carried out in the UK are due to vascular disease but an increasing proportion have diabetes mellitus.[1] The overall risk of amputation is six times higher in insulin-dependent people with diabetes compared with non-insulin-dependent people with diabetes. A global study group also reported a marked difference in the incidence of amputation between 10 centres in six different countries. Rates were highest in the North American and northern European centres and lowest in Spain, Taiwan and Japan. In the Navajo population, a very high prevalence of diabetes was thought to be the explanation for their high amputation rates.[2]

The National Amputee Statistical Database for the UK reported that dysvascularity is the most common reason for referral to prosthetic services centres following a lower limb amputation, accounting for 70% of all lower limb referrals in 2006–7.[3] In this group referred to the prosthetic centres in the UK, 53% were transtibial and 39% were transfemoral amputees. In this 1-year period there were a total of 4957 referrals to Prosthetic Services in the UK, of which 4574 were following lower limb amputation (92% of the total).[3]

There is some evidence that the impact of modern vascular surgery may reduce the incidence of amputation.[4] The Danish National Amputation Register has demonstrated a 27% fall in the number of major amputations due to peripheral vascular disease in the decade 1980–90. This decline was attributed to the increased use of infrainguinal bypass operations.[5] A paper from Finland also reported that it was possible to reduce amputation rates with an aggressive reconstruction policy in critical limb ischaemia.[6] However, the West Coast Vascular Surgeons Study Group in Sweden failed to demonstrate a negative correlation between amputation and revascularisation rates.[7]

Survival rates after an amputation depend upon the cause of the amputation rather than the amputation itself. Those who have amputations following trauma tend to have good long-term survival, but those from vascular disease (including diabetes) face a 30-day mortality rate reported to be between 9% and 15% and a long-term survival rate of 60% at 1 year, 42% at 3 years and 35–45% at 5 years.[8] Of people with diabetes who have lower limb amputation, up to 55% will require amputation of the second leg within 2–3 years.[9]

Indications for amputation

The decision to perform amputation seems straightforward where there is extensive tissue loss or no reasonable prospect of revascularisation. However, the precise role of amputation in the management of critical limb ischaemia remains controversial. If it is predicted that vascular reconstruction is likely to be unsuccessful, then primary amputation perhaps offers the best outcome in terms of quality of life and cost benefit.[10] Chapter 3 discusses the treatment of chronic lower limb ischaemia and covers these issues of economics and quality of life in more detail. Where patients with critical limb ischaemia also have coexisting disabilities or other medical conditions that would render them unable to make use of a salvageable limb, then primary amputation with appropriate rehabilitation offers the best option. Examples of such patients include those with severe dementia, dense hemiplegia or spinal paralysis, severe arthritis and severe cardiorespiratory disease.

Level selection

Selection of the ideal level of amputation depends on the healing potential, rehabilitation potential and prosthetic considerations. The potential for rehabilitation and likely goals can only be set by a holistic assessment of the patient by the specialist amputee rehabilitation team. This assessment should include other illnesses and disabilities, cognitive state and motivation, likely discharge destination, lifestyle, as well as the patient's own aspirations and wishes.

In general terms, the more proximal the level of amputation, the more difficult it will be for the patient to achieve independent walking. Therefore, the more distal the amputation site, the better the rehabilitation potential for walking, as this preserves more joints and hence more control of the prosthesis. **Figure 6.1** is an algorithm dealing with level selection.

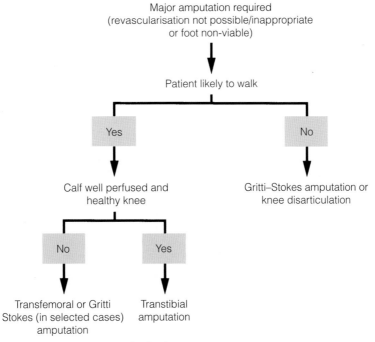

Figure 6.1 • Algorithm for the selection of amputation level.

Except in people with diabetes with good foot pulses (see Chapter 7), local amputation of single or multiple toes generally does not heal unless the foot can be revascularised. Transmetatarsal or ray amputation, if technically feasible, produces excellent functional results. Chopart's mid-tarsal amputation and Symes' through-ankle amputation are rare in chronic limb ischaemia and are not recommended because of the risks of developing an equinus deformity (in Chopart's), movement of the distal flap (in Symes'), poor long-term flap viability and considerable technical difficulties in prosthetic fitting. Thus, the commonest major levels of amputation in limb ischaemia are transtibial, knee disarticulation, Gritti–Stokes and transfemoral. Hip disarticulation and hindquarter amputation are rare and in 2006–7 accounted for just over 1% of all cases of lower limb amputations referred to the prosthetic centres in the UK. Dysvascularity was given as the cause for this level of amputation in only 19% of cases.[3] In our experience this level of amputation is mainly considered for people with neoplasia (usually sarcoma) or intravenous drug users (IVDUs). Preservation of the knee joint has enormous advantages in terms of mobility. In one study, 80% of transtibial amputees achieved unlimited household mobility or better, compared with 40% of above-knee amputees.[11] In a Sheffield study, only 26% of transfemoral vascular amputees achieved community ambulation, compared with 50% of transtibial vascular amputees at 1-year follow-up of a group of amputees who underwent prosthetic rehabilitation. In this study group, the figures for household mobility were 48% and 63%, respectively, for transfemoral and transtibial vascular amputees at 1-year follow-up.[12]

Transcutaneous oximetry (tcP_{O2}),[13] photoplethysmography,[14] laser Doppler velocimetry,[15] thermography[16] and isotope clearance rates[17] have all been shown to correlate with subsequent stump healing. However, while all these methods seem superior to Doppler ankle pressures,[18] a review concluded that sensitivities and specificities were inadequate to recommend their clinical use.[19]

The energy cost of walking with prostheses for vascular amputees is increased by 63% and 117%, respectively, in unilateral transtibial and transfemoral amputees compared with non-amputees. In bilateral transfemoral amputees, it is calculated that energy cost is 280% higher.[20] Therefore, it should not seem surprising that even in a selected group of bilateral transfemoral amputees who were successfully trained to walk with prostheses in an inpatient rehabilitation facility, the majority of them abandoned walking when they returned home and preferred to be wheelchair-dependent.[21]

Thus, for patients in whom major lower limb amputations are necessary, the following points should be remembered:

- Preserve the knee joint whenever possible if it is anticipated that the patient has the potential to achieve prosthetic walking or has the potential to use a prosthetic limb for assisting transfers from chair, bed, etc.
- In patients likely to remain chair- or bed-bound following amputation, a transtibial amputation risks non-healing and may become a hindrance to transfers if flexion contractures of the knee and hip joints develop. In such patients, knee disarticulation or Gritti–Stokes amputation seems a better option.
- Where there is a fixed knee flexion deformity of 25% or more and/or severe arthropathy, satisfactory fitting of a transtibial prosthesis for walking may not be possible. In such cases, a more proximal amputation should be undertaken.
- For patients likely to remain wheelchair- or bed-bound, including bilateral amputees, knee disarticulation or Gritti–Stokes amputation is preferable to transfemoral or transtibial as the longer lever lengths and larger surface areas are more conducive to transferring and provide a much better seating balance.
- In patients where a transtibial amputation is not possible but the patient has the potential to walk, most amputee rehabilitation units prefer a transfemoral rather than knee disarticulation or Gritti–Stokes amputation. This is because of problems of prosthetic fitting, which may compromise cosmetic appearance and function. Conversely some studies have demonstrated better functional outcomes in patients with a through knee amputation.

Surgical considerations

All amputations should be carried out by surgeons experienced in the procedure and should not be delegated to unsupervised and inexperienced junior staff. The following important general principles should be followed:

- tissues must be handled with care with good haemostasis;
- flaps should be oversized initially and then shaped and trimmed as required;
- good-quality sensate skin coverage of stump without any tension;

- bone edges should be smoothed off and bevelled;
- skin and muscle flaps should be trimmed and shaped to prevent dog ears, redundant tissue or a bulbous stump;
- creating the correct shape of the stump is the responsibility of the surgeon at the time of surgery;
- the use of a thigh tourniquet can reduce blood loss significantly during fashioning of muscle flaps.

Transfemoral amputation

Ensure adequate muscle (myoplastic) cover over the cut end of femur to prevent pain and discomfort and allow balanced action of flexors and extensors.[22] The technique of myodesis, where drill holes are made in the bone to fix muscles, may not be applicable in ischaemic limbs due to poor tissue quality. However, this minimises the risk of the muscles slipping off the end of the femur. The myoplasty and myodesis need to be performed with the hip joint in the neutral and naturally adducted position.

Allow at least 12 cm of clearance from the distal end of stump to knee-joint level in order to allow space for incorporating a prosthetic knee joint. This will prevent an unacceptable cosmetic and functional disability of a lowered knee centre in the prosthetic limb. The exact level of bone section will depend on thickness of the thigh muscles and subcutaneous tissue. With this in mind, a through-knee level should be considered in morbidly obese patients.

Through-knee amputation

Historically, this level of amputation was considered in those patients who were deemed incapable of walking. The longer stump assists transfers, sitting balance and maintains muscle attachment and proprioception. However, recent research articles including a systematic review and meta-analysis suggest that the primary outcome measure of Physical Component Score (PCS) of the short-form-36 measure of quality of life (SF-36) are much higher for through-knee amputation than transfemoral amputation. A significantly greater proportion of patients with through-knee amputation were able to walk 500 metres than those with transfemoral amputation. However, patients with a through-knee amputation wore their prosthesis significantly less and had significantly more pain than those with a transfemoral amputation.[23] Another study[24] has concluded that the through-knee amputation is associated with an acceptable primary healing rate and satisfactory functional outcome in patients with

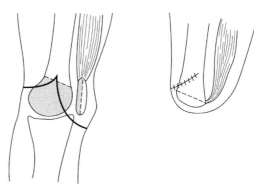

Figure 6.2 • Transection of the femur with a backward angle results in a more stable attachment of the patella in the modified Gritti–Stokes amputation.

peripheral arterial disease. This study concluded that the advantages of through-knee amputation over transfemoral amputation make it the preferred alternative for patients with vascular disease who are candidates for prosthetic rehabilitation.

The conventional through-knee amputation is associated with problems caused by the bulbous femoral condyles and leakage of synovial fluid. The modified Gritti–Stokes amputation avoids these problems and has fewer problems with wound healing than the alternative Mazet technique (**Fig. 6.2**). Limitations in prosthetic fitting due to a lowered knee centre, and limited availability of stance and swing phase control mechanisms in the prosthetic knee joint at this level, make the through-knee level unpopular with prosthetists, and further research is needed to develop suitable prosthetic devices. This may be prompted by the increasing use of the through-knee level for soldiers and civilians with extensive lower leg injuries caused by antipersonnel mines or improvised explosive devices (IEDs).

Transtibial amputation

Many surgeons now favour the skew flap technique[25] rather than the traditional Burgess long posterior flap.[26] The skewed skin flaps are based on the arteries that run with the long and short saphenous veins, which provide the main blood supply to the skin. In a small study of posterior flap and skew flap techniques, evaluation of flap hypoxia demonstrated that the posterior flap was associated with greater and more persistent reduction in tcP_{O_2}.[27]

> ✓✓ Randomised trials have shown little difference in healing between the skew flap and traditional Burgess long posterior flap, although exposure of the tibia occurs less often with skew flaps.[28] The time to limb-fitting and early mobility was shorter in the skew flap group due to a less bulbous stump (**Fig. 6.3**).

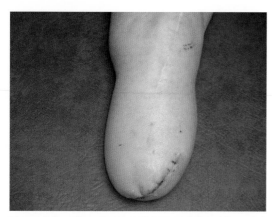

Figure 6.3 • Skew flap transtibial amputation at two and a half weeks showing a nicely shaped stump suitable for early limb fitting.

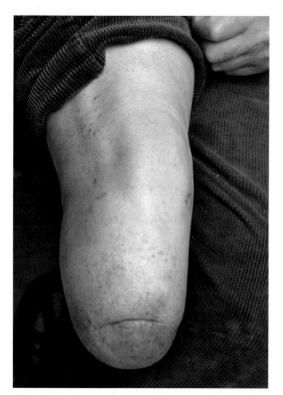

Figure 6.4 • An excellent transtibial amputation stump with a long posterior flap myoplasty.

The Burgess amputation still seems useful when skew flaps might be compromised by the medial skin incision of a failed femorodistal bypass graft or following fasciotomies (**Fig. 6.4**).

A tibial section at about 15 cm is considered ideal. The fibula should be divided around 1.5 cm proximal to the level of the tibial section. A short bevel and rounding off the sharp corners of the tibia must be undertaken. Much shorter transtibial stumps (up to 8 cm), though not ideal, can be fitted with additional suspension systems, e.g. pin and liner.

Foot amputation

Digital amputation is most commonly performed in people with diabetes because of their susceptibility to infection. In general, a digital amputation will only heal if foot pulses are present or can be restored. Therefore it is better to leave toes with partial dry gangrene alone. Amputation is best performed through the base of the proximal phalanx, leaving the wound open to heal by secondary intention. When infection extends beyond the proximal phalanx, a 'ray amputation' is indicated, especially in people with diabetes. After excision of the relevant toes, the line of excision is carried back through the infected tissue until healthy tissue is reached. The underlying metatarsal head is excised and the wound left open like a 'fish mouth'. Infection of the first or fifth metatarsophalangeal joint requires a 'tennis-racquet' incision; the handle of the racquet can usually be closed after excision of the metatarsal head. If osteomyelitis is present, a sample of the excised and retained bone should be sent for culture as the organisms causing the osteomyelitis are often different from those in the ulcer.

A transmetatarsal amputation can be useful when all the toes are gangrenous but when the plantar skin is still viable. A dorsal skin incision is made at mid-metatarsal level with a long plantar flap and bone transection through the metatarsal bases. As much soft tissue as possible should be preserved and consideration given to leaving the flaps open with delayed closure, as infection and gangrene of the flaps may occur if primary closure is attempted. Vacuum-assisted closure systems may facilitate the healing of such open-foot amputations.

Rehabilitation

The process of rehabilitation for vascular amputees, who are usually elderly and often have a number of other concurrent disabilities and illnesses, can pose a considerable challenge. A 'team approach' to amputee rehabilitation throughout the inpatient and prosthetic care pathway has now become the standard within the UK. The core members of the team should include a vascular surgeon, a specialist in rehabilitation medicine, a specialist physiotherapist, an occupational therapist and a prosthetist. Ready availability of a social worker, community nurses and a clinical psychologist is invaluable. Other services include wheelchair personnel, housing and adaptation officers, social services and orthotists. Close liaison and cooperation between all members of the team are vital. Counsellors and amputee volunteers, if available, can be very valuable.

> ✓ The British Society of Rehabilitation Medicine has recently updated and published standards and guidelines in amputee and prosthetic rehabilitation based on national consensus.[29]

Planning

A preamputation consultation by specialists in rehabilitation medicine and their team is ideal but impractical for every patient for whom an amputation is planned. However, a member of the amputee rehabilitation team (usually a therapist) should see all patients prior to amputation in order to make an initial assessment and prepare the patient for the likely programme to be implemented, instil realistic expectations and resolve any specific questions or anxieties. Other members of the multidisciplinary team may be involved at this stage if specially required. In our unit, specialist physiotherapists cover the boundary between the vascular and rehabilitation units and we find that this works extremely effectively. In cases where amputation is a treatment option rather than a necessity, and in situations where there is some uncertainty regarding level selection, we recommend that the surgical team obtain advice from an appropriate consultant in rehabilitation medicine.

Stump management

Tight or elasticated stump bandaging should not be used in vascular amputees as it can generate unacceptable pressures and cause tissue breakdown.[30] Rigid dressings of plaster of Paris are not generally used for vascular amputees in the UK, although some studies have suggested that they reduce the knee contracture rate following transtibial amputation. Adhesive clear-plastic film dressing applied postoperatively can be very useful as this allows easier and regular wound inspection. This type of dressing makes life easier for the physiotherapist when inspecting wounds before and after application of early walking aids. Where a more conventional dressing for the wound is required, an elasticated tubular bandage (e.g. Tubifast) is usually placed on the stump to hold these dressings in place. If the wound is healed or healing satisfactorily, then elasticated and graduated pressure stump shrinker socks (e.g. Juzo) are applied to the stump (**Fig. 6.5**). A survey of amputee physiotherapists in the UK (unpublished) revealed that the current practice is moving forward using the stump shrinker socks

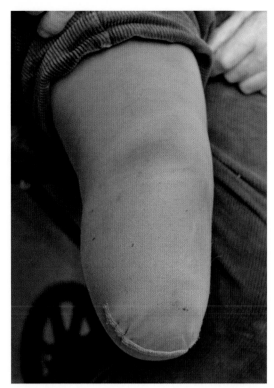

Figure 6.5 • A stump shrinker sock applied over a transtibial amputation stump.

earlier than previously. In Sheffield, if the vascular surgeons are satisfied with the below-knee stump wound and the patient is able to tolerate, the Juzo sock is applied on the fourth postoperative day. On the first day it is applied for 1 hour and then the wearing time is gradually increased over the next few days until the patient is wearing it all day and night. This process is carefully monitored by experienced staff. Stump supports are fitted to the wheelchair so that the patients can keep their below-knee stump elevated to prevent oedema and knee flexion. Sometimes, stump supports may also be necessary for long transfemoral or through-knee stumps. Specialist footwear may be required to protect the other foot from damage if it is vulnerable. In our centre we find pressure-relieving ankle-foot orthoses are effective for this purpose and also relieve pressure on the heel whilst lying down.

Pain management

Controlling stump and phantom pain is vital for the patient to participate successfully in a rehabilitation programme. Houghton et al.[31] found a significant relationship between preamputation pain and phantom pain in the first 2 years after amputation in vascular amputees. Nikolajsen et al.,[32] in a study of mostly vascular amputees, found a relationship between preoperative pain and incidents of phantom pain at 1 week and 3 months after amputation, but not after 6 months. Early involvement of the 'pain team' in such cases is most beneficial. Numerous medical interventions have been proposed over the years but tricyclic antidepressants and sodium channel blockers are currently considered to be the drugs of choice for neuropathic pain.[33] The anticonvulsant carbamazepine, a non-specific sodium channel blocker, has been reported to be effective in phantom pain.[34,35] The newer drug, pregabalin, has been found to be clinically effective in severe phantom pain.

In addition to the medical treatment of stump and phantom pains, various non-invasive treatments such as transcutaneous electrical nerve stimulation, vibration therapy, acupuncture, hypnosis and biofeedback can prove useful, although evidence of efficacy is limited.

Early postoperative rehabilitation

The occupational therapist and physiotherapist should work closely together to ensure an effective and timely rehabilitation programme. Following amputation the physiotherapist usually sees the amputee on the first postoperative day and will begin a programme of bed mobility, joint movements, transferring and wheelchair mobility, depending on the patient's general condition and pain control. Stump exercises, exercises for the remaining limb and upper limbs, muscle strengthening, maintaining range of movements of the proximal joints, sitting balance and improvement of general cardiovascular fitness will all be incorporated into the programme. Each amputee will be assessed for an appropriate wheelchair and cushion as early as possible to facilitate discharge. The amputee will be taught the skills necessary for independent use of the wheelchair. By around the 1-week assessment, the therapist is usually reasonably sure of a patient's potential ability to use a prosthesis or not. However, some amputees are too unwell at the early postoperative stage but later may recover sufficiently to benefit from prosthetic rehabilitation. Therefore appropriate follow-up assessment may need to be arranged for this group of amputees.

Extreme frailty, severe dementia, severe cardiorespiratory disease, gross fixed flexion contractures and severe arthritis are contraindications to prosthetic rehabilitation. In our experience elderly, vascular, bilateral transfemoral amputees do not achieve the ability to walk with a prosthesis. Assessing the home environment and adaptations, advice regarding driving, hobbies and employment also need addressing as an integral part of the rehabilitation.

> ✔ Evidence-based guidelines on the early rehabilitation phase have been published by the British Association of Chartered Physiotherapists in Amputee Rehabilitation.[36]

Primary prosthetic rehabilitation

All amputees who receive a prosthesis should undergo prosthetic rehabilitation to achieve the best prosthetic outcome. The role of the prosthetist in the fitting of a comfortable and functional prosthesis cannot be overemphasised. Prosthetic rehabilitation should aim to establish an energy-efficient gait based on normal physiological walking patterns. The physiotherapist should teach efficient control of the prosthesis through postural control, weight transfer, use of proprioception, and specific muscle strengthening and stretching exercises to prevent and correct gait deviations. Prosthetic rehabilitation will work towards the individual's own realistic goals, and should include functional activities relevant to that person and his or her lifestyle. All encouragement should be given to enable the individual to resume hobbies, sports, social activities, driving and return to work.

> ✔ The British Association of Chartered Physiotherapists in Amputee Rehabilitation have published useful evidence-based clinical guidelines for the physiotherapy of adults with lower limb prostheses.[37]

Sport activities for amputees

Amputation should not prevent an individual actively participating in sport. We often think of running, cycling, swimming and football, but there are others that may be more appropriate for the older, vascular amputee, including darts, snooker, bowls, fishing and golf.

Most sports will not require special prostheses and can be played alongside the able-bodied. Specialised componentry/prostheses are available for amputees who may want to run or swim. They may enable amputees to participate in more comfort and at a higher level than previously. Beach/water activity limbs do not assist the user to swim but allow an amputee to access in and around the water for activities such as windsurfing, sailing and canoeing, where not having the limb may prevent the activity. Previous and current fitness, concurrent disabilities (e.g. diabetic complications) and determination will all be important factors in the individual returning to or engaging in a new sport. Amputees may seek advice from professionals at their amputee rehabilitation centre, from peers, from groups such as British Amputee Les Autres Sports Association (BALASA) and, ever increasingly, the internet. Many local areas have groups who specialise in disabled sport and leisure that the amputee could access. The English Federation of Disability Sports (EFDS) keeps a list of all the disabled clubs nationally who deal with sports and leisure.

Prostheses

There are two main types of early walking aids used in the UK (**Figs 6.6** and **6.7**). The best known is the pneumatic postamputation mobility aid (PPAM Aid). The PPAM Aid is widely used and can be used for transtibial, through-knee and transfemoral levels of amputation. Until recently another type of early walking aid known as the amputee mobility aid (AMA), designed for transtibial amputation only, has been in use that allows amputees to flex and extend their knee during the gait cycle. It has a foot rather than a rocker end, allowing a more natural gait. Unfortunately the production of AMA has now ceased and no new ones are now available commercially. The Femurette is an excellent early walking aid for transfemoral amputees; it mimics

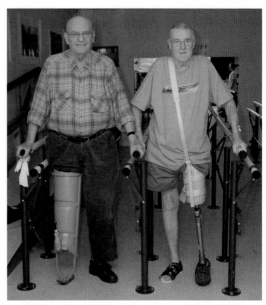

Figure 6.7 • A patient wearing Femurette (right) and a patient wearing PPAM Aid (left).

a definitive transfemoral prosthesis in terms of an ischial tuberosity-bearing socket configuration and knee joint and it also has a foot.[38] The early walking aids are excellent morale boosters and are also used as assessment tools to estimate an amputee's potential for walking. They allow stump desensitisation, assist in reduction of stump oedema and may promote wound healing, and allow re-education of postural reflexes, balance and gait. The early walking aids should be considered around 1 week after amputation, under the judicious supervision of experienced therapists. However, in some cases where wound healing is poor, introduction of early walking aids needs to be delayed.

Prosthetic developments

The lower limb prostheses used in the UK are mainly of endoskeletal modular construction (**Fig. 6.8**). This system allows much speedier manufacture, socket change, adjustments and repairs compared with old conventional exoskeletal prostheses. A new limb, from measurement to delivery, is usually available within 5 working days for primary patients. The standard prostheses usually incorporate thermoplastic materials like polypropylene or laminated plastics as socket materials and carbon fibre or lightweight alloy for fabrication of the weight-bearing components. Usually, vascular amputees are measured for their first prosthesis at about 6–8 weeks from amputation, although earlier fitting can take place subject to wound-healing status and

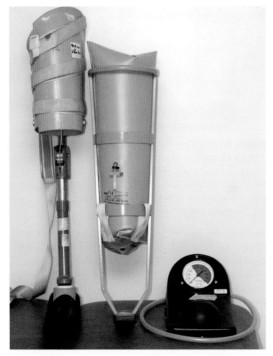

Figure 6.6 • A selection of early walking aids: Femurette (left) and pneumatic postamputation mobility aid (PPAM Aid; centre). A foot pump to inflate the PPAM Aid is shown on the right.

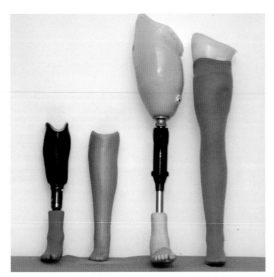

Figure 6.8 • Modular endoskeletal prostheses for transfemoral and transtibial amputation, with and without cosmetic covers.

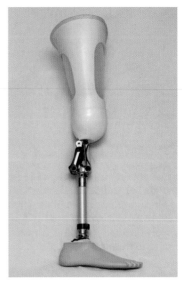

Figure 6.9 • A knee disarticulation prosthesis (without cosmetic cover) incorporating a four-bar linkage polycentric knee joint.

the general condition of the stump. It is not imperative that the stump be completely healed before a prosthesis can be provided.

Younger dysvascular transfemoral amputees may have good musculature of the stump and adequate hand function and agility to benefit from prostheses with suction socket fitting and sophisticated 'free knee' mechanisms like pneumatic or hydraulic swing phase controls. Microprocessor knee joints providing swing and stance phase control are also available for transfemoral amputees, although often the price is prohibitive in many NHS centres.[39] In the UK, most elderly and dysvascular transfemoral amputees, if they are accepted for a prosthetic rehabilitation programme, are provided with non-suction prostheses with some form of waist-belt suspension and a 'locked' knee (bends only to sit down). More active dysvascular transfemoral amputees may benefit from free knee designs including four-bar hydraulic, pneumatic or microprocessor knee units with suspending sockets.

For knee disarticulation, Gritti–Stokes or long transfemoral amputees, prosthetic options are limited. Use of polycentric knee joints like four-bar linkage knee mechanisms has eased some of the difficulties, though prostheses at these levels still create cosmetic as well as functional difficulties (**Fig. 6.9**).

For transtibial amputees there are various socket systems available to the prosthetist to achieve optimum fit and suspension. In addition to the anatomical system utilising a pelite liner and supracondylar suspension, the introduction of silicone or gel suspension systems using pin or valve locking

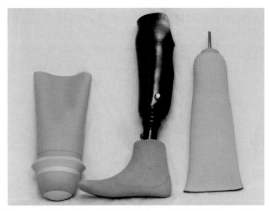

Figure 6.10 • From left to right: an ICEROSS liner with a distal locking pin which is applied by rolling onto the stump; a transtibial prosthesis on which the stump with the liner is inserted and locked in; and a Seal-in silicone liner that provides excellent suspension by suction without the necessity of a locking pin.

mechanisms has improved suspension as well as reducing friction and shear forces at the stump–socket interface[40] (**Fig. 6.10**). This type of prosthesis uses a silicone or gel sleeve directly on the stump, which is then locked into the prosthetic socket or uses a suction valve for suspension. There are many commercially available liners for use with pin suspension systems. Much shorter transtibial amputation stumps can now be fitted successfully, which was not possible previously with the traditional patellar tendon-bearing prosthesis. Computer-aided socket design and manufacture can be used, providing an alternative to casting.

Similar to prosthetic knee joints, there is a wide variety of commercially available prosthetic feet. They are categorised by their function. The most commonly prescribed foot in the UK is the multi-axis multiflex foot (Blatchfords), which provides movement through weight-bearing in the antero-posterior and mediolateral directions. Energy return feet can be considered for patients with higher activity levels and include Flexfoot, Elite, Epirius, Blade and Seattle. Energy storing feet are known to be less energy consuming for ambulant amputees.

✔✔ More recently energy return feet have also been found to offer significant help to transfemoral amputees.[41,42]

Other useful components include a patient-adjustable heel height device when shoes with different heel height are to be worn, torsion devices and vertical shock absorber in the shin of a prosthesis that absorbs vertical forces and rotational torque, turntables that allow sitting cross-legged on the floor, or individually created, highly lifelike silicone cosmetic cover, swimming or shower legs. Selection of the prostheses and components will be determined by clinical assessment and with consideration of the amputee's wishes, realistic goals, progress in rehabilitation and ability to benefit from a prescribed device.

Rehabilitation for the bariatric patient

Obesity is increasing in the UK, along with many countries. In 2006, 24% of adults were classified as obese. Following amputation the weight of the missing limb needs to be accounted for when making the calculation for the correct body mass index to be recorded. The health risks associated with being overweight are well known and include risk of diabetes, coronary heart disease, stroke and osteoarthritis. Weight gain also affects amputees in unique ways, which will have a negative impact on prosthetic rehabilitation.

- **Osteoarthritis.** Wearing a prosthesis puts an excessive strain on the joints of the residual limb and contralateral limb, causing pain and increased likelihood of osteoarthritis.
- **Cardiovascular effects.** As already discussed there is a greater energy expenditure when walking following amputation and any additional body weight would further compromise cardiac and pulmonary function.
- **Component selection.** There are currently many dozens of prosthetic components on the market, each having its own upper weight limit. As a person's weight increases, the choice of components will become limited. The heavy-duty components tend to be heavier, costlier and more difficult to obtain, and will increase the overall weight of the prosthesis.
- **Socket fit.** The comfort of the socket is vital; however, where there is an excess of soft tissue and the bony prominences are less well defined, it is difficult to obtain a firm stable fit with good suspension. Consequently the soft tissues are more prone to inflammation and ulceration.

Key points

- In the UK, 80% of all amputations carried out are due to vascular disease, and an increasing proportion have diabetes.
- Revascularisation may reduce the incidence of amputation.
- Selection of the ideal level of amputation depends on healing potential, rehabilitation potential and prosthetic considerations.
- Transtibial amputees have a much higher potential to achieve prosthetic mobilisation compared with those undergoing transfemoral amputation.
- For patients who are not likely to achieve prosthetic walking, a Gritti–Stokes amputation is preferable to the transfemoral level.
- A comprehensive and holistic assessment of amputees or prospective amputees, followed by multidisciplinary rehabilitation, is likely to provide the optimal outcome.
- Amputation surgery should be considered as a constructive procedure to create the best possible amputation stump and should therefore be carried out by surgeons who have had proper training in these procedures.

- Stump bandaging with elasticated bandages is not recommended.
- Appropriate use of early walking aids during the early postamputation period is an essential part of rehabilitation.
- Modern prostheses are modular and can be made quickly using modern materials technology.
- Increasingly, more sophisticated components are becoming available, although they tend to be applicable only for the more active amputee.
- The types of prostheses and their components will be determined by the amputee's realistic goals, progress in rehabilitation and ability to benefit.

References

1. Fyfe NCM. Amputation and rehabilitation. In: Davies AH, Beard JD, Wyatt MG, editors. Essential vascular surgery. London: WB Saunders; 1999. p. 243–51.

2. The Global Lower Extremity Amputation Study Group. Epidemiology of lower extremity amputation in centres in Europe, North America and East Asia. Br J Surg 2000;87:328–37.

3. Amputee Statistical Database for the United Kingdom 2006–07: Information Services Division. Edinburgh: National Health Service Scotland, Edinburgh; 2009.

4. Gutteridge W, Torrie P, Galland R. Trends in arterial reconstruction, angioplasty and amputation. Health Trends 1994;26:88–91.

5. Ebskov LB, Schroeder TV, Holstein PE. Epidemiology of leg amputation: the influence of vascular surgery. Br J Surg 1994;81:1600–3.

6. Luther M. The influence of arterial reconstruction surgery on the outcome of critical leg ischaemia. Eur J Vasc Surg 1994;8:682–9.

7. The West Coast Vascular Surgeons Study Group. Variations of rates of vascular surgical procedures for chronic critical limb ischaemia and lower limb amputation rates in Western Swedish counties. Eur J Vasc Endovasc Surg 1997;14:310–4.

8. Kuiken TA, Miller L. Lipschutz R, et al. In: Braddom RL, editor. Rehabilitation of people with lower limb amputation. Philadelphia, PA: Elsevier; 2007. p. 283–323.

9. Pandian G, Hamid F. Hammond M. In: Delisa JA, Gans BM, editors. Rehabilitation of the patient with peripheral vascular disease and diabetic foot problems. Philadelphia, PA: Lippincott-Raven; 1998.

10. Johnson B, Evans L, Datta D, et al. Surgery for limb threatening ischaemia. A reappraisal of costs and benefits. Eur J Vasc Endovasc Surg 1995;9:181–8.

11. Houghton AD, Taylor PR, Thurlow S, et al. Success rates for rehabilitation of vascular amputees: implications for preoperative assessment and amputation level. Br J Surg 1992;79:753–5.

12. Davies B, Datta D. Mobility outcome following unilateral lower limb amputation. Prosthet Orthot Int 2003;27:186–90.

13. Ratcliffe DA, Clyne CAC, Chant ADB, et al. Prediction of amputation wound healing: the role of transcutaneous pO_2 assessment. Br J Surg 1984;71:219–22.

14. Van Den Broek TAA, Dwars BJ, Rauwerda JA, et al. Photoplethysmographic selection of amputation level in peripheral vascular disease. J Vasc Surg 1988;8:10–3.

15. Karanfilian RG, Lynch TG, Zinsl VT, et al. The value of laser Doppler velocimetry and transcutaneous oxygen tension determination in predicting healing of ischaemic forefoot ulcerations and amputations in diabetic and non-diabetic patients. J Vasc Surg 1986;4:511–6.

16. Stoner HB, Taylor L, Marcuson RW. The value of skin temperature measurements in forecasting the healing of below-knee amputation for end-stage ischaemia of the leg in peripheral vascular disease. Eur J Vasc Surg 1989;3:355–61.

17. Moore WS, Henry RE, Malone JM, et al. Prospective use of xenon Xe-133 clearance for amputation level selection. Arch Surg 1981;166:86–8.

18. Welch GH, Leiberman DP, Pollock JG, et al. Failure of Doppler ankle pressure to predict healing of conservative forefoot amputations. Br J Surg 1985;72:888–91.

19. Savin S, Sharni S, Shields DA, et al. Selection of amputation level: a review. Eur J Vasc Surg 1991;5:611–20.
The authors reviewed the evidence for many tests (Doppler indices, segmental pressures, skin blood flow, skin perfusion pressure, tcP_{O_2}, thermography) to predict the likelihood of successful healing of an amputation stump. They concluded that the foremost requirement to raise the below-knee/above-knee ratio is to promote awareness among surgeons of the value of medical management and encourage the use of routinely available tests such as ankle–brachial pressure index and Doppler segmental pressures. The value of more specialised tests remains to be established.

20. Huang CT, Jackson JR, Moore NB, et al. Amputation: energy cost of ambulation. Arch Phys Med Rehabil 1979;60:18–24.

21. Datta D, Nair PN, Payne J. Outcome of prosthetic management of bilateral lower limb amputees. Disabil Rehabil 1992;14:98–102.

22. Chadwick SJD, Lewis JD. Above-knee amputation. Ann R Coll Surg Engl 1991;73:152–4.

23. Penn-Barwell JG. Outcomes in lower limb amputation following trauma: a systematic review and meta-analysis. Injury, Int J Care Injured 2011;42:1474–9.

24. Morse BC, Cull DL, Kalbaugh C, et al. Through knee amputation in patients with peripheral arterial disease: A review of 50 cases. J Vasc Surg 2008;48:638–43.

25. Robinson KP, Hoile R, Coddington T. Skew flap myoplastic below knee amputation: a preliminary report. Br J Surg 1992;69:554–7.

26. Burgess EM. The below knee amputation. Bull Prosthet Res 1968;10:19–25.

27. Johnson WC, Watkins MT, Hamilton J, et al. Transcutaneous partial oxygen pressure changes following skew flap and Burgess-type below knee amputations. Arch Surg 1997;132:261–3.

28. Ruckley CV, Stonebridge PA, Prescott RJ. Skewflap versus long posterior flap in below-knee amputations: multicenter trial. J Vasc Surg 1991;13:423–7.
A multicentre trial – 191 patients with end-stage occlusive vascular disease needing transtibial amputation were randomised to skew flap technique in 98 and long posterior flap technique in 93 patients. The two groups were well matched: 30-day mortality rate, state of wound at 1 week and need for surgical revision at the same or higher level were not statistically significant between the groups. Follow-up information at 6 months showed 64 (84%) of the skew flaps and 50 (77%) of the long posterior flaps were fitted with prostheses. Walking, alone or with support, was achieved in 59 (78%) and 46 (71%), respectively. None of these differences reached statistical significance.

29. British Society of Rehabilitation Medicine. Amputee and prosthetic rehabilitation standards and guidelines. 2nd ed. Report of the Working Party (chair Hanspal RS). London: British Society of Rehabilitation Medicine; 2003.

30. Isherwood PA, Robertson JC, Rossi A. Pressure measurements beneath below-knee stump bandages. Elastic bandaging, the Puddifoot dressing and a pneumatic bandaging technique compared. Br J Surg 1975;62:982–6.

31. Houghton AD, Nicholls G, Houghton AL, et al. Phantom pain: natural history and association with rehabilitation. Ann R Coll Surg Engl 1994;76:22–5.

32. Nikolajsen L, Ilkjaer S, Kroner K, et al. The influence of preamputation pain on postamputation stump and phantom pain. Pain 1997;72:393–405.

33. Nikolajsen L, Jensen TS. Phantom limb pain. Br J Anaesth 2001;87:107–16.

34. Elliott F, Little A, Milbrandt W. Carbamazepine for phantom limb phenomena. N Engl J Med 1976;295:678.

35. Patterson JF. Carbamazepine in the treatment of phantom limb pain. South Med J 1988;81:1101–12.

36. Broomhead P, Davies D, Hancock A, et al. Clinical guidelines for the pre and post operative physiotherapy management of adults with lower limb amputation. London: British Association of Chartered Physiotherapists in Amputee Rehabilitation; 2006.

37. Broomhead P, Dawes D, Hale C, et al. Evidence based clinical guidelines for physiotherapy management of adults with lower limb prostheses. London: British Association of Chartered Physiotherapists in Amputee Rehabilitation; 2003.

38. Ramsay EM. A clinical evaluation of the LIC Femurette as an early training device for the primary above knee amputee. Physiotherapy 1988;74:598–601.

39. Datta D, Howitt J. Conventional versus microchip controlled pneumatic swing-phase control for transfemoral amputees. Prosthet Orthot Int 1998;22:129–35.

40. Datta D, Vaidya S, Howitt J, et al. Outcome of fitting of ICEROSS prosthesis: views of transtibial amputees. Prosthet Orthot Int 1996;20:111–5.

41. Graham LE, Datta D, Heller B, et al. A comparative study – oxygen consumption and energy storing prosthesis in transfemoral amputees. Clin Rehabil 2008;22(10–11):896–901.
This experimental crossover trial established transfemoral amputees wearing Multiflex foot initially and then Variflex foot and concluded that a high functioning transfemoral amputee who wears an energy-storing prosthetic foot may have significantly reduced oxygen consumption at normal walking speed.

42. Graham LE, Datta D, Heller B, et al. A comparative study of conventional and energy storing prosthetic feet in high functioning transfemoral amputees. Arch Phys Med Rehab 2007;88(6):801–6.
In this study of the same subjects as in Ref. 41 it was shown that a transfemoral amputee who wears an energy-storing foot can have a more symmetrical gait in regard to some measures of spatial symmetry, kinetics and kinematics than one who wears a conventional prosthetic foot.

7

Revision vascular surgery

Jan Brunkwall
Michael Gawenda

Introduction

Revision of vascular reconstructions is frequently required beyond the first 6 weeks because of progressive atherosclerosis, graft occlusion, aneurysm formation or infection. Up to 40% of infrainguinal bypass surgery grafts require reintervention within 5 years.[1] The same is true for endovascular intervention, where it has been shown that up to 30% of patients need a reintervention within 5 years after endovascular aortic aneurysm reconstruction (EVAR).[2–6] Revision surgery requires experience and judgment; open surgery is technically more difficult because of fibrosis and the loss of easily definable tissue planes, which necessitates careful sharp dissection to gain arterial control. The anatomy may be altered by previous operations or interventions, and operating times, blood loss, infection rates and operative risk are therefore increased. Endovascular revision requires careful assessment with regard to when and how to intervene, and especially when to convert to open surgery.

Graft occlusion

Graft thrombosis usually presents acutely but is occasionally foreshown by increasing ischaemic symptoms, ranging from mild claudication to critical ischaemia; asymptomatic graft occlusion can also occur. Occasionally, simultaneous distal embolisation causes digital ischaemia (blue toe syndrome or gangrene). Graft thrombosis with loss of run-off due to distal embolisation is associated with a high risk of limb loss. Whereas graft thrombosis in the first 6 weeks is generally due to technical error or poor run-off, most late occlusions result from intimal hyperplasia within the bypass, progressive inflow or run-off disease (see Chapter 4). Graft stenoses are usually asymptomatic and occur in 20–30% of infrainguinal vein grafts, mostly in the first year.[7,8] Stenoses of greater than 70% (velocity >3 m/s or velocity ratio >3.0) compromise flow and often occlude if left untreated.[9]

Factors influencing graft occlusion

Local factors

These are essentially the quality of the inflow, the run-off and the conduit itself (see Chapter 4).

✓✓ Patency is better for suprainguinal than infrainguinal grafts and graft occlusion is more frequent in femorotibial than in femoropopliteal bypasses.[10] Infrainguinal bypass patency of autologous vein is better than Dacron, polytetrafluoroethylene (PTFE) or human umbilical vein.[11] Dacron and PTFE used in femoropopliteal bypass grafting did not differ at 5 years.[12] However, a recently published Scandinavian multicentre randomised trial revealed that a heparin-bonded PTFE graft significantly reduced the overall risk of primary graft failure by 37%. Risk reduction was 50% in femoropopliteal bypass cases and in cases with critical ischaemia.[13] Registry data acknowledged these results.[14]

In terms of technique, the results of reversed and in situ vein grafts are equivalent.[15,16] In a meta-analysis on the long-term primary and secondary patency and foot preservation after popliteal-to-distal bypass grafts, there was a superiority trend favouring reversed vein grafts.[17]

Arm veins are similar to the long saphenous vein provided that angioscopically detected defects are corrected.[18] Preoperative ultrasound mapping is important to identify the best autogenous conduit available.[19] A recently published retrospective study of infrainguinal bypasses for critical limb ischaemia (CLI) using arm vein conduits or prosthetic grafts revealed that arm vein conduits, even when spliced, are superior to prosthetic grafts in terms of midterm assisted primary patency, secondary patency, and leg salvage in infrapopliteal bypasses for CLI.[20]

✓✓ A recently published Cochrane Review demonstrated a clear primary patency benefit for autologous vein when compared to synthetic materials for above-knee bypasses. In the long term (5 years) Dacron confers a small primary patency benefit over PTFE for above-knee bypass. PTFE with a vein cuff improved primary patency when compared to PTFE alone for below-knee bypasses.[21]

The risks of ischaemic complications and the need for emergency limb revascularisation are greater with occlusion of prosthetic grafts compared to venous grafts. This is because the thrombus in the prosthetic graft extends into the outflow artery. Vein cuffs at the distal anastomosis reduce the risk of outflow impairment after thrombosis of PTFE grafts (**Fig. 7.1**).[22]

✓✓ While most studies demonstrate a clear advantage for vein, the Dutch BOA Study found no difference between venous and prosthetic graft material in the risk of amputation after infrainguinal bypass occlusion.[23]

The quality and number of run-off vessels appear to potentially identify patients at high risk for a poor initial outcome from infrainguinal bypass reconstructions.[24,25] Bypasses for gangrene are at higher risk of occlusion than those performed for other indications, probably related to the poorer run-off associated with worsening ischaemia.[26]

General factors

✓ Continued smoking after lower limb bypass surgery results in an at least threefold increased risk of graft failure.[27] Diabetes and renal failure compromise patient survival but not graft patency.[27–29]

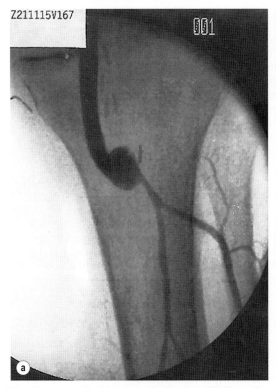
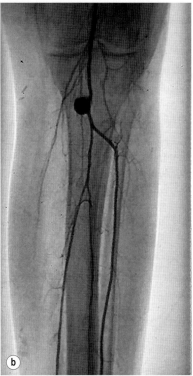

Figure 7.1 • Femoropopliteal bypass with venous cuff (Miller cuff) at the distal anastomosis. **(a)** Perioperative angiography. **(b)** Preservation of outflow vessels after thrombosis at 3 years.

Raised fibrinogen, hyperlipidaemia, thrombophilias (e.g. protein C, protein S or antithrombin III deficiency, antiphospholipid antibodies) and increased platelet aggregation favour graft thrombosis.[30] The role of factor V Leiden mutation is debatable.[31,32]

Black race and female gender are risk factors for adverse outcomes after vein bypass surgery for limb salvage, with graft failure and limb loss being more common events in black patients, and black women being a particularly high-risk group.[33] Hormone replacement therapy potentiates this increased risk.[34,35]

Prevention of graft thrombosis

✔✔ Antiplatelet therapy with aspirin had a slight beneficial effect on the patency of peripheral bypass grafts but seemed to have a lesser effect on venous graft patency compared with artificial grafts.[36]
The Dutch BOA trial revealed that aspirin is more effective for infrainguinal prosthetic grafts, whereas warfarin is better for vein grafts.[37] There is, however, no indication for routine warfarinisation.

In the CASPAR trial the combination of clopidogrel plus aspirin did not improve limb or systemic outcomes in the overall population of peripheral arterial disease (PAD) patients requiring below-knee bypass grafting. A subgroup analysis suggested that clopidogrel plus aspirin has benefit in patients with prosthetic grafts without significantly increasing major bleeding risk.[38]

Surveillance for suprainguinal bypass grafts does not seem to be cost-effective, offering relatively small clinical benefit. Occlusion is far more frequent after infrainguinal bypass grafting and since most of the occlusions occur within 2 years after the implantation, patients should be carefully followed during this time period. This includes medical history, clinical examination and Doppler pressure measurements. Additional duplex scanning is not effective after prosthetic bypass.

✔✔ Some published reports tend to argue in favour of duplex surveillance on the basis of patency alone.[39] In a recent large randomised trial, intensive surveillance with duplex scanning did not show any additional benefit in terms of limb salvage rates for patients undergoing femoropopliteal or femorocrural vein bypass graft operations.[40]

Management of graft stenosis (the failing graft)

Although there is some discussion about asymptomatic stenosis, it is clear that symptomatic graft stenosis should be treated by either angioplasty or surgical revision. Open surgical revision of infrainguinal vein grafts provides an increased freedom from further reinterventions or major amputation; however, early success rates for endovascular procedures are similar, particularly for non-occluded grafts. With time, endovascular revisions require an increasing number of reinterventions and manifested higher rates of failure.[41] Surgical revision is probably more durable in the longer term, but an endovascular approach is actually preferred because of the acceptable short-term patency and a low rate of complications, particularly for late graft stenosis (>3 months), short (<2 cm) and single stenoses.[42,43]

Short graft stenosis, whether midgraft or anastomotic, usually responds well to angioplasty with high inflation pressures (up to 2020 kPa; **Fig. 7.2**). Cutting balloons have been advocated, but seem to offer only small benefit at the expense of an elevated complication rate.[44–46] Stents (preferably self-expandable bare nitinol) should be used only selectively.[47]

✔✔ A randomised clinical study demonstrated that implantation of a polymer-free, paclitaxel-coated nitinol stent in patients with moderate-length lesions of the superficial femoral artery and proximal popliteal artery was safe and associated with a superior 12-month patency compared with both percutaneous transluminal angioplasty (PTA) and bare metal stent placement.[48]

Longer graft stenoses are best treated by open surgery and may be bypassed using the contralateral long saphenous or superficial femoral vein.[18] Tibial or distal popliteal anastomotic stenoses, resistant to angioplasty, are best treated by a jump graft to a fresh run-off vessel in order to avoid the scar tissue or adherent tibial veins (**Fig. 7.3**).

Management of the failed graft

If graft occlusion causes non-disabling claudication, a conservative approach is preferred. Acute subcritical ischaemia allows time for thrombolysis or elective surgery but an anaesthetic paralysed limb demands emergency revascularisation within a few hours (see Chapter 8).

Role of thrombolysis

✔ Local catheter-directed thrombolysis may be a valuable tool for a viable limb within 14 days of prosthetic graft occlusion provided that the patient has undergone surgery within 3 months.[49]

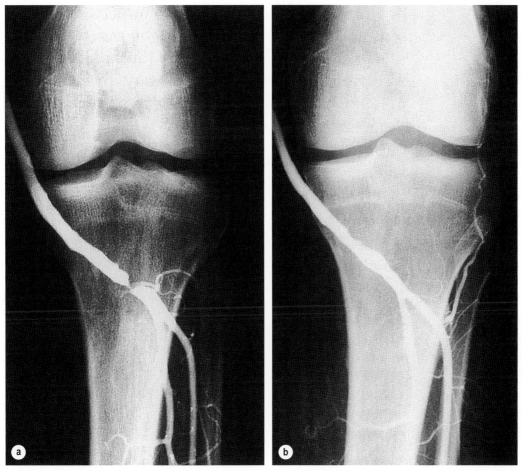

Figure 7.2 • Vein graft stenosis near the below-knee popliteal anastomosis **(a)**, successfully treated by balloon angioplasty **(b)**.

Although not applicable for suprainguinal grafts, thrombolysis is still frequently used for infrainguinal graft occlusion. The advantages are that redo surgery may be avoided and the graft will be cleared, allowing identification and simultaneous endovascular treatment of the underlying cause of thrombosis. The outflow vessels can also be cleared more effectively than with open surgery. Percutaneous mechanical thrombectomy or the use of high bolus therapy can reduce the duration of the procedure.[50,51] If thrombolysis is unsuccessful or reveals a problem that is not amenable to endovascular treatment, then open surgery can be performed with a clear knowledge of the cause of the problem and the state of the run-off. Although thrombolysis has a high initial success rate, it is also characterised by contraindications, haemorrhagic complications, poor long-term patency and persistent ischaemia.[52,53] Some therefore advocate reserving thrombolysis to those with associated extensive thrombosis of the outflow vessels.[54]

Suprainguinal graft thrombosis

A unilateral limb thrombosis of an aortobifemoral graft can often be thrombectomised through the groin even months after the occlusion. Thrombectomy is performed with Fogarty embolectomy catheters, an adherent clot catheter or a ring stripper. During these manoeuvres, the contralateral groin is compressed to avoid embolisation. The underlying cause is most frequently a stenosis at the distal anastomosis, which should be repaired by extension of the graft mostly into the profunda femoris artery (**Fig. 7.4**). Graft thrombectomy by a femoral approach is usually not possible in the case of bilateral graft occlusion, as the problem is more likely to be related to inflow. Here the graft should be replaced in situ or with an extra-anatomical bypass (axillobifemoral bypass).

The underlying cause of axillofemoral graft occlusion is most frequently an anastomotic or inflow vessel stenosis.[55] Thrombectomy can be performed

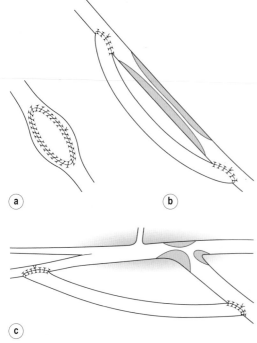

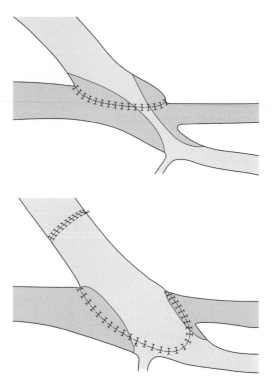

Figure 7.3 • Vein patch angioplasty **(a)**, bypass of long vein graft stenosis **(b)** and jump graft around stenosed distal anastomosis of a femoropopliteal bypass graft to the popliteal artery **(c)**.

Figure 7.4 • Extension graft to one limb of an aortobifemoral graft to treat a stenosis at the profunda femoris origin. In this case the superficial femoral artery is occluded.

from the groin, but most often an incision along the graft is needed. The underlying cause needs to be addressed. A new graft in unscarred tissues offers the best solution in cases of long-standing thrombosis or when thrombectomy is insufficient. For an occluded femorofemoral graft the same principles apply.

Infrainguinal graft thrombosis

In cases of chronic occlusion, the decision regarding revascularisation should be taken in the light of the clinical history, examination and results of investigations (Doppler, duplex scan, angiography).

In patients with acute ischaemia, an immediate decision should be taken regarding thrombolysis or open surgery. Prosthetic grafts can usually be thrombectomised by a groin approach if the occlusion is less than 1 week old. Anastomotic stenosis must be corrected, and inflow and outflow vessels need to be checked by perioperative angiography. If necessary, outflow vessels can be selectively approached by an infragenicular approach, and intraoperative thrombolysis may be an adjunct in selected cases (see Chapter 8).[56] Venous grafts are usually more difficult to thrombectomise. Here it may be wise to place a new graft, as is the case in prosthetic grafts where thrombectomy is

insufficient. If at all possible, a vein conduit should be used. Following thrombectomy for acute ischaemia, four-compartment fasciotomy should be considered to relieve pressure and improve distal perfusion, especially if there is any calf swelling or tenderness preoperatively.[57,58]

Graft infection

Graft infection is relatively uncommon (1–5%) but has a high amputation and mortality risk.[59] In a recent multicentre audit of 55 graft infections, 31% died, 33% underwent amputation and only 45% left the hospital alive without amputation.[60] Treatment has therefore to focus on patient survival, eradication of infection, and revascularisation by a method that is durable and does not predispose to further infection.

Causes

Graft infection is thought to occur most commonly by inoculation of bacteria from the patient's skin at the time of surgery (e.g. skin commensals) or by direct spread in the perioperative period, often secondary to wound breakdown.[61] Surgical site infection (SSI) after open surgery for lower extremity revascularisation is a serious complication that is associated with a more than twofold increased risk of early graft loss and re-operation.[62]

The risk of infection is higher in patients with gangrene, the elderly, obese and those undergoing re-operation during the same hospital admission. Preoperative shaving, open surgical drainage for more than 3 days, operations lasting over 4 hours, emergency surgery, redo surgery, female gender, diabetes, steroids, renal failure, recent angiography and wound haematoma are further risk factors.[62,63] Blood-borne bacteria from intravenous lines or systemic infections may also cause graft inoculation and sepsis.

Venous grafts are more resistant to infection than prostheses but direct bacterial erosion can occur, especially when exposed in an open wound.

Prevention

Patients should be admitted as near to surgery as possible and isolated from patients with known infections, especially methicillin-resistant *Staphylococcus aureus* (MRSA). Many hospitals are adopting a policy of screening elective surgical patients for MRSA colonisation before admission and eradicating any infection before proceeding with the surgery.

Strict aseptic technique and laminar air-flow theatres minimise infection rates. Iodine-impregnated adhesive drapes help isolate the operative field.

Prophylactic antibiotics (cephalosporin or co-amoxiclav) reduce wound and graft infection. There is no evidence for using more than three perioperative doses. Some surgeons add a single dose of gentamicin or vancomycin as cover for MRSA.

✔✔ Prophylactic systemic antibiotics reduce the risk of wound infection and early graft infection. Antibiotic prophylaxis for more than 24 hours appears to be of no added benefit. There was no evidence that prophylactic rifampicin bonding to Dacron grafts reduced graft infection at either 1 month or 2 years.[64] The same is true for silver-coated grafts.[65,66] There was no evidence of a beneficial or detrimental effect on rates of wound infection with suction groin-wound drainage[64] or of any benefit from a preoperative bathing or shower regimen with antiseptic agents.[67]

There is also little evidence regarding the need for prophylactic antibiotics before other surgical or dental procedures in the presence of prosthetic grafts.

Presentation

Wound infections after vascular surgery are classified according to the depth of tissue involvement: type 1 involves the skin only, type 2 the

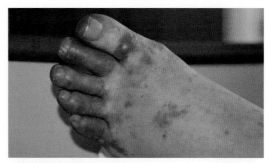

Figure 7.5 • Septic emboli at the foot as the presenting sign of aortofemoral graft infection.

subcutaneous tissue and type 3 the graft itself.[68] Prosthetic graft infection can present at any time from days to years after surgery with pyrexia, systemic sepsis, local abscesses and sinuses, graft exposure, thrombosis or anastomotic haemorrhage. On rare occasions septic emboli can be the first sign (**Fig. 7.5**). Septic erosion of exposed vein grafts can occur at any point.

Infrarenal aortic grafts can erode the third or fourth part of the duodenum causing an aortoduodenal fistula, which may present with one or two sentinel gastrointestinal bleeds before the inevitable catastrophic haemorrhage. Occasionally, an aortic graft can also erode any other part of the bowel, including the appendix, and also the ureter. Such aortoenteric erosion will lead to localised peritonitis with retroperitoneal or groin abscesses (**Fig. 7.6a, b**) and ultimately catastrophic bleeding. The mortality rate of aortoenteric complications is high (>50%), with recurrent infection or aortic stump blowout in over 25%.[69]

Bacteriology

Most graft infections are due to skin organisms.[70] *Staphylococcus epidermidis* is the least virulent, producing a biofilm or an infected seroma after months or years. It is difficult to culture, requiring homogenisation of explanted graft material to dislodge adherent bacteria. *Staphylococcus aureus* is more virulent and usually presents earlier. MRSA infections have a particularly high morbidity and mortality and the incidence unfortunately is increasing. Apart from staphylococci, there are a wide variety of organisms that can cause graft infection. Gram-negative species include *Escherichia coli* and *Pseudomonas aeruginosa*, the latter being recognised by a high tendency of anastomotic disruption and bleeding. It may be difficult or even impossible to culture the causative organism, particularly after prolonged periods of antibiotic therapy.

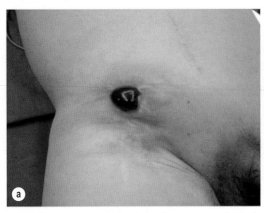
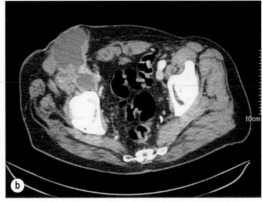

Figure 7.6 • Aortoenteric fistula leading to retroperitoneal and groin abscesses. **(a)** Aspect of the groin. **(b)** CT scan.

Diagnosis

In most cases there is a perigraft collection or sinus. Aspiration of frank pus or turbid fluid from around the graft and the subsequent culture of a causative organism are diagnostic. Computed tomography (CT), magnetic resonance imaging (MRI) or ultrasound usually demonstrate perigraft fluid and inflammation but can underestimate the extent of infection, especially if a sinus is present. A sinogram may be useful in very selective cases, though other modes of imaging will usually suffice. Aortic graft infection is often difficult to diagnose, requiring a high index of suspicion and aggressive investigation. Leucocyte count, erythrocyte sedimentation rate and C-reactive protein are often raised. Persistence of perigraft fluid or perigraft soft-tissue attenuation beyond 3 months or perigraft gas (**Fig. 7.7**)

beyond 4–7 weeks should be presumed to be infection. Perigraft fluid can be aspirated using an image-guided technique and characterised for pathogens, though this does pose a further infection risk.[71] One in four anastomotic aneurysms results from graft infection, but this is not always evident from CT. Where doubt exists, indium-labelled leucocyte or positron emission tomography (PET) scanning is occasionally helpful. In aortoenteric fistula, the graft may be seen eroding the duodenum at endoscopy (**Fig. 7.8**). Definitive confirmation of an infection is sometimes only made at the operation by the presence of pus around the graft and the absence of tissue incorporation (**Fig. 7.9**).

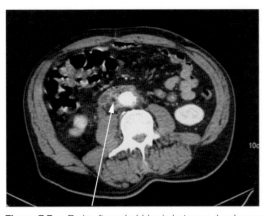

Figure 7.7 • Perigraft gas bubbles in between duodenum and aortic graft (see arrow).

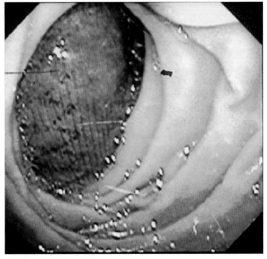

Figure 7.8 • Aortic graft, eroding the duodenum as seen during endoscopy.

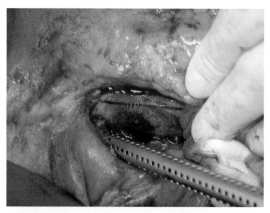

Figure 7.9 • Intraoperative situs with absence of tissue incorporation of the graft and discoloration by duodenal secretion.

Management

General principles

Once infection is confirmed, semi-urgent treatment is required to pre-empt catastrophic haemorrhage, graft thrombosis or systemic sepsis. An infected prosthesis acts as a foreign body, rendering bacteria inaccessible to antibiotics. Conservative measures (including prolonged antibiotic therapy, drainage and irrigation of abscesses, muscle flaps) may be helpful and can buy time, but they are rarely curative.

The mainstay of vascular graft infection management is as follows. First, excision of the graft, as this as a foreign body that may potentiate the infection. Second, wide and complete debridement of devitalised and infected tissue to provide a clean wound in which healing can occur. Third, establishing a vascular flow to the distal bed. Fourth, intensive and prolonged treatment with antibiotics, in order to reduce the risk for sepsis and secondary graft infection.[72]

Complete graft excision may be mandatory. Partial graft resection commonly requires later replacement.[73] Although contrary to conventional concepts, partial or complete graft preservation combined with aggressive drainage and groin wound debridement is an acceptable option for treatment of infection involving an entire aortic graft in selected patients with prohibitive risks for total graft excision.[74,75]

Simple graft excision without revascularisation can heal infection but usually results in major amputation, even in patients operated on initially for claudication. Revascularisation is traditionally performed by extra-anatomical bypass (axillofemoral graft for infrarenal aortic graft infection, obturator bypass for infection at the groin, lateral bypass for infection of a femoropopliteal graft).[59]

✅ There is growing evidence that in situ reconstruction produces equal or better results than graft excision and extra-anatomical bypass, with regard to reinfection rate and particularly late patency and amputation rates.[76,77] An autologous conduit is preferable for in situ reconstruction.[78]

Arterial allografts are an alternative but they may dispose to late complications such as stenosis, occlusion or aneurysmal degeneration.[76,79] There are a few encouraging reports on the use of rifampicin-bonded grafts or silver-impregnated grafts, but they should be reserved for patients with low-grade infections (e.g. *Staphylococcus epidermidis*).[80,81]

The duration of postoperative antibiotic therapy is still under discussion. Most authors will accept a period of 2–6 weeks, depending on the causative organism.[82]

Infrarenal aortic graft infection

Traditional management of aortic graft infection has comprised extra-anatomical bypass, specifically axillobifemoral bypass, with complete removal of the infected aortic graft. During the last two decades, methods have included debridement of infected tissue, with in situ replacement using cryopreserved allograft, autogenous vein or rifampicin-bonded prostheses (**Fig. 7.10**).

✅✅ A recent meta-analysis of in situ replacement methods found these alternative techniques overall to be superior to the traditional method in terms of rates of reinfection, conduit failure, and early and late mortality and amputation rates.[77] Rifampicin-bonded prosthetics were found to have the lowest rates of amputation, conduit failure and early mortality. However, the reinfection rate with rifampicin-impregnated grafts was higher than for other conduits. Autogenous vein had the lowest rate of reinfection, followed by cryopreserved allograft. Later mortality was lowest for autogenous vein and cryopreserved allograft reconstruction. When all outcomes were considered, in situ options for aortic graft infection have shown considerable promise.

An early study of silver-coated prosthetic grafts showed encouraging results for in situ management of aortic graft infection. That study showed the method to be safe and effective, with a 3.7% reinfection rate at 16 months. However, a later study showed results similar to other in situ methods and further studies are required.[80,83]

As an alternative for aortic reconstruction, the superficial femoral veins following total graft excision have been used.[84,85]

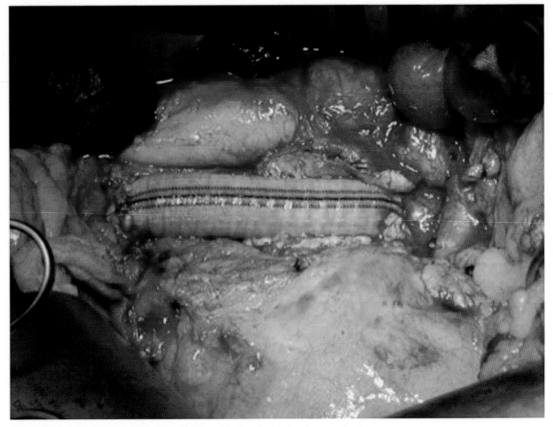

Figure 7.10 • In situ reconstruction with rifampicin-bonded polyester prosthesis.

It is agreed that in situ reconstruction with the superficial femoral veins represents a technically demanding and time-consuming operation. The operation has also been criticised because of the risk of venous hypertension in the lower limbs, though this can be prevented by the preservation of the profunda vein branches (**Figs. 7.11** and **7.12**), and an increased need for fasciotomy.[86] Within 30 days of the operation, 4.5% of the patients required a fasciotomy.[87]

Our preferred method is the use of an allograft (**Fig. 7.13**), using either fresh homograft or, more frequently, a cryopreserved allograft from the German Transplant Donor Organisation (DSO).

The thoracic aorta is most often provided, requiring construction of a bifurcation and adjustment for size discrepancy when anastomosing to the native aorta (Fig. 7.13a). It is wise to check for bleeding along the suture line before the graft is tunnelled. Furthermore, the length is more accurately judged when the allograft is stressed with arterial pressure. Sometimes, extension with saphenous vein or other native artery may be required (Fig. 7.13b).

The role of endovascular reconstruction in graft infection, and particularly infrarenal aortic graft infection, seems limited.

Endovascular repair is often successful in the short term, achieving favourable immediate outcome. In the presence of systemic infection, however, EVAR alone as an ultimate solution is often followed by repeat infection and bleeding.[88] A staged combination of EVAR treatment for acute bleeding and aggressive infection treatment with systemic and local antibiotics, surgical abscess revision and fistula tract closure may be an option in frail patients. For patients fit for open repair, EVAR can be used as a bridging procedure to definitive repair, particularly in the setting of systemic infection.[89]

Endograft infection occurs in less than 1% of endovascular grafts implanted[90–92] (**Fig. 7.14**). Approximately one-third of patients present with evidence of an aortoenteric fistula (although less than half of these present with gastrointestinal haemorrhage), one-third present with non-specific signs of low-grade sepsis (malaise, weight loss) and the remainder with evidence of severe systemic sepsis.[91] In one series, mortality was 18%

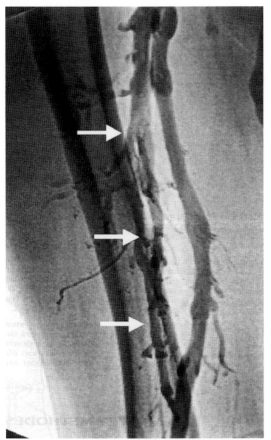

Figure 7.11 • Phlebography showing the femoral vein. Important collaterals of the profunda femoris vein (white arrows) protect from venous hypertension after harvest.

overall, 36.4% after conservative treatment and 14% after surgical treatment. Mortality was 16% after surgical treatment with extra-anatomical bypass vs. 5.8% for surgical treatment with in situ reconstruction.[90]

Graft aneurysms

True aneurysms

Following repair of a true aneurysm, the adjacent artery may also become aneurysmal. Aneurysms were frequent within some early PTFE grafts but manufacturing improvements have almost eliminated this. Biological grafts such as the human umbilical vein graft frequently became aneurysmal before the addition of a Dacron wrap.[93] Xenografts such as bovine mesenteric vein and cryopreserved venous or arterial allografts are particularly subject to aneurysmal degeneration.[76,79] Dacron undergoes late degradation and

dilatation, which becomes clinically significant in 2–3% of cases. After 5–10 years, disruption can occur at points of stress (e.g. under the inguinal ligament) causing false aneurysms,[94] which may present with haemorrhage or thrombosis. Distraction during shoulder abduction may cause spontaneous rupture or axillary anastomotic disruption of PTFE axillofemoral grafts.[95] Vein graft aneurysms are rare but more frequent in bypasses for popliteal aneurysms than for occlusive disease.[96] Information on the natural history of untreated graft aneurysms is lacking but repair is generally recommended and is essential to prevent rupture, thrombosis or embolism. Treatment is either with a covered endovascular stent or by graft replacement.

False aneurysms

False aneurysms are essentially pulsating haematomas, which may occur at the arterial puncture site after angiography (or intervention), following intra-arterial injection by intravenous drug users (IVDUs), after trauma (usually penetrating), due to primary arterial infection (e.g. salmonella and HIV) and at disrupted arterial anastomoses. Puncture-site aneurysms often thrombose spontaneously.

✔✔ Although limited, the present evidence appears to support the use of thrombin injection as an effective treatment for femoral pseudoaneurysm. A pragmatic approach may be to use compression (blind or ultrasound-guided) as first-line treatment, reserving thrombin injection for those in whom the compression procedure fails.[97]

Ultrasound-guided compression occludes over 80% and most others will thrombose following thrombin injection.[98] Direct surgical repair or a covered stent are rarely necessary. The management of infected (mycotic) aneurysms is dealt with in Chapter 13.

The incidence of anastomotic aneurysms is increasing, due primarily to the increased frequency of prosthetic vascular reconstructions involving groin anastomosis. The overall incidence following vascular anastomoses is about 2%, but this increases to 3–8% when the anastomosis involves the femoral artery. Although they are most common after prosthetic bypass, anastomotic aneurysms occasionally occur after vein bypass, semi-closed endarterectomy and open endarterectomy with a vein patch. Anastomotic aneurysms can occur anywhere, but they frequently develop near to a joint. About 80% occur at the groin, presumably due to movement-related strains.[99]

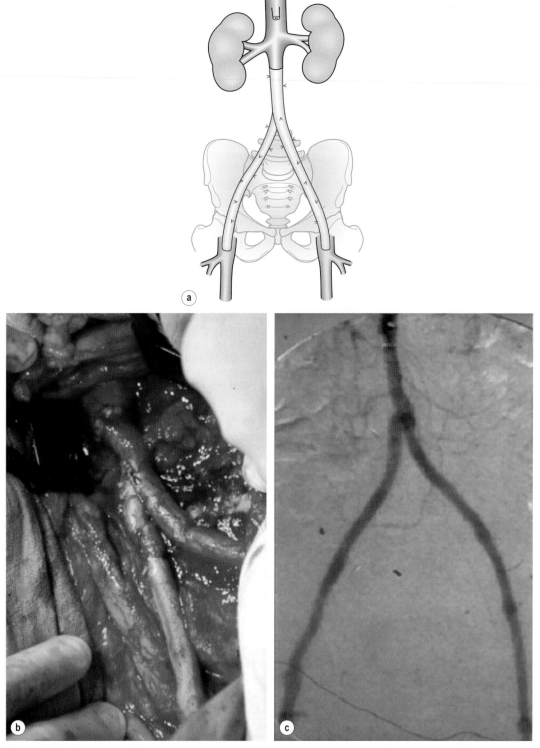

Figure 7.12 • The reversed Y technique for in situ reconstruction of an infected aortobifemoral graft. **(a)** Schematic drawing. **(b)** Perioperative view. **(c)** Postoperative angiography.

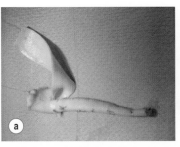
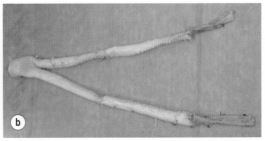

Figure 7.13 • Cryopreserved allograft from thoracic aorta. **(a)** Suturing a new bifurcation. **(b)** Peripheral extension with endarterectomised superficial femoral arteries.

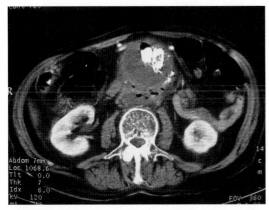

Figure 7.14 • CT scan demonstrating gas bubbles inside the aneurysm sac following EVAR with concomitant retroaortic abscess formation.

Aortic anastomotic aneurysms are not easily discovered by clinical examination, but when followed by CT the incidence may be as high as 4%.[100] Some feel this justifies the need for lifelong follow-up after open aortic reconstruction,[101] though few are revised due to the complexity of repair.

Anastomotic aneurysms at the femoral level are best treated by open surgery and graft interposition,[101] although there are anecdotal reports of endovascular reconstruction.[102] The treatment of choice for iliac anastomotic aneurysms is now stent graft placement from the groin (**Fig. 7.15**). This can be performed under local anaesthesia and mortality and morbidity is minimal. Late complications include endoleak and occlusion in a minority of cases.[103,104] Preoperative embolisation of the internal iliac artery is frequently required, which may lead to gluteal claudication[105] and other pelvic complications (see Chapter 13).

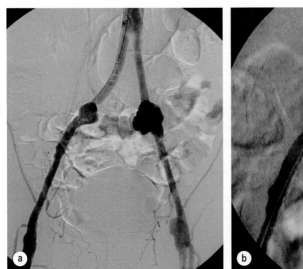
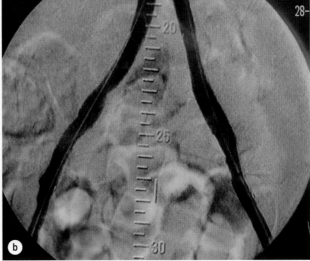

Figure 7.15 • Preoperative angiography with bilateral para-anastomotic iliac artery false aneurysm. **(a)** Preoperative angiography. **(b)** Angiography after placement of tubular endoprostheses.

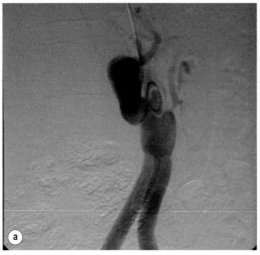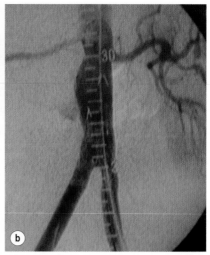

Figure 7.16 • Preoperative angiography with para-anastomotic false aneurysm of the aorta after interval of 4 years. **(a)** Preoperative angiography. **(b)** Angiography after placement of tubular endoprosthesis.

✅ Endovascular reconstruction is preferred if the patient has a suitable morphology (**Fig. 7.16**).[108,109] A comparative study confirmed reduced blood loss, procedural time and a shorter hospital stay in the endovascular group. The operative mortality was 19% in the surgical group vs. 10% in the endovascular series.[110] A recently published study demonstrated that endovascular repair of para-anastomotic aortic and iliac aneurysms after initial prosthetic aortic surgery is safe and durable in patients with an appropriate anatomy. The long-term follow-up showed fewer complications occurred after procedures with bifurcated stent grafts compared with procedures with tube grafts, aortouniiliac or iliac extension stent grafts.[111] Although a tubular stent graft from a technical point of view can exclude most aneurysms, it appears that a bifurcated graft may be more effective at midterm follow-up.[112]

Graft interposition for aortic anastomotic aneurysms unsuitable for endovascular repair is performed preferentially using a retroperitoneal approach. It is associated with a higher surgical risk than a primary vascular operation, with an elective mortality up to 17%, considerably higher if ruptured.[106,107]

Carotid artery

Infection

Revision of carotid artery surgery is required postoperatively during the first 48–72 hours either due to acute bleeding or thrombosis leading to hemispheric symptoms. These complications are dealt with extensively in Chapter 10 and will not be further discussed here. The risk of long-term patch infection is below 1%[113] and is higher when prosthetic material has been used (**Fig. 7.17**). The patient normally presents with a swelling or a sinus with a positive bacterial isolate. Revision surgery is required and should be performed under general anaesthetic. Frequently, the scar tissue is so dense that adequate distal control requires balloon occlusion of the external carotid artery and insertion of a Pruitt–Inahara shunt to the internal carotid artery. This also gains valuable extra length for subsequent patch closure using saphenous vein, preferably from the groin.[114]

Stents or stent grafts do not seem to play any definite role in the treatment of carotid artery infection, but may play a bridging role in haemorrhage control.

Aneurysm formation

Aneurysm formation following carotid endarterectomy (CEA) is most frequently encountered secondary to a 'low-grade' infection or pseudoaneurysm. Aneurysms should undergo surgical repair if they are over 2 cm in diameter, symptomatic or associated with patch infection. The surgical exposure is similar to standard CEA but it may be necessary to resect the artery and perform an interposition graft. There is no evidence for the use of carotid artery stenting (CAS) to treat aneurysm formation after CEA but it may be possible with covered stents if surgery is not possible.

Revision after CAS

The risk of complications is probably higher for CEA after CAS and if longer segments are stented. Operative treatment should be reserved for patients

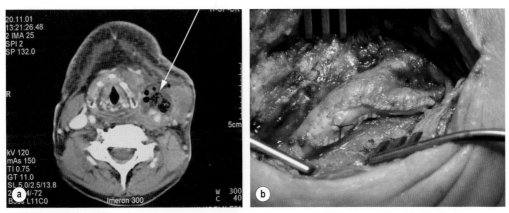

Figure 7.17 • Infection following CEA with patch. **(a)** CT scan (see arrow). **(b)** Intraoperative vein patch.

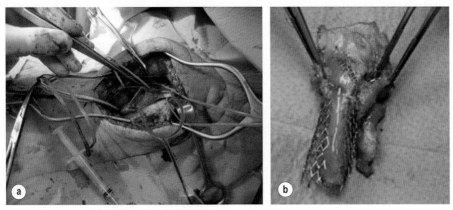

Figure 7.18 • CEA after CAS. **(a)** Intraoperative view. **(b)** Specimen following CEA.

who are neurologically symptomatic and unsuitable for further endovascular intervention. The surgical exposure is similar to standard CEA (Chapter 10). The dissection can be more difficult due to persistent inflammation and scarring. Should the stent penetrate the arterial wall, then it is often necessary to insert an interposition graft instead of doing a thrombo-endarterectomy. **(Fig.7.18)**.

Revision surgery after EVAR

EVAR is associated with a significant risk of late complications and reintervention, in some series occuring at a rate of 5–10% per annum, though this is decreasing. Endoleaks are the most frequent complication and are described in more detail in Chapter 13. Most complications can be treated by endovascular reintervention if required.[115] Surgical techniques such as laparoscopic clipping of the side branches and remodelling of the aneurysm have not generated much enthusiasm.[116,117] Open surgery, on the other hand, is well accepted for graft limb thrombosis, e.g. graft thrombectomy or femorofemoral crossover grafting.[115]

✅ A recently published review revealed that the rate of early conversion ranged from 0.8% to 5.9%; the latest studies carried lower rates of early conversion. Mortality rates of early conversion varied between 0% and 28.5%, with an average mortality of 12.4%. The rates of late conversion ranged from 0.4% to 22% with a mortality rate of 10%.[118]

Although the operation is more challenging, the procedure is essentially similar to primary aneurysm surgery. Dissection of the proximal infrarenal aortic neck may be more difficult because of periaortic inflammation related to the stent graft. Suprarenal and preferably supracoeliac clamping is frequently required, particularly in stent grafts with suprarenal fixation. Endografts with infrarenal fixation are easily removed once the aneurysm sac has been opened and the aorta is clamped below the renal arteries. In grafts with suprarenal fixation, particularly in those with hooks and barbs, it may be wise to leave the suprarenal portion in place and to amputate the infrarenal portion of the endoprosthesis by cutting the metal frame of the suprarenal attachment system.[119] The suprarenal fixation system is then incorporated into the proximal anastomosis, which is performed under supracoeliac aortic clamping. Preferably, the graft should be removed completely. In the usual case of a bifurcation graft this means that the iliac arteries have to be dissected and that the external and internal iliac arteries have to be clamped selectively in order to perform a reconstruction to the iliac bifurcation.

Although it is understood that conversion is associated with increased risk of mortality and morbidity, some have reported a 0% mortality rate for elective late conversion. Mortality rates for early conversion range from 7% to 25%, rising to 40% in cases of rupture.[120–122]

Revision after thoracic endovascular aortic repair (TEVAR)

Complications following TEVAR predominantly relate to endoleaks or migration of the stent graft, which may be treated endovascularly (see Chapter 14), though there are occasionally more complicated problems, including aortobronchial fistula, aorto-oesophageal fistula and stent graft infection.

Aortobronchial fistula

Aortobronchial fistula after TEVAR is rare. Statistically robust data are not available, but according to a national survey of 1113 TEVARs, the risk seems to be <2% when combined with aorto-oesophageal fistula.[123]

The symptoms prior to haemoptysis are vague, if they present at all. The typical patient will have some episodes of minor bleeding preceding a major haemorrhage, and diagnosis is often delayed.

Although a bronchoscopy may theoretically show the graft, sometimes the fistula is more peripheral in the lung tissue.

A new stent graft may serve as a bridging solution to stabilise the patient, but a more radical definitive and durable solution requires open replacement using a standard graft or preferably an allograft (**Fig. 7.19**).

Aorto-oesophageal fistula

The hooks or bare stent of an endoprosthesis may penetrate the oesophagus due to mechanical reasons, but an aorto-oesophageal fistula may also appear, even in patients where the stent graft is not in contact with the oesophagus. Aorto-oesophageal arterial branches may be occluded by the stent graft, thereby leading to an ischaemic necrosis. TEVAR could serve as a bridge to surgery for emergency cases only, with

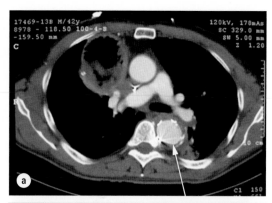
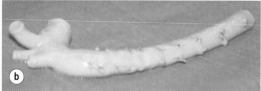
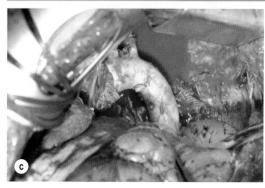

Figure 7.19 • Infection following TEVAR in a case of traumatic transection 4 years previously. **(a)** CT scan (see arrow). **(b)** Cryopreserved thoracic allograft. **(c)** Thoracic aortic reconstruction with allograft.

definitive open surgical correction of the fistula undertaken as soon as possible.[124] In addition to the aforementioned principles for the aorta, it is necessary to resect the oesophagus and later perform a new gastro-oesophageal anastomosis to restore the normal tract.

Infection

Stent graft infection occurs in 0.2–3% of endovascular grafts implanted.[74,91] The infected stent graft is a challenge where the definitive treatment is explantation of the device and replacement with an allograft of rifampicin-soaked graft. Although long-term antibiotic therapy may be an alternative for non-surgical candidates, it will rarely eradicate infection. As for several of the thoracic entities, there are no robust data, rather individual case reports or case series.[92]

Key points

- Late graft occlusion is caused by intimal hyperplasia or progression of atherosclerosis of the inflow or outflow.
- Graft stenoses occur in 20–30% of infrainguinal vein grafts. Symptomatic stenoses require treatment. Angioplasty offers excellent early results. In the long term, open surgery is probably better.
- Thrombolysis of occluded prosthetic infrainguinal grafts may be attempted in patients aged under 80 years with critical ischaemia provided that limb viability is not severely threatened, that the patient has not undergone surgery within 3 months and that the occlusion is less than 14 days old.
- Graft infection results from a breakdown of sterility at surgery, by extension from a superficial wound infection or from blood-borne bacteria.
- Prosthetic graft infections cause perigraft abscesses, sinuses and anastomotic haemorrhage, including aortoenteric fistula and erosion. Vein grafts may be eroded by infection, particularly in open wounds.
- *Staphylococcus epidermidis* is the most frequent cause of low-grade infection. *Staphylococcus aureus* and Gram-negative infections tend to present early and are more virulent. The incidence of MRSA infection has increased over recent years.
- Any perigraft fluid after 3 months, or gas beyond 4–7 weeks on CT or ultrasound, suggests infection. Aspiration or perigraft fluid pus can usually secure the diagnosis, though there are risks associated with this approach.
- Conservative measures, such as prolonged antibiotic therapy, drainage and irrigation, or covering exposed grafts with muscle or omental flaps are rarely curative. The same applies for partial graft excision.
- Simple graft excision without revascularisation usually causes severe ischaemia leading to amputation or death.
- Extra-anatomical revascularisation has been the 'gold standard' in the past. In situ revascularisation with autologous vein (e.g. femoral vein) has better patency and recurrent infection is rare. Arterial allografts are an alternative. The role of in situ reconstruction with silver-bonded or rifampicin-bonded Dacron grafts is debatable.
- Endoprostheses can buy time in cases of bleeding aortoduodenal fistula but recurrence of infection is high.
- True aneurysms can occur within prosthetic or vein grafts or adjacent to previous aneurysms.
- False aneurysms may result from anastomotic distraction or infection. Treatment of femoral false aneurysms is surgical. Endovascular treatment offers an excellent alternative in cases of non-infected iliac or aortic false aneurysms.
- Surgical conversion is rarely needed after endovascular treatment of abdominal aortic aneurysms, but can be performed with excellent results.

References

1. Dawson I, van Bockel JH. Reintervention and mortality after infrainguinal reconstructive surgery for leg ischaemia. Br J Surg 1999;86:38–44.

2. Blankensteijn JD, de Jong SE, Prinssen M, et al. Two-year outcomes after conventional or endovascular repair of abdominal aortic aneurysms. N Engl J Med 2005;352:2398–405.

3. Giles KA, Landon BE, Cotterill P, et al. Thirty-day mortality and late survival with reinterventions and readmissions after open and endovascular aortic aneurysm repair in Medicare beneficiaries. J Vasc Surg 2011;53:6–12, 3 e1.

4. Karthikesalingam A, Holt PJ, Hinchliffe RJ, et al. Risk of reintervention after endovascular aortic aneurysm repair. Br J Surg 2010;97:657–63.

5. Mertens J, Houthoofd S, Daenens K, et al. Long-term results after endovascular abdominal aortic aneurysm repair using the Cook Zenith endograft. J Vasc Surg 2011;54:48–57 e2.

6. Verhoeven BA, Waasdorp EJ, Gorrepati ML, et al. Long-term results of Talent endografts for endovascular abdominal aortic aneurysm repair. J Vasc Surg 2011;53:293–8.

7. Mills JL, Bandyk DF, Gahtan V, et al. The origin of infrainguinal vein graft stenosis: a prospective study based on duplex surveillance. J Vasc Surg 1995;21:16–25.

8. Mofidi R, Kelman J, Berry O, et al. Significance of the early postoperative duplex result in infrainguinal vein bypass surveillance. Eur J Vasc Endovasc Surg 2007;34:327–32.

9. Mills Sr. JL, Wixon CL, James DC, et al. The natural history of intermediate and critical vein graft stenosis: recommendations for continued surveillance or repair. J Vasc Surg 2001;33:273–80.

10. Norgren L, Hiatt WR, Dormandy JA, et al. Inter-Society Consensus for the Management of Peripheral Arterial Disease (TASC II). Eur J Vasc Endovasc Surg 2007;33 (Suppl. 1):S1–75.

11. Pereira CE, Albers M, Romiti M, et al. Meta-analysis of femoropopliteal bypass grafts for lower extremity arterial insufficiency. J Vasc Surg 2006;44:510–7.

12. Takagi H, Goto SN, Matsui M, et al. A contemporary meta-analysis of Dacron versus polytetrafluoroethylene grafts for femoropopliteal bypass grafting. J Vasc Surg 2010;52:232–6.

13. Lindholt JS, Gottschalksen B, Johannesen N, et al. The Scandinavian Propaten® trial – 1-year patency of PTFE vascular prostheses with heparin-bonded luminal surfaces compared to ordinary pure PTFE vascular prostheses – a randomised clinical controlled multi-centre trial. Eur J Vasc Endovasc Surg 2011;41:668–73.

14. Dorigo W, Pulli R, Castelli P, et al. A multicenter comparison between autologous saphenous vein and heparin-bonded expanded polytetrafluoroethylene (ePTFE) graft in the treatment of critical limb ischemia in diabetics. J Vasc Surg 2011;54:1332–8.

15. Moody AP, Edwards PR, Harris PL. In situ versus reversed femoropopliteal vein grafts: long-term follow-up of a prospective, randomized trial. Br J Surg 1992;79:750–2.

16. Wengerter KR, Veith FJ, Gupta SK, et al. Prospective randomized multicenter comparison of in situ and reversed vein infrapopliteal bypasses. J Vasc Surg 1991;13:189–99.

17. Albers M, Romiti M, Brochado-Neto FC, et al. Meta-analysis of popliteal-to-distal vein bypass grafts for critical ischemia. J Vasc Surg 2006;43:498–503.

18. Gibbons CP, Osman HY, Shiralkar S. The use of alternative sources of autologous vein for infrainguinal bypass. Eur J Vasc Endovasc Surg 2003;25:93–4.

19. Vauclair F, Haller C, Marques-Vidal P, et al. Infrainguinal bypass for peripheral arterial occlusive disease: when arms save legs. Eur J Vasc Endovasc Surg 2012;43(1):48–53.

20. Arvela E, Soderstrom M, Alback A, et al. Arm vein conduit vs prosthetic graft in infrainguinal revascularization for critical leg ischemia. J Vasc Surg 2010;52:616–23.

21. Twine CP, McLain AD. Graft type for femoro-popliteal bypass surgery. Cochrane Database Syst Rev 2010;CD001487.

22. Jackson MR, Belott TP, Dickason T, et al. The consequences of a failed femoropopliteal bypass grafting: comparison of saphenous vein and PTFE grafts. J Vasc Surg 2000;32:498–505.

23. Smeets L, Ho GH, Tangelder MJ, et al. Outcome after occlusion of infrainguinal bypasses in the Dutch BOA Study: comparison of amputation rate in venous and prosthetic grafts. Eur J Vasc Endovasc Surg 2005;30:604–9.

24. Seeger JM, Pretus HA, Carlton LC, et al. Potential predictors of outcome in patients with tissue loss who undergo infrainguinal vein bypass grafting. J Vasc Surg 1999;30:427–35.

25. Ulus AT, Ljungman C, Almgren B, et al. The influence of distal runoff on patency of infrainguinal vein bypass grafts. Vasc Surg 2001;35:31–5.

26. Nasr MK, McCarthy RJ, Budd JS, et al. Infrainguinal bypass graft patency and limb salvage rates in critical limb ischemia: influence of the mode of presentation. Ann Vasc Surg 2003;17:192–7.

27. Willigendael EM, Teijink JA, Bartelink ML, et al. Smoking and the patency of lower extremity bypass grafts: a meta-analysis. J Vasc Surg 2005;42:67–74.

28. Albers M, Romiti M, Braganca Pereira CA, et al. A meta-analysis of infrainguinal arterial reconstruction in patients with end-stage renal disease. Eur J Vasc Endovasc Surg 2001;22:294–300.

29. Wolfle KD, Bruijnen H, Loeprecht H, et al. Graft patency and clinical outcome of femorodistal arterial reconstruction in diabetic and non-diabetic patients: results of a multicentre comparative analysis. Eur J Vasc Endovasc Surg 2003;25:229–34.

30. Cheshire NJ, Wolfe JH, Barradas MA, et al. Smoking and plasma fibrinogen, lipoprotein (a) and serotonin are markers for postoperative infrainguinal graft stenosis. Eur J Vasc Endovasc Surg 1996;11:479–86.

31. Aleksic M, Jahn P, Heckenkamp J, et al. Comparison of the prevalence of APC-resistance in vascular patients and in a normal population cohort in Western Germany. Eur J Vasc Endovasc Surg 2005;30:160–3.

32. Sampram ES, Lindblad B. The impact of factor V mutation on the risk for occlusion in patients undergoing peripheral vascular reconstructions. Eur J Vasc Endovasc Surg 2001;22:134–8.

33. Nguyen LL, Hevelone N, Rogers SO, et al. Disparity in outcomes of surgical revascularization for limb salvage: race and gender are synergistic determinants of vein graft failure and limb loss. Circulation 2009;119:123–30.

34. Timaran CH, Stevens SL, Grandas OH, et al. Influence of hormone replacement therapy on graft patency after femoropopliteal bypass grafting. J Vasc Surg 2000;32:506–18.

35. Watson HR, Schroeder TV, Simms MH, et al. Association of sex with patency of femorodistal bypass grafts. Eur J Vasc Endovasc Surg 2000;20:61–6.

36. Brown J, Lethaby A, Maxwell H, et al. Antiplatelet agents for preventing thrombosis after peripheral arterial bypass surgery. Cochrane Database Syst Rev 2008;CD000535.

37. Dutch BOA trial. Efficacy of oral anticoagulants compared with aspirin after infrainguinal bypass surgery (the Dutch Bypass Oral Anticoagulants or Aspirin Study): a randomised trial. Lancet 2000;355:346–51.

38. Belch JJ, Dormandy J, Biasi GM, et al. Results of the randomized, placebo-controlled clopidogrel and acetylsalicylic acid in bypass surgery for peripheral arterial disease (CASPAR) trial. J Vasc Surg 2010;52:825–33, 33 e1–2.

39. Golledge J, Beattie DK, Greenhalgh RM, et al. Have the results of infrainguinal bypass improved with the widespread utilisation of postoperative surveillance? Eur J Vasc Endovasc Surg 1996;11:388–92.

40. Davies AH, Hawdon AJ, Sydes MR, et al. Is duplex surveillance of value after leg vein bypass grafting? Principal results of the Vein Graft Surveillance Randomised Trial (VGST). Circulation 2005;112:1985–91.

41. Berceli SA, Hevelone ND, Lipsitz SR, et al. Surgical and endovascular revision of infrainguinal vein bypass grafts: analysis of midterm outcomes from the PREVENT III trial. J Vasc Surg 2007;46:1173–9.

42. Carlson GA, Hoballah JJ, Sharp WJ, et al. Balloon angioplasty as a treatment of failing infrainguinal autologous vein bypass grafts. J Vasc Surg 2004;39:421–6.

43. Simosa HF, Pomposelli FB, Dahlberg S, et al. Predictors of failure after angioplasty of infrainguinal vein bypass grafts. J Vasc Surg 2009;49:117–21.

44. Garvin R, Reifsnyder T. Cutting balloon angioplasty of autogenous infrainguinal bypasses: short-term safety and efficacy. J Vasc Surg 2007;46:724–30.

45. Schneider PA, Caps MT, Nelken N. Infrainguinal vein graft stenosis: cutting balloon angioplasty as the first-line treatment of choice. J Vasc Surg 2008;47:960–6.

46. Vikram R, Ross RA, Bhat R, et al. Cutting balloon angioplasty versus standard balloon angioplasty for failing infra-inguinal vein grafts: comparative study of short- and mid-term primary patency rates. Cardiovasc Intervent Radiol 2007;30:607–10.

47. Duda SH, Bosiers M, Lammer J, et al. Drug-eluting and bare nitinol stents for the treatment of atherosclerotic lesions in the superficial femoral artery: long-term results from the SIROCCO trial. J Endovasc Ther 2006;13:701–10.

48. Dake MD, Ansel GM, Jaff MR, et al. Paclitaxel-eluting stents show superiority to balloon angioplasty and bare metal stents in femoropopliteal disease: twelve-month Zilver PTX randomized study results. Circ Cardiovasc Interv 2011;4:495–504.

49. Comerota AJ, Weaver FA, Hosking JD, et al. Results of a prospective, randomized trial of surgery versus thrombolysis for occluded lower extremity bypass grafts. Am J Surg 1996;172:105–12.

50. Braithwaite BD, Buckenham TM, Galland RB, et al. Prospective randomized trial of high-dose bolus versus low-dose tissue plasminogen activator infusion in the management of acute limb ischaemia. Thrombolysis Study Group. Br J Surg 1997;84:646–50.

51. Muller-Hulsbeck S, Order BM, Jahnke T. Interventions in infrainguinal bypass grafts. Cardiovasc Intervent Radiol 2006;29:17–28.

52. Aburahma AF, Hopkins ES, Wulu Jr JT, et al. Lysis/balloon angioplasty versus thrombectomy/open patch angioplasty of failed femoropopliteal polytetrafluoroethylene bypass grafts. J Vasc Surg 2002;35:307–15.

53. Richards T, Pittathankal AA, Magee TR, et al. The current role of intra-arterial thrombolysis. Eur J Vasc Endovasc Surg 2003;26:166–9.

54. Tiek J, Fourneau I, Daenens K, et al. The role of thrombolysis in acute infrainguinal bypass occlusion: a prospective nonrandomized controlled study. Ann Vasc Surg 2009;23:179–85.

55. Ricco JB, Probst H. Long-term results of a multicenter randomized study on direct versus crossover bypass for unilateral iliac artery occlusive disease. J Vasc Surg 2008;47:45–54.

56. Comerota AJ, Sidhu R. Can intraoperative thrombolytic therapy assist with the management of acute limb ischemia? Semin Vasc Surg 2009;22:47–51.

57. Gawenda M, Prokop A, Walter M, et al. The compartment syndrome with special reference to vascular surgery aspects. A patient sample of the Cologne University Clinic 1981 to 1991. Zentralbl Chir 1992;117:432–8.

58. Jensen SL, Sandermann J. Compartment syndrome and fasciotomy in vascular surgery. A review of 57 cases. Eur J Vasc Endovasc Surg 1997;13:48–53.

59. Yeager RA, Porter JM. Arterial and prosthetic graft infection. Ann Vasc Surg 1992;6:485–91.

60. Naylor AR, Hayes PD, Darke S. A prospective audit of complex wound and graft infections in Great Britain and Ireland: the emergence of MRSA. Eur J Vasc Endovasc Surg 2001;21:289–94.

61. Herscu G, Wilson SE. Prosthetic infection: lessons from treatment of the infected vascular graft. Surg Clin North Am 2009;89:391–401, viii.

62. Greenblatt DY, Rajamanickam V, Mell MW. Predictors of surgical site infection after open lower extremity revascularization. J Vasc Surg 2011;54:433–9.

63. Turtiainen J, Saimanen E, Partio T, et al. Surgical wound infections after vascular surgery: prospective multicenter observational study. Scand J Surg 2010;99:167–72.

64. Stewart A, Eyers PS, Earnshaw JJ. Prevention of infection in arterial reconstruction. Cochrane Database Syst Rev 2006;3:CD003073.

65. Gao H, Sandermann J, Prag J, et al. Prevention of primary vascular graft infection with silver-coated polyester graft in a porcine model. Eur J Vasc Endovasc Surg 2010;39:472–7.

66. Larena-Avellaneda A, Russmann S, Fein M, et al. Prophylactic use of the silver-acetate-coated graft in arterial occlusive disease: a retrospective, comparative study. J Vasc Surg 2009;50:790–8.

67. Webster J, Osborne S. Preoperative bathing or showering with skin antiseptics to prevent surgical site infection. Cochrane Database Syst Rev 2007; CD004985.

68. Szilagyi DE, Smith RF, Elliott JP, et al. Infection in arterial reconstruction with synthetic grafts. Ann Surg 1972;176:321–33.

69. Menawat SS, Gloviczki P, Serry RD, et al. Management of aortic graft-enteric fistulae. Eur J Vasc Endovasc Surg 1997;14(Suppl. A):74–81.

70. Hicks RC, Greenhalgh RM. The pathogenesis of vascular graft infection. Eur J Vasc Endovasc Surg 1997;14(Suppl. A):5–9.

71. Orton DF, LeVeen RF, Saigh JA, et al. Aortic prosthetic graft infections: radiologic manifestations and implications for management. Radiographics 2000;20:977–93.

72. Bunt TJ. Vascular graft infections: an update. Cardiovasc Surg 2001;9:225–33.

73. Becquemin JP, Qvarfordt P, Kron J, et al. Aortic graft infection: is there a place for partial graft removal? Eur J Vasc Endovasc Surg 1997;14(Suppl. A):53–8.

74. Calligaro KD, Veith FJ, Yuan JG, et al. Intra-abdominal aortic graft infection: complete or partial graft preservation in patients at very high risk. J Vasc Surg 2003;38:1199–205.

75. Hart JP, Eginton MT, Brown KR, et al. Operative strategies in aortic graft infections: is complete graft excision always necessary? Ann Vasc Surg 2005;19:154–60.

76. Kieffer E, Gomes D, Chiche L, et al. Allograft replacement for infrarenal aortic graft infection: early and late results in 179 patients. J Vasc Surg 2004;39:1009–17.

77. O'Connor S, Andrew P, Batt M, et al. A systematic review and meta-analysis of treatments for aortic graft infection. J Vasc Surg 2006;44:38–45.

78. Clagett GP, Valentine RJ, Hagino RT. Autogenous aortoiliac/femoral reconstruction from superficial femoral-popliteal veins: feasibility and durability. J Vasc Surg 1997;25:255–70.

79. Verhelst R, Lacroix V, Vraux H, et al. Use of cryopreserved arterial homografts for management of infected prosthetic grafts: a multicentric study. Ann Vasc Surg 2000;14:602–7.

80. Batt M, Magne JL, Alric P, et al. In situ revascularization with silver-coated polyester grafts to treat aortic infection: early and midterm results. J Vasc Surg 2003;38:983–9.

81. Nasim A, Hayes P, London N, et al. Vascular surgical society of Great Britain and Ireland: In situ replacement of infected aortic grafts with rifampicin-bonded prostheses. Br J Surg 1999;86:695.

82. Legout L, Sarraz-Bournet B, D'Elia PV, et al. Characteristics and prognosis in patients with prosthetic vascular graft infection: a prospective observational cohort study. Clin Microbiol Infect 2012;18:352–8.

83. Batt M, Jean-Baptiste E, O'Connor S, et al. In-situ revascularisation for patients with aortic graft infection: a single centre experience with silver coated polyester grafts. Eur J Vasc Endovasc Surg 2008;36:182–8.

84. Daenens K, Fourneau I, Nevelsteen A. Ten-year experience in autogenous reconstruction with the femoral vein in the treatment of aortofemoral prosthetic infection. Eur J Vasc Endovasc Surg 2003;25:240–5.

85. Nevelsteen A, Lacroix H, Suy R. Autogenous reconstruction with the lower extremity deep veins: an alternative treatment of prosthetic infection after reconstructive surgery for aortoiliac disease. J Vasc Surg 1995;22:129–34.

86. Modrall JG, Sadjadi J, Ali AT, et al. Deep vein harvest: predicting need for fasciotomy. J Vasc Surg 2004;39:387–94.

87. Nevelsteen A, Baeyens I, Daenens K, et al. Regarding "Deep vein harvest: predicting need for fasciotomy". J Vasc Surg 2004;40:403–4.

88. Danneels MI, Verhagen HJ, Teijink JA, et al. Endovascular repair for aorto-enteric fistula: a bridge too far or a bridge to surgery? Eur J Vasc Endovasc Surg 2006;32:27–33.

89. Antoniou GA, Koutsias S, Antoniou SA, et al. Outcome after endovascular stent graft repair of aortoenteric fistula: a systematic review. J Vasc Surg 2009;49:782–9.

90. Ducasse E, Calisti A, Speziale F, et al. Aortoiliac stent graft infection: current problems and management. Ann Vasc Surg 2004;18:521–6.

91. Hobbs SD, Kumar S, Gilling-Smith GL. Epidemiology and diagnosis of endograft infection. J Cardiovasc Surg (Torino) 2010;51:5–14.

92. Numan F, Gulsen F, Solak S, et al. Management of endograft infections. J Cardiovasc Surg (Torino) 2011; 52:205–23.

93. Nevelsteen A, Smet G, Wilms G, et al. Intravenous digital subtraction angiography and Duplex scanning in the detection of late human umbilical vein degeneration. Br J Surg 1988;75:668–70.

94. Van Damme H, Deprez M, Creemers E, et al. Intrinsic structural failure of polyester (Dacron) vascular grafts. A general review. Acta Chir Belg 2005;105:249–55.

95. White GH, Donayre CE, Williams RA, et al. Exertional disruption of axillofemoral graft anastomosis. 'The axillary pullout syndrome'. Arch Surg 1990;125:625–7.

96. Jones 3rd WT, Hagino RT, Chiou AC, et al. Graft patency is not the only clinical predictor of success after exclusion and bypass of popliteal artery aneurysms. J Vasc Surg 2003;37:392–8.

97. Tisi PV, Callam MJ. Treatment for femoral pseudoaneurysms. Cochrane Database Syst Rev 2009;CD004981.

98. Maleux G, Hendrickx S, Vaninbroukx J, et al. Percutaneous injection of human thrombin to treat iatrogenic femoral pseudoaneurysms: short- and midterm ultrasound follow-up. Eur Radiol 2003;13:209–12.

99. Szilagyi DE, Smith RF, Elliott JP, et al. Anastomotic aneurysms after vascular reconstruction: problems of incidence, etiology, and treatment. Surgery 1975;78:800–16.

100. Nevelsteen A, Suy R. Anastomotic false aneurysms of the abdominal aorta and the iliac arteries. J Vasc Surg 1989;10:595.

101. Gawenda M, Prokop A, Sorgatz S, et al. Anastomotic aneurysms following aortofemoral vascular replacement. Thorac Cardiovasc Surg 1994;42:51–4.

102. Derom A, Nout E. Treatment of femoral pseudoaneurysms with endograft in high-risk patients. Eur J Vasc Endovasc Surg 2005;30:644–7.

103. Curti T, Stella A, Rossi C, et al. Endovascular repair as first-choice treatment for anastomotic and true iliac aneurysms. J Endovasc Ther 2001;8:139–43.

104. Tielliu IF, Verhoeven EL, Zeebregts CJ, et al. Endovascular treatment of iliac artery aneurysms with a tubular stent-graft: mid-term results. J Vasc Surg 2006;43:440–5.

105. Pavlidis D, Hörmann M, Libicher M, et al. Buttock claudication after interventional occlusion of the hypogastric artery – a mid-term follow up. Vasc Endovascular Surg 2012;46:236–41.

106. Mii S, Mori A, Sakata H, et al. Para-anastomotic aneurysms: incidence, risk factors, treatment and prognosis. J Cardiovasc Surg (Torino) 1998;39:259–66.

107. Mulder EJ, van Bockel JH, Maas J, et al. Morbidity and mortality of reconstructive surgery of noninfected false aneurysms detected long after aortic prosthetic reconstruction. Arch Surg 1998;133:45–9.

108. Piffaretti G, Tozzi M, Lomazzi C, et al. Endovascular treatment for para-anastomotic abdominal aortic and iliac aneurysms following aortic surgery. J Cardiovasc Surg (Torino) 2007;48:711–7.

109. Sachdev U, Baril DT, Morrissey NJ, et al. Endovascular repair of para-anastomotic aortic aneurysms. J Vasc Surg 2007;46:636–41.

110. Gawenda M, Zaehringer M, Brunkwall J. Open versus endovascular repair of para-anastomotic aneurysms in patients who were morphological candidates for endovascular treatment. J Endovasc Ther 2003;10:745–51.

111. Ten Bosch JA, Waasdorp EJ, de Vries JP, et al. The durability of endovascular repair of para-anastomotic aneurysms after previous open aortic reconstruction. J Vasc Surg 2011;54:1571–8.

112. van Herwaarden JA, Waasdorp EJ, Bendermacher BL, et al. Endovascular repair of para-anastomotic aneurysms after previous open aortic prosthetic reconstruction. Ann Vasc Surg 2004;18:280–6.

113. Stone PA, Srivastava M, Campbell JE, et al. A 10-year experience of infection following carotid endarterectomy with patch angioplasty. J Vasc Surg 2011;53:1473–7.

114. O'Hara PJ, Hertzer NR, Krajewski LP, et al. Saphenous vein patch rupture after carotid endarterectomy. J Vasc Surg 1992;15:504–9.

115. Becquemin JP, Kelley L, Zubilewicz T, et al. Outcomes of secondary interventions after abdominal aortic aneurysm endovascular repair. J Vasc Surg 2004;39:298–305.

116. Kolvenbach R, Pinter L, Raghunandan M, et al. Laparoscopic remodeling of abdominal aortic aneurysms after endovascular exclusion: a technical description. J Vasc Surg 2002;36:1267–70.

117. van Nes JG, Hendriks JM, Tseng LN, et al. Endoscopic aneurysm sac fenestration as a treatment option for growing aneurysms due to type II endoleak or endotension. J Endovasc Ther 2005;12:430–4.

118. Moulakakis KG, Dalainas I, Mylonas S, et al. Conversion to open repair after endografting for abdominal aortic aneurysm: a review of causes, incidence, results, and surgical techniques of reconstruction. J Endovasc Ther 2010;17:694–702.

119. Lawrence-Brown MM, Hartley D, MacSweeney ST, et al. The Perth endoluminal bifurcated graft system – development and early experience. Cardiovasc Surg 1996;4:706–12.

120. Bockler D, Probst T, Weber H, et al. Surgical conversion after endovascular grafting for abdominal aortic aneurysms. J Endovasc Ther 2002;9:111–8.

121. Lifeline Registry. Lifeline registry of endovascular aneurysm repair: long-term primary outcome measures. J Vasc Surg 2005;42:1–10.

122. Verzini F, Cao P, De Rango P, et al. Conversion to open repair after endografting for abdominal aortic aneurysm: causes, incidence and results. Eur J Vasc Endovasc Surg 2006;31:136–42.

123. Chiesa R, Melissano G, Marone EM, et al. Aortooesophageal and aortobronchial fistulae following thoracic endovascular aortic repair: a national survey. Eur J Vasc Endovasc Surg 2010;39:273–9.

124. Jonker FH, Schlosser FJ, Moll FL, et al. Outcomes of thoracic endovascular aortic repair for aortobronchial and aortoesophageal fistulas. J Endovasc Ther 2009;16:428–40.

8

Management of acute lower limb ischaemia

Robert J. Hinchliffe
Johannes Lammer

Introduction

☑☑ The revised (2007) TASC Inter-Society Consensus defines acute leg ischaemia (ALI) as any sudden decrease in limb perfusion causing a potential threat to limb viability.[1]

Presentation is usually less than 2 weeks' duration. However, some overlap with chronic critical leg ischaemia is inevitable. The severity of ischaemia is best defined according to the SVS/ISCVS guidelines (Table 8.1),[2] which group patients into the following categories:

- I Viable.
- IIa Threatened (salvageable if promptly treated).
- IIb Threatened (salvageable if immediately treated).
- III Irreversible.

Data on the incidence of acute limb ischaemia are sparse. Epidemiological surveys would suggest that the incidence is in the region of 140 per million of the general population and this figure appears to be increasing.[1] There is evidence that the outcome is improved when patients are managed by a vascular service providing 24-hour cover.[3] ALI is associated with a high cost to the community because of the risk of amputation (10–30% at 30 days) and prolonged hospitalisation. Costs are minimised and outcome optimised by accurate clinical assessment and an understanding of the available therapeutic options.

Aetiology

ALI is the result of occlusion of a native artery or vascular/endovascular prosthesis. In situ thrombosis or embolism can cause native arterial occlusion (Box 8.1).

Embolism

Until about 30 years ago, embolism was the underlying cause of most cases of ALI. Emboli large enough to occlude major vessels usually arise in the heart. Rheumatic mitral valve disease was the most common cause, with large emboli forming in a dilated left atrium. Atrial fibrillation due to ischaemic heart disease is now the cardiac origin in 80% of embolic cases; mural thrombus following acute myocardial infarction causes most of the remainder.[4] Less commonly, embolisations from mural thrombi of the aorta, aortic aneurysms and iliac arteries are observed. Large emboli typically lodge at an arterial bifurcation, particularly in the common femoral or popliteal arteries (**Fig. 8.1**). Patients with cardiac embolism may also suffer from peripheral vascular disease as a result of the underlying process of atherosclerosis. This increases the difficulty in establishing the cause of the ischaemia and in planning revascularisation. In 20% of patients with ALI, a source for the embolus cannot be found.

Atheroembolism

Less common sources of emboli include proximal aneurysms or atherosclerotic plaques, usually located in the thoracic or abdominal aorta. Whereas cardiac

Table 8.1 • Suggested classification of acute limb ischaemia

| Category | Description | Capillary return | Muscle paralysis | Sensory loss | Doppler signals | |
					Arterial	Venous
I Viable	Not immediately threatened	Intact	None	None	Audible	Audible
IIa Threatened	Salvageable if promptly treated	Intact/slow	None	Partial	Inaudible	Audible
IIb Threatened	Salvageable if immediately treated	Slow/absent	Partial	Partial/complete	Inaudible	Audible
III Irreversible	Primary amputation	Absent staining	Complete tense compartment	Complete	Inaudible	Inaudible

Reprinted from Rutherford RB, Flanigan DP, Gupta SK et al. Suggested standards for reports dealing with lower extremity ischemia. J Vasc Surg 1986; 4:80–94, with permission from Society for Vascular Surgery.

Box 8.1 • Aetiology of acute lower limb ischaemia

Thrombosis
- Atherosclerosis
- Popliteal aneurysm
- Bypass graft occlusion
- Endovascular stent or stent graft occlusion
- Iatrogenic (localised arterial dissection post endovascular intervention, e.g. arterial closure device failure)
- Thrombotic conditions

Embolism
- Atrial fibrillation
- Mural thrombosis
- Vegetations
- Proximal aneurysms
- Atherosclerotic plaque

Rare causes
- Dissection
- Trauma (including iatrogenic)
- Illicit drug use
- External compression
- Popliteal entrapment
- Cystic adventitial disease
- Iliac endofibrosis

embolism usually consists entirely of platelet thrombus, embolism from proximal arteries can include atherosclerotic plaques or cholesterol-rich emboli. This has a much worse prognosis than cardiac embolism because embolectomy is less effective. Small particles of atheroembolism can pass to very distal vessels in the foot. This digital embolism can result in the 'acute blue toe syndrome'. In this condition,

the embolic source should be identified and treated if possible. Often this is a proximal arterial plaque that has ruptured and the emboli are a mixture of platelet thrombus and cholesterol (**Fig. 8.2**). Embolisation of cholesterol-rich atheroma can occur spontaneously, but also follows intravascular manipulation by endovascular intervention, or occasionally surgery (trash foot). This can be disastrous, since both large and small arteries are occluded and cannot be reopened with either surgery or thrombolysis. This often results in limb or end-organ damage, and is sometimes fatal (**Fig. 8.3**).

Thrombosis

In situ thrombosis in a native artery is now the commonest cause of ALI. It may be the result of rupture of an atherosclerotic plaque or critical flow arrest at the site of an atherosclerotic stenosis. The advancing age of the population and the commensurate increase in atherosclerosis explain the rising incidence of ALI. Acute native vessel arterial occlusion may be compounded by surgery (e.g. knee replacement destroying geniculate collateral vessels formed around a popliteal occlusion), heart failure or a thrombotic tendency (polycythaemia, dehydration, malignancy, etc.). Acute thrombosis of a popliteal aneurysm poses the highest risk to the leg. Typically, this occurs in elderly men in association with aneurysms elsewhere (50% have an aortic aneurysm) or generalised arterial ectasia. Popliteal aneurysms usually commence in the above-knee popliteal artery and extend distally to the tibial trifurcation. As they enlarge they can fill with lamellar thrombus, which may cause either acute thrombosis or distal embolisation that occludes the tibial vessels. The latter will place the leg in extreme jeopardy (50% limb loss).

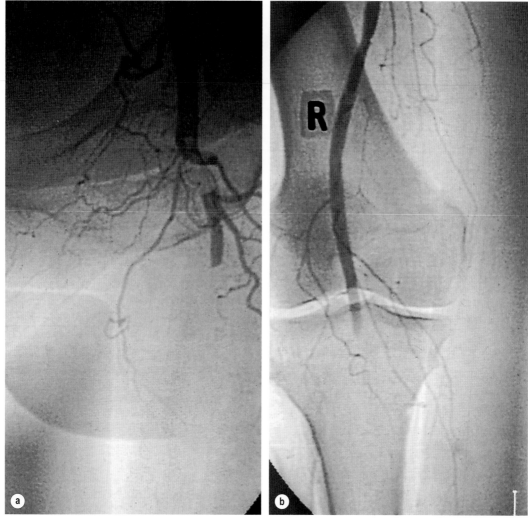

Figure 8.1 • Arteriogram demonstrating an embolus lodged in the bifurcation of the common femoral artery **(a)** with further emboli occluding the distal profunda and popliteal artery **(b)**.

Other causes

The increasing use of both open and endovascular techniques to revascularise ischaemic limbs means that surgeons often have to deal with acute thrombosis of bypass grafts and arteries that have previously undergone endovascular treatment. Grafts occlude for a variety of reasons. Graft occlusion within 1 month of insertion is usually the result of technical problems at the time of surgery or poor distal run-off. Graft occlusion within 1 year of placement is often caused by myointimal hyperplasia at an anastomosis or the development of stenoses within a vein graft. Occlusion after 1 year is usually due to progression of distal atherosclerosis. Prosthetic grafts have a higher occlusion rate than autogenous vein grafts (see Chapters 3 and 7).

Iliac limb occlusions are observed after aortobi-femoral bypass surgery if limbs become kinked or have poor outflow and after for similar reasons endovascular stent grafts are used to repair abdominal aortic aneurysms. Occlusion is more common when the iliac limb of the stent graft is extended in to the external iliac artery. Occlusion may occur any time after implantation in up to 5% of patients.[5]

A special group of iatrogenic occlusion of external iliac and femoral vessels is related to the mal-deployment or failure of arterial closure devices. These achieve closure of arteries after endovascular intervention using percutaneously delivered sutures or plugs. Inadvertently they can cause arrest of flow through direct closure or stenosis of the artery, or by dissection of the vessel. Presentation is usually in the early post-intervention period but may be delayed.

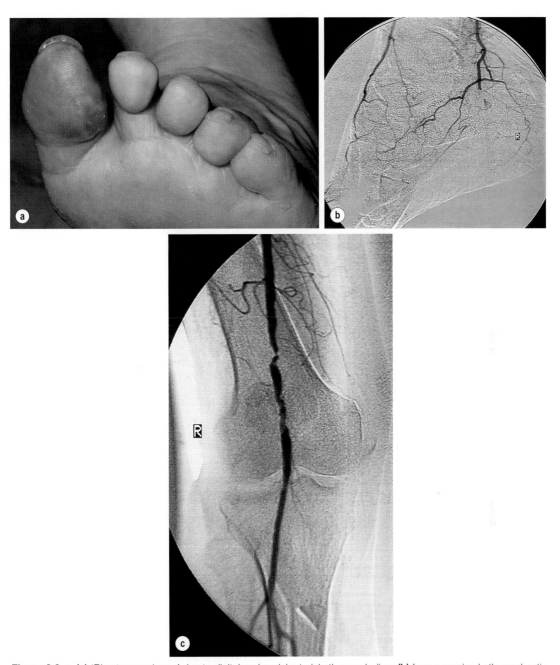

Figure 8.2 • (a) 'Blue toe syndrome' due to digital and pedal arterial atheroembolism **(b)** from a proximal atherosclerotic stenosis **(c)**. Note the acute cut-off of the posterior tibial artery. Ultrasonography excluded a popliteal aneurysm and the lesion was treated by balloon angioplasty.

Spontaneous native arterial thrombosis occasionally occurs without an underlying flow-limiting stenosis and these patients should be investigated for an intrinsic clotting abnormality/thrombophilia, e.g. antiphospholipid syndrome, activated protein C deficiency or malignancy.

Occasionally, acute arterial occlusion may be due to arterial dissection, trauma, extrinsic compression or illicit drug use (cocaine and 'crack' cocaine). In a young patient with acute popliteal artery occlusion, either popliteal entrapment or cystic adventitial disease should be considered (see chapter on chronic limb ischaemia).

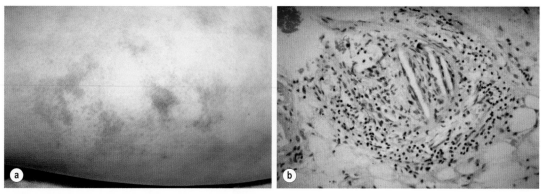

Figure 8.3 • Livedo reticularis **(a)** caused by cholesterol embolism **(b)**.

Recent changes

A number of factors may have changed the presentation of ALI. For example, many patients are now treated with risk factor-modifying drugs such as antiplatelet therapy and statins. Antiplatelet therapy probably reduces the risk of limb deterioration and the need for limb revascularisation in those patients with established peripheral arterial disease (PAD).[6] It is not yet clear whether this has had an effect on the incidence of ALI. Similarly, patients with atrial fibrillation are currently treated with prophylactic warfarin to prevent stroke according to their CHADS(2) risk score.[7] Whilst this does not entirely prevent peripheral embolisation, it can make the acute ischaemia easier to deal with, since there is less secondary thrombosis, particularly affecting small distal arteries.

Clinical features

The severity of ischaemia at presentation is the most important factor affecting outcome of the leg.[8,9] Complete occlusion of a proximal artery in the absence of preformed collateral vessels (as in cardiac embolism) results in the classical clinical presentation of pain, paralysis, paraesthesia, pallor, pulselessness and a perishingly cold leg. The pain is severe and frequently resistant to analgesia. Calf pain and tenderness with a tense muscle compartment indicates severe muscle ischaemia or necrosis and often irreversible ischaemia. Sensorimotor deficit including muscle paralysis and paraesthesia is indicative of muscle and nerve ischaemia with the potential for salvage if treated promptly. Initially the leg is white with empty veins but after 6–12 hours vasodilatation occurs, probably caused by hypoxia of the smooth muscle. The capillaries then fill with stagnant deoxygenated blood, resulting in a mottled appearance

that blanches on digital pressure (**Fig. 8.4**). If flow is not restored rapidly, the arteries distal to the occlusion fill with propagated thrombus and the capillaries rupture, resulting in a fixed blue staining of the skin that is a sign of irreversible ischaemia. These features are typical of an acute arterial occlusion in the absence of existing collaterals and suggest an embolic cause. When arterial occlusion occurs as part of a chronic process where collaterals have developed, typically the leg is less severely ischaemic. Patients with peripheral atherosclerosis deteriorate in a stepwise fashion as thrombosis supervenes on an existing arterial plaque. Patients often report a sudden change in symptoms, which progress over a few days: the foot often has a dusky hue with slow capillary return. Previous claudication or absent pulses in the contralateral foot help make a clinical diagnosis of in situ thrombosis. Palpation of a mass in either popliteal fossa suggests thrombosis of a popliteal aneurysm. Young patients (<50 years), those with an atypical history (e.g. severe back pain associated with aortic dissection) or recent endovascular intervention raise the possibility of non-atherosclerotic/embolic ALI.

Initial management

Patients presenting with ALI are often in poor general health, which contributes to the observed high mortality rate from associated cardiovascular disease. Dehydration, cardiac failure, hypoxia and pain should all be managed in the standard way. An intravenous infusion is required for rehydration and is also often the best means of providing analgesia with an infusion pump. If thrombolysis is an option, intramuscular analgesia should be avoided because of the risk of bleeding. Intravenous calcium heparin (5000 units) should be given immediately, followed by systemic heparinisation, principally to restrict

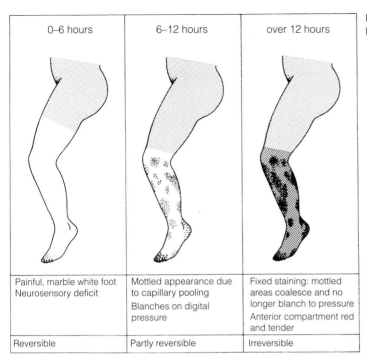

0–6 hours	6–12 hours	over 12 hours
Painful, marble white foot Neurosensory deficit	Mottled appearance due to capillary pooling Blanches on digital pressure	Fixed staining: mottled areas coalesce and no longer blanch to pressure Anterior compartment red and tender
Reversible	Partly reversible	Irreversible

Figure 8.4 • Clinical outcome after acute leg ischaemia.

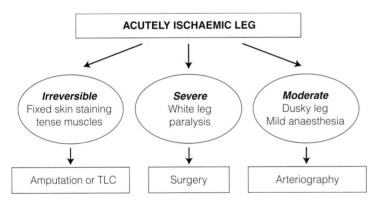

ACUTELY ISCHAEMIC LEG

Irreversible
Fixed skin staining
tense muscles

Severe
White leg
paralysis

Moderate
Dusky leg
Mild anaesthesia

Amputation or TLC

Surgery

Arteriography

Figure 8.5 • Clinical approach to the management of the acutely ischaemic leg.

propagation of thrombus, although there is also evidence that it improves the prognosis.[10] In many units low-molecular-weight heparins have replaced calcium heparin because of their more reliable effect on anticoagulation. Anticoagulation should be delayed if the patient is likely to need epidural anaesthesia. The short half-life of the latter, however, is helpful in this situation. In order to improve oxygenation, 24% oxygen should be given by face mask.

Venous blood should be taken for full blood count, urea, electrolytes and glucose. An electrocardiogram (ECG) and chest radiograph may be of value in diagnosing and managing cardiac arrhythmias and heart failure. If a primary thrombotic tendency is suspected, investigation of this should be delayed as the diagnostic tests are inaccurate in the face of fresh thrombus.

Revascularisation

The clinical assessment of the severity of limb ischaemia will largely dictate the most appropriate form of therapy (**Fig. 8.5**).

Irreversible (category III) leg ischaemia

A small number of patients will present in a moribund state or with irreversible leg ischaemia (muscle paralysis, tense swollen fascial compartments, fixed skin staining) and terminal care should be considered. For the irreversibly ischaemic leg, revascularisation is, by definition, inappropriate and may be dangerous. This includes the patient who develops ALI while being treated for another condition, usually as an inpatient on an elderly care ward. Prognosis is particularly dismal in this group.[11] Surviving patients should be resuscitated and stabilised before considering amputation.

Immediately threatened (category IIb ischaemia)

The acute white leg with sensorimotor deficit requires urgent intervention to prevent limb loss. Although the differentiation between thrombosis and embolus is often difficult, it is in this group of patients that embolism is more likely. An acute white leg with no prior history of claudication, normal contralateral pulses and a probable embolic source, such as atrial fibrillation, would indicate that embolisation is the likely cause. Urgent surgery is indicated in these patients, after resuscitation. Thrombolysis is inappropriate, given the potential delay in revascularisation using this method. Imaging may help guide revascularisation but should not be allowed to delay revascularisation. Many vascular and trauma centres now have rapid access to computed tomography (CT) angiography, which is a useful investigation especially when the femoral pulse is absent and alternative diagnoses such as aortic dissection are possible. An alternative approach is to perform on-table angiography at the same time as groin exploration. Duplex ultrasound imaging is often unhelpful because of the low-flow state in the limb arteries and the need for expert interpretation in the emergency setting.

Both groins and lower limbs should be prepared in theatre. If inflow cannot be re-established into the groin then a femoral crossover graft can be inserted (or aortic dissection managed according to Chapter 9).

Threatened (category IIa ischaemia)/viable (category I ischaemia)

The majority of patients presenting with ALI have acute onset of rest pain but no paralysis and no, or only mild, sensory loss. The cause is often acute thrombosis of either an atherosclerotic artery or graft. Because the leg is not immediately threatened, time is available to plan appropriate intervention after investigation. Conventionally, acute leg ischaemia was investigated using catheter (Fig. 8.6). The advantage was that imaging could be followed by therapeutic thrombolysis at the same sitting. There are now, however, non-invasive alternatives such as duplex imaging CT and MR angiography, both of which can provide enough information on which to plan intervention. The method of investigation will depend on the time of presentation and the available facilities. The two main alternatives in these patients are intervention with surgery or percutaneous thrombolysis. Thromboembolectomy is unlikely to reopen an artery occluded by thrombus and atherosclerotic plaque; formal arterial bypass is more likely to be needed. Nationwide registries suggest that surgical revascularisation is used three to five times more frequently than thrombolysis in everyday clinical practice for patients with ALI.[12] Logistics (multiple angiographies) and experience may account in part for this distribution.

Thrombolysis is arguably less invasive than revascularisation surgery. It has the capacity to open

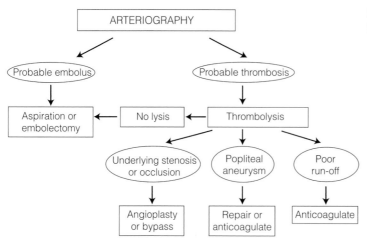

Figure 8.6 • Treatment pathways following arteriography.

small as well as large arteries. It may also uncover the cause of the in situ thrombosis, such as an arterial stenosis, which can be treated by angioplasty to produce a lasting outcome.

Some patients are admitted to hospital with acute thrombosis of a peripheral artery (usually the superficial femoral) but have only claudication and no ischaemic pain at rest. Thrombolysis might appear an attractive option to treat the claudication, but the risks are as high as in patients with limb-threatening ischaemia.[13] Initial anticoagulation followed by expectant management, depending on the progression of ischaemia, reduces the risk to both life and limb.[10] Some patients' symptoms improve and never require revascularisation. In others (especially those with short-distance claudication) it may be more appropriate to angioplasty the occluded arterial segment 6–12 weeks after the acute event, when the thrombus has organised and embolic risk is reduced.

Choice between surgery and thrombolysis: the evidence

There remains considerable controversy about the individual roles of surgery and thrombolysis for ALI. A review of 42 studies (most non-randomised) by Diffin and Kandarpa[14] suggested that thrombolysis was associated with substantially better limb salvage and mortality rates than surgery.

✓✓ There are three major randomised studies from which to draw harder evidence.[15–20] The New York study was the first to show that thrombolysis improves survival in patients with limb-threatening ischaemia of less than 14 days.[15] This study was small and the advantage was due to the high incidence of cardiorespiratory deaths following emergency surgery. The STILE study was much larger and included patients with ischaemia for longer than 14 days.[16] This study has been much criticised because of the failure to insert a catheter successfully for peripheral thrombolysis in one-third of cases. The study introduced the concept of amputation-free survival but failed to show any significant improvement in this primary end-point between the treatment groups. In the subgroup of patients with ischaemia for fewer than 14 days, thrombolysis reduced the rate of amputation. Subsequent analysis of patients from this study up to 1 year revealed that thrombolysis was a better initial treatment for graft occlusions, whereas surgery was more effective and durable for native vessel occlusions.[17,18] However, few of the patients in the STILE study had critical ischaemia. The TOPAS trial was designed, using lessons learned from the above studies, to try to settle this debate.

In the first phase, an optimal dose of thrombolytic therapy was selected (urokinase 4000IU/hour)[19] and in phase II this was compared with urgent surgery in 544 patients.[20] Amputation-free survival was similar in both groups at 6 months and 1 year (72% and 65% for urokinase vs. 75% and 70% for surgery, respectively), though thrombolysis reduced the need for open surgical procedures.

In conclusion, both surgery and thrombolysis seem effective and the choice should be made on an individual basis for each patient, taking into account the skills and experience available in the vascular unit.

Peripheral arterial thrombolysis

Thrombus dissolution is achieved by stimulating the conversion of fibrin-bound plasminogen into the active enzyme plasmin. Plasmin is a non-specific protease capable of degrading fibrin and producing thrombus dissolution.

In contrast to the thrombolytic treatment of acute myocardial infarction, systemic infusion of thrombolytic agents for ALI results in a poor success rate and unacceptable complications. By selectively placing a catheter within the thrombus via the percutaneous route and delivering the thrombolytic agent locally, the concentration of agent is maximised and plasmin is less likely to be neutralised by circulating antiplasmins. The dose of thrombolytic agent can be optimised to the minimum level that results in a local effect without producing systemic thrombolysis and the attendant complications.

Contraindications (Box 8.2)

Perhaps the only absolute contraindication to lysis is active internal bleeding. Most other contraindications

Box 8.2 • Contraindications to thrombolysis

- Active internal bleeding
- Pregnancy
- Stroke within 2 months
- Transient ischaemic attack within 2 months
- Known intracerebral tumour, aneurysm or arteriovenous malformation
- Severe bleeding tendency
- Craniotomy within 2 months
- Vascular surgery within 2 weeks
- Abdominal surgery within 2 weeks
- Puncture of a non-compressible vessel or biopsy within 10 days
- Previous gastrointestinal haemorrhage
- Trauma within 10 days

are relative, where the risk of complications from thrombolysis must be weighed against the potential benefits of limb salvage. The elderly (>80 years) are at particularly high risk of bleeding complications. It is unwise to consider thrombolysis within 2 weeks of surgery or within 2 months of a stroke. Dacron grafts may take 3 months to seal, and if they do not become fully incorporated they may become porous if thrombolytic therapy is employed. Care should be exercised when using thrombolysis to open Dacron grafts within the abdomen where manual compression is not possible should bleeding occur. The presence of cardiac thrombus theoretically increases the likelihood of systemic embolisation during thrombolysis, but there is no evidence that patient selection based on echocardiography affects management or outcome.

Technique

All patients should have adequate analgesia and a cannula inserted for venous access, analgesia and hydration. Patients should be managed in units where nursing and medical staff are experienced in thrombolysis and clear protocols exist to manage complications. A critical care environment is desirable for close monitoring during thrombolysis. The extent of occlusive disease needs to be defined by arteriography or duplex imaging before intervention. The number of arterial punctures should be kept to a minimum to reduce the risk of puncture-site bleeding during treatment. The initial diagnostic approach is tailored to the distribution of disease. If there is an absent femoral pulse in the affected leg but a palpable femoral pulse on the contralateral side, then it is reasonable to anticipate an iliac artery occlusion. In this situation, a contralateral femoral puncture will provide access for the diagnostic arteriogram and subsequently the iliac thrombosis can be approached from the same puncture site using a crossover technique (**Fig. 8.7**). If there is a normal femoral pulse on the side of acute ischaemia, then initial diagnostic information may be provided by CT angiography or duplex imaging. As long as adequate inflow can be confirmed using

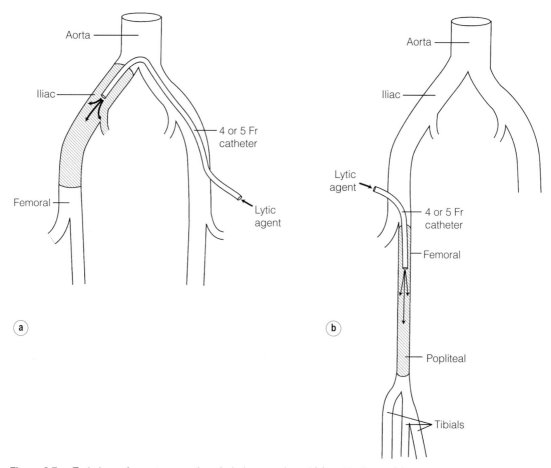

Figure 8.7 • Technique of percutaneous thrombolysis: contralateral **(a)** and ipsilateral **(b)** transfemoral approaches.

one of these methods, an antegrade puncture should be attempted to treat occlusions below the femoral bifurcation so that adjuvant procedures such as angioplasty or thrombus aspiration can be performed from the same side (Fig. 8.7). An occluded arterial bypass graft is optimally accessed from the native artery proximal to the graft so that any stenoses can be treated via the same puncture site. However, this is not always possible for technical reasons, although direct puncture of the most proximal accessible part of the graft results in a high success rate from thrombolysis. Once access has been achieved, a guidewire should be passed through the occlusion; indeed, the ability to do this implies the presence of soft thrombus and is a good predictor of success (guidewire traversal test). The catheter used to deliver the lytic agent is then placed within the thrombus.

Several techniques are described for delivering thrombolysis. The low-dose infusion method involves running the thrombolytic drug through the catheter over several hours. This may be combined with an initial high-dose bolus.

✔✔ More recently, high-dose techniques have been described that accelerate the rate of thrombus dissolution.[21] This may be achieved by administering a number of high-dose boluses sequentially or by using the 'pulse spray' technique.[18] The latter involves high-pressure injection of tiny pulses of lytic agent through a catheter with multiple side holes, and thus it combines enzymatic thrombolysis with mechanical disruption. The high-dose techniques accelerate thrombolysis and allow patients to be treated within the normal working hours of a radiology department.

Several randomised trials comparing low-dose and accelerated methods of thrombolysis have found that limb salvage rate and complication rates appear similar, though accelerated methods are quicker.[21–24]

Three drugs are currently available for peripheral thrombolysis: streptokinase, urokinase and tissue plasminogen activator (t-PA). Appropriate dose regimens are shown in Box 8.3.

✔✔ There are very few high-quality trials to determine which drug is most effective, but most agree that t-PA and urokinase are superior to streptokinase.[25] t-PA is the agent of choice in the UK; in North America, many vascular specialists preferred urokinase, but it has not been widely available due to manufacturing difficulties in the past few years.

Box 8.3 • Suggested drug regimens for thrombolysis

Slow infusion
- Streptokinase 5000 units/hour
- Tissue plasminogen activator (t-PA) 0.5 mg/hour
- Urokinase* 4000 IU/min for 2 hours, then 2000 IU/min for 2 hours, then 1000 IU/min

Pulsed spray
- t-PA 0.3 mg per pulse every 30 seconds
- Urokinase 5000 IU per pulse every 30 seconds

High-dose bolus
- t-PA 5-mg bolus every 10 min three times, then 3.5 mg/hour for up to 4 hours, then (if required) as for slow infusion

*Urokinase is not currently available.

The STILE trial suggested that urokinase and t-PA had equivalent activity,[16] and this was confirmed in unpublished manufacturers' data. Further randomised data would be helpful but cost considerations and availability largely determine the choice between urokinase and t-PA. A number of new agents such as staphylokinase and alfimeprase are under investigation, but as yet they have not been shown to be better than existing agents.

Heparin is often administered systemically before and after thrombolysis to counteract the associated prothrombotic tendency, although some data from trials of the thrombolytic treatment of acute stroke suggest that heparin may increase haemorrhagic complications. An alternative is concurrent administration of low-dose heparin (200 units/hour) via the proximal arterial sheath while delivering the thrombolytic agent via an end-hole catheter to an occlusion below the inguinal ligament. Heparin should be given routinely for 48 hours after completion of thrombolysis. Consideration will then be needed to determine whether individual patients need lifelong anticoagulation with warfarin. No data exist to guide appropriate therapy. Where contraindications exist to warfarin therapy, some clinicians use dual antiplatelet therapy, e.g. aspirin with clopidogrel, as an alternative. Thrombolysis should be considered a diagnostic process aimed at exposing the underlying flow-limiting lesion (**Fig. 8.8**). This should be found in the majority of patients using duplex ultrasonography of the suspect arterial segment. The majority of lesions can be managed by angioplasty or stent placement. Where the disease appears too extensive, surgical reconstruction may be required, particularly when an anastomotic stenosis results in graft occlusion.

ALI due to a popliteal aneurysm remains a difficult clinical problem. The bulk of thrombus within the aneurysm restricts the use of thrombolysis because

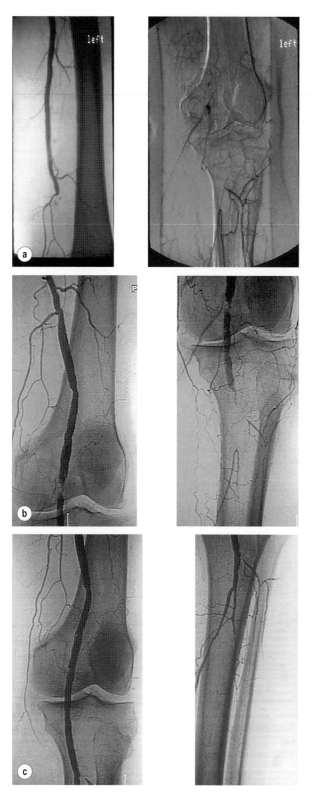

Figure 8.8 • (a) Arteriography demonstrates an occlusion of the popliteal artery extending into the tibial vessels. **(b)** Thrombolysis reveals a popliteal stenosis but persistent occlusion of the tibial trifurcation. **(c)** The stenosis was treated by balloon angioplasty and the thrombus aspirated from the tibial vessels using an aspiration catheter.

of the high risk of massive distal embolisation, the slow clearance and large amount of residual thrombus after recanalisation. If thrombolysis does have a role to play, then it is to open run-off vessels for distal bypass grafting. This is achieved by placing a catheter through the popliteal artery into a tibial vessel and then lysing it until a distal vessel becomes patent for bypass. Alternatively, urgent surgery may be performed with on-table angiography and thrombolysis to clear the run-off (see later).

Percutaneous thrombectomy devices

Percutaneous mechanical thrombectomy (PMT) devices have been developed to hasten thrombus removal and either replace the need for thrombolytic drugs or reduce the dose required.[26] The devices may be classified according to their mode of action. The most basic technique involves simply aspirating the thrombus by applying suction to a wide-bore catheter. Some devices simply macerate thrombus into particles so small that they are removed by natural fibrinolysis (e.g. Amplatz Thrombectomy™ Device). Others include a clot aspiration system based on the Bernoulii or Venturi principle to remove fragments of thrombus and prevent distal embolisation (e.g. Angiojet™). Ultrasound catheters use ultrasound energy to lyse thrombus (e.g. the Acolysis™ catheter). Thrombolysis is often required as a supplement after mechanical thrombectomy: in the Trellis Thrombectomy System, the occluded segment of artery is isolated by proximal and distal balloons. An oscillating wire fragments the thrombus while a thrombolytic infusion helps to dissolve it before the liquefied material is aspirated from the isolated segment. These devices are all expensive and disposable, and there is little consensus about their use. Few are licensed for use in peripheral arteries; manufacturers usually seek approval for thrombosed dialysis fistulas first. There is also the potential for further arterial damage during deployment, and large volumes of blood can be lost with the clot aspiration devices.

Complications

There are significant risks associated with percutaneous thrombolytic therapy, most of which can be attributed to the fragile health of the patients and their advanced systemic atherosclerosis. Myocardial infarction and stroke are the commonest causes of death. The rate of reported adverse outcomes is variable, depending on the condition of the patients treated. In the review by Diffin and Kandarpa, principally of North American articles, the mortality rate after thrombolysis was 4% at 30 days.[14] The British Thrombolysis Study Group (TSG) database, which includes over 1100 episodes of thrombolysis (mostly for limb-threatening ischaemia), records a 12.4% mortality rate at 30 days.[27] Other large series report intermediate results.[28,29] Major haemorrhage occurs in approximately 9% of patients, usually at a groin puncture site but occasionally retroperitoneal or intra-abdominal. If major haemorrhage occurs during thrombolysis, aprotinin is an effective plasmin inhibitor and the administration of whole blood, fresh frozen plasma and, in particular, fibrinogen concentrate will replenish the clotting factors. Stroke is seen in approximately 3% of patients (2.3% in the TSG database). Most occur after thrombolysis, during therapeutic anticoagulation. About half are thrombotic rather than haemorrhagic. If a stroke occurs, cerebral haemorrhage should be excluded by urgent CT. If haemorrhage is not the cause, then a clinical decision needs to be made whether to persist with thrombolysis to salvage the affected limb, with possible additional benefits to the intracerebral circulation.

Minor haemorrhage is common (approximately 40% of infusions) and usually occurs at the groin puncture site. It can be managed by direct compression or by exchanging the catheter system for a larger catheter or sheath. Distal embolisation during thrombolysis is a nuisance, occurring in 4% of patients, and is usually managed by either aspiration thromboembolectomy or continued lysis. Reperfusion damage has been reported in 2% and pericatheter thrombosis in 1%.

Outcome

Diffin and Kandarpa[14] report successful thrombolysis in 70% of treatments, with limb salvage in 93%, although many patients in the collected review did not have limb-threatening ischaemia. The TSG database records complete lysis in 45.5% and clinically useful lysis in a further 27.9% of infusions, leading to a limb salvage rate of 75.2%; 12.4% of patients required an amputation and 12.4% died.[30] Thrombolysis was similarly effective in bypass grafts and native vessels. The outcome seems dependent on the nature of the lesion treated and the clinical state of the patient. Patients with subcritical ischaemia appear less likely to need amputation than patients with critical ischaemia including a neurosensory deficit. In addition, the following are more likely to predict failure of thrombolysis: inability to traverse the occlusion with a guidewire or place a catheter within the thrombus, diabetes, multilevel disease, vein graft occlusion, advancing age and female sex.[28] In the long term, approximately 75% of successfully opened native vessels remain patent at 1 year and 55% at 2 years.[29,31] When an identifiable lesion is found after graft thrombolysis, the 2-year patency is approximately 85%. Long-term patency is less good where no underlying lesion is found in native vessels or grafts. In addition, successfully treated iliac occlusions and emboli have a better long-term outlook.[32,33]

The results of thrombolysis for vein graft occlusion have proved disappointing.[34] It is assumed that ischaemia of the vein graft reduces the chances of success. In contrast, the results of prosthetic graft thrombolysis are better. Where an underlying lesion is responsible for occlusion of a prosthetic graft, patency rates at 1 year are encouraging (86% vs. 37%).[35]

There is currently great interest in trying to improve the results of peripheral thrombolysis. It is unlikely that advances in techniques will make a significant difference as no one method can be shown to be superior.

✔✔ A consensus group has produced a document containing all the available evidence and made recommendations for thrombolytic treatment.[36]

Other scoring systems may be used to try to identify patients unlikely to survive after thrombolysis.[37] Detailed analysis of available data and large databases may help identify patients at greater risk of a poor outcome from thrombolysis. A detailed statistical analysis of the TSG database has shown that

the following factors were associated with reduced amputation-free survival: increasing patient age, increasing severity of ischaemia (Fontaine grade and presence of a sensorimotor deficit), shorter duration of ischaemia, and diabetes.[27] Being on warfarin at the time of the occlusion improved the chance of amputation-free survival. The risk of death after thrombolysis was highest in patients with an embolic occlusion, women, older patients and those with ischaemic heart disease. Amputation risk was highest in younger men, legs with a sensorimotor deficit, and graft and thrombotic occlusions.

Surgical management

With the increasing age of the population, underlying atherosclerosis often complicates ischaemia even if the cause is primarily embolic. Consequently, complex secondary procedures may well be necessary if initial balloon catheter embolectomy fails (**Fig. 8.9**). It is therefore advisable that an experienced vascular

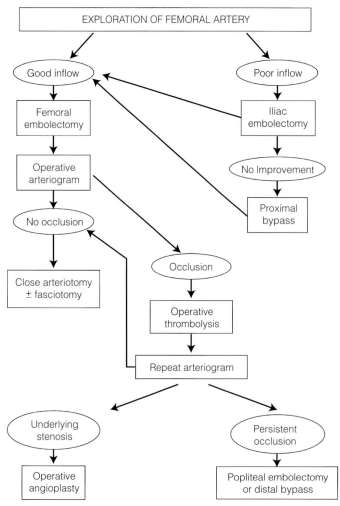

Figure 8.9 • Possible treatment pathway required when exploring the femoral artery.

surgeon performs or supervises the operation. Local anaesthesia may be considered in frail patients where a straightforward femoral embolectomy is considered likely, but an epidural is a better option. An anaesthetist should always be present to monitor the ECG and oxygen saturation, administer sedation or analgesia and convert to general anaesthesia if required.

Balloon catheter embolectomy

Both groins and the entire leg should be prepared to permit surgical access and arteriography. The foot should be placed in a sterile transparent bag for easy inspection. The common femoral artery bifurcation is exposed via a groin incision and the vessels controlled with silastic slings. Clamps should be avoided initially because they fragment thrombus that may otherwise be removed intact. A transverse arteriotomy is made in the common femoral artery proximal to the bifurcation, avoiding any obvious plaque (**Fig. 8.10**). A transverse arteriotomy is easier to close without narrowing and it can be converted to a diamond shape for proximal anastomosis if a bypass is required. Any thrombus at the bifurcation can be removed by gentle suction or forceps and momentary release of the sling or clamp. Some surgeons send the embolic material for histological and microbiological assessment, although there is little evidence to support this routinely.

If pulsatile inflow is not present, then a 4-Fr or 5-Fr balloon catheter is passed proximally up into the aorta, inflated and withdrawn. Pressure should be applied to the contralateral femoral artery during this procedure to prevent contralateral embolisation. If good inflow cannot be achieved, then a femorofemoral or axillofemoral bypass will be required. A saddle embolus can usually be retrieved by bilateral femoral embolectomy. Next, a 3-Fr or 4-Fr balloon catheter is passed as far distally as possible down both the profunda and superficial femoral arteries. Force should not be used if resistance is met as dissection or perforation may result. The balloon is inflated only as the catheter is withdrawn and the amount of inflation

adjusted to avoid excessive intimal friction. The procedure is repeated until no more thromboembolic material can be retrieved. Conventional embolectomy is performed blind and the surgeon has no control over the direction of the catheter past the popliteal trifurcation. Use of an 'over-the-wire' embolectomy catheter permits selective catheterisation of the tibial arteries under fluoroscopic control, which is preferable to performing an additional popliteal trifurcation exposure (**Fig. 8.11**).

Completion angiography

✔ A completion arteriogram should always be performed because persistent thrombus may be present even if the catheter passes to the foot;[38] back-bleeding is of no prognostic value as it may arise from established proximal collaterals. Modern vascular operating theatres now have excellent fluoroscopic facilities capable of high-quality arteriography. The distal arteries are flushed with heparin saline and if no thrombus is present on the arteriogram, the arteriotomy is repaired with 5/0 prolene. On removing the clamps the foot should become pink with palpable pulses.

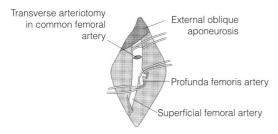

Transverse arteriotomy in common femoral artery

External oblique aponeurosis

Profunda femoris artery

Superficial femoral artery

Figure 8.10 • Exploration of the femoral artery using silastic slings to control the vessels and a transverse arteriotomy proximal to the common femoral bifurcation.

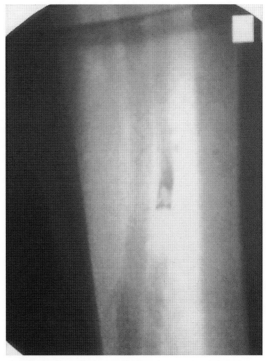

Figure 8.11 • Angiographically controlled balloon catheter embolectomy. The balloon occluding the lumen and the thrombus above it can be seen as negative images against the contrast-filled artery.

Failed embolectomy

If the arteriogram shows persistent occlusion, then 15 mg t-PA in 100 mL heparin saline can be infused via an umbilical catheter over 30 minutes and the arteriogram repeated (**Fig. 8.12**). This often results in complete lysis and reduces the need for popliteal exploration.[39] The technique may also be used to lyse residual thrombus in the tibial arteries during bypass of a popliteal aneurysm.[40] If an underlying stenosis of the superficial femoral artery is revealed, then on-table angioplasty may be attempted. Persistent distal occlusion requires exploration of the below-knee popliteal artery and either popliteal embolectomy or distal bypass. The origins of the anterior tibial artery and tibioperoneal trunk should be controlled with slings and selective embolectomy performed via a longitudinal arteriotomy. The popliteal arteriotomy requires repair with a vein patch to prevent stenosis.

Further management

Revascularisation of an ischaemic leg results in a sudden venous return of blood with anaerobic metabolites, low pH and a high potassium concentration. The anaesthetist must be prepared to correct these, as hypotension and arrhythmias may occur. Reperfusion of a large mass of ischaemic tissue results in a systemic inflammatory response. This may lead to multiple organ dysfunction and failure. Renal function may be further impaired by myoglobinuria, which is helped by maintaining a good diuresis.

✅ Revascularisation of ischaemic muscle can result in considerable swelling within the fascial compartments of the leg. This compartment syndrome will lead to further muscle and nerve damage if not relieved. In patients with a severely ischaemic limb or where the compartments are tense it is wise to perform a fasciotomy at the time of the initial revascularisation procedure. Diagnosis of compartment syndrome is a clinical one. Measurement of compartment pressures may be unreliable. All four muscle compartments should be decompressed via full-length skin and fascial incisions from knee to ankle if any muscle tenseness is present at the time of embolectomy or subsequently.[41] The anterior fasciotomy should be made about two finger-breadths lateral to the anterior border of the tibia, which avoids the peroneal nerve. The posterior fasciotomy incision is done in a line about two finger-breadths posterior to the medial condyle of the femur and the medial malleolus, which avoids the long saphenous vein. The defect can be closed later with sutures or a split-skin graft.

After embolectomy, anticoagulation with heparin and then warfarin is continued as this reduces the risk of recurrent embolism, especially if atrial fibrillation is present.[42–44] There is little guidance

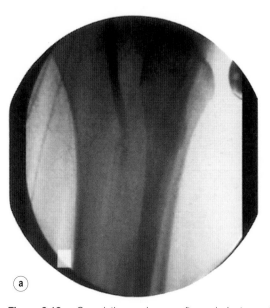 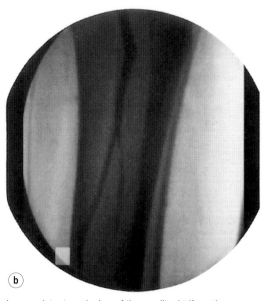

(a) (b)

Figure 8.12 • Completion angiogram after embolectomy showing persistent occlusion of the popliteal trifurcation **(a)** and complete lysis after intraoperative thrombolysis **(b)**.

about the role of anticoagulation in patients who are not fibrillating and have no other obvious cause. Results of a search for proximal sources of emboli using echocardiography and CT angiography may indicate the need for lifelong anticoagulation, but in many patients an individual decision will need to be made based on the risks of warfarinisation and the state of the distal circulation.

Overall prognosis

There has been little change in overall outcome from ALI because the improvements in radiological and surgical techniques have been balanced by increasing atherosclerotic arterial disease in ever older patients. Ten per cent of patients presenting with ALI will have an unsalvageable lower limb. A Swedish population study demonstrated that between 1965 and 1983 there was an increasing incidence of ALI, without any improvement in amputation rates or survival,[45] although outcome after treatment in a university hospital was better than in a district hospital.[46] A prospective survey by the Vascular Surgical Society of Great Britain and Ireland that included 539 episodes in 474 patients recorded a limb salvage rate of 70% and an overall mortality rate of 22%.[47] An analysis of patients taken from the National Inpatient Sample in the USA recorded an amputation rate of 12.7% and a mortality rate of 9%.[12] Patients with embolism have a higher mortality rate due to their underlying cardiac disease. In contrast, those with thrombosis are at increased risk of amputation. Patients with a high mortality rate after embolectomy are characterised by:[43]

- poor cardiac function;
- associated peripheral vascular disease;
- short duration of symptoms;
- the need for amputation.

The amputation risk appears higher in patients with a longer duration of ischaemia and poor preoperative and postoperative cardiac function.[48] Recently, an analysis of preoperative cardiac troponin T has suggested it can be used to predict outcome after embolectomy.[49] Patients with ALI are often elderly and within this group there is a cohort of individuals whose leg problem heralds the end of life. Patients with concomitant malignancy represent a very high risk population and most studies have found that these patients have a very poor prognosis. It is important to recognise this group and to offer appropriate palliative care rather than aggressive intervention.[50]

Conclusions

Although there have been huge changes in the therapeutic options for patients with ALI, there remains debate over the optimal management. Clinical trials in this area are difficult to organise and are often flawed by the great variation in the condition of the patients and their legs. However, further stratification of existing data could help define which occlusions are most suitable for thrombolysis or surgery. A clear comparison between the different drugs available and delivery techniques would help. New drugs will undoubtedly become available with improved safety profiles. In future, thrombolysis combined with other endovascular techniques may enhance its effectiveness.

Key points

- Patients with ALI have high morbidity and mortality rates.
- Optimal management is based on the severity of the ischaemia at presentation.
- Randomised trials have failed to show superiority of thrombolysis or surgery as primary management for all cases.
- The best results are achieved when management is agreed jointly by a team consisting of vascular surgeon and interventional radiologist using available expertise and local guidelines.
- Further research is required to identify which patients with salvageable legs at presentation may be better managed by primary amputation rather than futile attempts at revascularisation.
- For some patients ALI heralds end of life and palliative care should be instituted.

References

1. Norgeren L, Hiatt WR, Dormandy JA, et al. Inter-Society Consensus for the management of peripheral arterial disease. Eur J Vasc Endovasc Surg 2007;33:S1–75.
   Latest definitive standards for scientific research.

2. Rutherford RB, Flanigan DP, Gupta SK, et al. Suggested standards for reports dealing with lower extremity ischemia. J Vasc Surg 1986;4:80–94.

3. Clason AE, Stonebridge PA, Duncan AJ, et al. Acute ischaemia of the lower limb: the effect of centralising vascular surgical services on morbidity and mortality. Br J Surg 1989;76:592–3.

4. Earnshaw JJ. Demography and aetiology of acute leg ischaemia. Semin Vasc Surg 2001;14:86–92.

5. Mehta M, Sternbach Y, Taggert JB, et al. Long-term outcomes of secondary procedures after endovascular aneurysm repair. J Vasc Surg 2010;52(6):1442–9. Epub 2010 Aug 17.

6. Wong PF, Chong LY, Mikhailidis DP, et al. Antiplatelet agents for intermittent claudication. Cochrane Database Syst Rev 2011;11:CD001272.

7. Sandhu RK, Bakal JA, Ezekowitz JA, et al. Risk stratification schemes, anticoagulation use and outcomes: the risk–treatment paradox in patients with newly diagnosed non-valvular atrial fibrillation. Heart 2011;97(24):2046–50.

8. Earnshaw JJ, Hopkinson BR, Makin GS. Acute critical ischaemia of the limb: a prospective evaluation. Eur J Vasc Surg 1990;4:365–8.

9. Jivegard L, Holm J, Schersten T. Acute limb ischaemia due to arterial embolism or thrombosis: influence of limb ischaemia versus pre-existing cardiac disease on postoperative mortality rate. J Cardiovasc Surg (Torino) 1988;29:32–6.

10. Blaisdell FW, Steele M, Allen RE. Management of lower extremity arterial ischaemia due to embolism and thrombosis. Surgery 1978;84:822–34.

11. Davies B, Braithwaite BD, Birch PA, et al. Acute leg ischaemia in Gloucestershire. Br J Surg 1997;84:504–8.

12. Eliason JL, Wainess RM, Proctor MC, et al. A national and single institutional experience in the contemporary treatment of acute lower extremity ischemia. Ann Surg 2003;238(3):382–9.

13. Braithwaite BD, Tomlinson MA, Walker SR, et al. Peripheral thrombolysis for acute-onset claudication. Br J Surg 1999;86:800–4.

14. Diffin DC, Kandarpa K. Assessment of peripheral intraarterial thrombolysis versus surgical revascularization in acute lower limb ischemia: a review of limb salvage and mortality statistics. J Vasc Interv Radiol 1996;7:57–63.

15. Ouriel K, Shortell CK, DeWeese JA, et al. A comparison of thrombolytic therapy with operative revascularisation in the initial treatment of acute peripheral arterial ischaemia. J Vasc Surg 1994;19:1021–30.
    Intra-arterial thrombolysis was associated with a reduction in cardiorespiratory complications and a corresponding increase in survival.

16. The STILE Investigators. Results of a prospective randomized trial evaluating surgery versus thrombolysis for ischaemia of the lower extremity. Ann Surg 1994;220:1–68.
    There were similar outcomes at 30 days, but patients with ischaemia for less than 14 days had improved amputation-free survival after thrombolysis.

17. Comerota AJ, Weaver FA, Hosking JD, et al. Results of a prospective randomized trial of surgery versus thrombolysis for occluded lower extremity bypass grafts. Am J Surg 1996;172:105–12.
    Patients with ischaemia for less than 14 days did better after surgery, those with shorter-duration ischaemia did better after thrombolysis.

18. Weaver FA, Comerota AJ, Youngblood M, et al. Surgical revascularisation versus thrombolysis for nonembolic lower extremity native artery occlusions: results of a prospective randomized trial. J Vasc Surg 1996;24:513–23.
    Surgical revascularisation was more effective and durable than lysis for native vessel occlusions.

19. Ouriel K, Veith FJ, Sasahara AA, for the TOPAS investigators. Thrombolysis or peripheral arterial surgery: phase I results. J Vasc Surg 1996;23:64–75.
    This study was designed to find the optimum dose of urokinase for the second phase of the trial.

20. Ouriel K, Veith FJ, Sasahara AA, for the TOPAS investigators. A comparison of recombinant urokinase with vascular surgery as initial treatment for acute arterial occlusion of the legs. N Engl J Med 1998;338:1105–11.
    This was the largest of the thrombolysis studies and included 544 patients; the results were similar up to 1 year in both groups.

21. Braithwaite BD, Buckenham TM, Galland RB, et al. on behalf of the Thrombolysis Study Group. Prospective randomized trial of high-dose bolus versus low-dose tissue plasminogen activator infusion in the management of acute limb ischaemia. Br J Surg 1997;84:646–50.
    High-dose bolus therapy significantly accelerated thrombolysis without compromising outcome.

22. Yusuf SW, Whitaker SC, Gregson RHS, et al. Prospective randomised comparative study of pulse spray and conventional local thrombolysis. Eur J Vasc Endovasc Surg 1995;10:136–41.
    Pulse spray lysis was quicker.

23. Kandarpa K, Chopra PS, Arung JE. Intra-arterial thrombolysis of lower extremity occlusion: prospective randomized comparison of forced periodic infusion and conventional slow continuous infusion. Radiology 1993;188:861–7.
There was no difference in success or complication rates but forced periodic infusion was quicker.

24. Plate G, Jansson L, Forssell C, et al. Thrombolysis for acute lower limb ischaemia – a prospective, randomised multicenter study comparing two strategies. Eur J Vasc Endovasc Surg 2006;31:651–60.
Success rates were similar in the two groups.

25. Berridge DC, Gregson RHS, Hopkinson BR, et al. Randomized trial of intra-arterial recombinant tissue plasminogen activator, intravenous recombinant tissue plasminogen activator and intra-arterial streptokinase in peripheral thrombolysis. Br J Surg 1991;78:988–95.
Intra-arterial t-PA was safer and more effective than streptokinase.

26. Haskal ZJ. Mechanical thrombectomy devices for the treatment of acute peripheral arterial occlusions. Rev Cardiovasc Med 2002;3(Suppl. 2):S45–52.

27. Earnshaw JJ, Whitman B, Foy C, on behalf of the Thrombolysis Study Group. National Audit of Thrombolysis for Acute Leg Ischaemia (NATALI): clinical factors associated with early outcome. J Vasc Surg 2004;39:1018–25.

28. Hess H, Mietaschk A, Bruckl R. Peripheral arterial occlusions: a 6-year experience with local low-dose thrombolytic therapy. Radiology 1987;163:753–8.

29. Eliason JL, Wainess RM, Proctor MC, et al. A national and institutional experience in the contemporary treatment of acute lower extremity ischaemia. Ann Surg 2003;238:382–9.

30. Earnshaw JJ, Whitman B, Foy C, on behalf of the Thrombolysis Study Group. National Audit of Thrombolysis for Acute Leg Ischaemia (NATALI): clinical factors associated with early outcome. J Vasc Surg 2004;39:1018–25.

31. Ouriel K, Shortell CK, Azodo MVU, et al. Acute peripheral arterial occlusions: predictors of success in catheter-directed thrombolytic therapy. Radiology 1994;193:561–6.

32. McNamara TO, Bomberger RA. Factors affecting initial and six month patency rates after intra-arterial thrombolysis with high dose urokinase. Am J Surg 1986;152:709–12.

33. Durham JD, Rutherford RB. Assessment of long-term efficacy of fibrinolytic therapy in the ischaemic extremity. Semin Interv Radiol 1992;9:166–73.

34. Hye RJ, Turner C, Valji K, et al. Is thrombolysis of occluded popliteal and tibial bypass grafts worthwhile? J Vasc Surg 1994;20(4):588–96.

35. Gardiner Jr GA, Harrington DP, Koltun W, et al. Salvage of occluded arterial bypass grafts by means of thrombolysis. J Vasc Surg 1989;9(3):426–31.

36. Working Party on Thrombolysis in the Management of Limb Ischemia. Thrombolysis in the management of lower limb peripheral arterial occlusion: a consensus document. J Am Coll Cardiol 1998;81:207–18.
Recommendations from expert surgeons and radiologists.

37. Neary B, Whitman B, Foy C, et al. Value of POSSUM physiology scoring to assess the outcome after thrombolysis for acute leg ischaemia. Br J Surg 2001;88:1344–5.

38. Bosma HW, Jorning PJG. Intraoperative arteriography in arterial embolectomy. Eur J Vasc Surg 1990;4:469–72.

39. Beard JD, Nyamekye I, Earnshaw JJ, et al. Intraoperative streptokinase: a useful adjunct to balloon catheter embolectomy. Br J Surg 1993;80:21–4.

40. Thompson JF, Beard J, Scott DJA, et al. Intraoperative thrombolysis in the management of thrombosed popliteal aneurysm. Br J Surg 1993;80:858–9.

41. Ernst CB. Fasciotomy in perspective. J Vasc Surg 1989;9:829–30.

42. Hammarsten J, Holm J, Shersten T. Positive and negative effects of anticoagulant treatment during and after arterial embolectomy. J Cardiovasc Surg (Torino) 1978;19:373–9.

43. Ljungman C, Adami H-O, Bergqvist D, et al. Risk factors for early lower limb loss after embolectomy for acute arterial occlusion: a population-based case–control study. Br J Surg 1991;78:1482–5.

44. Campbell, Ridler BM, Szymanska TH. Two year follow-up after acute thromboembolic leg ischaemia: the importance of anticoagulation. Eur J Vasc Endovasc Surg 2000;19:169–73.

45. Ljungman C, Adami H-O, Bergqvist D, et al. Time trends in incidence rates of acute, non-traumatic extremity ischaemia: a population based study during a 19-year period. Br J Surg 1991;78:857–60.

46. Ljungman C, Holmberg L, Bergqvist D, et al. Amputation risk and survival after embolectomy for acute arterial ischaemia. Time trends in a defined Swedish population. Eur J Vasc Endovasc Surg 1996;11:176–82.

47. Campbell WB, Ridler BMF, Symanska TH, on behalf of the Vascular Surgical Society of Great Britain and Ireland. Current management of acute leg ischaemia: results of an audit by the Vascular Surgical Society of Great Britain and Ireland. Br J Surg 1998;85:1498–503.

48. Dreglid EB, Stangeland LB, Eide GE, et al. Patient survival and limb prognosis after arterial embolectomy. Eur J Vasc Surg 1987;1:263–71.

49. Rittoo D, Stahnke M, Lindesay C, et al. Prognostic significance of raised cardiac troponin T in patients presenting with acute limb ischaemia. Eur J Vasc Endovasc Surg 2006;32:500–3.

50. Braithwaite BD, Davies B, Birch PA, et al. Management of acute leg ischaemia in the elderly. Br J Surg 1998;85:217–20.

9

Vascular trauma

Jacobus van Marle
Dirk A. le Roux

Introduction

Fewer than 10% of patients with polytrauma have associated vascular injuries, but these injuries can cause significant morbidity and mortality.[1] In most European countries the majority of vascular trauma is caused by blunt (traffic accidents) and iatrogenic injuries.[2] In South Africa, injuries are mostly penetrating and have also changed from predominantly stab wounds to injuries caused by firearms.[3]

Complex vascular injuries have a high morbidity and mortality, and a clear understanding of the pathophysiology of vascular trauma and a logical approach to the management of those injuries are essential for a favourable outcome.

Mechanism of injury

Vascular injuries are classified according to the mechanism of the injury.

Blunt trauma

Direct trauma to the artery accounts for the majority of blunt vascular injuries. Indirect trauma is usually the result of shearing and distraction forces following dislocation of major joints, displaced long-bone fractures and acceleration/deceleration injuries as seen with high-speed motor vehicle accidents and falls from a height. Blunt trauma causes contusion of the arterial wall with disruption of the intima. This intimal tear may cause immediate obstruction due to an intimal flap or may predispose to thrombosis and delayed occlusion (**Fig. 9.1a–d**). As the vessel is stretched further, progressive layers of the media are disrupted until the continuity of the vessel is maintained only by the elastic adventitia or there is complete disruption.

Penetrating trauma

Penetrating trauma may result in partial or complete transection of a vessel. Bleeding is often brisk and distal flow may be interrupted. Stab and low-velocity missile injuries cause localised damage confined to the injury tract. High-velocity missiles cause total tissue destruction around the missile tract, surrounded by an area of doubtful tissue viability, causing extensive associated soft-tissue trauma. The shock wave of a high-velocity missile can also cause intimal injury.[4] The vessel may be macroscopically intact with minimal bruising, but on opening the vessel there is an intimal tear with superimposed thrombosis. Shotgun injuries cause extensive local tissue destruction with often multiple sites of perforation. Bomb blasts cause complex injuries due to the combination of extensive local tissue trauma, high-velocity fragments and thermal injury.

Iatrogenic injuries are becoming increasingly important and account for more than 40% of vascular trauma in many European countries.[2]

Sequelae of vascular injuries

Vascular injuries have significant sequelae (Box 9.1, **Figs 9.2** and **9.3**). A contused artery may be patent initially but thrombose later. Subsequent

140

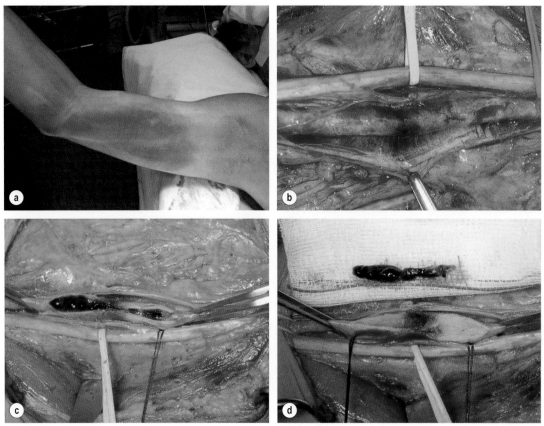

Figure 9.1 • Blunt injury to the arm **(a)** causing contusion of the brachial artery **(b)** predisposing to thrombosis **(c)** due to underlying intimal damage **(d)**.

Box 9.1 • Sequelae of vascular injuries

Acute haemorrhage
- Overt external bleeding
- Contained bleeding (e.g. in muscle compartment)
- Concealed bleeding (e.g. pleural cavity)

Hypovolaemia, shock

Haematoma with or without secondary infection

Delayed bleeding and rebleeding

Thrombosis: acute or delayed

Ischaemia: acute or delayed

Arteriovenous fistula (see **Fig. 9.2**)

Pseudoaneurysm formation (see **Fig. 9.3**)

propagation of thrombus may cause progressive ischaemia by obstructing essential collaterals. Acute ischaemia leads to degeneration and necrosis of muscle cells and Wallerian degeneration in nerves. Findings from large-animal studies indicate that early restoration of flow within 3 hours is associated with near-complete recovery, whereas delayed

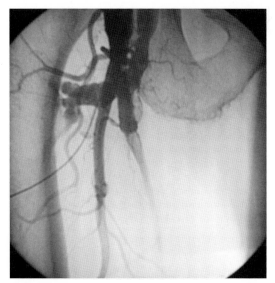

Figure 9.2 • Arteriovenous fistula of the right femoral vessels following iatrogenic injury after diagnostic cardiac catheterisation.

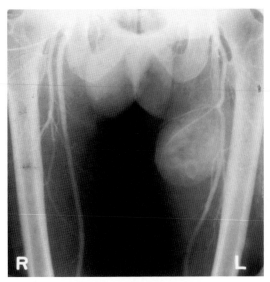

Figure 9.3 • False aneurysm of the left thigh after gunshot wound.

revascularisation at 6 hours was associated with significant muscle necrosis and nerve degeneration.[5]

Concomitant fractures, dislocations, injuries to accompanying veins and nerves, soft-tissue trauma and contamination of the wound with foreign material serve to compound vascular injury. Other determinants of the final outcome are the level of vascular injury, the quality of the collateral circulation and pre-existing occlusive arterial disease.

Clinical assessment

History

Information regarding the mechanism of the trauma, blood loss prior to hospital admission and underlying vascular disease should be obtained.

Examination

Initial assessment should be carried out according to advanced trauma life support (ATLS) principles and life-threatening conditions managed. Vascular injury may present with any of the sequelae listed in Box 9.1. Clinical signs of vascular injuries can be divided into hard and soft signs.

Hard signs of vascular injury:

- Active pulsatile bleeding.
- Shock with ongoing bleeding.
- Absent distal pulses.
- Symptoms and signs of acute ischaemia.
- Expanding or pulsating haematoma.
- Bruits or thrill over the area of injury.

Soft signs of vascular injury:

- History of severe bleeding.
- Diminished distal pulse.
- Injury of anatomically related structures.
- Small non-expanding haematoma.
- Multiple fractures and extensive soft-tissue injury.
- Injury in anatomical area of major blood vessel.

Distal pulses may be difficult to evaluate in patients with extensive soft-tissue trauma, swelling and multiple wounds. A diminished or absent pulse is due to arterial occlusion until proven otherwise and should not be attributed to vascular spasm, external compression or any other ill-defined factor.

Signs of acute arterial insufficiency (ischaemia) include pulse deficit (absent/diminished pulse), pain, pallor, paraesthesia and paralysis. Neurological deficit must be evaluated carefully in order to distinguish between ischaemic neuropathy and direct injury to the nerve.

Diagnosis

> ✔✔ The value and accuracy of a thorough clinical examination in predicting significant vascular injury has been reported in various series.[6]
>
> Arterial Doppler pressure measurement is a useful supplement to the clinical examination. An arterial pressure index (API) above 0.9 reliably excludes significant occult arterial injury.[7]

Special investigations should only be performed in patients who have been adequately resuscitated and who are haemodynamically stable. Haemodynamic instability, active bleeding and an expanding haematoma are indications for immediate surgery.

Resuscitation and initial management

ATLS guidelines are followed, keeping in mind that the resuscitation of the unstable patient in urgent need of surgery may be best conducted in the operating room.

> ✔✔ The amount and timing of fluid resuscitation is important. In uncontrolled haemorrhagic shock where bleeding has been temporarily stopped due to hypotension, vasoconstriction and thrombus formation, aggressive fluid resuscitation may lead to increased intravascular pressure, decreased blood viscosity and loss of the haemostatic plug, with resultant increased bleeding and mortality.[8]

Hypotensive resuscitation (permissive hypotension) aims at a systolic blood pressure of between 70 and 90 mmHg to maintain cerebral and renal perfusion until operative control of bleeding has been achieved.

Active bleeding is an indication for urgent exploration, but can usually be temporarily controlled by direct pressure. Blind clamping of vessels in the depth of a wound is discouraged, because of the danger of injuring adjacent nerves and vessels. Tourniquets should only be used under exceptional circumstances e.g., after traumatic lower leg amputation due to a mine or IED and then only for short periods.

Fractures must be stabilised during the period of resuscitation and diagnostic investigation in order to protect blood vessels and other soft tissue from further trauma. Preliminary reduction of a displaced fracture or dislocation may improve distal circulation.

Special investigations

Plain radiography

Plain radiographs are usually taken for associated skeletal injuries. A high index of suspicion for vascular trauma should exist with dislocations and displaced fractures (**Fig. 9.4**). Chest radiography is valuable in patients with chest trauma.

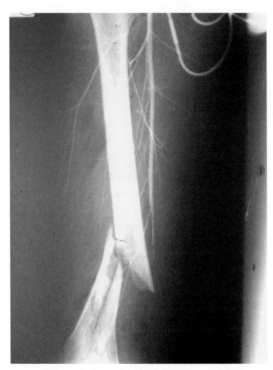

Figure 9.4 • Displaced fracture of the femur with injury to the superficial femoral artery.

Arteriography

✓✓ The routine use of arteriography for excluding vascular injury in the absence of hard clinical signs is no longer warranted, especially in extremity trauma.[9]

Catheter arteriography has largely been superseded by computed tomography angiography. It may still be indicated for selected conditions in haemodynamically stable patients, including multiple fractures, extensive soft-tissue injury, shotgun injuries, zone 1 and 3 neck injuries, thoracic and abdominal injuries.

Surgical intervention should not be delayed by arteriography where vascular injury is evident and the patient unstable or the limb is at ischaemic risk. On-table arteriography in the operating room should be performed in vascular injuries to the extremity where surgery cannot be delayed and the additional information is considered valuable.[10]

Ultrasound

Duplex Doppler examination is mostly used as a screening test, in the absence of hard signs, in extremity vascular trauma, neck and abdominal injuries, as well as for follow-up evaluation in patients managed expectantly.

Axial imaging

Computed tomographic angiography (CTA) is valuable in blunt cervical, abdominal and thoracic injuries. It can also be useful in the localisation and characterisation of limb trauma. The use of magnetic resonance angiography (MRA) in trauma is limited due to time constraints and inaccessibility to the patient during the examination.

General principles of management of vascular injury

Procedures are performed under general anaesthesia in a suitably equipped theatre. Blood products should be available and arrangements for intraoperative auto-transfusion should be made where further bleeding is expected. The value of prophylactic antibiotics in vascular surgery is established.

Adequate exposure is vital for obtaining proximal and distal control of injured vessels. This often requires inclusion of adjacent anatomical areas in the operative field, e.g. preparing the neck in thoracic injuries (and vice versa) and the abdomen in groin injuries. An uninjured leg is prepared for possible vein harvesting should bypass be required. Vascular control must be achieved proximally and distally before directly approaching the area of injury. Bleeding may be temporarily arrested by digital compression or by endovascular means until clamps have been applied.

In blunt and high-velocity trauma there is often extensive intimal damage, and careful debridement of the vessel is necessary until normal-appearing intima is found (**Fig. 9.5**). Antegrade and retrograde flow should be evaluated. Arteries are cleared of thrombus by careful passage of embolectomy catheters followed by irrigation with heparin/saline solution.

Simple laceration of the vessel wall is repaired by lateral suture, provided it does not lead to stenosis, when patch graft angioplasty is indicated. Where more than 50% of the circumference of a vessel wall is damaged, this area should be excised followed by end-to-end anastomosis. This requires mobilisation of the proximal and distal arterial stumps to achieve approximation without tension. Failing this, an interposition graft is indicated. Autogenous vein is the preferred conduit for reconstruction. Prosthetic material should only be used in exceptional circumstances due to the risk of graft infection.[11]

Where there is a mismatch in diameter between the vessel that needs to be repaired and the available autogenous vein, either a panelled or spiral vein graft should be used.

✔✔ Where complex arterial repair will result in delay in revascularisation, intraluminal shunts should be used to maintain antegrade flow during repair, thereby reducing ischaemic time.[12]

Completion angiography should be performed to document a technically perfect repair and to assess the distal arterial tree. Associated injuries are addressed once vascular repair has been completed. Wound debridement should be performed, with removal of all devitalised and contaminated tissue. Contaminated wounds are left open, but the vascular repair must be covered by soft tissue. Repeated wound inspections are performed, with delayed primary suture when the wound is clean.

Venous injuries

Venous injuries found during exploration for associated arterial injury should be repaired, if the repair

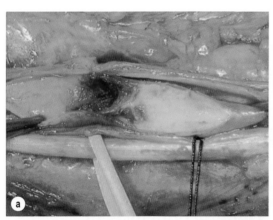
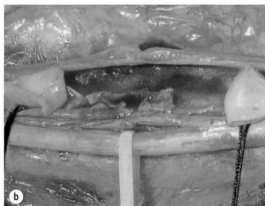
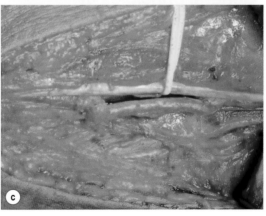

Figure 9.5 • Blunt injury of the intima **(a)**, resected **(b)** and replaced with a venous interposition graft **(c)**.

itself can be done simply (e.g. lateral suture repair) and only if it will not significantly delay treatment of associated injuries or destabilise the patient's condition. Complex venous repair or bypass should only be attempted if the patient is haemodynamically stable. All veins, including the inferior vena cava (IVC), can be tied off in cases of haemodynamic instability.

Endovascular management of vascular trauma

The application of endovascular techniques in the injured patient has many potential advantages. General anaesthesia is not required. Surgical trauma, with further blood loss, hypothermia, etc., as well as cross-clamping of major vessels, distal ischaemia and subsequent reperfusion injury, is avoided. The main advantage is the option of approaching complex arterial lesions in anatomically challenging locations from a remote site. A difficult exploration in an injured area is avoided, with less potential damage to surrounding structures, and preventing fresh bleeding.

Endovascular techniques are increasingly applied in vascular trauma, but still have certain limitations. These techniques are usually not applicable, mainly due to time constraints, in patients with active bleeding, in unstable patients or where there is end-organ ischaemia. Endovascular techniques are contraindicated where there are compression symptoms, infected wounds or where concomitant injuries require open exploration. Technical restrictions include inability to traverse the lesion by guidewire, where intraluminal thrombus prevents the safe passage of a guidewire due to the danger of distal embolisation or where luminal discrepancy exists between the proximal and distal involved segments.

Endovascular techniques are used to manage vascular trauma in three ways:

1. **To obtain haemostasis.** Damaged vessels are embolised using a variety of substances including haemostatic agents (gel foam), coils and balloons. This technique has become the standard treatment for managing significant bleeding following pelvic fractures, and is also a recognised option for treating lesions of non-essential, inaccessible vessels in the cervical, pelvic and limb regions.[13,14] It is also used to control bleeding due to penetrating and blunt trauma of the liver, kidneys and spleen.[15-17]

2. **To obtain vascular control.** Temporary balloon occlusion of a damaged vessel at the time of diagnostic angiography can prevent exsanguinating bleeding until surgical control is achieved. It is especially valuable in relatively inaccessible regions and allows limiting the extent of the exposure to obtain surgical control.[18] This technique is valuable in injuries in zones 1 and 3 of the neck, the abdominal aorta, proximal subclavian and iliac arteries.

3. **For vascular repair.** Covered stent grafts are used for repairing vessels in anatomically challenging locations and to avoid major surgical exposures, e.g. the thoracic aorta, thoracic outlet vessels, internal carotid and vertebral arteries (**Fig. 9.6**).[19-22] This will be discussed in

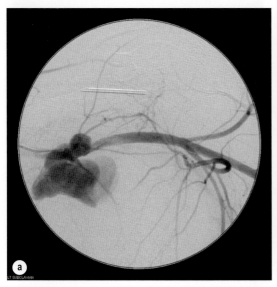
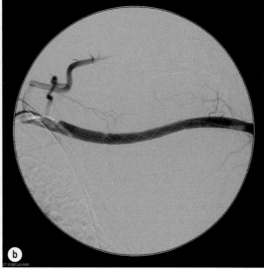

Figure 9.6 • False aneurysm of left subclavian artery after infraclavicular stab wound **(a)** repaired by means of a covered stent graft **(b)**.

more detail in the relevant sections. Covered stentgrafts may also be used as a temporary measure to allow stabilisation of the patient and definitive open repair later.

In-stent stenosis, graft migration, stent breakage and endoleaks are well-known complications of stent graft repair. Durability is therefore of concern in the younger population, who are the main victims of trauma. Early results are promising, but long-term follow-up and prospective randomised trials comparing standard surgery with endovascular repair are awaited.

Cervical vascular injuries

Carotid artery injuries

The cervical vessels are involved in 25% of patients with head or neck trauma. Carotid artery injury constitutes 5–10% of all arterial injuries.[23] The mortality for carotid injuries ranges from 10% to 31%, with permanent neurological deficit ranging from 16% to 60%.[24,25]

Mechanism

More than 90% of carotid injuries are caused by penetrating trauma. Blunt trauma is caused by a direct blow to the artery, hyperextension, hyper-rotation, or contusion by bone fragments associated with fractures of the mandible, temporal bone or cervical spine.

Penetrating injury may cause partial or complete transection of the vessel, pseudoaneurysm or arteriovenous fistula (**Fig. 9.7**). Pseudoaneurysm may have an acute or delayed onset, with progressive enlargement causing compression of the aerodigestive tract or brachial plexus. Blunt trauma may cause intimal flaps, intramural haematoma, dissection, complete disruption of arterial wall with pseudoaneurysms, arteriovenous fistulas and total occlusion (**Fig. 9.8**).

Neurological sequelae are caused by hypoperfusion (transected or thrombosed vessels) or embolisation from thrombus, pseudoaneurysm or arteriovenous fistula.

Clinical signs

Active external bleeding, rapidly expanding cervical haematoma, absent carotid pulse and a bruit or thrill are indicative of vascular injury. Signs that may indicate an associated vascular injury warranting further investigation include bleeding from wounds of the neck or the pharynx, a deficit of the superficial temporal artery pulse, ipsilateral Horner's sign, dysfunction of cranial nerves IX–XII, a widened mediastinum, fractures of the skull base and temporal bone, and fractures and dislocation of the cervical spine. Neurological deficit may be present, but obscured due to concomitant head injury, shock or the use of alcohol or drugs. About 50% of patients with established blunt injury to the carotid and vertebral arteries could initially be asymptomatic, but

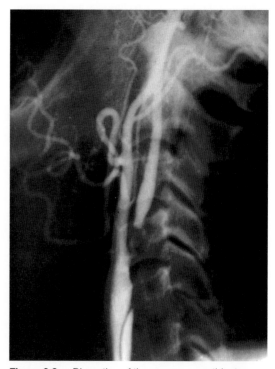

Figure 9.8 • Dissection of the common carotid artery with blunt trauma to the neck following a motor vehicle accident.

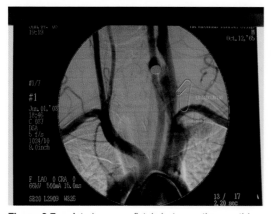

Figure 9.7 • Arteriovenous fistula between the carotid artery and internal jugular vein caused by gunshot wound.

43–58% of these will eventually develop neurological signs after hospital admission.[26]

Diagnosis

Only patients who are haemodynamically stable and have a patent airway should undergo further appropriate investigations.

The neck has been divided into three anatomical zones in order to standardise diagnosis and management of cervical vascular injuries (**Fig. 9.9**).

Anteroposterior chest radiography can provide valuable information regarding associated haemothorax or pneumothorax, widening of the mediastinum, surgical emphysema of the neck with concomitant aerodigestive tract injuries, etc.

> ☑ ☑ Duplex Doppler examination is useful for investigating zone 2 vascular injuries and is now the preferred diagnostic modality in experienced hands.[27,28]

Duplex scanning has limitations in zones 1 and 3, where arch angiography remains the gold standard for the diagnosis of vascular injuries. It is also important for proper planning of the surgical procedure and evaluation for possible endovascular treatment. Routine angiography is not indicated in asymptomatic patients.[29]

Computed tomography (CT) of the brain should be used to investigate patients with associated head trauma, bone injuries of the spine and skull, and neurological deficit. It is a good predictor of outcome: patients who have an infarct on initial CT on admission have a high mortality with poor chance of neurological recovery compared with those who have a normal CT on admission. MRA may be valuable in carotid artery and vertebral artery dissection.[30]

Management

Active external bleeding can be controlled in the emergency room by direct digital compression or a Foley catheter inflated in the wound tract to obtain balloon tamponade.[31]

Mandatory exploration of all penetrating neck injuries has been replaced by a selective approach.[32] Active pulsatile haemorrhage, expanding cervical haematoma and airway compromise are indications for urgent surgical exploration. Some low-velocity penetrating injuries may be managed expectantly with careful observation, provided there is no active bleeding and the distal circulation is normal.[33] These injuries include intimal defects, small pseudoaneurysms (<5 mm) and non-obstructive intimal flaps. The majority of penetrating carotid artery injuries, however, are best managed by primary arterial repair.[34] Neurological deficit is only a contraindication to surgical repair in a deeply comatose patient with a dense neurological deficit, arterial occlusion and a huge infarct on cerebral CT.[34] All other patients with associated neurological deficit would benefit from arterial repair, with improved mortality and final neurological status.

Most blunt injuries of the carotid and vertebral arteries result in intimal disruption, with dissection and/or thrombosis, and the immediate goal of management is to restore cerebral perfusion and to prevent embolisation. Systemic anticoagulation is therefore the treatment of choice, because it limits the formation, propagation and/or embolisation of the thrombus. Intravenous heparin is administered in the acute phase, followed by oral anticoagulation for at least 3 months.[35]

Operative technique

Detailed description of operative technique falls outside the scope of this chapter and the reader is referred to the standard textbooks on operative surgery.[36] The general principles of management include the following:

- The patient should be in a supine position with a bolster between the scapulae and with the neck extended and the head rotated to the contralateral side. The patient must be draped to allow access from the base of the skull to the xiphisternum.
- Zone 2 injuries are explored by the standard carotid incision overlying the anterior border of the sternocleidomastoid muscle.
- Zone 1 injuries may require a median sternotomy.
- Various techniques have been described to improve exposure of the distal internal carotid artery in zone 3 injuries, including subluxation of the mandible, mandibular osteotomy, excision of the styloid process, etc.

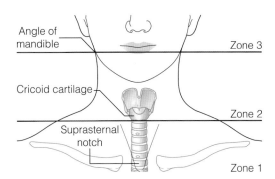

Angle of mandible

Cricoid cartilage

Suprasternal notch

Zone 3

Zone 2

Zone 1

Figure 9.9 • Zones of the neck.

- Some authors recommend routine shunting to maintain antegrade flow.
- Where simple repair is not feasible, a bypass should be performed. Saphenous vein should preferably be used in the internal carotid artery whereas polytetrafluoroethylene (PTFE) is used to repair the common carotid artery.
- The external carotid artery can be safely ligated if the internal carotid artery is patent. Internal carotid artery ligation is only recommended when the distal vessel is thrombosed with no back-bleeding following extraction of thrombus.
- Minor venous injuries can be managed by lateral suture repair, but complex venous repair is not indicated as there is a high occlusion rate and it increases the magnitude of the operative procedure. Ligation of the jugular vein can be performed without significant sequelae.[37]
- In the presence of associated injuries to the trachea and oesophagus, the vascular repair should be protected by soft-tissue interposition (sternocleidomastoid muscle).

Vertebral artery injuries

The occurrence of vertebral artery injury is low, with the reported incidence in penetrating neck trauma ranging from 1% to 7.4%. Gunshot wounds are the most common mechanism of injury.[38] Blunt injury of the vertebral artery is even less common and is caused by fractures of the lateral mass of the cervical vertebrae involving the foramen transversarium, vertebral fractures, ligamentous cervical spine injury, or severe and sudden rotation and/or hyperextension of the head. These injuries are seen with motor vehicle accidents, near-hanging injuries and after extreme chiropractic manipulation.[39]

The majority of patients with vertebral artery injuries have associated injuries of the cervical spine, spinal cord and other vascular structures in the neck or aerodigestive tract.[40] CTA has a high sensitivity and specificity for detecting injury of the vertebral artery and is being used increasingly in neck trauma.[41]

Angiographic embolisation is the treatment of choice in the majority of patients with vertebral artery injuries.[22] Operative management is only indicated for severe active bleeding or when embolisation has failed. Haemodynamically stable patients with a thrombosed vertebral artery do not need any intervention.

A detailed description of surgical approaches to, and management of, vertebral artery injuries is given by Hatzitheofilou et al.[42]

Endovascular management of cervical injuries

An important advantage of endovascular repair of extracranial cerebrovascular trauma is the avoidance of general anaesthesia and the ability to monitor neurological status during the procedure. Endovascular therapies are used in three ways in the management of cervical vascular trauma:

1. **Angiographic embolisation.** This is indicated for (a) persistent bleeding from external carotid artery branches (face, oro- and nasopharynx) and (b) injury to the vertebral artery in the osseus vertebral canal.[43]
2. **Temporary balloon occlusion.** This is used as an adjunct to support standard open vascular repair in neck zone 1 and 3 injuries. An occlusion balloon is placed via the femoral artery to provide proximal endoluminal control of the injured vessel, allowing surgical exposure in a more controlled fashion, and possibly avoiding sternotomy for proximal control.
3. **Covered stent grafts.** These are indicated for penetrating wounds, arteriovenous fistulas and pseudoaneurysms in (a) surgically inaccessible regions, e.g. distal carotid artery, and (b) in patients where extensive surgical exploration is to be avoided due to multiple trauma, local aggravating factors or high surgical risk due to medical comorbidities. This includes injuries to the brachiocephalic trunk, and proximal common carotid and subclavian arteries.[20,21,44]

Thoracic vascular injuries

Penetrating trauma is responsible for more than 90% of thoracic vascular injuries.[45] Blunt aortic injury is considered as the second most common cause of death in trauma patients;[46] 70–90% of patients sustaining these injuries will die before reaching a hospital. The site of insertion of the ligamentum arteriosum, just distal to the origin of the left subclavian artery, is the typical point of injury. Deceleration or compression injury may also involve the brachiocephalic trunk, the pulmonary veins and the vena cava.

Clinical presentation and initial management

Patients with penetrating thoracic vascular trauma are usually haemodynamically unstable, often with continuing haemorrhage into the pleural cavity or the mediastinum and should be taken for urgent thoracotomy. A precise diagnosis of vascular injury is only made intraoperatively. Patients with blunt thoracic trauma may initially be haemodynamically stable and the injury may not be immediately apparent due to the high incidence of concomitant trauma. The following clinical findings may be associated with underlying thoracic great vessel injury:

- shock/hypotension;
- difference in blood pressure or pulses between the two upper extremities;
- difference in blood pressure between upper and lower extremities (pseudocoarctation syndrome);
- expanding haematoma at the thoracic outlet;
- left flail chest;
- infrascapular murmur;
- palpable fracture of the sternum;
- palpable fracture of the thoracic spine;
- external evidence of major chest trauma;
- history indicating deceleration or compression injury to the chest.

Diagnostic studies

The number and type of diagnostic studies performed will be determined by the patient's haemodynamic stability and general status, as well as the type of aortic lesion and concomitant injuries.

Chest radiography

A frontal chest radiograph is an important screening tool and should be obtained in all patients with penetrating and suspected blunt thoracic trauma. Radio-opaque markers are useful for identifying entrance and exit sites.

A widened mediastinum on chest radiography is associated with more than 90% of thoracic aortic injuries, with a 90% sensitivity and 95% negative predictive value.[47] Other radiographic findings associated with blunt injuries of the descending aorta include the following:

1. Mediastinal findings:
   (a) widening of the mediastinum greater than 8 cm;
   (b) obliteration of the aortic knob contour;
   (c) depression of the left main stem bronchus greater than 140°;
   (d) loss of the paravertebral pleural line;
   (e) lateral displacement of the trachea;
   (f) deviation of a nasogastric tube;
   (g) calcium layering of the aortic knob.

2. Fractures of sternum, first and second ribs and thoracic spine. Scapular and clavicular fractures in a polytrauma patient.
3. Other findings on (a) anteroposterior chest radiograph: apical pleural haematoma (apical cap), massive left haemothorax/effusion, ruptured diaphragm; (b) lateral chest radiograph: anterior displacement of trachea, loss of the aorto-pulmonary window.

Positive findings on chest radiography are indications for further advanced diagnostic studies, mainly angiography and helical CT.

Angiography

CTA is indicated for penetrating trauma in haemodynamically stable patients with suspected injury to the innominate, carotid or subclavian arteries, and is preferred to conventional arteriography. It provides important information that may influence management, e.g. type of incision or possible endovascular therapy. The proximity of a missile trajectory to the brachiocephalic vessels may in itself be an indication for arteriography even without any physical findings of vascular injury.

> ✓✓ CTA is accepted as a definitive diagnostic procedure that recognises aortic injury and rupture.[48]

CTA is less invasive, faster to obtain and more readily available than catheter angiography, and has a further advantage that it can provide important information regarding associated lesions. However, the relative inaccessibility to the patient during examination limits its use in unstable patients.

Other imaging modalities

Transoesophageal echocardiography and intravascular ultrasound may be used as complementary modalities in selected patients, but routine use of these techniques is limited.

Treatment

Indications for urgent surgery are haemodynamic instability, increasing haemorrhage from chest tubes and radiographic evidence of an expanding haematoma. An initial large volume of blood drained from a chest tube (>1500 mL) or ongoing haemorrhage of more than 200–300 mL/hour may indicate great vessel injury that requires thoracotomy.

The current indications for delayed aortic repair are haemodynamically stable patients with trauma to the central nervous system and coma, respiratory failure from lung contusion, body surface burns, blunt cardiac injury, visceral injury that will undergo non-operative management, retroperitoneal haematoma, contaminated wounds, hypothermia, coagulopathy and other conditions that can be corrected to improve the outcome of operative repair, age 50 years or older and medical comorbidities.[49]

Certain minimal aortic lesions, for example intimal defects, small intimal flaps and pseudoaneurysms, may be managed non-operatively with close observation.[50] Patients selected for initial non-operative management should be closely monitored, with systolic blood pressure kept below 120 mmHg or mean arterial pressure below 80 mmHg. Intravenous beta-blockade, titrated to heart rate, was shown to be beneficial in patients with a blunt aortic injury and is currently included in many protocols.

Endovascular repair

Injuries to the arch outflow vessels can be successfully managed with endovascular stent grafting. (**Fig. 9.10**).[20,51]

✅✅ Endovascular stent grafting is currently the preferred method for treating traumatic rupture of the descending thoracic aorta. Mortality is significantly lower compared to open surgery (9% vs. 19%) with a decreased risk of spinal cord ischaemia, renal injury, graft and systemic infection.[52]

Surgical repair

Open surgery is reserved for unstable, hypotensive patients, for injuries of the ascending aorta and arch, and where endovascular treatment is not readily available. The basic surgical approaches are: median sternotomy, left anterolateral thoracotomy and left posterolateral thoracotomy. The reader is referred to the standard textbooks on thoracic surgery for a detailed description of these procedures.

Abdominal vascular injuries

Penetrating trauma accounts for 90–95% of abdominal vascular injuries (**Fig. 9.11**), with a high mortality due to the nature of these injuries as well as associated injuries to other intra-abdominal organs. It is important to consider intra-abdominal injury with all penetrating injuries from the nipples to the upper thighs.

Diagnosis

The unstable patient with a possible abdominal vascular injury requires immediate surgery. The stable patient should be investigated according to the injuries. Plain abdominal radiography using radio-opaque markers is of value in establishing the trajectory of missiles in penetrating injuries. Arteriography and CT have little if any role in the diagnosis of penetrating abdominal vascular injury.[53]

Management

Abdominal vascular injuries are usually associated with haemodynamic instability or concomitant bowel injuries requiring a laparotomy. The abdominal cavity should be entered rapidly at induction of anaesthesia. A generous laparotomy incision is required from xiphisternum to suprapubis.

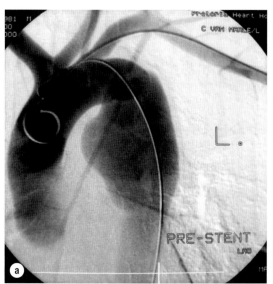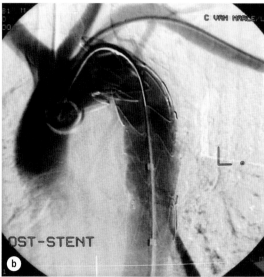

Figure 9.10 • Thoracic aneurysm after blunt injury to the chest **(a)** treated with a covered aortic stent graft **(b)**.

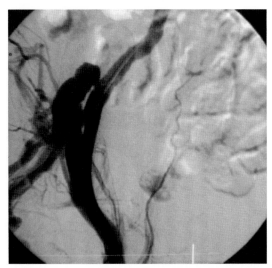

Figure 9.11 • Fistula of left common iliac artery after a penetrating injury (gunshot wound to the abdomen).

Four-quadrant packing of the abdomen is performed immediately and the proximal aorta is controlled at the diaphragmatic crus through the lesser sac. Once the vascular injury is controlled, resuscitation with blood products is started. Bowel injuries are temporarily controlled until vascular repair is effected.

The retroperitoneum is divided into three anatomical zones for purposes of treatment. Central retroperitoneal haematomas (zone 1) are formally explored due to the high incidence of associated major vascular, pancreatic or duodenal injuries, and the high morbidity and mortality if these are overlooked. Flank/perinephric haematomas (zone 2) caused by penetrating injuries should routinely be explored, whilst haematomas caused by blunt trauma can be left alone if they are not expanding and the urogram on contrast-enhanced CT scan is normal. Zone 3 injuries, which are confined to or originate from the pelvis, are most often associated with pelvic fractures; exploration in these cases can be hazardous and is usually avoided. Retroperitoneal haematomas following penetrating injuries are usually explored to exclude major vascular injuries.

Different surgical exposures are used for specific injuries:

- Medial visceral rotation of the left-sided viscera (Mattox manoeuvre), i.e. spleen, tail of the pancreas, left colon and kidney allows access to the supracoeliac aorta, coeliac axis with its branches to the left, superior mesenteric artery (SMA), inferior mesenteric artery, left renal artery and left iliac vessels.

- The Cattell–Braasch or extended Kocher manoeuvre (right-sided medial visceral rotation) allows access to infrahepatic inferior vena cava, right renal vein, portal system and right iliac vessels.
- The infrarenal aorta and IVC are exposed by reflecting the transverse colon superiorly and the small intestine to the right and then dividing the midline retroperitoneum.
- The iliac arteries are exposed via separate incisions lateral to the caecum and sigmoid respectively, avoiding injury to the ureters as they cross the common iliac arteries. The iliac veins may only be accessible after dividing the arteries that lie anterior to them.

Aortic injury

Direct repair is used for simple lacerations; this should be done transversely to avoid narrowing. An interposition polyester or PTFE graft may be necessary where there is extensive destruction, but should be avoided in a contaminated field.

✅✅ In the 'damage control' scenario, a temporary shunt using a sterile thoracostomy tube is placed in the aorta. Definitive repair is performed once the patient is stable and all physiological parameters are normal.[53]

In severe contamination, a graft made of panelled saphenous vein may be used, or the aorta is ligated and an extra-anatomical bypass (e.g. axillofemoral) performed.[54]

Abdominal aortic dissection after blunt trauma ('seat-belt aorta') is relatively uncommon, but endovascular repair has been described in such cases.[55]

Iliac injury

These injuries can be repaired using primary suturing or interposition grafting. In the case of severe contamination, ligation and femorofemoral bypass is an accepted technique.[54] A single internal iliac artery injury may be ligated.

Visceral artery injury

Injuries to the coeliac trunk and its branches are usually dealt with by primary ligation.[54] The superior mesenteric artery is divided into four zones.[56] Injuries to the first two zones (i.e. SMA trunk to the origin of the middle colic artery) should be repaired. Where primary repair is not possible due to extreme damage, bypass with saphenous vein or PTFE should be performed to maintain midgut viability. Isolated injuries to the inferior mesenteric artery can usually be ligated.

Renal artery injury

Blunt injury, usually caused by acceleration/deceleration, results in intimal disruption with subsequent thrombosis of the vessels. These injuries should be repaired within 12 hours, since renal viability after this period is very slim. Proximal injuries are approached from the midline through the base of the mesentery, while distal injuries are approached laterally. Repair is performed by either primary repair or interposition grafting using saphenous vein.

Traumatic renal artery dissection can be managed endovascularly with either bare metal stents or covered stent grafts.[57]

Inferior vena cava injury

The IVC consists of four parts: infrarenal, suprarenal, retrohepatic and intrapericardial. The retrohepatic and intrapericardial portions are usually affected by blunt trauma. Approximately 50% of patients die before reaching hospital and the in-hospital mortality ranges between 20% and 57%.[58]

Wounds in the infrahepatic IVC can be temporarily controlled by means of digital pressure or intraluminal balloon catheters. When clamps are applied, one should be aware of the abundant lumbar collateral circulation. Repair is effected by means of lateral suture or, when there are large defects, prosthetic material. The anterior laceration in a through-and-through lesion may need to be extended so that the posterior defect can be repaired first. In dire attempts to save an exsanguinating patient this part of the IVC may be ligated. The retrohepatic IVC should be approached with extreme caution. If haemorrhage can be controlled with packing this should be the method of treatment. Various strategies to repair these injuries have been described but the prognosis is still dismal, with a reported mortality of 70–90%.[59] The Shrock shunt, which is inserted through the right atrium, can be used to control these injuries temporarily. We use a modified technique by inserting an endotracheal tube through the infrahepatic IVC and inflating the balloon in the right atrium. Total hepatic isolation (Heany manoeuvre) is associated with a high mortality, especially in an exsanguinated patient. Venous repair is by means of ligation of hepatic veins or direct repair.

Emergency endovascular stent graft repair for traumatic injury of the inferior vena cava was described by Castelli et al.[60]

Pelvic vascular injury

Haemorrhage is the primary cause of death in patients with pelvic fractures. The major sources of bleeding are branches of the internal iliac artery and vein, bone and soft tissues. Bleeding can usually be controlled by external stabilisation of the pelvic ring. Persistent bleeding from branches of the internal iliac artery can be treated with trans-catheter embolisation.[13] The common iliac, external iliac and common femoral arteries and corresponding veins are the source of catastrophic blood loss in only about 1% of pelvic fractures. Initially these were managed by open surgery, but recent reports support a role for the endovascular management of iliac artery injuries in this setting.[61]

Extremity vascular trauma

The incidence of peripheral vascular injury depends on the extent and type of trauma, ranging from 0.6–3.6% for isolated extremity fractures to 25–30% for all penetrating injuries of the extremities.[1] The risk of limb loss is greatest following blunt trauma and injuries from high-velocity missiles or close-range shotgun wounds.

Diagnosis

Any extremity injury warrants a complete physical examination of the injured extremity and distal vessels. The absence of hard signs of vascular injury reliably excludes surgically significant arterial injury and does not require arteriography.[62] Arteriography for proximity injury is indicated only in patients with shotgun injuries and multiple fractures (**Fig. 9.12**).[63]

The occurrence of delayed thrombosis stresses the importance of regular reassessment of the peripheral circulation for at least 24 hours after orthopaedic injury. There may be a role for duplex Doppler studies in patients with soft signs of vascular injury or with proximity injuries.[64]

General principles of management

- Restoration of perfusion to an ischaemic extremity should be performed as quickly as possible. Classical teaching advised restoring perfusion within 6 hours for limb salvage. Contemporary studies, however, emphasise the importance of speedier restoration of perfusion (within 3–4 hours) to optimise neuromuscular recovery of the injured limb.[5] Adjunctive therapies such as hypertonic saline resuscitation, temporary intravascular shunts, fasciotomy, limb cooling and ischaemic reconditioning may reduce the severity of ischaemic injury.[5,65]
- Non-operative observation of asymptomatic non-occlusive arterial injuries is acceptable. These injuries can be defined as small pseudoaneurysms, intimal flaps or irregularities, small arteriovenous

fistulas, and haemodynamic insignificant narrowings of the vessels. Should subsequent repair of these injuries be required, it can be done without significant increase in morbidity.[6]

- Extremity arterial trauma is usually addressed by conventional open surgical techniques. Endovascular treatment usually consists of embolisation of non-essential vessels after penetrating trauma.

- Simple arterial repairs do better than grafts. If complex repair is required, vein grafts appear to be the best choice.[66] PTFE is an acceptable conduit when no vein is available and may even be used in a contaminated field.[11] Effort should be made to cover the graft with soft tissue.

- Temporary shunting is valuable for maintaining antegrade flow in order to allow stabilisation of unstable fractures and/or dislocations prior to definitive arterial repair (**Fig. 9.13**).[12]

- Early four-compartment lower leg fasciotomy should be applied liberally. Indications for fasciotomy include: (i) ischaemic time greater than 4–6 hours; (ii) signs of acute ischaemia; (iii) extensive soft-tissue injuries; (iv) combined arterial and venous injuries; (v) intracompartmental bleeding; and (vi) increased compartmental pressure. Measurement of compartment pressures may be useful but must be interpreted with caution, remembering that tissue perfusion is a balance between compartment pressure and blood pressure. Acceptable compartment pressures have been defined as absolute compartment pressures of less than 20 mmHg and at least 30 mmHg less than mean arterial pressure.[67]

- Completion arteriogram should be performed after arterial repair to assess patency and technical perfection of the repair.

- Although amputation rates increase with longer ischaemia times, quantifying the relationship is difficult, because amputation rates also depend on other factors such as extent of soft-tissue

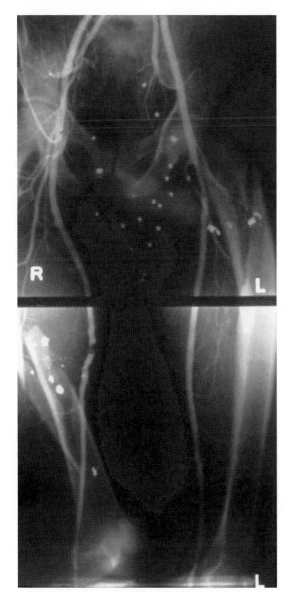

Figure 9.12 • Arteriogram of the pelvis and thighs to assess level of arterial injury after shotgun wound.

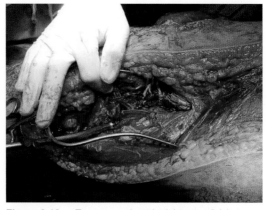

Figure 9.13 • Temporary shunt in right superficial femoral artery, allowing distal perfusion while external fixator is applied to the femur.

damage, the capacity of collaterals, pre-existing arterial disease and the vessels injured.[68]

- In certain cases primary amputation may be considered. Scoring systems such as the mangled extremity severity score (MESS) have been developed to help predict outcome of limb salvage procedures.[69] A MESS score of 7 or more has a predicted amputation rate of 100%. Given the significance of amputation, delaying the procedure even by a day or two is preferred as it allows careful examination of the limb and discussion with the patient and family.

- Measures should be taken to protect against the systemic effects of reperfusion injury and subsequent renal damage. A diuresis of at least 2–3 mL/kg per hour is maintained with the administration of adequate volumes of normal saline. This should be started during the operation and is continued postoperatively for as long as the serum myoglobin and creatine kinase remains elevated. Measures to treat hyperkalaemia may be required.

Vascular injuries to the upper extremity (Fig. 9.14)

The majority of injuries are to the brachial artery, and 90% of injuries are due to penetrating trauma.[70] Upper extremity vascular injuries are usually not life-threatening, but significant morbidity may occur. Return of function is often related to associated nerve injury. Venous injuries to the arm rarely require repair and even injuries to the brachial and axillary veins may be ligated because the collateral venous network is extensive.

Subclavian and axillary injuries

All patients with periclavicular trauma should be evaluated for possible vascular injury. Most of these injuries are caused by penetrating trauma. The presence of a peripheral pulse does not reliably exclude significant proximal arterial injury. A difference in blood pressure of more than 20 mmHg between the upper limbs or an API of less than 0.9 warrants further investigation. The brachial plexus is injured in about one-third of patients with subclavian or axillary artery injuries. A thorough neurological assessment should be performed.

Duplex ultrasound reliably assesses arterial and venous injuries but has certain limitations, for

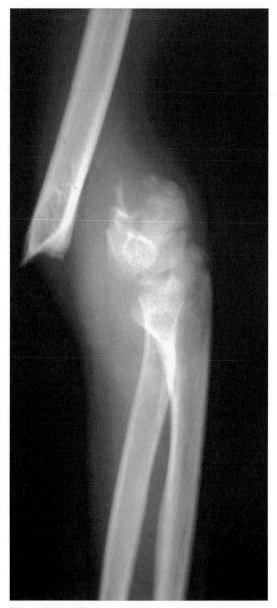

Figure 9.14 • Fractures of the supracondylar humerus are often associated with vascular injuries and should alert the physician to the possibility of a vascular injury.

example visualising the origin of the subclavian artery.[71] CT arteriography has a useful diagnostic role in evaluating superior mediastinal injuries, where duplex is inconclusive, and catheter arteriography has a therapeutic role in embolisation or stent graft repair.

Where surgical repair is required, the neck and chest should be included in the operative field. The patient is placed supine and the arm is draped free and abducted to 30°. The head is turned to the other side. The standard incision starts at the sternoclavicular joint and extends over the medial half of the clavicle, curving over the deltopectoral groove. For proximal subclavian artery injuries this incision can be combined with a median sternotomy, which gives excellent exposure of both proximal subclavian arteries.[36] The so-called 'trapdoor' incision (supraclavicular incision, upper third median sternotomy and left anterior thoracotomy) is not recommended due to significant postoperative morbidity.

The axillary artery is exposed through an infraclavicular incision between the clavicular and sternal parts of the pectoralis major muscle. Dividing the clavicle should be avoided whenever possible due to postoperative morbidity.

Promising results have been obtained with endovascular repair of pseudoaneurysms and arteriovenous fistulas in selected patients[20] (**Fig. 9.15a, b**). Most studies report a significant incidence of brachial plexus injury associated with surgical repair of subclavian artery injuries; this may be avoided with endovascular repair.[51]

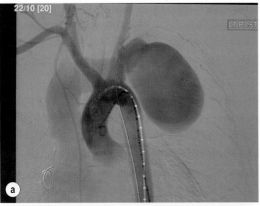

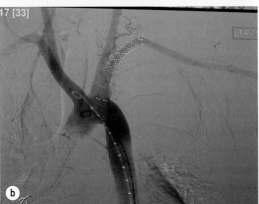

Figure 9.15 • Arteriovenous fistula of the subclavian artery **(a)** repaired by stent graft **(b)**.

Vascular injuries to the lower limb

These injuries are often associated with skeletal injuries, especially posterior dislocation of the knee, proximal tibial fractures and supracondylar femur fractures. Immediate arterial repair should be performed when the skeletal injury is stable and not significantly displaced. When there is instability, severe displacement and where extreme orthopaedic manipulation is anticipated, a temporary shunt should be placed to restore blood flow while the orthopaedic repair is completed, after which definite arterial repair is performed. Patients may have significant exsanguination from these injuries, which should be controlled with direct pressure.

Femoral vascular injuries
Bleeding from the femoral triangle can be difficult to control, particularly if both the artery and vein are injured. The suprainguinal region can be entered through a separate incision above the inguinal ligament to obtain proximal control of vessels.

✔✔ Common femoral artery injuries should always be repaired as ligation has a 50% amputation rate.[68]

Effort should be made to also repair the common femoral vein.

Iatrogenic injuries (pseudoaneurysms and arteriovenous fistula) secondary to attempted femoral access are fairly common. Primary treatment of femoral pseudoaneurysms consists of ultrasound-guided compression and thrombin injection.[72]

Popliteal vascular injury
Popliteal artery injury has an amputation rate of up to 16%.[68] The association between posterior knee dislocation and popliteal artery disruption is well known (**Fig. 9.16**). All patients with posterior knee dislocations should have a complete neurovascular examination of the affected limb. Most popliteal artery injuries present with hard signs of arterial injury. The absence of hard signs is usually sufficient to rule out injuries to the popliteal artery.[73]

✔✔ Selective arteriography following knee dislocation is safe as there is a strong correlation between results of serial physical examinations and the need for arteriography. Patients who are managed expectantly should be closely observed, with regular reassessment of the peripheral circulation.[74,75]

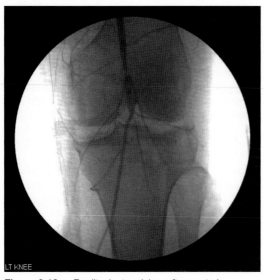

Figure 9.16 • Popliteal artery injury after posterior dislocation of the left knee.

Injury to popliteal veins should be repaired in order to minimise postoperative swelling and compartment syndrome and to improve the patency of arterial repairs.

Compartment syndrome is a major risk factor for amputation following popliteal artery injury.[76] There is evidence that fasciotomy performed at the time of arterial repair, but before the development of compartment syndrome (prophylactic fasciotomy), may lower amputation rates, particularly in patients with long preoperative delays, extensive injuries, injuries of the artery and vein, and venous injuries treated with ligation.

Single tibial vessels may be ligated if there is documented collateral flow distally.

Key points

- A high index of suspicion should be maintained regarding possible vascular injuries in the trauma patient.
- A thorough clinical examination is accurate in predicting significant vascular injury.
- Special investigations should only be performed in adequately resuscitated and haemodynamically stable patients.
- Haemodynamic instability, active bleeding and an expanding haematoma are indications for immediate surgery.
- The absence of hard signs of arterial injury justifies an expectant non-operative approach with careful observation.
- Restoration of arterial blood supply should be achieved as soon as possible; temporary intra-arterial shunts are valuable in this regard.
- Adequate surgical exposure is vital for proper management of vascular injuries.
- Fasciotomy should be applied liberally in lower-extremity vascular trauma.
- Endovascular treatment is useful in managing arterial lesions in anatomically challenging locations and is currently indicated for injuries of the descending thoracic aorta, proximal aortic arch branches, and distal internal carotid and vertebral arteries.

References

1. Herberer G, Becker HM, Ditmer H, et al. Vascular injuries in polytrauma. World J Surg 1983;7:68–79.

2. Fingerhut A, Leppäniemi AK, Androulakis GA, et al. The European experience with vascular injuries. Surg Clin North Am 2002;82:175–88.

3. Bowley DMG, Degiannis E, Goosen J, et al. Penetrating vascular trauma in Johannesburg, South Africa. Surg Clin North Am 2002;82:221–36.

4. Levien LJ. Ballistics of bullet injury. In: Champion HR, Robbs JV, Trunkey D, editors. Robb and Smith's operative surgery. 4th ed. London: Butterworths; 1989. p. 106–10.

5. Burkhardt GE, Gifford SM, Propper BW, et al. The impact of ischaemic interval on neuromuscular recovery in a porcine (Susscrofa) survival model of extremity vascular injury. J Vasc Surg 2011;53:165–75.

6. Dennis JW, Frykberg ER, Veldenz HC, et al. Validation of non-operative management of occult vascular injuries and accuracy of physical examination alone in penetrating extremity trauma: 5–10 year follow up. J Trauma 1998;44:243–53.
   A prospective study with 10-year follow-up proving the accuracy of clinical assessment and conservative management of occult vascular trauma.

7. Johansen K, Lynch K. Non-invasive vascular tests reliably exclude occult arterial trauma in injured extremities. J Trauma 1991;31:515–22.

In this prospective study it was shown that an API of more than 0.9 has a negative predictive value of 99% for excluding significant arterial trauma. Reserving arteriography for limbs with an API of less than 0.9 is safe, accurate and cost-effective.

8. Bickell WH, Wall MJ, Pepe PE, et al. Immediate vs delayed fluid resuscitation for hypotensive patients with penetrating torso injuries. N Engl J Med 1994;331:1105–9.

In a randomised controlled trial of patients with penetrating torso injuries, reduced mortality and complications were seen when fluid resuscitation was delayed until haemorrhage was controlled.

9. Weaver FA, Yellin AE. Is arterial proximity a valid indication for arteriography in penetrating extremity trauma? A prospective study. Arch Surg 1990;125:1256–60.

In this prospective study of 373 patients with penetrating extremity trauma it was found that arteriography rarely identified significant arterial injury in the absence of clinical signs, and that its routine use was not justified.

10. O'Gorman RB, Feliciano DV. Emergency centre arteriography in the evaluation of suspected peripheral vascular injuries. Arch Surg 1984;119:568–73.

11. Shah DM, Leather RP, Carson JD, et al. Polytetrafluoro-ethylene grafts in the rapid reconstruction of acute contaminated peripheral vascular injuries. Am J Surg 1984;148:229–33.

12. Barros D'Sa AAB. Complex vascular and orthopedic injuries. J Bone Joint Surg 1992;74:176–8.

This paper discusses the problems encountered with, and management of, complex vascular and orthopaedic injuries, advocating the use of temporary arterial and venous shunts for improving outcome.

13. Panetta T, Sclafani SJA, Goldstein AS, et al. Percutaneous transcatheter embolization for massive bleeding from pelvic fractures. J Trauma 1985;25:1021–9.

14. Coldwell DM, Stokes KR, Jakes WF. Embolotherapy: agents, clinical applications and techniques. Radiographics 1994;14:623–43.

15. Mervis SE, Pais SO. Trauma radiology: part 3. Diagnostic and therapeutic angiography in trauma. Intensive Care Med 1994;9:244–56.

16. Carrillo EH, Spain DA, Wohltmann D, et al. Interventional techniques are useful adjuncts in non-operative management of hepatic injuries. J Trauma 1999;46:619–22.

17. Sclafani SJ, Shafton GW, Scalea TM, et al. Non-operative salvage of CT diagnosed splenic injury: utilization of angiography for triage and embolization for hemostases. J Trauma 1995;39:818–25.

18. Scalea TM, Sclafani SJ. Angiographically placed balloons for arterial control: a description of a technique. J Trauma 1991;31:1671–7.

19. Lachat M, Phammatter T, Witzke H, et al. Acute traumatic aortic rupture: early stentgraft repair. Eur J Cardiothorac Surg 2002;21:956–63.

20. Du Toit DF, Strauss DC, Blaszczyk M, et al. Endovascular treatment of penetrating thoracic outlet arterial injuries. Eur J Vasc Endovasc Surg 2000;19:489–95.

The authors give an overview of the clinical problem and discuss the technique used.

21. Gomez CR, May AK, Terry JB, et al. Endovascular therapy of traumatic injuries of the extracranial cerebral arteries. Crit Care Clin 1999;15:789–809.

22. Demetriades D, Theodorou D, Asensio J. Management options in vertebral arteries injuries. Br J Surg 1996;83:83–6.

23. Kumar SR, Weaver FA, Yellin AE. Cervical vascular injuries: carotid and jugular venous injuries. Surg Clin North Am 2001;81:1331–44.

24. McKevitt EC, Kirkpatrick AW, Vertisi L, et al. Blunt vascular neck injuries: diagnosis and outcomes of extra-cranial vessel injury. J Trauma 2002;53:472–6.

25. Weaver FA, Yellin AE, Wagner WH, et al. The role of arterial reconstruction in penetrating carotid injuries. Arch Surg 1988;123:1106–11.

26. Biffl WL, Moore EE, Offner PJ, et al. Blunt carotid and vertebral arterial injuries. World J Surg 2001;25:1036–43.

27. Fry WR, Dot JA, Smith RS, et al. Duplex scanning replaces arteriography and operative exploration in the diagnosis of potential cervical vascular injury. Am J Surg 1994;168:693–5.

28. Corr P, Abdool-Carim AT, Robbs J. Colour-flow ultrasound in the detection of penetrating vascular injuries of the neck. S Afr Med J 1999;80:644–6.

This prospective study demonstrates the sensitivity of colour-flow ultrasound as a screening investigation to detect vascular injuries following penetrating neck trauma.

29. Demetriades D, Charalambides D, Lakhoo M. Physical examination and selective conservative management in patients with penetrating injuries of the neck. Br J Surg 1993;80:1534–6.

30. Levy C, Laissy JP, Raveau V, et al. Carotid and vertebral artery dissections: three-dimensional time-of-flight MR angiography and MR imaging vs conventional angiography. Radiology 1994;190:97–103.

31. Gilroy D, Lakhoo M, Sharalambides D, et al. Control of life-threatening haemorrhage from the neck: a new indication for balloon tamponade. Injury 1992;23:557–9.

32. Stain SC, Yellin AE, Weaver FA, et al. Selective management of non-occlusive arterial injuries. Arch Surg 1989;124:1136–40.

33. Frykberg ER, Crump JM, Dennis JW, et al. Non-operative observation of clinically occult arterial injuries: a prospective evaluation. Surgery 1991;109:85–96.

34. Robbs JV. Penetrating injury to the blood vessels of the neck and mediastinum. In: Branchereai A, Jacobs M, editors. Vascular emergencies. New York: Futura; 2003. p. 39–48.

35. Fabian TC, Pattern Jr. JH, Croce MA, et al. Blunt carotid injury. Importance of early diagnosis and anticoagulation therapy. Ann Surg 1996;223:513–25.

36. Robbs JV. Injuries to the vessels of the neck and superior mediastinum. In: Champion HR, Robbs JV, Trunky D, editors. Robb and Smith's operative surgery. 4th ed. London: Butterworths; 1989. p. 529–38.

37. Nair R, Robbs JV, Muckart D. Management of penetrating cervico-mediastinal venous trauma. Eur J Vasc Endovasc Surg 2000;19:65–9.

38. Demetriades D, Theodorou D, Cornwill E, et al. Evaluation of penetrating injuries of the neck: prospective study of 223 patients. World J Surg 1997;21:41–8.

39. Nadgir RN, Loevner LA, Ahmed T, et al. Simultaneous internal carotid and vertebral artery dissection following chiropractic manipulation: case report and review of the literature. Neuroradiology 2003;45:311–4.

40. Biffl WL, Moore E, Elliot J, et al. The devastating potential of blunt vertebral artery injuries. Ann Surg 2000;231:672–81.

41. Munera F, Solo J, Palacio D, et al. Diagnosis of arterial injuries caused by penetrating trauma to the neck: comparison of helical CT angiography and conventional angiography. Radiology 2000;216:556–62.

42. Hatzitheofilou C, Demetriades D, Melissas J, et al. Surgical approaches to vertebral artery injuries. Br J Surg 1988;75:234–7.

43. Mwipatyi BP, Jeffery P, Benningfield SJ, et al. Management of extra-cranial vertebral artery injuries. Eur J Vasc Endovasc Surg 2004;27:156–62.

44. Duane TM, Parker F, Stokes GK, et al. Endovascular carotid stenting after trauma. J Trauma 2002;52:149–53.

45. Mattox KL, Feliciano DV, Burch J, et al. Five thousand seven hundred and sixty cardiovascular injuries in 4459 patients. Epidemiologic evolution 1958–1978. Ann Surg 1989;209:698–707.

46. Clancy TV, Gary-Maxwell J, Covington BI, et al. A statewide analysis of level I and II trauma centers for patients with major injuries. J Trauma 2001;51:346–57.

47. Patel NH, Stephens KE, Mirvis SE, et al. Imaging of acute thoracic aortic injury due to blunt trauma: a review. Radiology 1998;209:335–48.

48. Gavant ML, Menke PG, Fabian T, et al. Blunt traumatic aortic rupture: detection with helical CT of the chest. Radiology 1995;197:125–33.
Helical CT is compared to conventional arteriography in a series of 1518 patients with blunt chest trauma. CT sensitivity and specificity were 100% and 82%, respectively, vs. 94% and 96% for conventional arteriography.

49. Magissano R, Nathens A, Alexandrova NA, et al. Traumatic rupture of the thoracic aorta: should one always operate immediately? Ann Vasc Surg 1995;9:44–52.

50. Fischer RG, Oria RA, Mattox KL, et al. Conservative management of aortic lacerations due to blunt trauma. J Trauma 1990;30:1562–6.

51. Carrick MM, Morrison CA, Pham HQ, et al. Modern management of traumatic subclavian artery injuries. A single institution's experience in the evolution of cardiovascular repair. Am J Surg 2010;199:28–34.

52. Lee WA, Matsumura MD, Mitchell RS, et al. Endovascular repair of traumatic thoracic aortic injury: clinical practice guidelines for the Society for Vascular Surgery. J Vasc Surg 2011;53:187–92.
A systematic review of 7768 patients from 139 studies.

53. Aucar JA, Hirshberg A. Damage control for vascular injuries. Surg Clin North Am 1997;77:853–62.
A good review of the different techniques in vascular damage control.

54. Asensio JA. Abdominal vascular injuries. Surg Clin North Am 2001;81:1395–416.

55. Fontaine AB, Nichols SC, Barsa J, et al. Seatbelt aorta: endovascular management with a stentgraft. J Endovasc Ther 2001;8:83–6.

56. Fullen WD, Hunt J, Altemeier WA. The clinical spectrum of penetrating injury to the superior mesenteric arterial circulation. J Trauma 1972;12:656–64.

57. Lee JT, White RA. Endovascular management of blunt traumatic renal artery dissection. J Endovasc Ther 2002;9:354–8.

58. Burch JM, Feliciano DV, Mattox KL. Injuries to the inferior vena cava. Am J Surg 1998;156:548–52.

59. Buckman RF, Bradley M. Injuries to the inferior vena cava. Surg Clin North Am 2001;81:1431–48.

60. Castelli P, Caronno R, Pifaretti G, et al. Emergency endovascular repair for traumatic injury of the inferior vena cava. Eur J Cardiothorac Surg 2005;28:906–8.

61. White R, Krajcer Z, Johnson M, et al. Results of a multicentre trial for the treatment of traumatic artery injury with a covered stent. J Trauma 2006;60:1189–95.

62. Frykberg ER, Dennis JW, Bishop K, et al. The reliability of physical examination in the evaluation of penetrating extremity trauma for vascular injury: results at one year. J Trauma 1991;31:502–11.

63. Frykberg ER, Crump JM, Vines FS, et al. A reassessment of the role of arteriography in penetrating proximity trauma: a prospective study. J Trauma 1989;29:1041–52.

64. Schwartz M, Weaver F, Yellin A, et al. The utility of color flow Doppler examination in penetrating extremity arterial trauma. Am Surg 1993;59:375–8.

65. Percival TJ, Rasmussen TE. Reperfusion strategies in the management of extremity vascular injury with ischaemia. BJS 2012;99(Suppl. 1):66–74.

66. Keen RR, Meyer JP, Durham JR, et al. Autogenous vein graft repair of injured extremity arteries: early and late results with 134 consecutive patients. J Vasc Surg 1991;13:664–8.

67. Mabee JR, Bostwick TL. Pathophysiology and mechanisms of compartment syndrome. Orthop Rev 1993;22:175–81.

68. Hafez HM, Woolgar J, Robbs JV. Lower extremity arterial injury: results of 550 cases and review of risk factors associated with limb loss. J Vasc Surg 2001;33:1212–9.

   The authors review the factors associated with limb loss in their extensive experience of more than 500 cases.

69. Johansen K, Daines M, Howey T, et al. Objective criteria accurately predict amputation following lower extremity trauma. J Trauma 1990;30:568–72.

70. Hunt CA, Kingsley JR. Upper extremity trauma. South Med J 2000;93:466–8.

71. Demetriades D, Ascensio JA. Subclavian and axillary vascular injuries. Surg Clin North Am 2001;81:1357–73.

72. Lonn L, Olmarker A, Geterud K, Risberg B. Prospective randomized study comparing ultrasound-guided thrombin injection to compression in the treatment of femoral pseudo-aneurysms. J Endovasc Ther 2004;11:570–6.

73. Miranda FE, Dennis JW, Frykberg ER, et al. Confirmation of the safety and accuracy of physical examination in the evaluation of knee dislocation for injury of the popliteal artery: a prospective study. J Trauma 2000;49:247–52.

74. Stannard JP, Shiels TM, Lopez-Ben RR, et al. Vascular injuries in knee dislocations: the role of physical examination in determining the need for arteriography. J Bone Joint Surg 2004;86:910–4.

75. Holtis JD, Daley BJ. 10-year review of knee dislocations: is arteriography always necessary? J Trauma 2005;59:672–6.

76. Fainzilber G, Roy-Shapira A, Wall Jr MJ, et al. Predictions of amputation for popliteal artery injuries. Am J Surg 1995;170:568–70.

10

Extracranial cerebrovascular disease

A. Ross Naylor
Sumaira Macdonald

Introduction

Stroke is the third commonest cause of death and the principal cause of neurological disability. It is defined as an acute loss of focal cerebral function with symptoms exceeding 24 hours (or leading to death), with no apparent cause other than that of a vascular origin. A transient ischaemic attack (TIA) has the same definition but lasts <24 hours. In the UK, the annual incidence of stroke is 2 per 1000 and 125 000 patients will suffer their first stroke each year.[1] Half of all strokes affect patients >75 years of age. Stroke patients use 10% of inpatient beds and 5% of healthcare expenditure.[2] Although mortality has diminished by about 20%, attributed to improved survival rather than a decline in incidence, the incidence of stroke could increase by 30% by 2033 because of the ageing population.[3] About 36 000 patients will suffer a TIA each year, giving an annual UK incidence of 0.5 per 1000. TIA incidence increases with age from 0.9 per 1000 (55–64 years) to 2.6 per 1000 (75–84 years).[4]

Aetiology and risk factors

About 80% of strokes are ischaemic, the remainder haemorrhagic (intracerebral/subarachnoid). Approximately 80% of ischaemic strokes affect the carotid territory. Risk factors include increasing age, smoking, hypertension, ischaemic heart disease, cardioemboli, previous TIA, diabetes, peripheral vascular disease, high plasma fibrinogen and hypercholesterolaemia. The principal causes of ischaemic, carotid territory stroke are: thromboembolism of the internal carotid artery (ICA) or middle cerebral artery (MCA) (50%); small-vessel intracranial disease (25%); cardiac embolism (15%); haematological disorders (5%); and non-atheromatous disease (5%).[4]

Large-vessel thromboembolism

The commonest cause is thromboembolism of the ICA and/or MCA. Haemodynamic failure accounts for <2% of strokes. Stenoses develop at the ICA origin because of a region of low shear stress, flow stasis and flow separation that predisposes to atherosclerotic plaque formation. Should the plaque undergo acute disruption (rupture, ulceration, intraplaque haemorrhage), the core of subendothelial collagen is exposed, triggering thrombus formation and embolism.

Small-vessel disease

Occlusion of penetrating end-arterioles causes lacunar infarcts. The occlusive process follows fibrinoid necrosis (hypertensive encephalopathy), lipohyalinosis and micro-atheroma (chronic hypertension) or microcalcinosis (diabetes). The commonest sites for lacunar infarction include the basal ganglia, thalamus and internal capsule.

Cardiogenic brain embolism

Sources include ventricular mural thrombus (post-myocardial infarction, cardiomyopathy), left atrial thrombus (atrial fibrillation) and valvular lesions (vegetations, prostheses, calcified annulus, endocarditis).

Haematological disorders

Myeloma, sickle-cell disease, polycythaemia, the oral contraceptive pill and related prothrombotic disorders predispose towards stroke.

Non-atheromatous carotid diseases

Fibromuscular dysplasia (FMD)

FMD is a rare disorder of unknown aetiology affecting medium-sized arteries, including the renal (60–75%) and carotid arteries (25–30%), in young to middle-aged women. The commonest presentation is hypertension. FMD is classified as: (i) intimal fibroplasia; (ii) medial dysplasia (medial fibroplasia, perimedial fibroplasia, medial hyperplasia); and (iii) adventitial (periarterial) fibroplasia. The commonest is medial fibroplasia (75–80% of cases), characterised by alternating stenotic webs and dilatation/aneurysm formation (**Fig. 10.1**). In up to 60%, FMD is bilateral. Patients with carotid FMD may be asymptomatic or symptomatic (TIA/stroke, dissection, false aneurysm). Although management tends to be conservative in asymptomatic individuals, surveillance is recommended. Once symptomatic, patients should be treated as for symptomatic atherosclerotic disease. Options include resection and interposition bypass, open graduated internal dilatation or (more commonly) percutaneous angioplasty.

Arteritis (see also Chapter 12)

Takayasu's arteritis (TA) is a transmural, granulomatous inflammatory condition, ultimately causing occlusion through fibrosis. TA predominantly affects younger females (female to male ratio 7:1) and presentation may be a relatively innocuous illness comprising malaise, fever and arthralgia/myalgia. In the acute phase, there is a granulomatous vasculitis with medial disruption, followed by transmural fibrosis. Occasionally, focal aneurysms form as a consequence of disruption of the internal elastic lamina and media.

Neurological symptoms follow occlusion or are via renovascular hypertension. Type I TA (arch branches) and type IIa (ascending aorta, aortic arch, arch branches) present with cerebral vascular/ocular symptoms or asymptomatic stenoses. Type III TA (arch vessels plus abdominal aorta and its branches) accounts for 65% of cases and is associated with stroke, renovascular hypertension and mesenteric ischaemia.

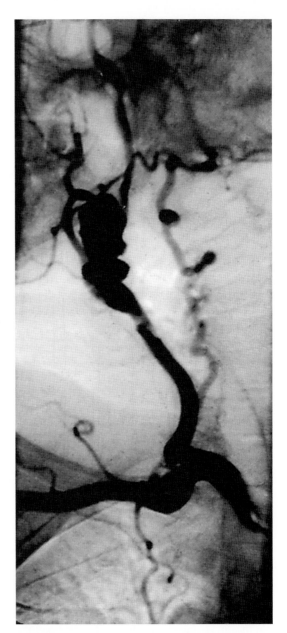

Figure 10.1 • Example of fibromuscular dysplasia causing early aneurysm formation in the carotid artery.

The mainstay of management is immunosuppression (steroid/cyclophosphamide/methotrexate). Surgery should be avoided in the acute phase. Neither endarterectomy nor angioplasty/stenting is really an option with involvement of the carotid vessels because of the long segments of fibrotic disease. If surgery becomes necessary, bypass is the preferred option and the inflow should be taken from the ascending aorta (as opposed to the subclavian artery) as the latter may be involved in the disease process.

Giant-cell arteritis (GCA) is the most common primary vasculitis in adults and primarily affects older females (female to male ratio 4:1). There are three recognised subtypes (systemic inflammatory syndrome, cranial arteritis and large vessel arteritis). The intracranial vessels are unaffected. The commonest presentation is generalised malaise, headache and myalgic pain. Jaw claudication occurs in 50%, while 50% will develop pain over the temporal artery. Stroke is rare, the commonest presentation being transient/permanent blindness. Ocular symptoms (blindness, corneal ulcers/cataracts) can occur up to 6 months after initial presentation. Treatment is corticosteroid therapy.

Carotid aneurysm

Carotid aneurysms are rare (<4% of peripheral aneurysms). The accepted definition is a diameter >150% of the common carotid artery (CCA) or twice the diameter of the distal ICA. The aetiology is unknown, but may be 'atherosclerotic' or follow trauma/infection. Presentations include pulsatile swelling (with/without pain), Horner's syndrome, thrombosis, dissection, rupture or embolisation (TIA/stroke). Treatment involves exclusion and primary re-anastomosis or interposition bypass. Endovascular exclusion is the preferred option in patients with distal ICA aneurysms.

Carotid dissection

Dissection causes 2% of strokes, increasing to 20% in young adults (**Fig. 10.2**). One-fifth of trauma patients with an unexplained neurological deficit will have suffered a dissection and 25% will be bilateral. Dissection can be spontaneous (fibromuscular dysplasia), iatrogenic (rarely following angioplasty/stenting), be part of a central dissection (type A thoracic dissection) or follow blunt trauma (direct crushing, forced hyperextension or forced rotation) with crushing of the ICA between the mastoid process and the transverse process of C2.

Type I dissections involve irregularity but no significant stenosis; type II involves a 70–99% stenosis and/or a >50% dilatation, while type III dissections present with the characteristic 'flame'-shaped occlusion about 2–3 cm distal to the bifurcation. The latter appearance is due to compression of the true lumen by thrombus in the false channel.

The commonest presentation is ipsilateral head/neck pain (70%), but 50–75% of patients will then present with TIA/stroke (usually embolic), pulsatile tinnitus, syncope, ocular signs or cranial nerve palsies (III, IV, VI, VII, IX, X, XII). Cranial nerve signs probably follow mechanical compression from mural haematoma or stretching. Up to

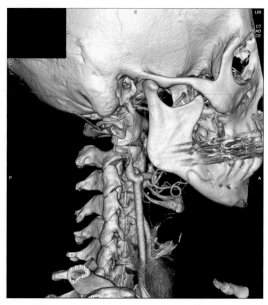

Figure 10.2 • Three-dimensional CT angiogram showing typical features of an acute dissection of the right ICA. The dissection starts 2–3 cm above the true bifurcation and blood in the false lumen compresses the true lumen (the narrow channel extending up to the skull base).

60% with spontaneous dissection will have ocular signs (oculo-sympathetic paresis, amaurosis fugax (aggravated by sitting/standing), hemianopia, ischaemic optic neuropathy and painful Horner's syndrome). The latter follows segmental ischaemia of the postganglionic fibres distal to the superior cervical ganglion and may persist in 50%.

> ✅ Recognition of ocular symptoms in patients with suspected dissection is important as up to 25% will suffer a stroke within 7 days.

Patients suspected of having a dissection should undergo ultrasound and computed tomography (CT) or magnetic resonance angiography (MRA). This typically shows the dissection to start 2–3 cm beyond the origin of the ICA (Fig. 10.2). The distal limit is variable (occasionally as high as the petrous segment) with varying combinations of stenosis, dilatation, intimal flaps and occlusion in the intervening segment. The majority are managed conservatively. The aim is to reduce the risk of thrombosis and embolism.

> ✅ Most are treated with anticoagulation (heparin then warfarin), but systematic reviews suggest that there is no evidence that this is preferable/safer to antiplatelet therapy.[5]

Endovascular intervention is reserved for complex trauma cases (usually type II), but may be indicated in patients with recurrent cerebral events despite medical therapy. Overall, dissection carries a 20% mortality and a 30% rate of persisting disability.

Carotid body tumour

The carotid body is located within the adventitia of the posterior aspect of the carotid bifurcation and is responsible for monitoring blood gases/pH. A carotid body tumour (CBT) is derived from cells originating from the neural crest ectoderm (chemoreceptor cells), is typically located in the space between the ICA and external carotid arteries (ECA), and consists of nests of neoplastic epithelioid chief cells. As it enlarges, the bifurcation splays (**Fig. 10.3a**) and the patient becomes aware of a neck swelling. Other presentations include pain, invasion/compression causing hoarseness, cranial nerve palsies and Horner's syndrome. CBTs rarely present with cerebral ischaemia, but can present as a hormonally mediated syndrome comprising flushing, dizziness, arrhythmias and hypertension.

Diagnosis requires awareness, supplemented by ultrasound and MRA/CT angiography. Overall, 5% are bilateral and 5% are malignant. Treatment involves excision, although a conservative approach may be preferable in elderly patients with small asymptomatic tumours. Preoperative embolisation or insertion of a covered stent into the proximal ECA may reduce intraoperative bleeding, but this is probably only necessary in large tumours.

Differential diagnoses include glomus vagale/glomus jugulare tumours. The glomus vagale tumour arises from chemoreceptor cells within the vagus nerve and can be differentiated from a CBT because the bifurcation is not splayed. Instead, the tumour causes deviation of the ICA above the bifurcation (**Fig. 10.3b**). It is important to consider a glomus vagale tumour preoperatively as resection leads to swallowing problems (injury to motor fibres) and hoarseness (recurrent laryngeal nerve) and the patient has to be warned of this possibility.

Presentation of carotid disease

Asymptomatic cerebrovascular disease

Four per cent of patients >45 years will have a bruit, increasing to 12% in those >60 years.[6] One-third of patients with a 70–99% ICA stenosis will not have a bruit, increasing to 60% for those with 90–99%

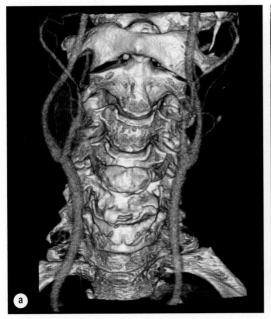
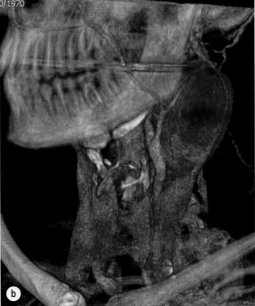

Figure 10.3 • (a) Three-dimensional reconstruction of a CT angiogram of a highly vascular right carotid body tumour causing splaying of the bifurcation. In addition to providing information about the size and location of the tumour, this type of imaging is useful to exclude bilateral involvement (present in 5%). Note that the majority of the tumour circulation arises from branches of the ECA. **(b)** Three-dimensional CT angiogram of a probable glomus vagale tumour. Note that the tumour does not splay the bifurcation, but it pushes between the ECA and ICA from a posterior location higher up in the neck.

stenoses. Paradoxically, up to 30% of patients with an ICA occlusion will still have an audible bruit. The commonest reasons for a false-positive bruit are systolic cardiac murmurs, haemodynamic causes and bruits arising from the vertebrals or ECA.

> ✔ The presence/absence of a bruit and the quality of the bruit does not correlate with the degree of stenosis.

Symptomatic cerebrovascular disease

Carotid territory

'Classical' carotid territory symptoms include: (1) hemimotor/sensory signs, (2) transient monocular blindness (TMB) and (3) higher cortical dysfunction (Box 10.1). TMB usually develops over a few seconds and clears within a few minutes. Failure to resolve within 24 hours is analogous to a stroke.

> ✔ A history of TMB in the absence of a source of embolisation should prompt referral to an ophthalmologist to exclude anterior ischaemic optic neuropathy (microvascular disease of the posterior ciliary arteries), which causes acute ischaemia of the optic nerve head.

Differential diagnoses for carotid territory events include epilepsy, tumour, giant aneurysm, hypoglycaemia and migraine (i.e. stroke mimics). Where TIAs are precipitated by a heavy meal, hot bath or exercise, a haemodynamically critical ICA stenosis should be suspected.

Box 10.1 • 'Classical' carotid and vertebrobasilar features

Carotid territory
Hemimotor/hemisensory signs
Monocular visual loss (amaurosis fugax)
Higher cortical dysfunction (dysphasia, visuospatial neglect, etc.)
Vertebrobasilar
Bilateral blindness
Problems with gait and stance
Hemi- or bilateral motor/sensory signs
Dysarthria
Homonymous hemianopia
Diplopia, vertigo and nystagmus (provided it is not the only symptom)

Conventional teaching has been that the risk of stroke after suffering a TIA/minor stroke is 1–2% at 7 days and 2–4% at 30 days. This, in conjunction with a reluctance to perform carotid surgery within the hyperacute period (because of concerns about increased procedural risks), has led to there being no real urgency regarding referral, investigation and management. However, there is now compelling evidence (Table 10.1) that the risk of stroke may be as high as 10% within 7 days of the index event,[7,8] with almost half of these strokes occurring within the first 24 hours.[9] The stroke risk may be as high as 20% at 7 days in TIA patients with a 50–99% carotid stenosis.[10] There is good evidence that the early risk of stroke can be predicted from the ABCD[2] score[11] (see below).

With increasing awareness that TIAs should be investigated and treated urgently, single-visit,

Table 10.1 • Early risk of stroke after presenting with a TIA

	6 h	12 h	24 h	48 h	72 h	7 days	14 days	28 days
Conventional teaching						1–2%		2–4%
Meta-analysis (face to face)[7,8]				6.7%		10.4%		
Single-centre series (very early period)[9]	1.2%	2.1%	5.1%					
Single centre (ICA stenosis 50–99%)[10]					17%	22%	25%	
ABCD[2] 0–3[11]				1.0%		1.2%		
ABCD[2] 4–5[11]				4.1%		5.9%		
ABCD[2] 6–7[11]				8.1%		11.7%		
Infarction on CT/MRI + ABCD[2] score 0–3[12]						2.3%		
+ ABCD[2] score 4–5[12]						8.9%		
+ ABCD[2] score 6–7[12]						15.0%		
No infarction on CT/MRI + ABCD[2] score 0–3[12]						0.2%		
+ ABCD[2] score 4–5[12]						1.4%		
+ ABCD[2] score 6–7[12]						3.3%		

Table 10.2 • ABCD^2 scoring system for predicting the 7-day risk of stroke after TIA

Parameter		Score	Max. score
Age >60 years		1	1
Systolic >140 mmHg or diastolic >90 mmHg		1	1
Clinical features	Unilateral weakness	2	
	Speech disturbance, no weakness	1	2
	Other	0	
Duration of symptoms	>60 min	2	
	10–59 min	1	2
	<10 min	0	
Diabetes	Yes	1	1

Data derived from Johnston SC, Rothwell PM, Nguyen-Huynh N et al. Validation and refinement of scores to predict very early stroke risk after transient ischaemic attack. Lancet 2007; 369:283–92.

rapid-access clinics have been established. In most UK centres, referrals are triaged using the ABCD^2 scoring system (Table 10.2). The decision to refer should never be influenced by the presence/absence of a carotid bruit.[12] The 'ABCD^2' scoring system[11] allocates a score based on five bedside parameters (A = age, B = blood pressure, C = clinical features, D = duration of symptoms, D = diabetes), with '7' being the maximum). The early risk of stroke increases rapidly as the ABCD^2 score increases (Table 10.1).

✔ It is not logistically possible to see every suspected TIA patient within <24 hours of referral. The ABCD^2 scoring system enables patients with the lowest 7-day risks of stroke (0–3) to be triaged and seen within 7 days. However, anyone with an ABCD^2 score of 4–7 should be seen the same day or the following morning.

A recent modification to the ABCD^2 score has been the inclusion of whether or not there is CT/magnetic resonance imaging (MRI) evidence of infarction.[13] In a prospective, multicentre series (4574 patients), the presence of CT/MRI infarction increased the early risk of stroke, irrespective of the ABCD^2 score (Table 10.1). Specifically, patients with CT/MRI infarction and a low ABCD^2 score had a similar early risk of stroke to patients with no evidence of infarction but a high ABCD^2 score.

Vertebrobasilar

Vertebrobasilar (VB) symptoms (Box 10.1) include bilateral blindness, problems with gait/stance, hemilateral/bilateral motor or sensory impairment (10% will have hemisensory/motor signs), dysarthria, homonymous hemianopia, nystagmus, dizziness, diplopia and vertigo (provided the latter three are not isolated).

✔ VB TIAs carry early stroke risks comparable to carotid territory events, especially if they have an ipsilateral 50–99% stenosis (20–30% stroke risk within 90 days[14]). Patients reporting VB symptoms need to be treated urgently.

Non-hemispheric

The term 'non-hemispheric' is allocated to patients with isolated syncope (blackout, drop attack), presyncope (faintness), isolated dizziness, isolated double vision (diplopia) and isolated vertigo.

✔ 'Non-hemispheric' symptoms should never be considered to be carotid or VB in origin unless other 'classical' symptoms are present. It is very important to exclude a cardiac or inner ear pathology.

Investigation of carotid disease

✔ NICE recommendation: patients who have a suspected TIA with an ABCD^2 score of 4–7 should undergo specialist assessment and investigation within 24 hours of onset of symptoms.[15]

NICE recommendation: patients who have a suspected TIA with an ABCD^2 score of 0–3 should undergo specialist assessment and investigation within 7 days of onset of symptoms.[15]

Every centre should have clear guidelines as to which measurement method is being used to measure stenosis severity (ECST/NASCET).

These recommendations focus attention on three important issues. (i) What is the best single and/or combination imaging strategy? (ii) How do imaging strategies for carotid artery stenting (CAS) and carotid endarterectomy (CEA) differ? (iii) Can these imaging strategies be provided within a 24-hour window in symptomatic patients?

Duplex ultrasound

The degree of stenosis is usually first evaluated using duplex ultrasound, which combines B-mode (real-time) imaging with waveform analysis using pulsed-wave Doppler. Advantages include (i) low cost; (ii) accessibility within 'single-visit' clinics and (iii) being non-invasive. There are recognised limitations to duplex, mostly relating to the expertise of the practitioner. With highly experienced sonographers, however, duplex can identify up to 95% of lesions responsible for carotid territory symptoms. In most UK centres, the majority of CEA procedures are planned on the basis of duplex alone.

✔ The Society of Radiologists in Ultrasound Consensus Conference[16] noted that duplex 'is often performed inconsistently within a given laboratory and there is non-uniformity in practice from one laboratory to the next. In many settings, interpretive criteria for carotid stenosis are either indiscriminately applied or the interpreters are uncertain about exactly how to make the diagnosis of carotid stenosis.'

Duplex can only insonate the cervical portion of the extracranial carotid artery and is therefore relatively unreliable at excluding disease elsewhere.

In diabetic patients, the incidence of tandem distal ICA stenoses varies between 14% and 21.3%, while 17–24% will have tandem intracranial disease.[17] Any suspicion of additional lesions requires alternative imaging (e.g. MRA).

The Society of Radiologists in Ultrasound Consensus Conference[16] developed consensus criteria for diagnosing the severity of carotid disease based on the North American Symptomatic Carotid Endarterectomy Trial (NASCET) measurement method (Table 10.3).

The identification of the 'vulnerable plaque', i.e. those more likely to cause thromboembolic complications, has proved difficult to achieve with ultrasound. The Gray–Weale classification[18] classifies plaques according to whether they are echolucent (type 1), predominantly echolucent (type 2), predominantly echogenic (type 3) or echogenic (type 4). Unfortunately, correlation with histology and clinical risk is variable. An objective ultrasound parameter, the grey-scale median (GSM), has been shown to reliably differentiate between plaques associated with retinal and cerebrovascular symptomatology and asymptomatic status.[19] There are, however, conflicting reports regarding the correlation between plaques considered to be vulnerable on the basis of a GSM ≤25 and increased procedural risk during CAS.[20,21]

Catheter angiography

In the modern era of high-quality non-invasive imaging there is no role for routine catheter angiography. Arch angiography is employed in some CAS centres as a means of assessing anatomic suitability for CAS and the status of the aortic arch/ arch origins of the great vessels. It is associated

Table 10.3 • Society of Radiologists in Ultrasound Consensus Conference on ultrasound criteria for measuring carotid stenosis using the NASCET measurement method

Degree of stenosis (%)	Primary parameters		Additional parameters	
	ICA PSV (cm/s)	Plaque estimate (%)*	ICA/CCA PSV ratio	ICA EDV (cm/s)
Normal	<125	None	<2.0	<40
<50	<125	<50	<2.0	<40
50–69	125–230	>50	2.0–4.0	40–100
≥70 but less than near occlusion	>230	>50	>4.0	>100
Near occlusion	High, low, or undetectable	Visible	Variable	Variable
Total occlusion	Undetectable	Visible, no detectable lumen	Not applicable	Not applicable

Reproduced from Grant EG, Benson CB, Moneta GL et al. Carotid artery stenosis: gray-scale and Doppler US diagnosis – Society of Radiologists in Ultrasound Consensus Conference. Radiology 2003; 229:340–6. With permission from the Radiological Society of North America.
*Plaque estimate (diameter reduction) with grayscale and colour Doppler US.

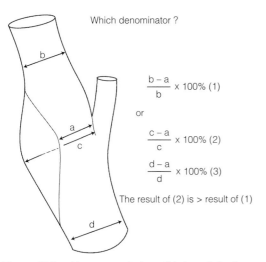

Which denominator ?

$$\frac{b-a}{b} \times 100\% \quad (1)$$

or

$$\frac{c-a}{c} \times 100\% \quad (2)$$

$$\frac{d-a}{d} \times 100\% \quad (3)$$

The result of (2) is > result of (1)

Figure 10.4 • Measurement of carotid stenosis by the ECST, NASCET and common carotid methods.

Table 10.4 • Correlation between ECST and NASCET measured carotid stenoses

NASCET (%)	ECST (%)
30	65
40	70
50	75
60	80
70	85
80	90
90	95

In reality, a 50% NASCET stenosis broadly corresponds to a 75% ECST, while a 70% NASCET stenosis is equivalent to an 85% ECST stenosis.

with a much lower rate of stroke than selective angiography.[22]

There are three methods for measuring stenosis severity, each using the luminal diameter at the point of maximum stenosis as the numerator (**Fig. 10.4**). Stenoses measured using the ECST method generate higher grades than those using the NASCET method (Table 10.4). However, while the CCA method may be the most reproducible, most cerebrovascular centres now use the NASCET measurement method.

✔✔ In ACAS, selective catheter angiography incurred a stroke/death risk of 1.5% (>50% of the overall surgical risk).[23] It is no longer part of the routine work-up of a TIA patient.

Magnetic resonance angiography

MRA uses flowing blood (time of flight) or gadolinium (contrast-enhanced MRA, CEMRA) as the contrast agent. CEMRA is not so dependent on vessel orientation and the field of view can be extended to include the arch of aorta and intracranial vessels (**Fig. 10.5**).

Although many studies comparing MRA with catheter angiography are methodologically flawed, a few are worthy of mention. One compared 71 bifurcations in 39 symptomatic patients with ultrasound, CEMRA and digital subtraction angiography (DSA).[24] For the detection of 'surgically appropriate' lesions, CEMRA was found to have a sensitivity of 95% and a specificity of 79%, with 10% false-positive and 2.5% false-negative rates. Ultrasound had similar accuracy.

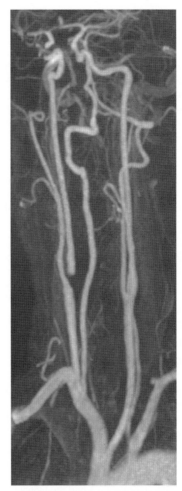

Figure 10.5 • CEMRA in the right anterior oblique orientation providing overview anatomical imaging, i.e. from the arch origin to the circle of Willis. There is an extremely tight stenosis (>95%) at the right carotid bulb/proximal internal carotid artery.

However, if ultrasound and CEMRA were concordant (80% of cases), then all 70–99% stenoses were correctly identified and there were only 8.4% false-positive results. These 'false positives' were in the 60–65% category of stenoses. A second study (50 patients) found that CEMRA misclassified 24% of surgically amenable lesions (ultrasound misclassified 36%), but when CEMRA and ultrasound were concordant (48% of lesions) there was 100% sensitivity and only 17% of lesions were misclassified.[25]

✅✅ Non-invasive imaging modalities for the evaluation of carotid stenosis were compared with DSA in a recent systematic review.[26] CEMRA had the highest sensitivity (0.94, 95% confidence interval (CI) 0.88–0.97), specificity and least heterogeneity, followed by ultrasound (0.89, 95% CI 0.85–0.92).

✅ If MRA is to be used to non-invasively image the carotid arteries, current data would suggest that this is best done in conjunction with ultrasound. There are no studies describing the accuracy of MRA in assessing arch disease.

If duplex ultrasound is used to plan CEA, the HTA recommend that a second corroborative scan be performed by a different technologist using a second duplex machine.[26]

Whilst MRA is non-invasive and does not involve the use of ionising radiation, gadolinium has recently been identified as the cause of nephrogenic systemic fibrosis (NSF).

✅ NSF is a systemic scleroderma-like condition that affects 3–5% of patients with pre-existing renal impairment exposed to gadolinium-based compounds. Five per cent of affected individuals exhibit a rapidly progressive course.

Computed tomography angiography (CTA)

Multidetector computed tomography (MDCT) angiography permits the rapid acquisition of large amounts of cross-sectional data that can be reformatted into any plane.

✅✅ In a systematic review on the performance of non-invasive imaging modalities in the assessment of a 70–99% stenosis, CTA had the highest specificity (0.94, 95% CI 0.91–0.97), followed by CEMRA (0.93, 95% CI 0.89–0.96), then ultrasound (0.84, 95% CI 0.77–0.89).[26] Unfortunately only single-detector row CT was evaluated in this review.

The principal advantages of CTA include: (i) minimally invasive (i.v. injection of iodinated contrast); (ii) overview anatomical imaging possible (short scan times and thinner 'slices' mean fewer artifacts); (iii) more accessible than MRA; and (iv) generally well tolerated. Disadvantages include: (i) requirement for iodinated contrast load; (ii) radiation burden; (iii) inability to impart dynamic information, i.e. 'trickle flow' not reliably identified; and (iv) heavy calcification can increase the difficulty of reliable estimates of stenosis severity.

✅ The National Clinical Guideline for Stroke 2004[27] recommends that duplex findings be confirmed by MRA (or second duplex). If the 'second' duplex option is adopted, it is good practice to ensure that this is performed by a second practitioner.

The Society of Radiologists in Ultrasound Consensus[16] recommends that vascular laboratories should have a system for quality assurance and that the NASCET measurement method is used.

Management of cerebrovascular disease

'Best medical therapy'

All patients benefit from optimisation of risk factors, antiplatelet/statin therapy and exclusion of important comorbidity. Everyone should undergo an electrocardiogram (ECG) to exclude occult cardiac pathology. Baseline blood tests will exclude diabetes, arteritis, polycythaemia, anaemia, thrombocytosis, sickle-cell disease and hyperlipidaemia.

✅✅ Table 10.5 summarises recommendations from the European Stroke Initiative[28] regarding what should constitute 'best medical therapy' in patients with symptomatic and asymptomatic carotid disease.

Angina therapy should be optimised as the principal cause of late death is cardiac. Blood pressure (BP) should be maintained <140/90 mmHg. Systematic reviews suggest that reducing diastolic BP by 5 mmHg lowers the relative risk of stroke by 35%, while the relative risk of myocardial infarction (MI) falls by 25%.[29] However, evidence suggests that only 60% with known hypertension will receive treatment prior to suffering their first stroke and only half will have a documented diastolic BP <90 mmHg.[30] The Heart Protection Study[31] has provided level 1, grade A evidence for the role of statin therapy in patients with cerebrovascular disease.

Table 10.5 • European Stroke Initiative[28] recommendations for what constitutes 'best medical therapy' in patients with asymptomatic and symptomatic carotid disease

Treatment	Level of evidence Asymptomatic	Symptomatic
BP <140/90 mmHg or <130/80 mmHg in diabetics	Level I	Level I
Glycaemic control to prevent other diabetic complications	Level III	Level III
Statin therapy	Level I	Level I
Stop smoking	Level II	Level II
Avoid heavy consumption of alcohol	Level I	Level I
Regular physical activity	Level II	Level II
Low salt, low saturated fat, high fruit and vegetable diet rich in fibre	Level II	Level II
If BMI elevated, reduce weight	Level II	Level II
HRT should not be used for stroke prevention in women	Level I	Level I
Aspirin	To prevent MI, level IV	Level I
Aspirin and dipyridamole	Not recommended, level IV	Level I
Clopidogrel	Not recommended, level IV	Level I

BMI, body mass index; BP, blood pressure; HRT, hormone replacement therapy; MI, myocardial infarction.

✔✔ The British Heart Protection Study showed that patients randomised to statin had a 25% relative risk reduction (RRR) in (i) any major coronary event, (ii) any stroke and (iii) the need for revascularisation at 5 years. This benefit was irrespective of age, gender or presenting cholesterol level.[31]

Antiplatelet therapy should be commenced in all patients unless contraindicated.

✔✔ In its latest guidance,[32] NICE recommends the following:
- Ischaemic stroke – aspirin 300 mg for up to 14 days and then clopidogrel 75 mg daily indefinitely.
- Ischaemic TIA – aspirin 300 mg followed by aspirin 75 mg + dipyridamole SR 200 mg b.d. indefinitely.
- OR aspirin 300 mg followed by clopidogrel 75 mg indefinitely if dipyridamole intolerant.

There has been controversy over aspirin dosage during CEA. NASCET reported that patients receiving high-dose aspirin (650–1300 mg) had a lower perioperative risk than patients taking 0–325 mg aspirin daily.[33] This was an unplanned analysis and a randomised trial of 2849 patients subsequently showed that the risks of stroke, MI and death within 30 and 90 days of CEA were significantly lower in patients receiving 80–325 mg as opposed to 650–1300 mg.[34] This suggests greater evidence for prescribing low-dose aspirin.

✔ Dual antiplatelet therapy may increase the risk of bleeding during CEA. Surgeons must liaise with their stroke physicians regarding the optimal antiplatelet strategy in symptomatic patients being considered for urgent CEA. A clear policy should be available regarding the use of routine, single-dose or loading-dose clopidogrel.

All patients being considered for CAS require dual antiplatelet therapy.

The early risk of stroke after suffering a TIA is higher than previously thought. This has led to a review of practice regarding the timing of surgery (see later), but also regarding the benefit of very early implementation of 'best medical therapy'. The EXPRESS study evaluated early stroke risk in two cohorts of TIA patients. In the first cohort (2002–2004), patients were seen in a dedicated daily TIA clinic (appointment based, usual referral delays, etc.) with treatment recommendations being faxed to the referring doctor. The patient then contacted their doctor to obtain their prescription, but an average of 19 days elapsed before these medications were started. In the second cohort (2004–2007), there was a daily 'walk-in' service and statin, antiplatelet therapy was started in the outpatient clinic.[35] The 90-day risk of stroke fell from 10.3% in the first cohort to 2.1% in the second. This reduction in risk was independent of age and gender, and rapid commencement of therapy was not associated with an increased risk of haemorrhagic stroke.

✅ Rapid institution of 'best medical therapy' significantly reduces the risk of early stroke and should be started in the TIA clinic.

Surgical management of carotid disease

Symptomatic carotid artery disease

The Carotid Endarterectomy Trialists Collaboration (CETC) combined data from ECST, NASCET and the Veteran's Affairs (VA) trials, having remeasured the pre-randomisation angiograms using the NASCET measurement method. This unique database[36-38] includes 5-year outcomes in >6000 patients (Table 10.6).

✅ Notwithstanding criticisms of the 'historical' nature of these trials, the 5-year CETC data should now be quoted in preference to the constituent studies.

✅✅ CEA is not indicated in symptomatic patients with a 0–50% NASCET stenosis. CEA confers modest (but significant) benefit in the recently symptomatic (<6 months) with a 50–69% NASCET stenosis (ECST 70–85%). CEA confers maximum benefit in the recently symptomatic (<6 months) with a 70–99% NASCET stenosis, excluding those with the 'string sign'.

Following the publication of ECST/NASCET, there were concerns that the results may not be generalisable into clinical practice. For example, <0.5% of patients undergoing CEA in North America in 1988–9 were randomised into NASCET.

At present, 94% of CEAs in the USA are performed in non-NASCET hospitals with a mortality significantly higher than observed in NASCET.[39] The controversial issue regarding the relationship between hospital volume and outcome has been addressed in a systematic review of death/stroke after 936 436 CEAs.[40]

✅✅ This meta-analysis concluded that there was a significant relationship between volume and outcome, with the critical volume threshold (per hospital) being 79 CEAs per annum.[40]

Low-volume surgeons had similar results to higher-volume surgeons provided they worked in higher-volume centres. The question as to where CEA should be performed has always been a provocative subject, but the evidence from this meta-analysis, together with the drive towards faster (perhaps more risky) surgery, means that surgeons cannot simply ignore this controversial issue.

✅ Surgeons must know and quote their own results rather than justifying practice on the basis of ECST and NASCET.

ECST/NASCET have published over 50 papers since 1991, most being secondary analyses that have increased knowledge about the role of CEA in patients with symptomatic cerebral vascular disease.[41] These data should not be used to *exclude* patients from intervention, but rather to identify clinical and imaging predictors of increased risk of stroke on 'best medical therapy' (Box 10.2) and who derives the 'least' and 'greatest' benefit from CEA (Table 10.7). One of the most topical issues facing practitioners of both CEA and CAS is the effect of delay to intervention. Previously, there

Table 10.6 • Carotid Endarterectomy Trialists Collaboration: 5-year risk of any stroke (including 30-day stroke/death) from the combined VA, ECST and NASCET trials

Trial	Stenosis	n	30-day CEA risk	5-year risk Surgery	Medical	ARR	RRR	NNT	Strokes prevented per 1000 CEAs
CETC	<30%	1746	No data	18.36%	15.71%	− 2.6%	N/b	N/b	None at 5 years
CETC	30–49%	1429	6.7%	22.80%	25.45%	+ 2.6%	10%	38	26 at 5 years
CETC	50–69%	1549	8.4%	20.00%	27.77%	+ 7.8%	28%	13	78 at 5 years
CETC	70–99%	1095	6.2%	17.13%	32.71%	+ 15.6%	48%	6	156 at 5 years
CETC	String	262	5.4%	22.40%	22.30%	− 0.1%	N/b	N/b	None at 5 years

ARR, absolute risk reduction; N/b, no benefit conferred by CEA; NNT, number needed to treat; RRR, relative risk reduction; strokes prevented per 1000 CEAs, number of strokes prevented at 5 years by performing 1000 CEAs.
Data derived from the CETC[36-38] with all pre-randomisation angiograms remeasured using NASCET method.

was no great impetus for expediting intervention other than recommending that CEA should be performed 'as soon as reasonably possible'.

Box 10.2 • Which patients with symptomatic 70–99% stenoses are at higher risk of suffering a stroke on 'best medical therapy'?

Clinical features

Male versus female gender

Increasing age (especially >75 years)

Hemispheric versus ocular symptoms

Cortical versus lacunar stroke

Recurrent symptoms for >6 months

Increasing medical comorbidity

Symptoms within 1 month

Imaging features

Irregular versus smooth plaques

Increasing stenosis but not near occlusion

Contralateral occlusion

Tandem intracranial disease

No recruitment of intracranial collaterals

Adapted from Naylor AR, Rothwell PM, Bell PRF. Overview of the principal results and secondary analyses from the European and the North American randomised trials of carotid endarterectomy. Eur J Vasc Endovasc Surg 2003; 26:115–29. With permission from Elsevier.

✓ This approach has been challenged because of indisputable evidence that (a) the most vulnerable patients are probably suffering strokes before they can undergo surgery and (b) the long-term benefit of surgery diminishes rapidly following onset of the index event.

The CETC published compelling evidence that 'delays to surgery' significantly reduced benefit to the patient.[12,36–38] By implication, the same applies to CAS. **Table 10.8** presents a reanalysis of CETC data in patients with NASCET 50–99% stenoses (i.e. ECST 70–99%) undergoing CEA, specifically: (i) the ARR in ipsilateral stroke conferred by CEA stratified for delay to surgery; (ii) the number needed to treat (NNT) to prevent one ipsilateral stroke at 5 years; (iii) the number of ipsilateral strokes prevented/1000 CEAs at 5 years; and (iv) the number of 'uneccessary' procedures per 1000 CEAs at 5 years.

✓✓ Maximum benefit, regarding late stroke prevention, was observed when surgery was performed within 2 weeks. If surgery was delayed beyond 12 weeks, only eight ipsilateral strokes were prevented at 5 years by performing 1000 CEAs.[12,36–38]

Table 10.7 • Predictors of relative benefit conferred by CEA

'Lower' benefit conferred by CEA		'Higher' benefit conferred by CEA	
Clinical: imaging parameter	**CVA/1000**	**Clinical: imaging parameter**	**CVA/1000**
Symptomatic female (50–69%) + CEA >4 weeks	0 at 5 years	Symptomatic, 70–99%, aged >75 years	333 at 2 years
Symptomatic + string sign (subocclusion)	0 at 5 years	Symptomatic, 70–99%, high comorbidity	333 at 2 years
'All' asymptomatic females	2 at 5 years	Symptomatic, 70–99%, recurrent TIAs >6 months	333 at 2 years
Asymptomatic (anyone) with op. risk 6%	22 at 5 years	Symptomatic, 70–99%, operation < 2 weeks	333 at 3 years
Asymptomatic (anyone) with op. risk 2.8%	53 at 5 years	Symptomatic, 80–99%, + intracranial disease	333 at 3 years
Symptomatic (all) 50–69% stenosis	67 at 3 years	Symptomatic, 90–99%, no string sign	370 at 3 years
Symptomatic (female) 70–99%, op. 2–4 weeks	67 at 3 years	Symptomatic, 70–99%, female + CEA < 2 weeks	417 at 3 years
Symptomatic (all) 70–99% + lacunar stroke	91 at 3 years	Symptomatic, 70–99%, + contralateral occlusion	500 at 2 years
Symptomatic (all) 70–99% + age < 65 years	100 at 2 years	Symptomatic, 90–99% + plaque ulceration	500 at 2 years

CVA/1000, number of strokes prevented per 1000 patients treated.
Derived from secondary analyses from ECST, NASCET, ACAS, ACST and CETC.

Table 10.8 • Effect of 'delay to CEA' on 5-year prevention of ipsilateral stroke in patients with NASCET 50–99% stenoses

	< 2 weeks	2–4 weeks	4–12 weeks	>12 weeks*
ARR conferred by CEA at 5 years	18.5%	9.8%	5.5%	0.8%
NNT	5	10	18	125
Strokes prevented per 1000 CEAs	185	98	55	8
'Unnecessary' procedures	815	902	945	992

* Delay refers to time from randomisation to CEA. In the constituent studies, the average time from randomisation to CEA was about 7 days (P.M. Rothwell, personal communication).
Data derived from a reanalysis of the CETC data.[36–38]

However, this is only one side of a complex argument. It is also important to consider that early CEA might incur increased procedural risks. In a review of 1046 symptomatic patients undergoing CEA in New York, the 30-day death/stroke rate was three times higher (5.1%) if CEA was performed within 4 weeks as compared with 1.6% if surgery was deferred for >4 weeks.[42] Data like these have been used as a reason to delay interventions in order to get the 'lowest' procedural risks. However, an alternative analysis of the CETC data (**Fig. 10.6**) shows that even if a surgeon were to operate in <2 weeks with a 10% risk, he/she would still probably prevent more strokes in the long term than if the surgeon deferred any intervention for 4 weeks and then operated with a 0% risk.[12]

> ✅ Evidence suggests that more strokes will be prevented in the long term through rapid intervention, even if the procedural risk is increased. Future guidelines must consider whether it is reasonable to accept a slightly higher procedural risk if the operation is carried out early.

More controversial is the effect of 'delay to surgery' relative to gender[12,38] (**Fig. 10.7**). As can be seen, males gain considerable (and durable) benefit irrespective of delays to surgery or degree of stenosis. However, the CETC data suggest that the benefit conferred in women diminishes very rapidly after 4 weeks.

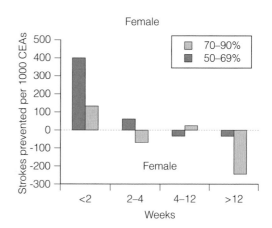

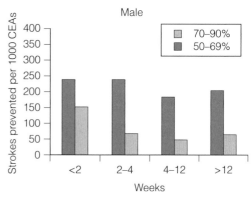

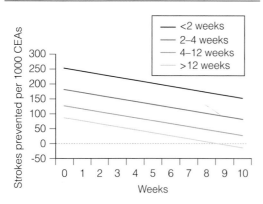

Figure 10.6 • Strokes prevented per 1000 CEAs at 5 years stratified for: **(i)** delay from last event to randomisation and **(ii)** 30-day death/stroke risk. Reproduced from Naylor AR. Time is brain! Surgeon 2007; 5:23–30. With permission from the Royal College of Surgeons of Edinburgh and Ireland.

Figure 10.7 • Strokes prevented per 1000 CEAs at 5 years stratified for stenosis severity and gender. Reproduced from Naylor AR. Time is brain! Surgeon 2007; 5:23–30. With permission from the Royal College of Surgeons of Edinburgh and Ireland.

Table 10.9 • Five- and 10-year outcomes from ACAS and ACST[22,43,4]

	n	Surgery	BMT	ARR	RRR	NNT	Number of strokes prevented per 1000 CEAs
		5-year stroke risk					
ACAS	1662	5.1%	11.0%	5.9%	54%	17	59
ACST	3120	6.4%	11.8%	5.4%	46%	19	54
		10-year stroke risk					
ACST	3120	13.4%	17.9%	4.6%	26%	22	46

ACAS, reported rates of 'ipsilateral stroke'; ACST, reported rates of 'any stroke'; ARR, absolute risk reduction; BMT, best medical therapy; NNT, number need to treat to prevent 1 stroke at either 5 or 10 years; RRR, relative risk reduction.

✅ Symptomatic women gain less benefit from CEA than men and maximum benefit is only conferred if surgery is performed as soon as possible. Excessive delays to treatment could mean that female patients face all the risks of intervention with little prospect of gaining benefit.

Asymptomatic carotid artery disease

Five randomised trials have compared CEA plus 'best medical therapy' (BMT) with BMT alone, but only two (ACAS and the Asymptomatic Carotid Surgery Trial (ACST)) influenced practice.[21,43,44] The 5- and 10-year outcomes from ACAS/ACST are summarised in Table 10.9.

✅✅ The 2011 American Heart Association (AHA) guidelines continue to retain the recommendation that intervention should be considered in 'highly selected' average risk patients with an asymptomatic 60–99% stenosis.[45]

The AHA is highly influential in determining international guidelines of practice and it is likely that other countries will adopt similar recommendations. However, the management of asymptomatic disease remains controversial. Those who feel it is time to rethink management strategies cite the following observations. (i) The overall benefit conferred by CEA (and CAS) is small. At 10 years, only 46 strokes are prevented per 1000 operations (Table 10.9). (ii) In a recent audit, 50% of clinicians around the world would not offer CEA/CAS to patients fulfilling AHA criteria.[46] (iii) The AHA recommends treating 'highly selected' patients, but never defined what this meant. (iv) The majority of patients were never destined to suffer a stroke. At 5 years, 88% treated medically were stroke free, with 82% stroke free at 10 years (Table 10.9). (v) Up to 94% of interventions in asymptomatic patients are ultimately unnecessary, costing US health providers $2 billion annually.[47] (vi) There is accumulating evidence that the stroke risk on medical therapy has declined over the last 20 years.[47]

Conversely, those who believe that guidelines should remain unchanged cite the following reasons for adopting this position. (i) The AHA guidelines are based on level I, randomised trial evidence. (ii) The procedural risks associated with CEA and CAS have reduced significantly and will further increase the benefit accrued to the patient. (iii) CEA/CAS offers the only chance of preventing stroke in the 80% of stroke victims who will not have suffered a prior TIA. (iv) The alleged decline in stroke risk is based on flawed data because it includes some studies with subsurgical (50–60%) stenoses.

The most controversial issue is the apparent decline in stroke risk over the last decade. This has been consistent across all stenosis severities and was also evident in ACAS and ACST.[47] In 1995, the 5-year risk of 'any' stroke in ACAS was 17.5% (3.5% p.a.) in patients randomised to BMT. When ACST reported in 2004, the first 5-year risk of 'any' stroke had fallen to 11.8% (2.4% p.a.). When ACST reported its 10-year data, the second 5-year risk of 'any' stroke was now only 7.2% (1.4% p.a.). In effect, the 5-year risk of 'any' stroke has declined by 60% since 1995. There is an identical trend for 'ipsilateral' stroke. In 1995, ACAS reported 5-year rates of 'ipsilateral' stroke in medically treated patients of 11.0% (2.2% p.a.). By 2004, ACST reported 5-year risks of ipsilateral stroke of 5.3% (1.1% p.a.), while in years 6–10, the 5-year risk of 'ipsilateral stroke' had fallen to 3.6% (0.7% p.a.). This represents a 70% decline in the 5-year risk of ipsilateral stroke since 1995.[8] It is hoped that future randomised studies in asymptomatic patients will include a third arm for 'best medical therapy' so as to determine whether the observed decline in stroke risk in non-randomised studies is a real phenomenon or not.

✅ It is inevitable that a smaller cohort of asymptomatic patients will benefit from intervention. It is essential that more research is performed to identify a 'higher or lower risk for stroke' cohort in whom to either target or avoid CEA/CAS. Until then, most guidelines continue to recommend the 2011 AHA guidelines, if only for medicolegal protection.

An overview[47] suggests that a number of imaging modalities could be used to identify high-risk patients for evaluation in future studies (spontaneous embolisation on transcranial Doppler, computerised plaque analysis (GSM, Activity Index), silent infarction on CT/MRA, and MRI evidence of intraplaque haemorrhage).

CEA/CAS and coronary bypass

Symptomatic patients who are unable to undergo CEA/CAS because of unstable cardiac disease should undergo staged or synchronous CEA/CAS plus coronary bypass as soon as possible. This is because the risk of stroke is highest in the early period after onset of symptoms. In reality, this only applies to <5% of cardiac surgery patients.[48] The role of prophylactic CEA/CAS in patients undergoing coronary artery bypass grafting (CABG) with an asymptomatic carotid stenosis remains an enduring controversy. In the USA, about 96% of staged/synchronous interventions are undertaken in patients with asymptomatic carotid disease, the majority with unilateral disease.[48] So what is the evidence supporting intervention in these patients?

✅✅ In a meta-analysis of 190 449 patients undergoing CABG,[49] the risk of stroke was 1.7% (95% CI 1.5–1.9).

The meta-analysis observed that three 'carotid' factors were predictive of post-CABG stroke: (i) carotid bruit; (ii) a prior history of stroke or TIA; and (iii) the presence of a severe carotid stenosis or occlusion.[49]

The stroke risk in 4674 duplex-screened patients undergoing CABG was 1.8% in patients with no significant carotid disease, 3.2% in those with unilateral 50–99% stenoses, 5.2% in those with bilateral 50–99% stenoses and 7–11% in patients with carotid occlusion.[49]

✅ In an updated meta-analysis (which excluded symptomatic patients, those with bilateral stenoses and patients with unilateral carotid occlusion), patients undergoing isolated coronary bypass in the presence of a unilateral, asymptomatic stenosis incurred a 2% risk of procedural stroke. It is unlikely that prophylactic CEA/CAS could confer significant benefit, although it would still be appropriate to consider prophylactic intervention in cardiac surgery patients with bilateral severe asymptomatic disease.[50]

Table 10.10 details the 30-day rates of death/stroke derived from meta-analyses[51] regarding the roles of synchronous/staged CEA or CAS in patients undergoing coronary artery bypass (CAB). As can be seen, morbidity and mortality rates were considerably higher than when either CEA/CAS are performed on their own.

✅ Once a decision has been made to undertake staged or synchronous CEA/CAS, there is no evidence that either strategy is safer.

Table 10.10 • Systematic review and meta-analysis of 30-day rates of death, stroke and MI after staged or synchronous CEA/CAS and coronary bypass

	30-day death	30-day death/stroke	30-day death/stroke/MI
Synchronous CEA + CABG (CEA pre bypass)	4.5%	8.2%	11.5%
Synchronous CEA + CABG (CEA done on bypass)	4.7%	8.1%	9.5%
Synchronous CEA + CABG (CABG done off pump)	1.5%	2.2%	3.6%
Staged CEA then CABG	3.9%	6.1%	10.2%
Reverse staged CEA then CABG	2.0%	7.3%	
CAS + CABG	5.5%	9.1%	9.4%

CABG, coronary artery bypass graft; CAS, carotid artery stenting; CEA, carotid endarterectomy.
Data derived from Naylor et al.[51]

Emergency CEA

In the 1960s, emergency CEA for acute stroke was associated with significant mortality and morbidity, mainly due to haemorrhagic transformation of ischaemic infarction. This led to the abandonment of this strategy and a recommendation that patients suffering a stroke should wait 6 weeks before undergoing CEA in order to stabilise the area of infarction. This is clearly at odds with current recommendations to expedite CEA. However, a meta-analysis suggests that procedural risks for early CEA in patients with minor stroke with recovery are similar to those in whom surgery is deferred.[52]

> ✓ Emergency CEA (i.e. immediate) should be reserved for patients suffering thrombotic stroke in the early period after CEA/CAS. Urgent CEA (<24 hours) is recommended in patients with stroke in evolution, stuttering hemiplegia or crescendo TIAs. There remains no evidence that patients with extensive neurological deficits should be considered for early intervention.

Vertebral artery revascularisation

The vertebrobasilar (VB) territory is affected in 15–25% of ischaemic strokes, but there have been no completed randomised trials similar to ECST/NASCET to guide practice. In the past, it was believed that the majority of VB strokes were haemodynamic. However, the New England Posterior Circulation Registry observed that 40% will be embolic (cardiac 60%, artery to artery 40%), 32% will be haemodynamic, while 28% had miscellaneous causes (trauma, dissection, aneurysm, arteritis, osteophyte compression).[53] Of those TIAs secondary to vertebral/basilar artery stenoses/occlusions, 62% were located within the extracranial vertebral artery (origin 39%, near VA origin 30%, V2/V3 segment 31%), 30% affected the intracranial vertebral artery, while 8% affected the basilar artery. The VIST trial is comparing vertebral artery stenting with 'best medical therapy' in patients suffering a VB stroke within the preceding 6 months and who have a 50–99% vertebral artery stenosis (www.vist.sgul.ac.uk).

In the past, most VB reconstructions involved open surgery (vein bypass or transposition on to the CCA). However, angioplasty with/without stenting is assuming an increasing role, especially in the upper limits of the extracranial vertebral artery and intracranial vessels. A meta-analysis of 993 patients (27 studies) undergoing vertebral artery angioplasty (99% stented) showed a technical success rate of 99%, a 30-day stroke rate of 1.1% and a 1% risk of recurrent VB stroke at 2 years. Re-stenosis rates were three times higher in patients receiving bare metal stents, compared with drug-eluting stents.[54] These exceptional results are unlikely to reflect 'real world' practice, but they do support a strategy wherein endovascular interventions are considered the first-line intervention.

Three VB-related syndromes are worthy of mention. An occlusion/severe stenosis at the subclavian artery origin may cause reversed flow down the ipsilateral vertebral artery to perfuse the arm (subclavian steal). Arm exercise may precipitate forearm claudication or dizziness. Intervention is usually recommended in patients with symptomatic lesions, especially involving the dominant arm. Both surgery and endovascular intervention carry a small risk of procedural stroke. At present, the latter is generally the first choice intervention.

A similar syndrome (coronary steal) occurs in patients who have undergone coronary bypass using the internal mammary artery (usually the left). Should a proximal subclavian stenosis be missed preoperatively (or develop subsequently) angina can be precipitated by arm exercise. In this situation, the angina can be treated by carotid–subclavian bypass or angioplasty/stenting. There is no evidence that either strategy is preferable.

Third, it is traditionally believed that rotational (positional) dizziness/vertigo follows osteophyte compression of the extracranial VA. Recent evidence suggests that this is almost always never the case[55] and an alternative aetiology should be sought.

Surgical management of carotid disease – carotid endarterectomy

Anaesthesia

CEA under locoregional anaesthesia is the only reliable method for predicting who needs a shunt, but it will not prevent thromboembolism (main cause of intraoperative stroke).

> ✓✓ The GALA trial randomised >3500 CEAs to locoregional or general anaesthesia. There was no difference in 30-day outcomes. Surgeons may use either anaesthetic strategy according to their preference.[56]

Technique

CEA is usually performed using loupe magnification with the extended head turned away from the side of operation and placed on a rubber ring. An incision is made over the anterior border of the sternomastoid and dissection continued down to the carotid bifurcation after division of the common facial vein.

✔✔ Some surgeons infiltrate the carotid sinus with 1% lignocaine to prevent reflex hypotension or bradycardia. Four randomised controlled trials (RCTs) have found no clear evidence of benefit regarding this practice.

The distal ICA is mobilised 1 cm beyond the upper limit of the plaque, facilitated by ligation and division of the sternomastoid vessels that tether the hypoglossal nerve, with/without division of the digastric. If surgeons are worried about the need to proceed higher in the neck, access can be facilitated (preoperatively) by nasolaryngeal intubation or temporomandibular subluxation. The latter must be planned in advance as it cannot be performed once the operation has started. The main cranial nerves (hypoglossal, vagus) are identified. With high dissections, the glossopharyngeal nerve is at risk. Contrary to classical teaching, however, most postoperative swallowing problems do not follow glossopharyngeal nerve injury but are secondary to damage to the motor branches of the vagus that cross the ICA anteriorly, just distal to the hypoglossal nerve.

✔ Any patient who has undergone a contralateral CEA, neck dissection or thyroidectomy must undergo a preoperative check of recurrent laryngeal and hypoglossal nerve function. Bilateral injuries can be fatal.

Following systemic heparinisation, clamps are applied to the ICA, CCA and ECA. A longitudinal arteriotomy is made across the plaque and into the distal ICA. If a shunt is to be deployed it is inserted now (**Fig. 10.8**). The endarterectomy plane is developed using a Watson–Cheyne dissector and it is conventional to divide the plaque proximally and then mobilise it towards the distal ICA. The upper end usually feathers, but can be tacked down. Loose intimal fragments are removed in a radial, as opposed to axial, direction. An alternative technique is 'eversion' endarterectomy. Here the origin of the ICA is transected and reimplanted after eversion of the atheromatous core.

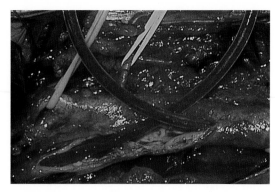

Figure 10.8 • An arteriotomy has been made across the carotid stenosis and a Pruit–Inahara shunt inserted. This type of shunt is held in place with balloons.

✔✔ Systematic reviews suggest that eversion endarterectomy confers similar benefits to traditional endarterectomy provided the arteriotomy is closed with a patch.

Patch or primary closure?

✔✔ The 2009 Cochrane Review of 10 RCTs[57] showed that routine patching was preferable to routine primary closure, with a threefold reduction in perioperative stroke, thrombosis and re-stenosis. No RCT has compared routine with selective patching and there is no evidence that patch type influences stroke rates, mortality or re-stenosis.

Routine, selective or never shunt?

✔✔ The Cochrane overview suggests that routine shunting does not influence outcome.[58]

Perioperative monitoring

The aim of monitoring is to prevent cerebral ischaemia before permanent neurological injury occurs. The simplest is a subjective assessment of ICA backflow or stump pressure, but this may bear little relation to intracranial perfusion in the presence of circle of Willis abnormalities. Transcranial Doppler (TCD) is probably the most versatile of methods and uses a low-frequency (2 MHz) pulsed-wave ultrasound beam directed through the temporal bone. This permits insonation of the MCA, which receives 80% of ICA inflow. The quality of the signal depends on the thickness of the cranium and an inaccessible window may be present in about 10% of patients.

A single monitoring modality, however, is no guarantee of protection. During CEA, TCD fulfils only four roles: (i) diagnosing embolisation during carotid dissection (unstable plaque); (ii) ensuring mean MCA velocity remains >15 cm/s; (iii) ensuring the shunt is working; and (iv) diagnosing the very rare case of on-table thrombosis following flow restoration. Neurological activity can be monitored using locoregional anaesthesia and this is the 'gold standard' for determining who needs a shunt. However, it will not prevent thromboembolic complications. Neurological activity can be evaluated indirectly by electroencephalogram (EEG) or sensory-evoked potential (SEP) measurement. Once perfusion falls below 18 mL/100 g brain per minute there is loss of high-frequency activity on the EEG, whereas below 15 mL/100 g brain per minute the EEG becomes isoelectric.[59]

✓ The surgeon should remember that just because the EEG is flat, it does not mean that a neurological injury is inevitable, as this only occurs once perfusion falls below 10 mL/100 g brain per minute.[59] Thus, loss of EEG function is a warning that insertion of a shunt or elevation of systemic blood pressure may be beneficial.

The advantage of SEP measurement is that it reflects the function of the afferent pathway from peripheral nerve (usually median nerve) to the somatosensory cortex. Ischaemia causes a reduction in the amplitude of the primary cortical wave and prolongation of central conduction time.

Completion assessment

The role of completion assessment is to identify technical error (incomplete endarterectomy, intimal flaps, luminal thrombus, residual stenoses and wall irregularities). The most important is exclusion of luminal thrombus, which originates from bleeding from the endarterectomised vasa vasorum.[60] Quality control techniques include TCD, completion angiography, duplex ultrasound, continuous-wave Doppler and angioscopy. TCD ensures optimal shunt function and is the only method capable of diagnosing embolisation, on-table thrombosis and postoperative occlusion. Angiography (which must be biplanar) provides anatomical data, but requires ionising radiation and can only be performed after restoration of flow (i.e. any thrombus could be swept distally). The latest colour duplex probes are smaller and more accessible because of the development of L-shaped probes but usually require the presence of a technician in theatre. The principal advantage of angioscopy is that it is performed *prior*

to restoration of flow. Its main role is to identify the 3–5% of patients with residual luminal thrombus and the 1% with large intimal flaps.

Operative complications

Cranial nerve injuries

✓✓ Cranial nerve injury is an important source of morbidity. In a detailed review, Forsell et al.[61] observed that up to 50% of patients will suffer some degree of cranial nerve injury.

In NASCET, the incidence of injury to the mandibular branch of the facial nerve was 2.2%, to the vagus 2.5%, to the spinal accessory nerve 0.2% and to the hypoglossal 3.7%. The overall rate of cranial nerve injury was 8.6%, although 92% were minor and fully recovered within 4 weeks.[62] In CREST, the risk of cranial nerve palsy following CEA was 4.7% (2% unresolved at 30 days), compared to 0.3% after stenting.[63] By 1 year, cranial nerve injury did not impact on quality of life in patients randomised to CEA in CREST.

Wound complications

In NASCET, 132 CEA patients (9.3%) developed wound complications, of which 76 (58%) were minor, 52 (39%) moderate, while only 4 (3%) were classed as severe.[62] Early vein patch rupture complicates <1% of CEAs, but is virtually abolished provided saphenous vein is harvested from the groin.

Perioperative stroke

Perioperative stroke is classed as intraoperative if the patient recovers from anaesthesia with a new deficit and postoperative if the event occurs thereafter. In historical series, intraoperative stroke predominated and was more likely to affect patients with a combination of cerebral infarction and partial/total haemodynamic compromise. This suggests that high-risk patients are more vulnerable to otherwise minor changes in perfusion or emboli, so that the margin for technical error is reduced or possibly non-existent.

Intraoperative stroke has been virtually abolished at the Leicester Royal Infirmary (0.3% in 1600 cases[60]), a feature attributed to removing luminal thrombus (identified by angioscopy) prior to flow restoration. The commonest causes of postoperative stroke are: (i) ICA thrombosis (especially in the first 6 postoperative hours); (ii) hyperperfusion syndrome; and (iii) intracranial haemorrhage (ICH). ICH and the hyperperfusion syndrome complicate 1–2% of CEAs and are more common in patients with severe bilateral extracranial disease in association with impaired cerebral vascular reserve, defective autoregulation and poor collateral flow patterns.[63]

> ✔ It is essential that emergency medical units recognise the importance of rapid BP treatment in the CEA patient who presents with seizures, usually 5–7 days after surgery. These patients have a high risk of suffering ICH and the mainstay of management is control of seizures and aggressive blood pressure control.[62]

The strategy for managing perioperative stroke depends on: (i) timing (intraoperative/postoperative); (ii) whether it follows thrombosis, embolism or haemorrhage; and (iii) the severity of the deficit. The more extensive the deficit, the more likely that the ICA/MCA has occluded. For those without access to TCD or duplex, the surgeon has to assume that any deficit following recovery from anaesthesia or in the first 24 hours is thromboembolic and the patient re-explored. Although re-exploration will not benefit patients with MCA branch embolism or haemodynamic stroke, this cannot be avoided. For those with access to TCD, decision-making is easier. The immediate priority is to identify patients with ICA thrombosis, as they require immediate exploration. Provided flow is restored within 1 hour, good neurological recovery can be expected.

> ✔ TCD features of early carotid thrombosis include flow reversal in the ipsilateral anterior cerebral artery, enhanced flow in the ipsilateral posterior cerebral artery and, most importantly, flow velocities in the ipsilateral MCA that mimic those observed during carotid clamping.

It would be preferable to *prevent* thrombosis from happening. Evidence from three continents has shown that early postoperative carotid thrombosis is preceded by 1–2 hours of increasing embolisation, which can be diagnosed using TCD,[64] and that 50–60% of patients with sustained embolisation will progress to thrombotic stroke.[64] In the past, it was necessary to monitor everyone in the early postoperative period and administer dextran to those with increasing rates of embolisation. However, research suggests that patients vulnerable to early postoperative thromboembolism have platelets that are more sensitive to ADP. The administration of 75 mg clopidogrel the night before surgery (in addition to aspirin) is sufficient to virtually abolish postoperative thromboembolic stroke.[65] In Leicester, postoperative TCD monitoring is no longer performed following the introduction of preoperative dual antiplatelet strategy.[66]

Long-term follow-up and re-stenosis

The annual risk of late ipsilateral and contralateral stroke after CEA is 1–2%.

> ✔✔ Meta-analyses suggest that the average annual risk of recurrent stenosis (50–100%) is 1.5–4.5%,[67] with the highest risk being the first 12 months. The association between recurrent stenosis and ipsilateral stroke is tenuous.

Some surgeons recommend serial clinical and duplex surveillance with the intention of performing repeat CEA in patients with recurrent stenoses >70%. However, there is little evidence to support this practice.

> ✔ If one focuses on outcomes from RCTs (independent neurological verification, pre-planned follow-up strategy), there is no evidence that recurrent stroke correlates with recurrent stenosis. In ACAS, the risk of late stroke was unrelated to the presence of a recurrent stenosis and only one patient (0.15%) suffered a stroke and had a severe recurrent stenosis.[68]

There seems to be little clinical or cost-based evidence for undertaking surveillance after CEA. Most can be discharged at 6 weeks and told to report back should they develop symptoms. Exceptions might be those who have undergone vein bypass (higher re-stenosis rate) or those who developed neurological complications during test clamping under locoregional anaesthesia or who had MCA velocities <15 cm/s on TCD during carotid clamping (unlikely to tolerate carotid occlusion).

Patch infection

Patch infection complicates <1% of all CEAs.

> ✔ No abscess overlying a CEA wound should be incised before being seen by a vascular surgeon.

If infection is suspected, the CCA must be controlled below the original incision. The prosthetic patch should be removed and replaced (where possible) with vein (bypass/patch). Ligation should only be considered as a last resort (uncontrollable haemorrhage) and preferably if some form of monitoring (e.g. TCD, awake neurological testing at the original procedure) suggests that collateral flow is satisfactory.

Endovascular treatment of carotid disease

Results of CAS

Thirteen RCTs have compared CEA with CAS in 7480 patients. Five were single-centre studies, 10 recruited symptomatic patients, one randomised a symptomatic patients, while two randomised symptomatic and asymptomatic patients. Six stopped early, one of which was never published. Some were performed prior to the era of stenting, dual antiplatelet therapy or protection devices (making them somewhat historical), leaving EVA-3S, SPACE, ICSS and CREST as the most influential of the contemporary RCTs in average risk patients to influence practice.[63,69–72] These studies, which reported after 2004, randomised 5932 patients.

Table 10.11 summarises the procedural risks from the Carotid Stenting Trialists Collaboration (CSTC), which performed an individual patient meta-analysis from patients recruited to EVA-3S, SPACE and ICSS,[70–72] along with those from CREST.[63] There have been many interpretations of the RCT data, but important findings are worthy of mention. (1) CAS was associated with a near twofold excess risk of procedural death/stroke in symptomatic patients (compared with CEA), even when historical studies were excluded.[73,74] (2) Using a clinical definition of MI (as in ICSS/SPACE), there was no difference in procedural MI between CEA and CAS.[72] (3) In CREST, MI was defined by a creatinine kinase MB or troponin level that was twice the upper limit of normal or higher according to the centre's laboratory in addition to either chest pain symptoms consistent with ischaemia or ECG evidence of ischemia. Using this definition of perioperative MI, CEA was associated with a twofold excess risk of MI73.[4] Using the CREST definition of MI within 30-day death/stroke/MI, outcomes were similar between CEA/CAS for symptomatic and asymptomatic patients.[73] (5) The 30-day rate of death/stroke after CAS in patients aged <70 years was similar to those after CEA. However, death/stroke was higher after CAS in older patients.[73,74] (6) Following successful CAS long-term stroke risks were similar to CEA, i.e. successful CAS was durable.[75] (7) Re-stenosis rates were higher following CAS, but not associated with an increased risk of late ipsilateral stroke.[75] (8) CEA was associated with a higher rate of cranial nerve injury. (9) Filter protected CAS in symptomatic patients was associated with a fivefold excess risk of new/persisting MRI lesions[76] compared with CEA.

The 2011 AHA guidelines[45] were primarily driven by CREST and, despite being the largest RCT in symptomatic patients (and published 1 year before CREST), the AHA did not refer at all to ICSS in its 2011 guidelines. Table 10.12 summarises the 2011 AHA recommendations for CEA/CAS in 'average risk' and 'high risk for CEA' patients.

Ongoing controversies

Is CEA or CAS safer in the hyperacute period after onset of symptoms?

In the CSTC meta-analysis,[74] patients undergoing CAS within 14 days of their most recent symptom were almost three times more likely to suffer a procedural stroke (compared with CEA). However, there is evidence that CAS can be performed in the hyperacute period with results comparable to CEA in specialist centres using reverse-flow protection devices.[77] It remains to

Table 10.11 • Summary of 30-day risk data from the Carotid Stenting Trialists Collaboration (individual patient meta-analysis of EVA-3S, SPACE, ICSS) and CREST

Trial	Symptom	CEA D/S	CAS D/S	OR 95% CI	CEA D/S/MI	CAS D/S/MI	OR 95% CI
CSTC[74] n = 3433	Symptomatic	5.8%	8.9%	1.5 (1.2–2.0)			
CREST[63] n = 1321	Symptomatic	3.2%	6.2%	1.9 (1.1–3.2)	5.4%	6.7%	1.3 (0.8–2.0)
CREST[63] n = 1181	Asymptomatic	1.4%	2.5%	1.9 (0.8–4.4)	3.6%	3.5%	1.0 (0.6–1.9)

CAS, carotid artery stenting; CEA, carotid endarterectomy; D/S = 30-day death or stroke; D/S/MI = 30-day death/stroke or MI; OR, odds ratio.

Table 10.12 • 2011 American Heart Association Guidelines for the management of average risk symptomatic and asymptomatic patients[45]

Type of patient	Level of evidence for CEA	Level of evidence for CAS
Average risk, 50–69% TIA/stroke <6 months	Class I/Level B	Class I/ Level B
Average risk, 70–99% stenosis TIA/stroke <6 months	Class I/ Level A	Class I/ Level B
'High risk for CEA', 70–99% stenosis TIA/stroke <6 months		Class IIb/Level B
Average risk, asymptomatic 60–99% (angiography), 70–99% (non-invasive)	Class IIa/Level A	Class IIb/Level B
'High risk for CEA', asymptomatic 60–99% (angiography), 70–99% (non-invasive)		Class IIb/Level C; role 'uncertain'

be seen whether this can be offered routinely to the majority of patients.

✓✓ Patients presenting with TIA/minor stroke benefit from rapid intervention. Provided CAS centres can offer expedited CAS with results comparable to CEA, CAS can be offered to patients in this situation. Otherwise, patients should undergo urgent CEA. It is not appropriate to delay interventions in order to get better procedural results.

Importance of perioperative MI

A surgeon's perspective

The AHA liberalised guidelines for CAS in average-risk patients (Table 10.12), primarily because when CREST included perioperative MI within the primary end-point there was no difference in risk between CEA and CAS (Table 10.11). CREST was the first RCT in average-risk patients to observe that MI was significantly more common following CEA and that patients suffering a perioperative MI faced a fourfold reduction in life expectancy.[78] However, no data were provided on whether reduced life expectancy was related to cardiac events. More importantly, it is often assumed that the reduction in life expectancy in CREST was attributable to a greater proportion of CEA patients dying during the course of follow-up. In fact, CREST reported the opposite. A greater proportion of CAS patients suffering a perioperative MI died during the course of follow-up (6/22; 27%) as compared with CEA (7/40; 18%), i.e. the fourfold poorer long-term survival in patients suffering a perioperative MI in CREST was not due to excess deaths in CEA patients. Perioperative MI should certainly

inform the debate, but the evidence does not suggest that it is of greater (equivalent) importance than (for example) the proportionally greater benefits conferred to the patient through rapid intervention. Thirteen patients (0.5%) randomised within CREST died 'prematurely' following a perioperative MI. By contrast, up to 10% will suffer a stroke in the first seven days[7] after onset of symptoms, perhaps even higher in the presence of a severe ipsilateral stenosis.[10] From the surgeon's perspective, the benefits of intervening in the hyperacute period outweigh the very low risk of dying prematurely following a procedural MI.

An interventionist's perspective

The NIH superiority analysis detailed in the CREST publication[78] used a classical clinical definition of MI: 'MI was defined by a creatinine kinase MB or troponin level that was twice the upper limit of normal range in addition to either chest pain symptoms consistent with ischaemia or ECG evidence of ischaemia, including new ST-segment depression or elevation of more than 1 mm in two or more contiguous leads'. The FDA pre-specified Abbott analysis (a non-inferiority construct) included 'enzyme rise only' as a definition of MI, in addition to a classical definition. Both 'enzyme rise only' and 'classical MI' peri-procedural (i.e. 30-day) rates were significantly higher for CEA than CAS and both (regardless of definition) impacted significantly on 4-year mortality.

That early intervention after the index event is a valid and evidence-based imperative is accepted, but there are no hard data to support the premise (either from CREST or other trials formulated to compare CAS and CEA) that CAS (in experienced units) is associated with excess harm. There is arguably still room for improvement for the tried and tested procedure of CEA, despite 60 years of evolution, in terms of a small but real excess MI risk and its legacy, and there is clear room for improvement for CAS in terms of minor stroke excess, accepting that minor stroke (the main stroke differential between treatment limbs) neither impacted on late neurological deficit nor late mortality. CAS and CEA should be seen as complementary rather than competitive procedures and both should be allowed to continue to evolve.

New ischaemic lesions on MRI

A systematic review of non-randomised studies observed that CAS was associated with a sixfold increase in new ischaemic lesions on MRI.[79] This was corroborated by ICSS,[76] which observed that CAS was associated with a fivefold increase in new ischaemic lesions in the immediate postoperative period and which persisted at 30 days (compared with CEA). There were more (smaller) lesions following CAS and fewer (larger) lesions following CEA, such that the median affected brain volume was similar for CEA and CAS. In 17% of the CAS-related new diffusion-weighted MRI lesions, there were persistent signal abnormalities on FLAIR imaging compared with 53% of the CEA-associated new diffusion-weighted MRI lesions. The fate and clinical relevance of these lesions remains uncertain as many remain subclinical and a substantial proportion fade on follow-up imaging.[80] The latest analysis of cognitive function between patients with florid new white lesions (during filter-protected CAS) and those with far fewer lesions following CEA does not provide compelling evidence of adverse clinical sequelae.[81]

Within the ICSS substudy,[76] five centres used filter-type embolic protection devices (EPDs) in the majority of patients, while two centres did not routinely employ EPDs. The new white lesion rate was 73% following filter protection and 34% for unprotected CAS ($P = 0.019$). Two small RCTs have compared control of microembolic burden during CAS with the MoMa flow arrest device and filter protection. The first (53 patients with lipid-rich plaque on CTA) demonstrated significantly more microembolic signals with filters than with MoMa and substantially more diffusion-weighted MRI new lesions.[82] The second trial recruited 62 patients and demonstrated an 87% new white matter lesion rate following filter-protected CAS compared with 45% following MoMa-protected CAS. This differential in favour of proximal protection was maintained regardless of symptomatic or octogenarian status.[83]

Prospective studies show consistent discrepancies between proximal and distal filter devices in favour of proximal protection. Schmidt observed a significant reduction in total embolus counts in CAS patients using the MoMa device, 57 ± 41 versus 196 ± 84 for the filter ($P < 0.0001$). Sheath

and/or protection device placement and retrieval were universally emboligenic stages.[84] In the PROOF analysis of the MICHI system (high-flow rate reversed flow via a mini-incision in the ipsilateral CCA, thus avoiding catheterisation of the arch and great vessels), the diffusion-weighted MRI new white lesion rate was 17%, similar to the new white lesion rate for CEA within ICSS.[85]

> ✅ Filter-protected CAS is associated with a significant increase in new ischaemic lesions on MRI (compared with CEA) but there is no evidence this translates into worsening cognitive function. Proximal protection devices appear to reduce the overall microembolic burden.

Assessing suitability for CAS

Careful case selection is mandatory for safe practice and most patients being considered for CAS require 'overview' anatomical imaging (arch to the circle of Willis). Absolute contraindications include an occluded ICA or visible thrombus. A difficult origin to the brachiocephalic artery/left CCA or severe CCA tortuosity are relative contraindications. Tortuosity of the ICA above the stenosis (**Fig. 10.9**) may prevent use of filter type or distal occlusive protection systems. This tortuosity could be turned into a kink or occlusion by a stent.

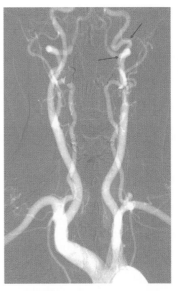

Figure 10.9 • Tortuosity of the distal left ICA may preclude the use of distal protection devices (filters and distal balloons), but the neuroprotection device from Gore (Flagstaff, AZ) and the MoMa system from Medtronic (Minneapolis, USA), both proximal embolic protection systems, could be used.

Many experienced CAS specialists do not now perform overview imaging, preferring to undertake angiography with a view to proceeding if appropriate. A number of novel carotid catheters have been developed and these tend to render most challenging anatomies relative rather than absolute contraindications.

✅ Once anatomical suitability for CAS is confirmed, the decision to intervene by CAS is best made in a multidisciplinary environment.[86]

A multispeciliality Delphi consensus provides recommendations for case selection based on anatomical criteria, and is aimed specifically at the novice (a practitioner with <50 CAS experience). The expected level of difficulty is presented as a traffic-light table (green for straightforward and red for high level of expected difficulty).[87]

Dual antiplatelet therapy

It is routine practice to employ dual antiplatelet therapy prior to CAS; 75 mg of clopidogrel is commenced 1 week prior to intervention in addition to 75 mg aspirin daily. In recently symptomatic patients, 300–600 mg clopidogrel (depending on body weight) is given at least 15 hours pre-intervention. The dual antiplatelet regime should continue for 28 days post-procedure, i.e. the presumed time-frame for endothelialisation of the stent.

✅✅ Randomised trials have confirmed the benefit of perioperative dual antiplatelet therapy prior to CAS.[88]

CAS technique

The femoral artery is the commonest access point. Brachial, radial or direct carotid approaches are alternatives if there is a difficult arch ('type III' or 'bovine'). In a type III arch, the origin of the brachiocephalic is significantly lower than a horizontal line drawn across the highest point of the arch. In a 'bovine' arch, there is a conjoint origin to the brachiocephalic and left CCA.

Unfractionated heparin (5000–7500 u) is administered following arterial access. An additional bolus (2000 u) is given if the procedure lasts >1 hour. Lesion access depends on anatomy, experience and choice of protection. Methods include: (i) exchange technique (ipsilateral ECA accessed with a selective catheter and hydrophilic guidewire with subsequent exchange for supportive exchange-length guidewire over which a long sheath is advanced); (ii) co-axial technique (advancement of a dedicated catheter and long 6 F sheath over a wire into the CCA, thus avoiding interaction with the bifurcation); and (iii) 'direct probing' with an 8 F guiding catheter that is positioned just beyond the ostium of the great vessel of interest, and which is therefore slightly more vulnerable to catheter prolapse and loss of secure access during the procedure.

Atropine (0.6–1.2 mg) or 200 μg glycopyrrolate (synthetic derivative with less cardioaccelerator effect) is delivered either via the sheath or intravenously to block the carotid sinus baroreceptors.

✅ Atropine/glycopyrrolate will cause short-term unilateral mydriasis if administered via the arterial sheath. Staff looking after the patient upon return to the ward should be notified about this harmless finding.

The stenosis is then either crossed with a distal embolic protection device or by a 0.014-inch wire after deployment of proximal protection (see 'Embolic protection devices').

Stent delivery systems are mostly 5-Fr or 6-Fr compatible (<2 mm diameter). Occasionally it is possible to cross the lesion with the delivery system without predilatation, but plaque 'snow-ploughing' must be avoided. Severe stenoses (80–90%) require 3 mm predilatation in order to permit safe passage of the stent-delivery system. The stent is delivered across the stenosis using road-mapping when filter protection is employed or by reference to a 'control' image with bony anatomy once flow arrest/flow reversal has been established. It is advisable to discontinue the road-map function for stent deployment. Once deployed, the stent can be dilated to ensure good apposition against the arterial wall. It is important to avoid aggressive postdilatation as emboli are generated during this phase of the procedure. Many practitioners are comfortable with leaving some degree of residual stenosis. This is on the understanding that most Nitinol stent systems will continue to expand after deployment and because the 'potato masher effect' should be avoided.

Angiography is performed in at least two planes after completion of the procedure with attention directed towards excluding plaque prolapse into the lumen through stent interstices (or platelet/thrombus aggregates) (**Fig. 10.10**). This requires gentle re-ballooning or 'double scaffolding' (placement of a second stent inside the first). Spasm (usually well tolerated) is managed by careful cephalad movement of the filter, the administration of diluted nitroglycerine

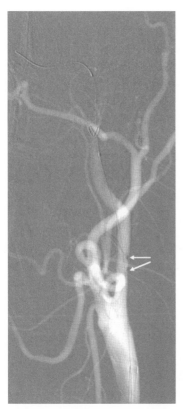

Figure 10.10 • Plaque prolapse through the interstices of a closed-cell stent (the Abbott XAct; white arrows). This was treated by placing a second stent inside the first, i.e. 'double scaffolding'.

(100–200 µg) into the long sheath and timely completion of the procedure. A full filter (causing sluggish flow) requires aspiration with a 0.014-inch compatible rapid-exchange system. Proximal EPD devices avoid these issues, but a proportion of patients are intolerant, leading to yawning, lack of responsiveness, obtundation or seizure. This can be dealt with by either intermittent flow reversal or by stopping flow reversal and using a distal filter.[89]

A recent evaluation of 627 protected CAS procedures yielded important findings regarding the timing of procedural complications.[90] At 30 days there were 10 major strokes (two fatal), 18 minor strokes (2.9%) and one cardiac death. Four major strokes occurred in phase 1 (catheterisation of the arch, target vessel and CCA) and six in phase 3 (stent deployment, pre- and postdilatation). It was concluded that a large proportion of major strokes (4/10) during CAS occurred during catheterisation and that these could not have been prevented by the use of a protection device.

Embolic protection devices

No RCTs have determined whether protection devices reduce the risk of post-CAS stroke, but a recent systematic review concluded that embolic protection was associated with significantly fewer procedural strokes than unprotected CAS.[91] There are three types of embolic protection device.

Distal balloon occlusion

Although the rationale is simple, there are a number of disadvantages. Angulated lesions may be difficult to cross, the balloon can damage the arterial wall, 10% of patients are intolerant of ICA occlusion and the stenosis cannot be imaged whilst the ICA is occluded. The 'FiberNet' filters down to 40 µm and employs a dual strategy of flow stagnation and tight filtration (aspiration of the 'standing column' in the ICA being an integral part of the protection mechanism).

Distal filters

Most filters require the lesion be crossed with a constrained filter that is then deployed above the stenosis or crossed with a 0.014-inch guidewire onto which the filter is loaded whilst flow is antegrade. The filter is retrieved following final stent dilatation. There is the potential for filter through-flow (controlled by pore size) and filter peri-flow. Self-limiting spasm of the ICA is relatively common (**Fig. 10.11a–c**).

Flow reversal/flow arrest (endovascular clamping)

Flow reversal in the ICA is achieved by occluding flow in the CCA using a balloon on the guide catheter and another in the ECA using a separate balloon occlusion system. In the Gore flow reversal system, the side arm of the working sheath is connected percutaneously to the common femoral vein, producing reversed flow through an arteriovenous fistula. The MoMa device causes flow arrest and three 20-mL syringes of blood are aspirated from the standing column in the ICA and sieved to check for visible debris before release. The MICHI system involves high-flow-rate flow reversal via a mini CCA incison between the heads of sternomastoid and does not require occlusion of the ipsilateral ECA in order to ensure flow reversal into the femoral vein. This is achieved by means of low-resistance, wide-bore dialysis tubing that completes the extracorporeal circuit.

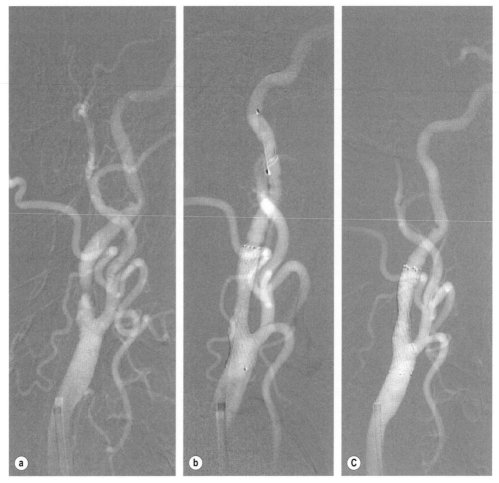

Figure 10.11 • An example of non-flow-limiting spasm. **(a)** Pre-stenting appearance of the lesion. **(b)** Post-stenting appearances (EV3 Protégé) with a filter in place (EV3 SpideRx). Spasm extends from the leading stent struts to the base of the filter. The patient remained asymptomatic. **(c)** Appearance after retrieval of the filter and the administration of 250 µg of isosorbide dinitrate into the arterial sheath.

Does stent design influence outcome?

A systematic review of 32 studies (1363 procedures) found that closed-cell stents significantly reduced new white lesions on diffusion-weighted MRI, compared with open-cell stents.[79] A small RCT comparing Wallstent and the expanded polytetrafluoroethylene (ePTFE)-covered Symbiot stent (stopped early due to excessive re-stenosis in the covered stent limb) demonstrated significantly fewer microemboli with the covered stent.[91] The Belgian/Italian registry detailed outcomes following 3179 procedures in a mixed population (largely asymptomatic) and found that stent 'free cell area' impacted on stroke/death rates. There was a statistically significant benefit for the XAct, the WallStent and the NexStent compared with the open-cell Precise, Protégé, Acculink and Exponent.[92] A 'rival' European registry sought to refute these findings, but demonstrated a similar trend towards a lower rate of procedural events when a closed-cell stent was used in symptomatic patients.[93] Lastly, in the SPACE trial, the use of the closed-cell WallStent was associated with significantly better outcomes than use of the open cell Acculink or Precise.[94]

Periprocedural haemodynamic problems

Haemodynamic depression

Haemodynamic instability is common during CAS and is baroreceptor mediated. Early CAS literature suggested that without anticholinergic prophylaxis, the incidence of intraprocedural hypotension was 17–22%, while 28–71% develop intraprocedural bradycardia.

Postprocedural hypotension is common (usually lasting about 24 hours) but is usually benign. Treatment is reserved for symptomatic patients or those in whom sustained hypotension may cause cardiovascular compromise (patients awaiting coronary artery bypass grafting or aortic valve replacement). Treatment in symptomatic or 'at-risk' patients includes antimuscarinic and/or selective alpha agonists. A recent study evaluated the use of vasopressors in the critical care unit (CCU) for treatment of persistent post-CAS hypotension in 623 patients.[95] The authors concluded that in those with a systolic BP of ≤90 mmHg, especially those protracted cases where the BP was low for ≥24 hours, there was a significant increase in the risk of stroke/death/MI.[95] Furthermore, compared with the the mixed alpha/beta agonist dopamine, the more selective alpha agonists (norepinephrine and phenylephrine) were associated with a shorter infusion time and reduced CCU length of stay and fewer major adverse events.

Hyperperfusion

A total of 54 cases of CAS-associated ICH have been reported and a pooled analysis suggests that the incidence of ICH is 0.63% (95% CI 0.38–0.97%).[96] The incidence of ICH is 2.01% (9/448; 95% CI 0.98–3.65%) in patients treated with glycoprotein IIb/IIIa inhibitors.[97] Factors predictive of ICH include symptomatic lesions, severe stenosis (≥90%) and pre-existing cerebral infarction. The interval between CAS and ICH ranges from immediately after the procedure to 6 days. In 33 of 47 reported cases (70%), the interval between CAS and ICH was ≤24 hours. In 13 cases, the interval was ≤1 hour. In two cases, there was sustained hypotension prior to suffering the ICH (contrary to expectation) and in 9 of 21 patients (43%) there were no prodromal symptoms. Prophylactic pharmacotherapy (short-acting beta-blockers) are considered in patients deemed high risk, and may reduce the incidence of hyperperfusion syndrome and ICH.[97] The incidence of ICH is not significantly different following CEA, despite the exacting antiplatelet regime mandated by CAS.

> ✅ Intraprocedural haemodynamic instability is an important cause of stroke. Baseline systolic BP >180 mmHg in a patient without prior good control of BP is an independent risk factor for an increased incidence of intra- and periprocedural hypotension/hypertension. If hypotension develops, the magnitude of BP drop correlates linearly with the severity of subsequent neurological insult.[98] Permissive tolerance of an elevated systolic BP in patients with good BP control is supportive during CAS procedures with proximal protection. Withholding angiotensin-converting enzyme inhibitors and calcium antagonists prior to the procedure generally allows a pressure that will withstand 'endovascular clamping'. A procedural systolic BP of ≥160 mmHg generally supports the use of proximal embolic protection.

Post-CAS care

Following CAS, patients should be monitored to ensure they remain free of neurological, haemodynamic and puncture-site complications. BP monitoring should continue after discharge for at least 2 weeks and patients should be advised to return immediately should severe headache develop.

Achievement and maintenance of competence

> ✅✅ The RCR[99] recommends the following as being indicative of 'competence':
> • a minimum number of 30 diagnostic cervicocerebral angiograms;
> • 100 diagnostic angiograms;
> • 50 non-neurological selective angiograms;
> • 25 peripheral or coronary stents;
> • microcatheter techniques;
> • neuroimaging (carotid Doppler, MRA, CTA, catheter angiography).

Key points

- Best medical therapy and risk factor control is mandated in everyone.
- There is compelling evidence that recently symptomatic patients benefit from treatment (medical therapy and intervention) in the hyperacute period after onset of symptoms.

- The beneficial role of CEA is supported by level 1 evidence in selected asymptomatic and symptomatic patients. It is dependent on being performed early with a low operative risk, and requires surgeons to quote their operative risk rather than trial data.
- Since the last edition, randomised trials have shown that CAS has emerged as an alternative to CEA in selected patients. The decision as to which treatment strategy should be implemented in individual patients will depend on unit experience, speed to treatment and overall cardiovascular risk.
- Interventions should not be delayed in order to achieve a lower procedural risk. The highest risk of stroke is in the first few days after onset of symptoms.

References

1. Bamford J, Sandercock P, Dennid M, et al. A prospective study of acute cerebro-vascular disease in the community. The Oxfordshire Community Stroke Project 1981–1986. (I) Methodology, demography and incident cases of first ever stroke. J Neurol Neurosurg Psychiatry 1988;51:1373–80.

2. Dunbabin D, Sandercock P. Stroke prevention. Hosp Update 1992; July: 540–5.

3. Malmgren R, Bamford J, Warlow CP, et al. Projecting the number of patients with first ever strokes and patients newly handicapped by stroke in England and Wales. Br Med J 1989;298:656–60.

4. Dennis MS, Bamford JM, Sandercock PAG, et al. Incidence of transient ischaemic attacks in Oxfordshire, England. Stroke 1989;20:333–9.

5. Menon R, Kerry S, Norris JW, et al. Treatment of cervical artery dissection: a systematic review and meta-analysis. J Neurol Neurosurg Psychiatry 2008;79(10):1122–7.

6. Hammond JH, Eisinger RP. Carotid bruits in 1000 normal subjects. Arch Intern Med 1962;109:563–5.

7. Giles MF, Rothwell PM. Risk of stroke after transient ischaemic attack: a systematic review and meta-analysis. Lancet Neurol 2007;6:1063–72.

8. Wu CM, McLaughlin K, Lorenzetti DL, et al. Early risk of stroke after transient ischaemic attack: a systematic review and meta-analysis. Arch Intern Med 2007;167:2417–22.

9. Chandratheva A, Mehta Z, Geraghty OC, et al. Population based study of risk and predictors of stroke in the first few hours after a TIA. Neurology 2009;72:1941–7.

10. Ois A, Cuadrado-Godia E, Rodriguez-Campello A, et al. High risk of early neurological recurrence in symptomatic carotid stenosis. Stroke 2009;40:2727–31.

11. Johnston SC, Rothwell PM, Nguyen-Huynh N, et al. Validation and refinement of scores to predict very early stroke risk after transient ischaemic attack. Lancet 2007;369:283–92.

12. Naylor AR. Time is brain! Surgeon 2007;5:23–30.

13. Giles MF, Albers GW, Amarenco P, et al. Early stroke risk and ABCD2 score performance in tissue versus time defined TIA: a multicentre study. Neurology 2011;77:1222–8.

14. Marquardt L, Kuker W, Chandratheva A, et al. Incidence and prognosis of > or = 50% symptomatic vertebral or basilar stenosis: prosepctive population based study. Brain 2009;132:982–8.

15. NICE. Stroke: diagnosis and initial management of acute stroke and transient ischaemic attack. CG68, issued July 2008.

16. Grant EG, Benson CB, Moneta GL, et al. Carotid artery stenosis: gray-scale and Doppler US diagnosis – Society of Radiologists in Ultrasound Consensus Conference. Radiology 2003;229:340–6.

17. Vidak V, Hebrang A, Brkljacic B, et al. Stenotic occlusive lesions of internal carotid artery in diabetic patients. Coll Antropol 2007;31:775–80.

18. Gray-Weale AC. Carotid artery atheroma: comparison of pre-operative B-mode ultrasound appearance with carotid endarterectomy specimen pathology. J Cardiovasc Surg (Torino) 1988;29:676–81.

19. Tegos TJ, Sohail M, Sabetai MM, et al. Echomorphic and histopathologic characteristics of unstable carotid plaques. AJNR Am J Neuroradiol 2000;21:1937–44.

20. Biasi GM, Froio A, Diethrich EB, et al. Carotid plaque increases the risk of stroke in carotid stenting: the Imaging in Carotid Angioplasty and Risk of Stroke (ICAROS) study. Circulation 2004;110:756–62.

21. Reiter M, Bucek RA, Effenberger I, et al. Plaque echolucency is not associated with the risk of stroke in carotid artery stenting. Stroke 2006;37:2378–80.

22. Berczi V, Randall M, Balamurugan R, et al. Safety of arch aortography for assessment of carotid arteries. Eur J Vasc Endovasc Surg 2006;31:3–7.

23. Executive Committee for the Asymptomatic Carotid Atherosclerosis Study. Endarterectomy for asymptomatic carotid artery stenosis. JAMA 1995;273:1421–61.

24. Borisch I, Horn M, Butz B, et al. Preoperative evaluation of carotid artery stenosis: comparison of contrast-enhanced MR angiography and duplex sonography with digital subtraction angiography. AJNR Am J Neuroradiol 2003;24:1117–22.

25. Johnston DC, Eastwood JD, Nguyen T. Contrast-enhanced magnetic resonance angiography of carotid arteries. Utility in routine clinical practice. Stroke 2002;33:2834–8.

26. Wardlaw JM, Chappell FM, Stevenson M, et al. Accurate, practical and cost-effective assessment of carotid stenosis in the UK. Health Technol Assess 2006;10:iii–iv, ix–x, 1–182.

27. Intercollegiate Stroke Working Party. National clinical guidelines for stroke, 2nd ed, , Section 3.5.6f, 2004.

28. The European Stroke Initiative Executive Committee and the EUSI Writing Committee. European Stroke Initiative recommendations for stroke management – Update 2003. Cerebrovasc Dis 2003;16:311–37.

29. MacMahon S. Antihypertensive drug treatment: the potential, expected and observed effects on vascular disease. J Hypertens 1990;8(Suppl.):S239–44.

30. Kalra L, Perez I, Melbourn A. Stroke risk management: changes in mainstream practice. Stroke 1998;29:53–7.

31. Heart Protection Study Collaborative Group. MRC/BHF Heart Protection Study of cholesterol lowering with simvastatin in 20536 high-risk individuals: a randomised placebo controlled trial. Lancet 2002;360:7–22.

32. NICE Technology Appraisal Guidance 90: clopidogrel and modified release dipyridamole for the prevention of occlusive vascular events, www.nice.org.uk/guidance/TA210; [accessed 11.08.12].

33. North American Symptomatic Carotid Endarterectomy Trial Collaborators. Beneficial effect of carotid endarterectomy in symptomatic patients with high grade stenosis. N Engl J Med 1991;325:445–53.

34. Taylor DW, Barnett HJM, Haynes RB, et al. Low dose and high dose acetylsalicylic acid for patients undergoing carotid endarterectomy: a randomised trial. Lancet 1999;353:2179–84.

35. Rothwell PM, Giles MF, Chandratheva A, et al. Effect of urgent treatment of transient ischaemic attack and minor stroke on early recurrent stroke (EXPRESS Study): a prospective population based sequential comparison. Lancet 2007;370:1–11.

36. Rothwell PM, Eliasziw M, Gutnikov SA for the Carotid Endarterectomy Trialists Collaboration. Analysis of pooled data from the randomised controlled trials of endarterectomy for symptomatic carotid stenosis. Lancet 2003;361:107–16.

37. Rothwell PM, Eliasziw M, Gutnikov SA, for the Carotid Endarterectomy Trialists Collaboration. Endarterectomy for symptomatic carotid stenosis in relation to clinical subgroups and timing of surgery. Lancet 2004; 363:915–24.

38. Rothwell PM, Eliasziw M, Gutnikov SA. Sex difference in the effect of time from symptoms to surgery on benefit from carotid endarterectomy for transient ischaemic attack and minor stroke. Stroke 2004;35:2855–61.

39. Wennberg DE, Lucas FL, Birkmeyer JD, et al. Variation in carotid endarterectomy mortality in the Medicare population. JAMA 1998;279:1278–81.

40. Holt PJE, Poloniecki J, Loftus IM. The relationship between hospital case volume and outcome from carotid endarterectomy in England from 2000 to 2005. Eur J Vasc Endovasc Surg 2007;34:646–54.

41. Naylor AR, Rothwell PM, Bell PRF. Overview of the principal results and secondary analyses from the European and the North American randomised trials of carotid endarterectomy. Eur J Vasc Endovasc Surg 2003;26:115–29.

42. Rockman CB, Maldonado T, Jacobowitz GR, et al. Early endarterectomy in symptomatic patients is associated with poorer perioperative outcomes. J Vasc Surg 2006;44:480–7.

43. Halliday A, Mansfield A, Marro J, et al. Prevention of disabling and fatal strokes by successful carotid endarterectomy in patients without recent neurological symptoms: randomized trial. Lancet 2004;363:1491–502.

44. Halliday A, Harison M, Hayter E, et al. 10 year stroke prevention after successful carotid endarterectomy for asymptomatic carotid stenosis (ACST-1): a multicentre randomised trial. Lancet 2010;376:1074–84.

45. Furie KL, Kasner SE, Adams RJ, et al. Guidelines for the prevention of stroke in patients with stroke or transient ischaemic attack: a guideline for healthcare professionals from the American Heart Association/American Stroke Association. Stroke 2011;42:227–76.

46. Autumn Klein A, Caren G, Solomon CG, et al. Management of carotid stenosis – polling results. N Engl J Med 2008;358:e23.Available at http://www.nejm.org/clinical%2Ddecisions/20080410/#commentbox; [accessed 19.07.12].

47. Naylor AR. Time to rethink management strategies in asymptomatic carotid artery disease. Nat Rev Cardiol 2011;9(2):116–24.

48. Timaran CH, Rosero EB, Smith ST, et al. Trends and outcomes of concurrent carotid revascularization and coronary bypass. J Vasc Surg 2008;48:355–61.

49. Naylor AR, Mehta Z, Rothwell PM. Stroke during coronary artery bypass surgery: a critical review of the role of carotid artery disease. Eur J Vasc Endovasc Surg 2002;23:283–94.

50. Naylor AR, Bown MJ. Stroke after cardiac surgery and its association with asymptomatic carotid disease: an updated systematic review and meta-analysis. Eur J Vasc Endovasc Surg 2011;41:607–24.

51. Naylor AR, Mehta Z, Rothwell PM. A systematic review and meta-analysis of 30-day outcomes following staged carotid artery stenting and coronary bypass. Eur J Vasc Endovasc Surg 2009;37:379–87.

52. Bond R, Rerkasem K, Rothwell PM. Systematic review of the risks of carotid endarterectomy in relation to the clinical indication for and timing of surgery. Stroke 2003;34:2290–301.

53. Caplan LR, Wityk RJ, Glass TA, et al. New England Medical Centre Posterior Circulation Registry. Ann Neurol 2004;56:389–98.

54. Stayman AN, Nogueria RG, Gupta R. A systematic review of stenting and angioplasty of symptomatic extracranial vertebral artery stenosis. Stroke 2011;42:2212–6.

55. Sultan MJ, Hartshorne T, Naylor AR. Extracranial and transcranial ultrasound assessment of patients with suspected positional vertebrobasilar iscaehemia. Eur J Vasc Endovasc Surg 2009;38:10–3.

56. GALA Trial Collaborative Group. General anaesthesia versus local anaesthesia for cartoid surgery (GALA): a multicentre randomised controlled trial. Lancet 2008;372:2132–45.

57. Rerkasem K, Rothwell PM. Patch angioplasty versus primary closure for carotid endarterectomy. Cochrane Database Syst Rev 2009;(4):CD000160.

58. Rerkasem K, Rothwell PM. Routine or selective carotid artery shunting for carotid endarterectomy (and different methods of monitoring in selective shunting). Cochrane Database Syst Rev 2009;(4):CD000190.

59. Astrup J, Siesjo BK, Symon L. Thresholds in cerebral ischaemia: the ischaemic penumbra. Stroke 1981;12:723–5.

60. Sharpe R, Sayers RD, McCarthy MJ, et al. The war against error: a 15 year experience of completion angioscopy following carotid endarterectomy. Eur J Vasc Surg 2012;43:139–45.

61. Forsell C, Bergqvist D, Bergentz SE. Peripheral nerve injuries in carotid artery surgery. In: Greenhalgh RM, Hollier LH, editors. Surgery for stroke. London: WB Saunders; 1993. p. 217–34.

62. Ferguson GG, Eliasziw M, Barr HWK, et al. The North American Symptomatic Carotid Endarterectomy Trial: surgical results in 1415 patients. Stroke 1999;30:1751–8.

63. Silver FL, Sergentanis TN, Tsivgoulis G, et al. Safety of stenting and endarterectomy by symptomatic status in the Carotid Revascularization Endarterectomy Versus Stenting Trial (CREST). Stroke 2011;42:675–80.

64. Naylor AR, Evans J, Thompson MM, et al. Seizures after carotid endarterectomy: hyperperfusion, dysautoregulation or hypertensive encephalopathy? Eur J Vasc Endovasc Surg 2003;26:39–44.

65. Naylor AR, Hayes PD, Allroggen H, et al. Reducing the risk of carotid surgery: a seven year audit of the role of monitoring and quality control assessment. J Vasc Surg 2000;32:750–9.

66. Payne DA, Jones CI, Hayes PD, et al. Beneficial effects of clopidogrel combined with aspirin in reducing cerebral emboli in patients undergoing carotid endarterectomy. Circulation 2004;109:1476–81.

67. Sharpe R, Sayers RD, McCarthy MJ, et al. Dual antiplatelet therapy prior to carotid endarterectomy reduces post-operative embolisation and thromboembolic events: post-operative transcranial Doppler monitoring is now unnecessary. Eur J Vasc Endovasc Surg 2010;40:162–7.

68. Frericks H, Kievit J, van Baalen JM. Carotid recurrent stenosis and risk of ipsilateral stroke. A systematic review of the literature. Stroke 1998;29:244–50.

69. Moore WS, Kempczinski RF, Nelson JJ, et al. Recurrent carotid stenosis: results of the Asymptomatic Carotid Atherosclerosis Study. Stroke 1998;29:2018–2025.

70. Mas J-L, Chatellier G, Beyssen B, et al. Endarterectomy versus stenting in patients with severe symptomatic stenosis. N Engl J Med 2006;355:1660–71.

71. SPACE Collaborators. Stent Protected Angioplasty versus Carotid Endarterectomy in symptomatic patients: 30 days results from the SPACE Trial. Lancet 2006;368:1239–47.

72. ICSS Investigators. Carotid artery stenting compared with endarterectomy in patients with symptomatic carotid stenosis: interim analysis of a randomised controlled trial. Lancet 2010;375:985–97.

73. Brott TG, Hobson RW, Howard G, et al. Stenting versus endarterectomy for treatment of carotid-artery stenosis. N Engl J Med 2010;363:11–23.

74. Carotid Stenting Trialists Collaboration. Short term outcome after stenting versus carotid endarterectomy for symptomatic carotid stenosis: preplanned meta-analysis of individual patient data. Lancet 2010;376:1062–73.

75. Economoupoulos KP, Sergentanis TN, Tsivgoulis G, et al. Carotid artery stenting versus carotid endarterectomy: comprehensive meta-analysis of short- and long-term outcomes. Stroke 2011;42:687–92.

76. Bonati LH, Jongen LM, Haller S, et al. New ischaemic brain lesions on MRI after stenting or endarterectomy for symptomatic carotid stenosis: Substudy of the ICSS. Lancet Neurol 2010;9:353–62.

77. Iwata T, Mori T, Tajiri H, et al. Safety and effectiveness of emergency carotid artery stenting for a high grade carotid stenosis with intraluminal thrombus under proximal flow control in hyperacute and acute stroke. J Neurointerv Surg 2011;Dec 14. Epub ahead of print.

78. Blackshear JL, Cutlip DE, Roubin GS, et al. Myocardial infarction after carotid stenting and endarterectomy: results from the Carotid Revascularization Endarterectomy versus Stenting Trial. Circulation 2011;123:2571–8.

79. Schnaudigel S, Groschel K, Pilgram SM, et al. New brain lesions after carotid stenting versus carotid endarterectomy: systematic review of the literature. Stroke 2008;39:1911–9.

80. Palombo G, Faraglia V, Stella N, et al. Late evaluation of silent cerebral ischemia detected by diffusion-weighted MR imaging after filter-protected carotid artery stenting. AJNR Am J Neuroradiol 2008;29:1340–3.

81. Altinbas A, van Zandvoort MJ, van den Berg J, et al. Cognition after carotid endarterectomy or stenting: a randomized comparison. Neurology 2011;77:1084–90.

82. Montorsi P, Caputi L, Galli S, et al. Microembolization during carotid artery stenting in patients with high-risk, lipid-rich plaque. A randomized trial of proximal versus distal cerebral protection. J Am Coll Cardiol 2011;58(16):1656–63.

83. The PROFI trial. Presented by Bijuklic K et al. Late breaking trials TCT, San Francisco; November 2011.

84. Schmidt A, Diederich KW, Scheinert S, et al. Effect of two different neuroprotection systems on microembolization during carotid artery stenting. J Am Coll Cardiol 2004;44:1966–9.

85. Pinter L, Ribo M, Loh C, et al. Safety and feasibility of a novel transcervical access neuroprotection system for carotid artery stenting in the PROOF study. J Vasc Surg 2011;54:1317–23.

86. NICE. IPG389: Carotid artery stent placement for symptomatic extracranial carotid stenosis: Guidance. 27 April 2011.

87. Macdonald S, Lee R, Williams R, et al., Delphi Carotid Stenting Consensus Panel. Towards safer carotid artery stenting: a scoring system for anatomic suitability. Stroke 2009;40:1698–703.

88. McKevitt FM, Randall MS, Cleveland TJ. The benefits of combined anti-platelet treatment in carotid artery stenting. Eur J Vasc Endovasc Surg 2005;29:522–7.

89. Verzini F, Cao P, De Rango P, et al. Appropriateness of learning curve for carotid artery stenting: an analysis of periprocedural complications. J Vasc Surg 2006;44:1205–1211.

90. Garg N, Karagiorgos N, Pisimisis GT, et al. Cerebral protection devices reduce periprocedural strokes during carotid angioplasty and stenting: a systematic review of the current literature. J Endovasc Ther 2009;16:412–27.

91. Schillinger M, Dick P, Wiest G, et al. Covered versus bare self-expanding stents for endovascular treatment of carotid artery stenosis: a stopped randomized trial. J Endovasc Ther 2006;13:312–9.

92. Bosiers M, de Donato G, Deloose K, et al. Does free cell area influence the outcome in carotid artery stenting? Eur J Vasc Endovasc Surg 2007;33:135–41.

93. Schillinger M, Gschwendtner M, Reimers B, et al. Does carotid stent cell design matter? Stroke 2008;39(3):905–9.

94. Jansen O, Fiehler J, Hartmann M, et al. Protection or nonprotection in carotid stent angioplasty: the influence of interventional techniques on outcome data from the SPACE Trial. Stroke 2009;40:841–6.

95. Nandalur MR, Cooper H, Satler LF. Vasopressor use in the critical care unit for treatment of persistent post-carotid artery stent induced hypotension. Neurocrit Care 2007;7:232–7.

96. Hyun-Seung K, Han MH, Kwon O-Ki, et al. Intracranial hemorrhage after carotid angioplasty: a pooled analysis. J Endovasc Ther 2007;14:77–85.

97. Abou-Chebl A, Reginelli J, Bajzer CT, et al. Intensive treatment of hypertension decreases the risk of hyperperfusion and intracerebral hemorrhage following carotid artery stenting. Catheter Cardiovasc Interv 2007;69:690–6.

98. Howell M, Krajcer Z, Dougherty K, et al. Correlation of periprocedural systolic blood pressure changes with neurological events in high-risk carotid stent patients. J Endovasc Ther 2002;9:810–6.

99. Advice from the Royal College of Radiologists concerning training for carotid artery stenting (CAS). Ref. No. BFCR (06)6.

11

Vascular disorders of the upper limb

Jean-Baptiste Ricco
Fabrice Schneider

Introduction

Arterial diseases of the upper limb are relatively rare in comparison with those involving the lower extremity. The good collateral supply around the shoulder and elbow explains why chronic occlusive disease is commonly asymptomatic, but acute occlusion due to embolism can result in limb-threatening ischaemia. In addition, thoracic outlet syndrome, axillo-subclavian vein thrombosis and occupational vascular problems need to be considered. In this chapter we do not review vasospastic disorders, connective tissue disease, vasculitis and Raynaud's disease, as these are covered in Chapter 12, nor vascular trauma, which is covered in Chapter 9. The main causes of upper limb vascular disease are summarised in Box 11.1.

Clinical examination

Vascular assessment of the upper limb should include the thoracic outlet. Palpation and auscultation of the supraclavicular region may help to detect a cervical rib, a subclavian stenosis or aneurysm. The arm pulses should be examined with the arm placed in the neutral position and then in abduction and external rotation (surrender position) in order to detect arterial thoracic outlet compression. Pulse palpation is important and must include the axillary, brachial, radial and ulnar pulses. The blood pressure should be measured in both arms, preferably using a hand-held Doppler. A difference of more than 15% is abnormal.

Examination in cases of hand ischaemia is not complete unless Allen's test is performed. The examiner compresses the radial and ulnar arteries at the wrist. The examiner then asks the subject to clench the fist in order to empty the hand of blood. The radial artery is then released and the hand is observed for return of colour. The test is then repeated for the ulnar artery. The test is normal if refilling of the hand is complete within less than 10 seconds from either side. Any portion of the hand that does not blush is an indication of incomplete continuity of the palmar arch. The nail folds should be examined for infarcts and splinter haemorrhages.

Occlusive disease

Occlusive lesions of the brachiocephalic and subclavian arteries occur in relatively young patients with mean ages ranging from 50 to 60 years. These lesions are much less frequent than those involving the carotid bifurcation.[1] Atherosclerosis is the predominant cause in Europe, with Buerger's disease and Takayasu's arteritis seen rarely. The symptoms of occlusive disease of the upper extremities include muscle fatigue and ischaemic rest pain. Digital necrosis or atheroembolisation is less common than in the lower extremities, accounting for no more than 5% of patients with limb ischaemia.[2]

Brachiocephalic artery

Stenotic lesions of the brachiocephalic artery are uncommon and may be asymptomatic in 13–22%

Box 11.1 • Causes of upper limb vascular diseases

Arterial obstruction

Large artery
Atherosclerosis
Radiotherapy
Thoracic outlet syndrome
Arteritis (giant cell, Takayasu's)

Small artery
Atherosclerosis
Connective tissue disease
Myeloproliferative disease
Buerger's disease
Vibrating tools

Arterial vasospasm

Large artery
Ergot-containing medications and other pharmacological causes

Small artery
Raynaud's disease
Vibrating tools

Embolism: proximal sources
Heart
Ulcerated arterial plaques (aortic arch, brachiocephalic and subclavian arteries)
Aneurysm (brachiocephalic, subclavian, axillary, brachial, ulnar arteries)
Thoracic outlet syndrome

Subclavian–axillary vein thrombosis
Primary: Paget–Schroetter syndrome (thoracic outlet syndrome)
Secondary: catheter, hypercoagulable states

Hypercoagulable states
Heparin antibodies
Deficiencies of antithrombin III, proteins C and S
Antiphospholipid syndrome
Malignancy
Cryoglobulinaemia

Aneurysms

of patients.[3,4] Symptomatic patients may present with ischaemia of the right upper extremity, carotid territory symptoms or vertebrobasilar symptoms.[5] The diagnosis is suspected by physical examination (i.e. right supraclavicular/cervical bruit, absent right subclavian or axillary pulse) and confirmed by duplex scanning, conventional angiography, or computed tomography (CT) or magnetic resonance angiography (MRA). Most patients (61–84%) with brachiocephalic artery occlusion have multiple lesions of the aortic arch vessels.[6] Stenotic lesions of

the brachiocephalic artery may be approached by median sternotomy with direct bypass grafting from the aortic arch, or indirectly by extra-anatomical bypass such as subclavian–subclavian, contralateral carotid–carotid or subclavian–carotid bypass.

Aorto-brachiocephalic bypass

✔✔ Extra-anatomical bypasses have a lower morbidity and mortality but direct bypasses from the aortic arch are more durable. In total, the combined postoperative death and stroke rate for direct reconstruction of the supra-aortic trunks ranges from 2.6% to 16% (Table 11.1). The primary patency is about 90% with a 72% survival rate at 10 years.[7]

A median sternotomy is used with extension into the neck. The left brachiocephalic vein is identified (**Fig. 11.1a**). A partial occluding clamp is applied to the ascending aorta proximal to the brachiocephalic artery in order to avoid the risk of fracturing atheromatous plaque (**Fig. 11.1b**). An 8–10 mm prosthetic graft is anastomosed at this site with deep suture placement in the aortic wall (**Fig. 11.1c**). Once the anastomosis is completed, a clamp is applied across the graft and systemic heparin is given. The brachiocephalic artery is clamped, sectioned and the proximal stump oversewn. The patent distal artery is spatulated and the graft attached in an end-to-end fashion (**Fig. 11.1d**). Air is evacuated from the graft by back-bleeding the subclavian artery, then flow is released into the arm and then into the carotid artery. The mortality of direct bypass ranges from 5.8% to 8% in Kieffer's and Berguer's series, with a primary patency rate at 5 years of 94% in both series.

Brachiocephalic endarterectomy

The proximal location of the disease with extension into the aortic arch makes this technique hazardous in some patients. Attempts to remove an orifice lesion may initiate an aortic dissection or distal embolisation. For this reason bypass or endovascular therapy are preferred for all brachiocephalic lesions where treatment is indicated, except perhaps for those located in the distal segment.

Endovascular treatment

Percutaneous transluminal angioplasty (PTA) and stenting of the brachiocephalic artery is being performed with increased frequency. The approach may be percutaneous from either the femoral or brachial artery or through an anterolateral cervical approach with clamping of the right common carotid artery to avoid atheroembolisation during the angioplasty. Because of a relatively small number of cases, most papers concerning angioplasty of the

Table 11.1 • Direct reconstruction of the supra-aortic vessels: complications and late patency

Authors, year	Patients	Mean follow-up (months) [range]	Complications (%)	Primary patency (%)
Takach et al.,[8] 2005	113	61.2 ± 6 [3–264]	Death: 2.7 Stroke: 2.7	10 years:[†] 94.4 ++ 4
Berguer et al.,[4] 1998	100	51 ± 4.8 [1–184]	MI:* 1.8 Stroke + death: 16 Morbidity: 27	5 years:[‡] 94±3
Uurto et al.,[7] 2002	76	158 [6–136]	Death: 2.6 Morbidity: 19.7	1 year: 95 5 years:[§] 91; 15 years:[§] 89

* MI, myocardial infarction.
† 22 patients were followed at 10 years.
‡ 34 patients followed at 5 years.
§ 54 patients followed at 5 years and 25 at 15 years.

brachiocephalic artery include results for the subclavian artery. Only three series report PTA of the brachiocephalic artery alone[9–11] (Table 11.2). The benefit of adjuvant stenting is not well established.[9,10] Open surgery gives better mid-term results but angioplasty is much less invasive.

Subclavian artery

Symptomatic lesions of the subclavian artery are associated in 72% of cases with concomitant lesions of carotid and vertebral vessels.[1] The indications for intervention are those of vertebrobasilar insufficiency and marked upper extremity ischaemia. Atheroembolisation is quite common in this location.[12] If surgery is contemplated and the ipsilateral common carotid artery is healthy, carotid–subclavian bypass or carotid–subclavian transposition is the method of choice.

Carotid–subclavian bypass

Access is achieved by a horizontal supraclavicular incision with division of both heads of the sternomastoid muscle. Scalenus anterior and the phrenic nerves are exposed, and then scalenus anterior is divided near its insertion into the first rib (Fig. 11.2a). On the left side, the thoracic duct is ligated. The carotid sheath is opened, safeguarding the vagus nerve. After heparinisation, the common carotid artery is clamped as low as possible. A vein or polytetrafluoroethylene (PTFE) graft is then anastomosed to the lateral aspect of the common carotid artery in an end-to-side fashion (Fig. 11.2b). Use of a prosthetic graft seems to give better results than the vein graft in this location.[13] The graft under arterial tension is then passed behind the jugular vein. Graft length should be cautiously estimated and the graft anastomosed end-to-side to the superior aspect of the distal subclavian artery. If the proximal subclavian lesion is ulcerated, it should be excluded by proximal ligation. If the distal subclavian artery is too diseased for distal implantation, the graft should be passed behind the clavicle and implanted on the axillary artery exposed via a short infraclavicular incision.

> ✔✔ Prosthetic carotid–subclavian bypass has an excellent patency. Postoperative mortality is less than 1%, with a primary patency of 95% at 10 years.[14,15]

Carotid transposition

Reimplantation of the subclavian artery into the common carotid artery is an alternative that avoids graft material but requires a more extensive cervical dissection. Dissection should avoid the recurrent laryngeal nerve, which is closely related to the posterior aspect of the subclavian artery. A curved clamp is applied across the subclavian artery, which is transected and the proximal stump oversewn. The site of anastomosis to the common carotid artery should be chosen to avoid kinking and angulation of the vertebral artery. The clamps on the common carotid artery should be rotated anteriorly to present the posterolateral surface for anastomosis with the subclavian artery (Fig. 11.3). An ellipse is excised from the wall of the common carotid artery and the subclavian artery anastomosed in end-to-side fashion.

> ✔✔ Subclavian–carotid reimplantation is an excellent technique that seems to give better results than the subclavian–carotid bypass in the series of Cinà et al.[16] (Table 11.3). Postoperative mortality is less than 1%, with a long-term patency of 100% in the series of Sandmann et al.[17] and Kretschmer et al.[18]

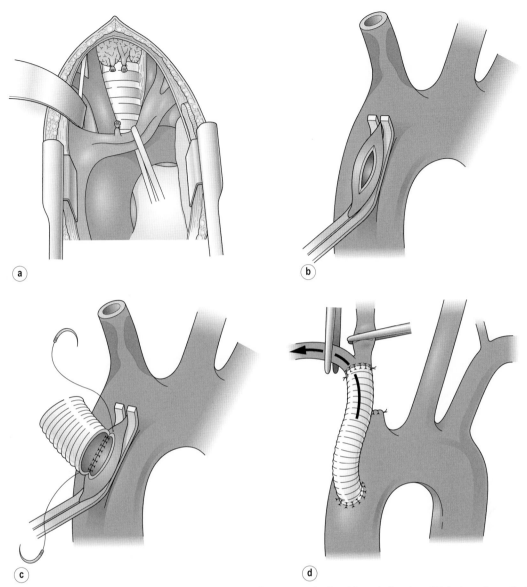

Figure 11.1 • (a) The left brachiocephalic vein is retracted to expose the brachiocephalic artery. **(b)** A clamp is applied laterally to the ascending aorta. **(c)** A polyester graft is implanted on the ascending thoracic aorta proximal to the brachiocephalic artery. **(d)** Completed bypass. Flow is released into the arm and then into the common carotid artery.

Crossover grafts

Subclavian revascularisation may also be achieved by crossover subclavian–subclavian or axilloaxillary bypass. These grafts are relatively simple to construct, although their greater length and reversed angle of take-off may reduce durability. Furthermore, problems may arise if subsequent median sternotomy is needed for coronary bypass. The donor and recipient arteries are exposed by a short supraclavicular incision on either side (**Fig. 11.4**). A tunnel is created from one side of the neck to the other passing behind the sternomastoid muscles and anterior to the carotid vessels. Crossover axilloaxillary bypass is easier to perform but the graft has to pass subcutaneously over the sternum, with risks of compression or erosion. The postoperative death rate for crossover axilloaxillary bypass is 1.6% with a 5-year primary patency of 86.5% in the series of Mingoli et al.[19]

Table 11.2 • Angioplasty of the brachiocephalic artery: postoperative complications and late patency

Authors, year	Patients	Mean follow-up (months) [range]	Complications (%)	Primary patency (%)	Secondary patency (%)
Paukovits et al.[9], 2010	72	42.3 [2–103]	Total: 8.3 Death: none TIA: 2.6 Access site bleeding:5.2	12 months: 100 24 months: 98 ± 1.6 96 months: 69.9 ± 8.5	12 months: 100 24 months: 100 96 months: 81.5 ± 7.7
Van Hattum et al.[10], 2007	30	Not available Median=24 [4 weeks–92]	Total: 10.0 Death: none TIA: 4.0	24 months: 79	Not available
Hüttl et al.,[11] 2002	89	Not available [12–117]	Neurological: 5.6 Local: 3.0	6 months: 98 ± 2 1 year: 95 ± 3	100 98 ± 2

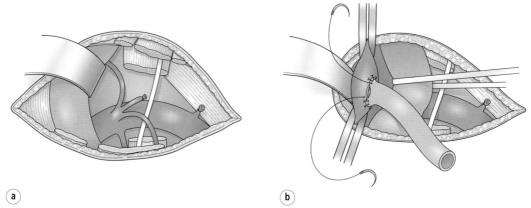

Figure 11.2 • (a) Cervical approach for carotid–subclavian bypass. The sternomastoid muscle is divided and the subclavian artery is exposed by sectioning the scalenus anterior. (b) A PTFE graft is anastomosed to the lateral aspect of the left common carotid artery.

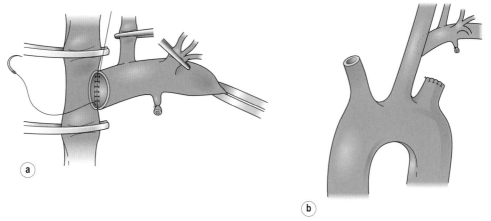

Figure 11.3 • Carotid–subclavian transposition: (a) clamps on the common carotid artery are rotated anteriorly to present the posterolateral surface for anastomosis with the subclavian artery; (b) end-to-side anastomosis completed.

Table 11.3 • Carotid transposition: postoperative complications and late patency

Authors, year	Patients	Mean follow-up (months) [range]	Complications (%)	Primary patency (%) at mean follow-up
Cinà et al.,[16] 2002	27	25 ± 21	Morbidity: 11.1	100
Schardey et al.,[13] 1996	108	70 [1–144]	Stroke: 1.8 Morbidity: 15	100*

* 84 patients followed.

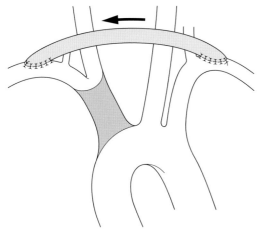

Figure 11.4 • Brachiocephalic artery occlusion. Revascularisation by a cross-subclavian PTFE graft. Tunnelisation is done behind the sternomastoid muscles and anterior to the carotid vessels.

Endovascular treatment

PTA of subclavian artery stenoses is a relatively safe and often simple procedure to perform. Access is usually obtained from the femoral artery or from the brachial artery and the lesion dilated to 5–8 mm (**Fig. 11.5**). Because there is usually retrograde flow in the vertebral artery, stroke is rare. When there is not retrograde flow, an occlusion balloon may be placed in the vertebral artery from the arm while the stenosis is dilated. Simple stenoses are adequately dilated by balloon. Occlusions are more difficult to cross and less frequent in most endovascular series;[20,21] they often require catheterisation from the brachial artery with the use of balloon or self-expandable stents.

> ✅✅ PTA with or without stenting is an appropriate treatment for symptomatic patients with localised subclavian artery stenosis with a 2-year primary patency of 90% in most series[20,21] (Table 11.4), but a long-term patency inferior to that obtained with carotid–subclavian bypass or transposition.

Upper arm arteries

Patients with chronic atherosclerotic occlusion of the axillary or brachial arteries usually present with fatigue on using the arm. Many of these patients have radiation-induced occlusive disease. Severe ischaemia with rest pain or digital necrosis is uncommon unless there have been repeated episodes of embolism due to proximal ulceration or aneurysmal degeneration. Direct reconstructive surgery is feasible since the occlusive lesions tend to be segmental with preserved distal patency. Axillobrachial occlusions can be managed by a bypass procedure if symptoms justify it. These sites can usually be approached by limited incisions and the bypass tunnelled subcutaneously between the two incisions (**Fig. 11.6**). Autogenous saphenous vein is the preferred graft material. When unavailable, the basilic or cephalic vein may be considered. Upper limb bypass using saphenous vein has a 5-year patency rate of 60–90%.[22] PTFE has a lower patency rate at this level.

Lower arm and hand arteries

The causes of chronic occlusion in the forearm or hand vessels include atherosclerosis, Buerger's disease, immunological and connective tissue disorders (see Chapter 12), and occupational trauma. Arch angiography, to exclude proximal embolic disease, and selective arteriography are essential in evaluating these patients with distal disease. Most of these patients with distal disease and severe digital ischaemia can be managed conservatively. Avoidance of cold and abstinence of tobacco are essential. Vasodilator or sympatholytic agents may also be employed. Patients with digital necrosis may require local debridement or amputation if gangrene is extensive. Some patients with radial, ulnar or palmar arch occlusion and critical ischaemia may be managed, if run-off is present, by vein graft bypass using microsurgical techniques. Cervicodorsal sympathectomy by thoracoscopy may also be considered in patients with severe distal forearm ischaemia. However, results of sympathectomy have often been disappointing, particularly in patients with diffuse arteritis.

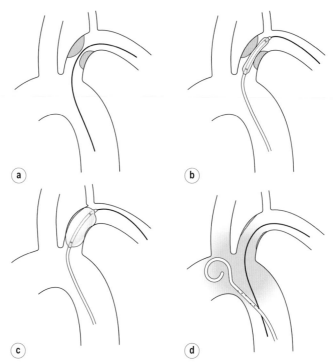

Figure 11.5 • Retrograde approach from the brachial artery by percutaneous puncture, or cut-down if stenting is necessary: **(a)** the guidewire is placed through the subclavian stenosis; **(b)** balloon is advanced over the guidewire and balloon angioplasty performed; **(c)** arteriography completed by withdrawing the balloon with the same catheter; **(d)** more accurate arteriographic control can be achieved by using a second transfemoral pigtail catheter positioned in the aortic arch. From Schneider PA. Endovascular skills, 2003. Reproduced by permission of Informa Healthcare.

Table 11.4 • Angioplasty of the subclavian artery: postoperative complications and late patency

Authors, year	Patients	Mean follow-up (months) [range]	Complications (%)	Primary patency (%)
De Vries et al.,[20] 2005	110	34 [3–120]	Stroke + death: 4.5 Local: 3.6	2 years:* 89 3 years:† 89
Berger et al.[21] 2011	72	82 [3–299]	Death: 19.6 Local: 4.9 Transient monoplegia: 1.5	10 years: 85.2

* 64 patients followed at 2 years.
† 36 patients followed at 3 years.

Aneurysmal disease

True aneurysms of the upper limb arteries are un-common. The subclavian artery is the most frequent site, usually caused by thoracic outlet compression. These patients may present with distal ischaemia, embolisation or acute thrombosis. False aneurysms from trauma or infection often produce motor or sensory impairment as a result of brachial plexus compression. Subclavian artery aneurysms are best managed by a combined supraclavicular and infraclavicular approach (see later). Aneurysms of the brachiocephalic artery are rare. In the series of Kieffer et al.[23] the perioperative death rate was 11%, most deaths occurring in patients operated in an emergency setting.

An aberrant right subclavian artery arising from the descending thoracic aorta is a common anom-aly. Rarely, the artery compresses the oesophagus against the trachea, producing a condition de-scribed as dysphagia lusoria. Aneurysmal degenera-tion, known as Kommerell's diverticulum, may also occur. The largest experience has been reported by Kieffer et al.[24] Because of the possibility of rupture,

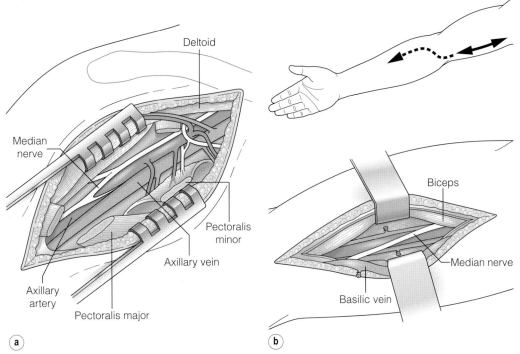

Figure 11.6 • **(a)** Axillary artery approach. The pectoralis minor muscle is divided and the neurovascular bundle is exposed. If access to the axillobrachial junction is needed, the pectoralis major tendon should also be resected. **(b)** Brachial artery approach. Incision along the medial border of the biceps. If necessary, the bicipital aponeurosis is divided to expose the brachial artery division.

resection of the aneurysmal artery with aortic prosthetic reconstruction via a thoracic approach is recommended. As this technique carries a high postoperative mortality, hybrid procedures with aortic stent grafts are feasible.

Upper arm artery aneurysms

Axillary artery aneurysms are usually caused by blunt or penetrating trauma. Degenerative or congenital aneurysms are rare in this location. False aneurysms of the axillary artery occur with humeral fractures and anterior dislocation of the shoulder. These aneurysms can lead to neurological complications because of compression of the brachial plexus. Duplex scan and arteriography allow an accurate diagnosis. The axillary artery is exposed by a deltopectoral incision with division of the pectoralis minor. The aneurysm is resected followed by interposition of a reversed saphenous vein graft. Stent grafts have been used for emergency control of upper limb aneurysms but their long-term integrity is often compromised by compression between the first rib and clavicle or by excessive arterial flexion.[25]

Lower arm and hand artery aneurysms

Radial artery aneurysms are usually due to inadequate compression or infection following removal of intra-arterial blood pressure cannulae. If the Allen test shows good filling of the hand from the ulnar artery, then the radial artery can simply be ligated above and below the aneurysm. If not, reconstruction using a vein graft is required.

Ulnar artery aneurysm or hypothenar hammer syndrome

It is important to recognise an ulnar artery aneurysm because it may lead to digital necrosis. The condition known as hypothenar hammer syndrome develops in workers who suffer repetitive trauma to their hands, including carpenters and pipe fitters. Those who play sports such as volleyball or karate are also at risk. The pathophysiology is related to the vascular anatomy of the hand. The distal ulnar artery is vulnerable to external trauma between the distal margin of Guyon's canal and the palmar aponeurosis. Over this short distance, the artery lies anterior to the hook of the hamate bone and is covered only by the palmaris brevis muscle and the skin. Trauma of the ulnar artery at this level causes thrombosis or aneurysm formation and distal embolisation in the fourth and fifth fingers, with pain, coldness and cyanosis. The thumb is always spared because of its radial blood supply. Angiography with magnification is essential in these patients.

When the ulnar artery is chronically thrombosed, calcium channel blockers may be helpful. In all cases, patients should avoid further hand trauma.

✔✔ Surgical therapy includes microsurgical arterial reconstruction with or without adjunctive preoperative thrombolytic therapy to restore patency to digital arteries. Resection of the aneurysm with placement of an interposition vein graft is the treatment of choice. Satisfactory long-term results have been reported by Vayssairat et al. using this approach.[26]

Upper limb embolism

Embolic arterial occlusion is the major cause of acute upper limb ischaemia; upper limb emboli represent 20–32% of major peripheral emboli.[27] A cardiac origin is found in 90% of cases and is related to arrhythmia, myocardial infarction, valvular disorder or ventricular aneurysm. Non-cardiac sources include ulcerative atherosclerotic plaques or aneurysms in the arch or subclavian–axillary arteries and thoracic outlet compression. The brachial bifurcation is the most frequently involved site for an embolus to lodge. Clinical examination and duplex scan can locate the level of the arterial occlusion. Preoperative conventional angiography or CT angiography is indicated in order to exclude a proximal arterial embolic lesion if a cardiac source is not evident or if the subclavian pulse is either absent (due to dissection or occlusion) or unduly prominent (due to a subclavian aneurysm or underlying cervical rib). Immediate systemic heparinisation is essential to limit the propagation of thrombus and to prevent recurrent embolism.

Most emboli can be retrieved through a distal brachial transverse arteriotomy. This site has the advantage that both forearm arteries can be directly cannulated. An S-shaped incision is made under local anaesthesia in the antecubital fossa and the brachial artery division exposed by dividing the bicipital aponeurosis. A transverse arteriotomy is made proximal to the bifurcation. It is important to clear both forearm vessels with a 2-Fr Fogarty catheter (**Fig. 11.7**). Heparin saline is then instilled distally, and after confirming proximal patency the arteriotomy is closed with 6/0 prolene interrupted sutures. Completion on-table angiography should be performed. If there

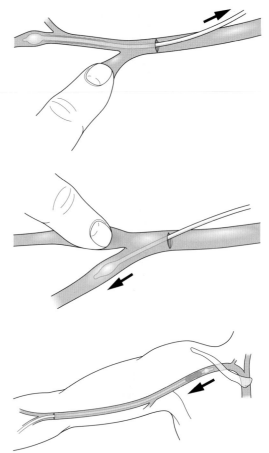

Figure 11.7 • Brachial artery embolectomy. A transverse arteriotomy is performed. A Fogarty catheter is directed into the radial and ulnar arteries in turn, using alternate digital compression and/or silastic slings. A subclavian–axillary embolectomy is carried out by retrograde catheterisation from the antecubital fossa.

is retained distal thrombus, the ulnar and radial artery can be opened at the wrist and a 2-Fr Fogarty catheter passed distally. Alternatively, intraoperative thrombolysis can be used (see Chapter 8). Emboli in the axillary or subclavian arteries may also be removed by the same approach, using transbrachial retrograde catheterisation. However, sometimes a large proximal embolus cannot be removed via the brachial arteriotomy, in which case an axillary or subclavian embolectomy will be required. Percutaneous thromboaspiration via a femoral approach has also been used in this situation.

Other causes of acute ischaemia

The pharmacological causes of upper extremity ischaemia are summarised in **Box 11.2**. Inadvertent arterial injection by drug abusers often results in

Ergot poisoning
Beta-blockers
Drug abuse, cocaine use
Dopamine overdose
Cytotoxic drugs

intense vasospasm due to particulate microembolism. Intra-arterial infusion of prostacyclin analogues such as iloprost or other vasodilators may help. Forearm compartment syndrome is rare except in this situation and requires fasciotomy. Limb loss is common.

Thoracic outlet syndrome

Thoracic outlet syndrome describes a variety of symptoms caused by compression of the brachial plexus or subclavian vessels at the thoracic outlet. In more than 90% of all cases of thoracic outlet syndrome,[28] symptoms are neurological with pain and weakness resulting from C8 or T1 root compression. Arterial or venous symptoms resulting from compression are uncommon, accounting for 5% of cases in large published series.[29]

Neurogenic thoracic outlet compression syndrome (N-TOCS)

The neurovascular bundle may be compressed between the first rib and the clavicle as a result of a low-lying shoulder girdle or loss of muscle tone. Other anatomical factors include congenital fibromuscular bands crossing the thoracic outlet that tent up the brachial plexus, and abnormalities/hypertrophy of the scalene muscles. Bony lesions may also be the cause. These include cervical ribs, a broad first rib, and fracture or exostoses of the first rib or clavicle. The scalene triangle is the commonest site of nerve compression. It contains the brachial plexus and the subclavian artery. N-TOCS probably represents a repetitive stress injury as there are well-defined at-risk occupations (e.g. typists) and sports (e.g. swimming). Most patients with N-TOCS are in the 25- to 45-year age group and 70% of them are women. The symptoms are arm pain, paraesthesia and weakness, with involvement of all the nerves of the brachial plexus or with specific patterns related to the upper plexus (median nerve) or lower plexus (ulnar nerve).

Diagnosis

Positive findings on clinical examination include supraclavicular tenderness and paraesthesia in the ipsilateral upper extremity in response to pressure over the scalene muscles. Rotating the head and tilting the head away from the involved side often produces radiating pain in the upper arm. Abducting the arm to 90° in external rotation and repeated slow finger clenching in this position often reproduces the symptoms (Roos' test). Diagnostic tests include a scalene muscle block, and a good response to this test correlates well with successful surgical decompression.[30] Neurophysiology testing is helpful in excluding other sites of nerve compression, e.g. cervical root and carpal tunnel. Duplex scanning is a useful surrogate marker if it shows arterial compression in the stress position. Cervical spine films may detect cervical or abnormal first ribs but will not detect non-bony causes of compression. Magnetic resonance imaging is more useful for excluding cervical disc lesions than confirming N-TOCS.

Treatment

Therapy for N-TOCS should always begin with non-operative treatment, including postural exercises and physiotherapy. Patients should avoid heavy lifting and working with the arm above shoulder level. Conservative treatment should be continued for several months. The majority of patients will improve significantly and will not require surgery. Indications for surgery include failure of conservative therapy after several months and persisting disabling symptoms that interfere with work and activities of daily living. The goal of surgery is to decompress the brachial plexus. A cervical rib can usually be removed via a supraclavicular approach. In the absence of a cervical rib, a first rib resection is required.

Transaxillary resection of first rib

The technique described by Roos[31] is indicated for neurogenic complications of N-TOCS and can be summarised as follows. The patient is placed in the lateral position leaving the arm free. The assistant elevates the shoulder by applying upward traction on the upper arm. This manoeuvre opens up the costoclavicular space and pulls the neurovascular bundle away from the first rib. A horizontal skin incision is made at the lower border of the axillary line over the third rib (**Fig. 11.8**). The intercostal nerve emerging from the second intercostal space should be preserved. The fascial roof of the axilla is opened to expose the anterior portion of the first rib. Scalenus anterior is separated from the artery and sectioned at its attachment to the first rib (**Fig. 11.9**). The tendon of the subclavius muscle is divided with care because of its close relation with the subclavian vein. The scalenus medius is then pushed off the rib. The intercostal muscles are similarly detached from

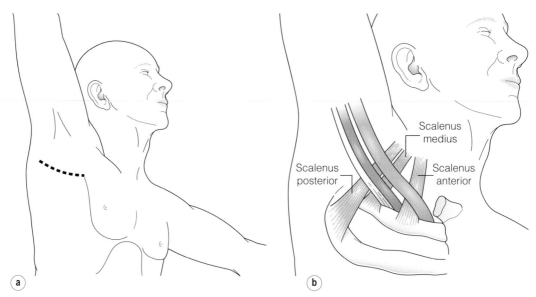

Figure 11.8 • Transaxillary resection of the first rib: **(a)** operative position and skin incision; **(b)** the neurovascular bundle is pulled away from the first rib by traction on the arm.

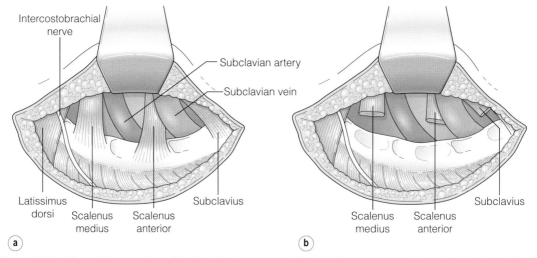

Figure 11.9 • Transaxillary resection of the first rib: **(a)** exposure of the first rib, scalene muscles and subclavian–axillary vessels; **(b)** detachment of the scalenus anterior, medius and subclavius muscles from the first rib.

the lower part of the rib. The rib is then sectioned at the chondrocostal junction and maintained by bone-holding forceps to distance it from the neurovascular bundle (**Fig. 11.10**). The T1 root is displaced medially. The rib is then divided and excised to within 1–2 cm of the vertebral transverse process using rongeurs. The stump must be smooth since sharp bony spicules may lacerate the plexus. Serum saline is then injected in the wound to ensure that the pleura is intact. The wound is closed in the usual way with suction drainage.

Complications of transaxillary rib resection include subclavian vein or artery injury, extrapleural haematoma or brachial plexus injury caused by traction of the arm or damage to the T1 root retraction. Good illumination and visualisation are crucial to this approach and a laparoscope can help with both.

Other operative techniques for N-TOCS include a supraclavicular approach. Axelrod et al.[32] reported the results of surgery in 170 patients operated for N-TOCS. No major operative complication occurred in those patients who underwent

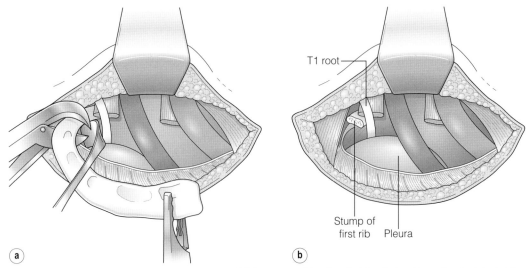

Figure 11.10 • Transaxillary resection of the first rib. **(a)** Exposure of the first rib. The rib has been disarticulated at the chondrocostal junction. T1 root is protected by a retractor. **(b)** Extraperiosteal resection of the first rib is complete.

decompression via a supraclavicular approach. Only 11% of patients experienced minor complications, most commonly the need for chest tube placement as a result of pneumothorax. At short-term follow-up (10 months), most patients had improved pain levels (80%) and range of motion (82%). However, at long-term follow-up (47 months), residual symptoms were present in 65% of patients, and 35% took medication for pain. Nonetheless, 64% said they were satisfied with the result. Scali et al.[33] performed a long-term follow-up after first rib resection (average 8.7 years). An equivalent or better functional outcome was observed in 72.7% of the patients. Gordobes-Gual et al.[34] showed the importance of a precise questionnaire (DASH) to evaluate the functional recovery after N-TOCS surgery.

> ✔ Controversy still exists concerning the surgical treatment of N-TOCS, and a randomised study of thoracic outlet surgery versus conservative treatment is lacking for this indication.

Arterial thoracic outlet compression syndrome

Arterial complications are often associated with bony abnormalities, including a complete cervical rib or fracture callus of the first rib or clavicle. The initial arterial lesion is fibrotic thickening with intimal damage and poststenotic dilation, leading to aneurysmal degeneration with mural thrombus and the risk of embolisation. Most emboli are small and localised in the hand vessels, with pallor, paraesthesia and coldness suggestive of Raynaud's

syndrome. If unrecognised, severe digital ischaemia with gangrene may occur. Early recognition of this condition is essential and a duplex scan should be performed in all patients with unilateral Raynaud's syndrome and asymptomatic patients with a cervical bruit. Loss or reduction of the radial pulse during Adson's manoeuvre (abduction and external rotation of the shoulder) is not very reliable as it is found in 9–53% of healthy volunteers.[28] The arteriographic changes may be obvious but sometimes minimal, with moderate dilation beyond a bony abnormality at the thoracic outlet and radiological evidence of distal embolisation (**Fig. 11.11**). Subclavian stenosis is not always evident on anteroposterior view and oblique stress views are often necessary.

Surgical management

Subclavian lesions associated with cervical ribs can usually be repaired via a supraclavicular approach, after excision of the cervical rib or by a combined supraclavicular and infraclavicular approach.

Combined supraclavicular and infraclavicular approach

The combined supraclavicular and infraclavicular approach offers a complete exposure. The infraclavicular dissection is commenced first with an S-shaped incision. Pectoralis major is detached from the upper sternum and clavicle (**Fig. 11.12**). The subclavius is resected and the artery and the axillary vein are then freed behind the clavicle. Via a supraclavicular incision, the clavicular head of the sternomastoid and the external jugular vein are divided to expose the scalenus anterior and the phrenic nerve. The scalenus anterior is then sectioned near the

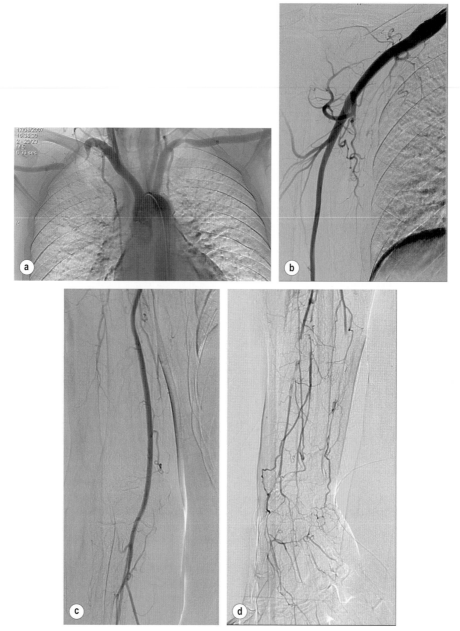

Figure 11.11 • Angiography of a thoracic outlet compression syndrome with arterial compression. **(a)** Right subclavian artery compression when the arm is abducted to 90° in external rotation. **(b)** Poststenotic dilatation of the right subclavian artery. **(c)** Right brachial artery. **(d)** Distal arterial embolisation.

first rib. The subclavian artery and vein are freed (**Fig. 11.13**). The intercostal muscles are detached from the first rib and the rib is disarticulated at the costochondral junction. The rib is then sectioned without attempting to reach the posterior segment. Access to the rib stump is achieved via the supra-clavicular exposure by reflecting the brachial plexus

laterally and the artery medially. The scalenus medius is then detached from the first rib and, after protecting the T1 root, the rib is sectioned near the transverse process.

In patients with aneurysm or poststenotic dilation secondary to first rib or cervical rib, there is often sufficient length of artery to permit resection of the

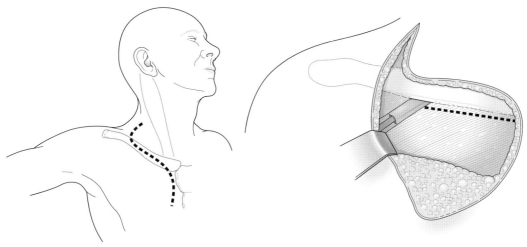

Figure 11.12 • Combined supraclavicular and infraclavicular approach for first rib resection when extensive arterial or venous reconstruction is required. Skin incision and section of the pectoralis major from the clavicle.

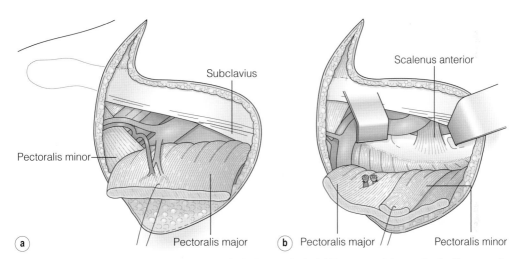

Figure 11.13 • Combined supraclavicular and infraclavicular approach. **(a)** Exposure of the proximal axillary vessels. The axillary vessels are held aside with a retractor to show the first rib and insertion of the scalenus anterior. **(b)** The infraclavicular dissection with detachment of the intercostal muscles from the first rib. The anterior portion of the rib will be removed and the first rib stump will be shortened via the supraclavicular exposure, not shown here.

arterial lesion and direct anastomosis (**Fig. 11.14**). When arterial lesions are more extensive, graft replacement is required using reversed great saphenous vein or PTFE if no vein is available. Intraoperative angiography is recommended in all cases. In patients with a recent distal embolic event, catheter embolectomy should be attempted. If embolectomy is impossible, a distal bypass using the great saphenous vein may be needed in an attempt to revascularise one of the forearm arteries. Additional sympathectomy may also be considered where there is extensive long-standing distal embolic occlusion. Difficulty in clearing the distal arterial bed accounts

for the incomplete revascularisation observed in advanced cases with disabling ischaemic sequelae.

> ✅✅ Arterial reconstruction and first rib or cervical rib resection are indicated in all patients with arterial complications of thoracic outlet syndrome.

Subclavian–axillary vein thrombosis

Spontaneous or effort-related venous thrombosis in a fit young patient is known as Paget–Schroetter

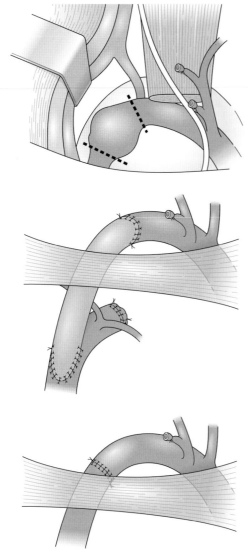

Figure 11.14 • Combined supraclavicular and infraclavicular approach. Exposure of the subclavian and axillary vessels. Depending on the extent of arterial resection, end-to-end anastomosis or graft replacement is done.

syndrome, the first cases being published separately by these two authors over a century ago. Hughes, who in 1949 collected 320 cases and recognised the distinct entity, coined the eponym. As the indications for central venous access have increased, so has the incidence of catheter-related subclavian–axillary vein thrombosis (SVT).[35]

Acute deep venous thrombosis (DVT) of the upper limb has many causes, with treatment and prognosis depending on the specific cause. SVT can be divided into two groups, primary and secondary.

Primary SVT (Paget–Schroetter syndrome) is due to anatomical venous compression in the thoracic outlet during exercise (V-TOCS) and comprises about 25% of all cases. Secondary SVT is the result of multiple aetiological factors, although in most series trauma due to central venous catheters dominates this category (40% of all cases of SVT). SVT is responsible for 1–4% of all cases of DVT. Monreal et al.[36] reported a 15% incidence of pulmonary emboli in 30 consecutive patients with SVT who were investigated with ventilation–perfusion scanning.

Primary SVT

In a review of the literature, Hurlbert and Rutherford[37] reported a male to female ratio of 2:1, with an average age of 30 years for patients with primary SVT that represents only 3.5% of all cases of thoracic outlet compression syndrome (TOCS). Venous thrombosis is seen three times more frequently in the right than the left upper limb, but bilateral venous compression also occurs frequently. Thrombosis is probably caused by repetitive trauma from compression. Virtually every patient with primary SVT has some degree of upper extremity swelling associated with pain that worsens with exertion. Some patients may have cyanosis of the arm. Unlike lower-extremity DVT, symptoms in the upper extremity are more related to venous obstruction than reflux. Venous outflow through the collateral vessels is limited, resulting in venous hypertension, swelling and occasionally venous claudication. Venous gangrene is an extremely rare complication of SVT.

Diagnosis
Clinically, the arm may be swollen and cyanosed, with dilated shoulder girdle collateral veins. Duplex is the first-line investigation and has a sensitivity of 94% and a specificity of 96% compared with venography.[38] MRA has poor sensitivity for non-occlusive thrombi and short-segment occlusion. CT has been used to diagnose upper-extremity DVT but its specificity and sensitivity are undetermined. Venography is still considered as the reference in evaluating SVT (**Fig. 11.15**). The basilic vein is the preferred site for injection, with the arm abducted at 30°. The catheter used for the venogram should be left in position as it can be used for subsequent thrombolysis and/or heparin infusion. The cephalic vein is not used because it joins directly with the subclavian vein and may miss an axillary vein thrombosis.

Treatment
For many years, treatment of SVT relied on rest and elevation of the upper limb with anticoagulant therapy. However, the morbidity associated with this conservative treatment is high. More recently,

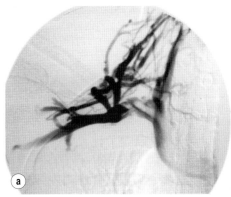
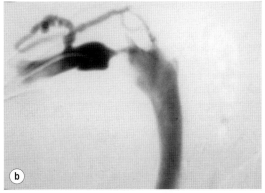

Figure 11.15 • (a) Venogram via basilic vein demonstrating SVT with collaterals. **(b)** Thrombolysis revealed an underlying stenosis of the subclavian vein. This was treated by excision of the first rib and vein patch.

investigators have realised that many patients with SVT have compression at the thoracic outlet. Initially, in patients with primary SVT, subclavian vein patency was restored by open thrombectomy associated with first rib resection.[39] Although now supplanted by thrombolysis, open thrombectomy has proved effective and should be considered in patients with contraindications or failure of thrombolysis therapy. Catheter-directed techniques of thrombolysis allow for immediate venous evaluation and assess extrinsic compression with positional venography after thrombolysis.[40] However, Sheeran et al.[41] have shown that recanalisation of the vein by thrombolysis without decompression of the thoracic outlet has poor outcome, with 55% of patients remaining symptomatic. Conversely, Machleder[42] reported the success of combined treatment, with 86% of 36 patients becoming asymptomatic. The appropriate time interval between thrombolysis and thoracic outlet decompression is still under discussion. Machleder waited 3 months, whereas Lee et al.[43] recommended immediate first rib resection within 4 days after thrombolysis. Waiting too long risks rethrombosis, whereas operating immediately risks bleeding due to the thrombolytic agent.

☑☑ Patients with thoracic outlet syndrome and SVT should have early treatment with thrombolysis followed by first rib resection.[44]

Specific problems may arise in some patients after thrombolysis. In a small group, no residual lesion or compression is seen on positional venography after thrombolysis. In these cases, anticoagulation therapy is recommended without thoracic outlet decompression. In other patients, intrinsic stenosis is seen on venography after thrombolysis (Fig. 11.15). In these cases operative vein bypass or patch angioplasty with

first rib resection is needed and should be performed in the days after thrombolysis because the risk of rethrombosis appears to be quite high. In this setting, percutaneous balloon venoplasty with or without stenting has been suggested. The results of this technique without thoracic outlet decompression are poor, with a primary patency of 35% at 1 year.[45] Obviously, this technique does not obviate the need for surgery because thoracic outlet decompression is still needed. Even after thoracic outlet decompression, some venous stenoses are resistant to dilation or present intrinsic elastic recoil. Various types of stents have been used to treat residual stenoses, but are associated with a worse prognosis than balloon angioplasty alone after vein decompression.[46]

☑☑ Stenting in primary SVT is not appropriate. As surgery is usually needed for thoracic outlet decompression, it seems logical to repair the subclavian vein with patch angioplasty or a short autogenous bypass at the same time.

In a significant number of patients, seen more than 10 days after the onset of primary upper-limb DVT, late thrombolysis fails. Most of these patients should be treated conservatively with anticoagulation unless the occlusion is short. In these cases, open thrombectomy with vein reconstruction and first rib resection can be done with acceptable results.[47] The technique involves internal jugular vein transposition or cephalic vein bypass with a temporary arteriovenous fistula. Prosthetic bypass has shown inferior results in this location.

Secondary SVT

The main cause of secondary SVT is central venous catheterisation (CVC). Overall, one-third of patients with central-line catheters develop SVT, although only

15% of them are symptomatic. The aetiology of catheter-associated thrombosis is multifactorial, but may be related to the fibrin sheath that forms around the catheter. The method of insertion, size, composition and duration of use of the catheter are also important. A reduced rate of thrombosis has been found with soft and more flexible catheters. Large catheters used for haemodialysis have a higher incidence of SVT. Another risk factor is the type of fluid infused through the catheter. Cancer chemotherapeutic agents are aggressive to vascular endothelium and may increase the risk of thrombosis. Furthermore, many patients with central-line catheters also have systemic risk factors for thrombosis, i.e. malignancy, sepsis, congestive heart failure and prolonged bed rest.

Symptomatic patients have oedema and distended veins around the shoulder. Pulmonary embolism is not uncommon, with 16% of patients positive on ventilation–perfusion scan.[48] Therapy guidelines are based on observational reports as no controlled studies are available. In all cases, anticoagulation using intravenous heparin via the affected arm is indicated to prevent clot extension until the catheter is removed. Thrombolytic therapy has a role in reopening thrombosed catheters. Prevention of thrombus formation has been emphasised, and for high-risk patients it may be advantageous to administer low-dose coumadin[49] or low-molecular-weight heparin to reduce the risk of catheter-associated thrombosis. A further discussion about CVC management can be found in Chapter 16.

Key points

- Vascular diseases of the upper limb are rare in comparison to those involving the lower limbs, with the exception of arterial embolism.
- Clinical examination, including the Allen test, is important.
- There are good mid-term results of endovascular treatment of supra-aortic trunk stenoses.
- The long-term results of carotid bypass or carotid transposition are excellent.
- It is important to consider arterial disease in the work environment, e.g. hypothenar hammer syndrome.
- There is controversy concerning the diagnosis and treatment of N-TOCS.
- The combined supraclavicular and infraclavicular approach for first rib resection and arterial bypass is of value in the treatment of patients with arterial thoracic outlet compression syndrome.
- Early thrombolytic therapy followed by surgical thoracic outlet decompression is indicated in patients with primary SVT.

References

1. Fields WS, Lemak NA. Joint study of extracranial artery occlusion. Subclavian steal. A review of 168 cases. JAMA 1972;222:1139–43.

2. McCarthy WJ, Flinn WR, Yao JST. Results of bypass grafting for upper limb ischemia. J Vasc Surg 1986;3:741–6.
   Between 1978 and 1984, the authors performed 33 bypass grafts to relieve hand and forearm ischaemia in 27 patients. A reversed saphenous vein graft was used in 22 cases and PTFE in the remaining 11 procedures. Follow-up of 31 grafts from 6 to 72 months (mean 35.5 months) revealed an overall patency rate of 73% at 2 years and 67% at 3 years. More proximal grafts fared better: the 2-year patency rate was 83% for grafts at or above the brachial artery but only 53% for bypass distal to the brachial bifurcation.

3. Kieffer E, Sabatier J, Koskas F. Atherosclerotic innominate artery occlusive disease: early and long term results of surgical reconstruction. J Vasc Surg 1995;20:326–37.
   During a 20-year period (1974–93), the authors operated on 148 patients with brachiocephalic (innominate) artery atherosclerotic occlusive disease. Approach was through a median sternotomy in 135 (91%) patients. Endarterectomy was performed in 32 (22%) patients, whereas 116 (78%) patients underwent bypass. Eight (5.4%) patients died in the perioperative period. There were five (3.4%) perioperative strokes. Mean follow-up was 77 months. Survival was 51.9% at 10 years. The probability of freedom from ipsilateral stroke was 98.6% at 10 years. The primary patency rate was 98.4% at 10 years. In conclusion, surgical reconstruction of brachiocephalic artery atherosclerotic occlusive disease yields acceptable rates of perioperative complications with excellent long-term patency and freedom from neurological events and reoperation.

4. Berguer R, Morasch M, Kline R. Transthoracic repair of innominate and common carotid artery disease. Immediate and long-term outcome of 100 consecutive surgical reconstructions. J Vasc Surg 1998;27:34–41.

5. Cherry KJ, McCullough JL, Hallett JW, et al. Technical principles of direct innominate artery revascularization. A comparison of endarterectomy and bypass grafts. J Vasc Surg 1989;9:718–24.

6. Reul GL, Jacobs MJHM, Gregoric ID, et al. Innominate artery occlusive disease. Surgical approach and long-term results. J Vasc Surg 1991;14:405–12.

7. Uurto IT, Lautamati V, Zeitlin R, et al. Long-term outcome of surgical revascularization of supra-aortic vessels. World J Surg 2002;26:1503–6.

8. Takach TJ, Reul GJ, Cooley DA, et al. Brachiocephalic reconstruction I: Operative and long-term results for complex disease. J Vasc Surg 2005;42:47–54.

9. Paukovits TM, Lukacs L, Berczi V, et al. Percutaneous endovascular treatment of innominate artery lesions: a single-center experience on 77 lesions. Eur J Vasc Endovasc Surg 2010;40:35–43.

10. Van Hattum ES, de Vries J-P, Lalezari F, et al. Angioplasty with or without stent placement in the brachiocephalic artery: feasible and durable? A retrospective cohort study. J Vasc Interv Radiol 2007;18:1088–93.

11. Hüttl K, Nemes B, Simonffy A, et al. Angioplasty of the innominate artery in 89 patients: experience over 19 years. Cardiovasc Intervent Radiol 2002;25:109–14.

12. Rapp JH, Reilly LM, Goldstone J, et al. Ischemia of the upper extremity. Significance of proximal arterial disease. Am J Surg 1986;152:122–6.

13. Schardey HM, Meyer G, Rau HG, et al. Subclavian carotid transposition: an analysis of a clinical series and a review of the literature. Eur J Vasc Endovasc Surg 1996;12:431–6.

14. Vitti MJ, Thompson BW, Read RC. Carotid–subclavian bypass. A twenty-two years experience. J Vasc Surg 1994;20:411–8.
A retrospective review of 124 patients who underwent carotid–subclavian bypass from 1968 to 1990 was done to assess primary patency and symptom resolution. Graft conduits were PTFE in 44 (35%) and Dacron in 80 (65%) cases; 30-day mortality was 0.8%, 30-day primary patency was 100%. Primary patency rate was 95% at 10 years. Survival rate was 59% at 10 years. Symptom-free survival rate was 87% at 10 years. Carotid–subclavian bypass appears to be a safe and durable procedure for relief of symptomatic occlusive disease of the subclavian artery.

15. AbuRahma AF, Robinson PA, Jennings TG. Carotid–subclavian bypass grafting with polytetra-fluoroethylene grafts for symptomatic subclavian artery stenosis or occlusion: a 20-years experience. J Vasc Surg 2000;32:411–9.

16. Cinà CS, Safar HA, Langanà A, et al. Subclavian carotid transposition and bypass grafting: consecutive cohort study and systematic review. J Vasc Surg 2002;35:422–9.

17. Sandmann W, Kniemeyer HW, Jaeschock R, et al. The role of subclavian–carotid transposition in surgery for supra-aortic occlusive disease. J Vasc Surg 1987;5:53–8.

18. Kretschmer G, Teleky B, Marosi L, et al. Obliterations of the proximal subclavian artery. To bypass or to anastomose? J Cardiovasc Surg (Torino) 1991;32:334–9.

19. Mingoli A, Sapienza P, Felhaus RJ, et al. Long-term results and outcomes of crossover axillo-axillary bypass grafting: a 24-year experience. J Vasc Surg 1999;29:894–901.

20. De Vries JPPM, Jagger LC, van den Berg JC, et al. Durability of percutaneous transluminal angioplasty for obstructive lesions of proximal subclavian artery: long-term results. J Vasc Surg 2005;41:19–23.

21. Berger L, Bouziane Z, Felisaz A, et al. Long-term results of 81 prevertebral subclavian artery angioplasties: a 26-year experience. Ann Vasc Surg 2011;25:1043–9.

22. Brunkwall J, Berqvist D, Bergentz SE. Long term results of arterial reconstruction of the upper extremity. Eur J Vasc Surg 1994;8:47–53.

23. Kieffer E, Chiche L, Koskas F, et al. Aneurysms of the innominate artery: surgical treatment of 27 patients. J Vasc Surg 2001;34:222–8.

24. Kieffer E, Bahnini A, Koskas F. Aberrant subclavian artery: surgical treatment in thirty-three adult patients. J Vasc Surg 1994;19:100–10.
The authors reviewed their experience with surgery for aberrant subclavian arteries (ASA). During a 16-year period they surgically treated 33 adult patients with ASA. Twenty-eight patients had a left-sided aortic arch with a right ASA, whereas five had a right-sided aortic arch with a left ASA. Eleven patients had dysphagia caused by oesophageal compression, five patients had ischaemic symptoms, 10 patients had aneurysms of the ASA and seven patients had an ASA arising from an aneurysmal thoracic aorta. In all cases the distal subclavian artery was revascularised, most often by direct transposition into the ipsilateral common carotid artery. The cervical approach was combined with a median sternotomy or a left thoracotomy in 17 patients. Aortic cross-clamping was required in 12 patients to perform the transaortic closure of the origin of the ASA with patch angioplasty or prosthetic replacement of the descending thoracic aorta. Cardiopulmonary bypass was used in six patients. Four patients died after operation. Satisfactory clinical and anatomical results were obtained in the remaining 29 patients. Provision should be made for cardiopulmonary bypass in patients with aneurysm of ASA or associated aortic aneurysm.

25. Sullivan TM, Bacharach JM, Perl J. Endovascular management of unusual aneurysms of the axillary and subclavian arteries. J Endovasc Surg 1996;3:389–95.

Aneurysms of the upper extremity arteries are uncommon and may be difficult to manage in emergency with standard surgical techniques. The authors report the exclusion of three axillary–subclavian aneurysms with covered stents. Palmaz stents were covered with either PTFE (two cases) or brachial vein and deployed to exclude pseudoaneurysms in one axillary and two left subclavian arteries. Endovascular exclusion of axillary and subclavian aneurysms with covered stents may offer a useful alternative to operative repair in patients with ruptured aneurysm or significant comorbidities.

26. Vayssairat M, Debure C, Cormier J-M. Hypothenar hammer syndrome. Seventeen cases with long-term follow-up. J Vasc Surg 1987;5:838–42.

The authors report 17 patients who had either ulnar thrombosis or ulnar aneurysm; most also had embolic occlusions of the digital arteries. Main pathological findings were thrombosis on the intima and fibrosis in the media. The authors adopted a surgical procedure consisting of resection with end-to-end reconstruction for patent aneurysms to avoid downstream emboli and more conservative treatment when the ulnar artery was thrombosed. No patient required digital amputation and all except one improved and were able to live and work normally.

27. Haimovici H. Cardiogenic embolism of the upper extremity. J Cardiovasc Surg (Torino) 1982;23:209–15.

28. Sanders RJ, Hammond SL, Rao NM. Diagnosis of thoracic outlet syndrome. J Vasc Surg 2007;46:601–4.

29. Sanders RJ, Cooper MA, Hammond SL, et al. Neurogenic thoracic outlet syndrome. In: Rutherford RB, editor. Vascular surgery. 5th ed. Philadelphia: WB Saunders; 2000. p. 1184–99.

30. Sanders RJ, Haug CE. Thoracic outlet syndrome: a common sequela of neck injuries. Philadelphia: JB Lippincott; 1991.

31. Roos DB. Thoracic outlet and carpal tunnel syndrome. In: Rutherford RB, editor. Vascular surgery. 2nd ed. Philadelphia: WB Saunders; 1984. p. 708–24.

32. Axelrod DA, Proctor MC, Geisser ME. Outcomes after surgery for thoracic outlet syndrome. J Vasc Surg 2001;33:1220–5.

This study determined whether there is an association between psychological and socio-economic characteristics and long-term outcome of operative treatment for patients with sensory N-TOCS. Multivariate logistic regression models were developed as a means of identifying independent risk factors for postoperative disability. Operative decompression of the brachial plexus via a supraclavicular approach was performed for upper-extremity pain and paraesthesia, with no mortality and minimal morbidity in 170 patients. After an average follow-up period of 47 months, 65% of patients reported improved symptoms and 64% of patients were satisfied with their operative outcome. However, 35% of patients remained on medication and 18% of patients were disabled. Preoperative factors associated with persistent disability include major depression, being unmarried and having less than a high-school education. Operative decompression was beneficial for most patients. The impact of the preoperative treatment of depression on the outcome of TOCS decompression should be studied prospectively.

33. Scali S, Stone D, Bjerke A, et al. Long-term functional results for the surgical management of neurogenic thoracic outlet syndrome. Vasc Endovascular Surg 2010;44:550–5.

34. Gordobes-Gual J, Lozano-Vilardell P, Torreguitart-Mirada N, et al. Prospective study of the functional recovery after surgery for thoracic outlet syndrome. Eur J Endovasc Surg 2008;35:79–83.

35. Rutherford RB, Hurlbert SN. Primary subclavian–axillary vein thrombosis. Consensus and commentary. Cardiovasc Surg 1996;4:420–3.

Fifteen multiple-choice questions concerning options in the management of primary subclavian–axillary vein thrombosis were discussed by a panel of experts and then voted upon by 25 attending vascular surgeons with experience in subclavian–axillary vein thrombosis. The large majority favoured or agreed upon: (i) early clot removal for active healthy patients with a need/desire to use the involved limb in work or sport; (ii) catheter-directed thrombolysis as initial therapy; (iii) further therapy based on follow-up positional venography; (iv) surgical relief of demonstrated thoracic outlet compression after a brief period of anticoagulant therapy; (v) conservative therapy if post-lysis venogram showed either no extrinsic compression or a short residual occlusion; and (vi) intervention for residual intrinsic lesions with over 50% narrowing.

36. Monreal M, Lafoz E, Ruiz J. Upper extremity deep venous thrombosis and pulmonary embolism. Chest 1991;99:280–3.

The authors prospectively evaluated the prevalence of pulmonary embolism in 30 consecutive patients with proved DVT of the upper extremity. Ten patients had primary DVT and 20 patients had catheter-related DVT. Ventilation–perfusion lung scans were routinely performed at the time of hospital admission in all but one patient. Lung scan findings were normal in 9 of 10 patients with primary DVT. In contrast, perfusion defects were considered highly suggestive of pulmonary embolism in four patients with catheter-related DVT. The authors conclude that pulmonary embolism is not a rare complication in upper-extremity DVT and that patients with catheter-related DVT seem to be at higher risk.

37. Hurlbert SN, Rutherford RB. Subclavian–axillary vein thrombosis. In: Rutherford RB, editor. Vascular surgery. 5th ed. Philadelphia: WB Saunders; 2000. p. 1208–21.

38. Koksoy C, Kuzu A, Kutlay J, et al. The diagnostic value of colour Doppler ultrasound in central venous catheter related thrombosis. Clin Radiol 1995;50:687–9.

39. DeWeese JA, Adams JT, Gaiser DL. Subclavian venous thrombectomy. Circulation 1970;42:158–63.

40. Lokanathan R, Salvian AJ, Chen JC, et al. Outcome after thrombolysis and selective thoracic outlet decompression for primary axillary vein thrombosis. J Vasc Surg 2001;33:783–8.

41. Sheeran SR, Hallisey MJ, Murphy TP, et al. Local thrombolytic therapy as part of a multidisciplinary approach to acute axillo-subclavian vein thrombosis (Paget–Schroetter syndrome). J Vasc Interv Radiol 1997;8:253–60.

42. Machleder HI. Evaluation of a new treatment strategy for Paget–Schroetter syndrome: spontaneous thrombosis of the axillary–subclavian vein. J Vasc Surg 1993;17:305–17.

43. Lee MC, Grassi CJ, Belkin M. Early operative intervention following thrombolytic therapy for primary subclavian vein thrombosis. An effective treatment approach. J Vasc Surg 1998;27:1101–8.
The authors conducted a study to determine an acceptable treatment approach to primary subclavian vein thrombosis. A retrospective review evaluated 11 patients in an 8-year period. All patients with occlusion received urokinase therapy and underwent surgical decompression within 5 days of thrombolytic therapy. Five percutaneous transluminal angioplasties were attempted before operative intervention. Eleven decompressions were performed. All patients received coumadin for 3–6 months after the operation. Urokinase therapy established wide venous patency in 9 of 11 extremities treated, with the remaining two requiring thrombectomy. One patient who underwent transluminal angioplasty before the operation had rethrombosis, and the remaining four showed no improvement in venous stenosis after the intervention. Eight of nine extremities treated by first rib resection and one of two treated by scalenectomy were free of residual symptoms at follow-up. The authors conclude that preoperative use of percutaneous balloon angioplasty is ineffective and should be avoided in this setting. Surgical intervention within days of thrombolysis enables patients to return to normal activity sooner.

44. Urschel HC, Razzuk MA. Paget–Schroetter syndrome: what is the best management. Ann Thorac Surg 2000;69:1663–9.
The authors evaluated the results of 312 extremities in 294 patients with Paget–Schroetter syndrome to provide the basis for optimal management. Group I (35 extremities) was initially treated with anticoagulants only. Twenty-one developed recurrent symptoms after returning to work, requiring transaxillary resection of the first rib. Thrombectomy was necessary in eight. Group II (36 extremities) was treated with thrombolytic agents initially, with 20 requiring subsequent rib resection after returning to work. Thrombectomy was necessary in only four. Of the most recent 241 extremities (group III), excellent results accrued using thrombolysis plus prompt first rib resection for those evaluated during the first month after occlusion (199). The results were only fair for those seen later than 1 month (42). The authors conclude that early diagnosis (less than 1 month), expeditious thrombolytic therapy and prompt first rib resection are critical for the best results.

45. Glanz S, Gordon DH, Lipkowitz GS, et al. Axillary and subclavian vein stenosis. Percutaneous angioplasty. Radiology 1988;168:371–3.

46. Illig KA, Doyle AJ. A comprehensive review of Paget–Schroetter syndrome. J Vasc Surg 2010;51:1538–47.

47. Sanders RJ, Cooper MA. Surgical management of subclavian vein obstruction, including six cases of subclavian vein bypass. Surgery 1995;118:856–63.

48. Monreal M, Raventos A, Lerma R, et al. Pulmonary embolism in patients with upper extremity DVT associated with venous central lines. A prospective study. Thromb Haemost 1994;72:548–50.

49. Bern MM, Lokich JJ, Wallach SR. Very low doses of warfarin can prevent thrombosis in central venous catheters. Ann Intern Med 1990;112:423–8.
The goal of this study was to determine whether very low doses of warfarin are useful in thrombosis prophylaxis in patients with central venous catheters. Patients at risk for thrombosis associated with chronic indwelling central venous catheters were prospectively and randomly assigned to receive, or not to receive, 1 mg of warfarin beginning 3 days before catheter insertion and continuing for 90 days. Subclavian, innominate and superior vena cava venograms were done at onset of thrombosis symptoms or after 90 days in the study. A total of 121 patients entered the study and 82 patients completed the study. Of 42 patients completing the study while receiving warfarin, four had venogram-proven thrombosis. All four had symptoms from thrombosis. Of 40 patients completing the study while not receiving warfarin, 15 had venogram-proven thrombosis and 10 had symptoms from thrombosis ($P<0.001$). In conclusion, very low doses of warfarin can protect against thrombosis without inducing a haemorrhagic state. This approach may be applicable to other groups of patients.

12

Primary and secondary vasospastic disorders (Raynaud's phenomenon) and vasculitis

Jill J.F. Belch
Matthew A. Lambert

Introduction

There are many inflammatory and vasospastic disorders that can present with ischaemia and thus come to the attention of the vascular clinician. These include Raynaud's phenomenon (RP) plus any associated connective tissue disorder, and the group of conditions known as 'vasculitis' (the vasculitides). Because of the systemic nature of these diseases, medical practitioners of all disciplines will be involved in their management at some stage in their career. Unfortunately, there is considerable overlap in the presenting features of these conditions and this can make diagnosis difficult. Although recent advances in immunopathological testing now allow the majority of disorders to be classified, the discovery of new autoantibodies makes the study of these disorders more difficult for the non-specialist. The aim of this chapter is to provide the vascular clinician with a grounding of knowledge in these disorders so that the initial diagnosis can be made. It describes the most common manifestations of these diseases, outlines their investigation (with particular emphasis on diagnostic autoantibody tests) and briefly delineates their treatment, with emphasis on recent advances.

Raynaud's phenomenon

Vasospasm is the key feature of RP. Maurice Raynaud's original description was of episodic digital ischaemia induced by cold and emotion.[1] The classical manifestation of pallor preceding cyanosis and rubor reflects the initial vasospasm, followed by deoxygenation of the static venous blood (cyanosis) and then reactive hyperaemia (rubor) with the return of blood flow. The full triphasic colour change is not essential for the diagnosis of RP, and a history of cold-induced blanching with subsequent reactive hyperaemia can still reflect significant vasospasm. In addition, other stimuli can provoke an attack, for example chemicals (including drugs and those in tobacco smoke[2]), trauma and hormones. In addition to the digits, the vasospasm may involve the nose, tongue, ear lobes and nipples. A decrease in lung,[3] oesophageal[4] and myocardial[5] perfusion has been shown after cold challenge, which suggests systemic vasospasm, and these patients have a higher incidence of migraine, irritable bowel syndrome and angina.[6]

The prevalence of primary RP varies between populations. Data from the Framingham Heart Study offspring cohort showed prevalence rates of 11% in women and 8% in men.[7] Primary RP usually develops in the second or third decade. Familial and monozygotic twin studies have indicated a hereditary factor but a search for candidate genes has been unsuccessful so far.[8] The prevalence of secondary RP (see below) depends on the prevalence of the underlying disorder, which itself varies between populations.

Inconsistent terminology is a major problem for clinicians managing RP. Europeans use RP as a blanket term for all cold-related vasospasm, with secondary Raynaud's syndrome (RS) being associated with another disease, and primary Raynaud's disease (RD) where it occurs in isolation. However, American and Australasian researchers use the syndrome and phenomenon interchangeably,[9] and differentiate the types of RP by indicating whether it is primary RP or secondary RP. The former classification has been used in this chapter.

Many patients with mild disease never present to their general practitioners but of those who do, most will have primary RD. Patients with more severe disease are likely to be referred to a hospital specialist, and an early marker for secondary RS is the severity of vasospastic attacks,[10] although the RP may precede associated systemic disease by more than 20 years.[11] Hospital practitioners are therefore more likely to see a higher proportion of RS, and the important challenge is to differentiate between the primary and secondary conditions in order to facilitate early management of the underlying associated disorder.

The secondary associations of RS are shown in Box 12.1. Of the connective tissue diseases (CTDs), systemic sclerosis is the most frequent association. In the hyperviscosity syndromes, such as myeloma, the prevalence is similar to the normal population but the symptomatology tends to be more severe.

Box 12.1 • Conditions associated with Raynaud's phenomenon

Connective tissue diseases

Systemic sclerosis

Systemic lupus erythematosus

Rheumatoid arthritis

Mixed connective tissue diseases

Sjögren's syndrome

Dermatomyositis/polymyositis

Obstructive

Atherosclerosis (especially thromboangiitis obliterans)

Microemboli

Thoracic outlet syndrome (especially cervical ribs)

Drug therapy

Beta-blockers

Cytotoxics, e.g. bleomycin

Ciclosporin

Ergotamine and other antimigraine therapies

Sulfasalazine

Occupational

Vibration white finger disease

Vinyl chloride disease

Ammunition workers (outside work)

Frozen food packers

Miscellaneous

Hypothyroidism

Cryoglobulinaemia

Reflex sympathetic dystrophy

Malignancy

Occupational RS is also well recognised and a relatively common form is hand–arm vibration syndrome (HAVS; previously known as vibration white finger). As the name suggests, it occurs in workers exposed to vibrating instruments such as chainsaws, pneumatic road drills and buffing machines. An estimated 4.2 million men and 667 000 women in Great Britain have occupational exposure to hand-transmitted vibration.[12] Before these tools were regulated 90% of exposed workers developed symptoms of HAVS. Among American shipyard workers, 71% of full-time pneumatic grinders complained of white fingers[13] and in Japan 9.6% of forest workers had symptoms of this syndrome.[14]

> ✅ By using lighter chainsaws and reduced vibration, the frequency of clinical problems in Finnish forest workers was reduced from 40% to 5%.[15]

The duration of exposure is important, with a latent period of often less than 5 years of full-time work. The severity of symptoms correlates with the length of exposure.[15] Vasospasm is not limited to the hands and has also been described in the toes (**Fig. 12.1**).[16] It is likely that vibration-induced damage of the endothelium underlies this condition.[17] In approximately one-quarter of cases, the symptoms may resolve if a job change is effected early in the course of the disease.[18]

In the UK, HAVS has been a proscribed industrial disease since 1985. Patients may be eligible for industrial injuries disablement benefits if they fulfil certain criteria.[19] Specific daily time limits for different machines have been proposed and are being implemented opportunistically, often by use of a points system.

Recently it has been suggested that prolonged exposure to vibrating computer game controls could cause HAVS. Other occupation-related causes of RP include vinyl chloride disease, which is estimated to

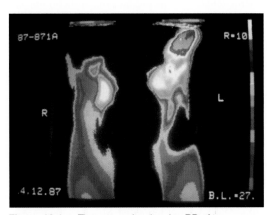

Figure 12.1 • Thermography showing RP of toes.

occur in 3% of workers exposed to this chemical. Ammunition workers also develop RP outside their work environment when the vasodilatory effects of nitrates are removed.

Atherosclerotic obstructive arterial disease is a common cause of RP in those over 60 years of age, particularly in men, and screening and treatment of known risk factors, such as hyperlipidaemia, are recommended. Various drugs may precipitate or exacerbate RP (e.g. beta-blockers for angina) and alternative drug therapies may be more appropriate (e.g. calcium channel blockers such as nifedipine). Vasospasm is also a feature of reflex sympathetic dystrophy and thoracic outlet syndrome, particularly occurring in the presence of a cervical rib (see Chapter 11).

Pathophysiology

The precise mechanism that causes Raynaud's is unknown but four aetiological factors are considered to be important: (i) neurogenic; (ii) interactions between blood cells and the blood vessel wall; (iii) inflammatory and immunological responses; and (iv) genetic factors. It is likely that these mechanisms are interdependent and interact closely to produce the symptoms.

Neurogenic

Most studies have focused on the peripheral nervous system. In patients with RP, α-adrenergic receptor sensitivity and density are increased[20] and the responsiveness of β-adrenergic presynaptic receptors in the peripheral vessels is also increased.[2] It has been suggested that the central nervous system may contribute to vasospasm but this is a difficult area to research and there is little direct evidence to support its influence.

Interactions between blood and blood vessel walls

Microcirculatory flow depends on a functioning endothelium, plasma factors and the cellular elements of blood. Activated platelets aggregate and form clumps that can obstruct flow. They may also release vasoconstrictors such as thromboxane A_2 and serotonin, causing further platelet aggregation. Red blood cells (RBCs) appear less deformable in RP and cold temperatures further increase RBC stiffness.[21] Rigid RBCs and white blood cells (WBCs) may impede the microcirculation, and activated WBCs aggregate and adhere within the microcirculation and can narrow the vascular lumen. Additionally, WBC activation increases the formation of free radicals, which may be prothrombotic.[22] Elevated fibrinogen and globulin levels increase plasma viscosity and reduce blood flow. Increased platelet aggregation,

rigid RBCs and activated WBCs have all been reported in patients with RS, together with raised plasma viscosity and reduced fibrinolysis.[23]

The intact endothelium is a functioning organ that produces many substances important in maintaining blood flow. Damage to it may impair blood flow in RP. Factor VIII von Willebrand factor (VWF) antigen is released following vascular damage and is increased in patients with RP.[24] VWF is active in the clotting cascade and platelet activation and may contribute to reduced blood flow. Tissue plasminogen activator is active in fibrinolysis and levels are reduced in RP, with a subsequent reduction in fibrinolysis.[23]

Endothelial vasoconstrictor/vasodilator production may also be impaired.[25-32] Most of these abnormalities are seen in patients with RS except for the increase in VWF, which occurs in the primary disease also. It is possible therefore that these are a consequence rather than the cause of the disorder. Nevertheless, they may still augment the impairment of blood flow and their correction by drug therapy may produce clinical benefit.

Inflammatory and immunological mechanisms

Most cases of severe RS occur when associated with CTD, and disordered immunology and inflammation are found in these patients. Interestingly, however, abnormal WBC behaviour also occurs in HAVS,[33,34] which has no clear immunological/inflammatory basis. The interested reader is referred to the scientific literature.[35-37]

Genetic factors

The link of genetic factors to RP has been suggested and primary RP has been found in monozygotic twins.[33] A twin study of 2852 women found a significantly higher concordance rate between monozygotic twins compared to dizygotic twins, suggesting a role of genetics in pathogenesis.[38]

Clinical features

The initial features of demarcated blanching of extremities produced in response to cold, temperature change and emotion are episodic. Digital artery spasm is the cause of this pallor, although many people may complain of cold hands with some mild poorly delineated colour changes. They do not necessarily have RP but probably cold-induced closure of the arteriovenous shunts in the skin, which decreases cutaneous blood flow and limits body heat loss. Patients with RP subsequently experience the cyanotic phase and/or the redness of the reactive hyperaemia phase. This last phase may be associated with rewarming paraesthesia and pain. RP is therefore characterised by being biphasic or triphasic, and usually affects the fingers and toes though finger symptoms tend to be more prominent. This may be asymmetrical in that, for example, only one or two digits may be affected on each hand, although all digits may be equally affected. As documented earlier, other extremities such as the ears, tongue and nose may also be affected, but a bluish discoloration in isolation is due to acrocyanosis and not RP. The occurrence of other skin-related problems (e.g. digital ulcers (**Fig. 12.2**) and recurrent chilblains), an onset in children under 10 years of age, an older adult onset (>30 years) and perennial attacks suggest secondary RP.

Investigations

These should be directed at confirming the diagnosis of RP, if appropriate, and differentiating between the primary and secondary disease with elucidation of the underlying cause. In the majority of patients, the diagnosis of RP is made clinically from the history and examination if they present during a Raynaud's attack. Objective measures of blood flow are not usually required unless the clinical findings are vague. There are a variety of techniques available, many involving cold challenge, but there is no gold standard because of practical difficulties and interindividual differences.

The test we use most involves the measurement of digital systolic blood pressure changes before and after local cooling at 15 °C. A pressure drop of >30 mmHg is considered to be significant, but precautions are required to avoid false-negative results. Ideally, patients should not be tested if they have had a Raynaud's attack earlier in the day as they may still be in the reactive hyperaemia stage and relatively protected from further vasospasm. In practice, the test may be carried out 2–3 hours after an attack if

there is good clinical recovery. All vasoactive medication should be stopped for 24 hours before testing, and testing should be avoided during mid-cycle in premenopausal women as poor flow can occur during ovulation. Patients should be warm and not vasoconstricted prior to baseline measurements and this is best done by resting in a temperature-controlled laboratory for 30 minutes prior to testing. In warmer weather, additional total body cooling may be required as a warm body may protect a patient from the vasospastic effects of localised digital cooling.

Strain gauge plethysmography is the usual method of measuring digital systolic blood pressure. Considerable operator skill is required and flow cannot be measured. Photoplethysmography with more sophisticated Doppler ultrasound equipment allows the measurement of the pressure at which blood flow returns.

Computerised thermography uses skin temperature as an indicator of finger blood flow. This technique allows dynamic measurement of all phases of the attack but results must be interpreted with care as skin temperature is also dependent on venous and arterial blood temperature.

Associated diseases should be sought by carrying out screening blood tests. A full blood count, urea and electrolytes, and urinalysis should detect anaemia of chronic disease and renal disease, and thyroid function tests detect hypothyroidism. Erythrocyte sedimentation rate (ESR) or plasma viscosity and rheumatoid antibody and antinuclear antibody tests help to detect associated CTD. Other tests, for example for cryoglobulins, may be carried out if appropriate. A chest radiograph may show basal fibrosis associated with CTD and a bony cervical rib.

Nail-fold capillaroscopy can be performed using an ophthalmoscope at high power. Normal vessels are not visualised but abnormally enlarged vessels, for example as seen in systemic sclerosis, will be seen quite easily (**Fig. 12.3**). These may also be examined by formal high-power microscopy but it should be noted that nail-fold changes also occur with trauma and in diabetes mellitus. The combination of abnormal nail-fold vessels and an abnormal immunological test has a 90% prediction value for later CTD.[9] Using structured classification systems, nail-fold patterns may be useful in assessing progression of the CTD.[39]

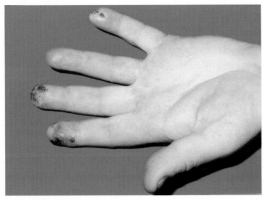

Figure 12.2 • Digital ulceration.

> ✔ The diagnostic value of nail-fold capillaroscopy is now fully recognised with a clear diagnostic pattern seen for associated CTD: dilatation and tortuosity of the capillary with patches of so-called 'drop-out' where the vessel has been obliterated by the CTD process.[40]

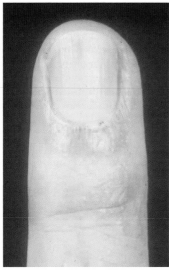

Figure 12.3 • Enlarged nail-fold capillaries in a patient with systemic sclerosis.

Other tests, such as laser Doppler flowmetry, are used as research tools but are not helpful in making the diagnosis.[41]

Management

A proportion of patients with mild disease will not require drug treatment. Associated disorders such as hypothyroidism should be treated and causative drug therapy (e.g. beta-blockers) changed. Good symptomatic relief can be achieved in many patients despite the current lack of cure. A suggested management plan is shown in **Fig. 12.4**.

General measures
Explanation of the disorder and reassurance is important in these patients, who are often apprehensive about their condition. The Raynaud's and Scleroderma Association in the UK issues free information booklets, and local self-help groups can be invaluable for support.

Smokers should stop cigarette smoking. Pocket-sized thermochemical warming agents are available and convenient to use. Electrically heated gloves and socks are ideal for some and provide warmth for up to 3 hours. Newer designs are available with the batteries inserted in a pocket on the gloves or socks themselves and should be more acceptable for many patients than the older garments that required heavy, cumbersome batteries. Nevertheless, patients should be warned that the heat may irritate existing skin ulcers. 'Abel' shoes, available from surgical appliance suppliers, are padded and broad fitting and therefore

warm while relieving pressure around the toes. Good ulcer care with early and adequate treatment of infection is important. It should be noted that the usual signs of infection, i.e. warmth, erythema and pus formation, may be absent because of poor blood flow. A high index of suspicion is required.

Drug therapy
This should be offered when symptoms are severe enough to interfere with work or lifestyle. Most patients with RS and some with RD will fall into this category. A selection of the drugs used in the treatment of RP is shown in Box 12.2.

Calcium channel blockers
These drugs are vasodilatory. Nifedipine is the gold standard and the most frequently prescribed drug, and has additional antiplatelet[42] and anti-WBC activity. However, its use is limited by the vasodilatory effects of flushing, headache and ankle swelling. These will be attenuated by using the slow-release, or 'retard', preparations and starting with 10 mg once daily, gradually increasing to a maximum of 20 mg t.d.s. if required. Apart from ankle swelling, the vasodilatory adverse effects often abate with continued use. Nifedipine has no licence for use in pregnancy and patients should be advised accordingly. Other potentially useful calcium blockers include amlodipine,[43] diltiazem[44] and isradipine.[45] These tend to have fewer

---

Box 12.2 • Commonly used drugs in the treatment of Raynaud's phenomenon

Nifedipine
Slow-release or retard preparation preferred, 10 mg b.d. then t.d.s.
Change to 20 mg b.d. then t.d.s. if required
Capsule as 'rescue medication' crushed under tongue if chronic dosing not tolerated
Can be combined at low dose (e.g. 10 mg once daily) with vasodilator if higher dose not tolerated

Naftidrofuryl
Initially 100 mg t.d.s. then 200 mg t.d.s. if required

Inositol nicotinate
Start at 500 mg t.d.s. increasing to forte 750 mg b.d. if required
Maximum dose is 1 g q.i.d.
Administer for a 3-month trial

Pentoxifylline
400 mg b.d. increasing to t.d.s. if required

Moxisylyte (thymoxamine)
40 mg q.d.s. increasing to 80 mg q.d.s.
Discontinue if no response in 2 weeks

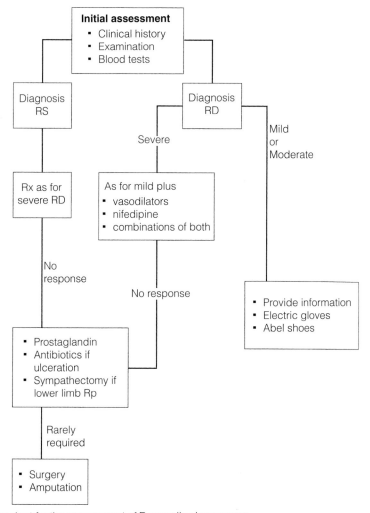

Figure 12.4 • Flow chart for the management of Raynaud's phenomenon.

vasodilatory effects but at the expense of efficacy. Verapamil and ketanserin are ineffective.

Other vasodilators

Naftidrofuryl oxalate (Praxilene) is a mild peripheral vasodilator with a serotonin receptor antagonist effect. An oral dose of 200 mg t.d.s. has been evaluated in many studies and mild improvement can be expected in terms of severity of pain and duration of attacks.

It is our experience that patients with primary RD respond better to vasodilators than those with RS, the limiting factor often being adverse effects at higher doses. Occasionally, we also find that a combination of a low-dose calcium blocker with a vasodilator such as naftidrofuryl can produce benefit while minimising the adverse effects seen with higher doses of either drug given in isolation.

Prostaglandins

Prostaglandins such as PGI_2 and PGE_1 have potent vasodilatory and antiplatelet effects but are both very unstable and require intravenous administration. Iloprost is a stable prostacyclin analogue that is effective in RP.[46] It is given intravenously for 6 hours daily for 3–5 days per treatment. The dose is gradually increased during each 6-hour period to a maximum tolerated dose, which should never be greater than 2 ng/kg per min. It is often less than this, particularly in women, because of flushing, headache or rarely hypotension. The same maximum dose is used each day. It is probably equipotent with nifedipine but remains a second choice in Europe because of its parenteral mode of administration and lack of licence in some countries. A study of oral iloprost in Raynaud's syndrome[47] has been encouraging, and a trial in those with RP secondary to systemic sclerosis has shown a significant benefit compared to placebo.[48] Oral beraprost seems to be ineffective.

Other drugs

Case reports and pilot studies suggest interesting areas for future work. Sildenafil improved pulmonary hypertension and peripheral blood flow in a patient with scleroderma-associated lung fibrosis and RP,[49] while *Ginkgo biloba* extracts[50] may also be effective in some cases. Cilostazol, a synthetic phosphodiesterase III inhibitor that reversibly inhibits platelet aggregation, is used for the treatment of intermittent claudication, and was tested in a randomised controlled trial in RP patients. Treatment was associated with vasodilation of the brachial arteries and conduit vessels.[51] However, the drug had no effects on microvascular blood flow or on the frequency and severity of RP attacks in both primary and secondary RP.

Sympathectomy

This involves the injection of phenol into the sympathetic chain. Lumbar sympathectomy has an important role in intractable RP of the feet and is often worth considering. Cervical sympathectomy has a poor response and a high relapse rate and is no longer indicated for upper limb RP. The more selective digital sympathectomy is popular in some specialised centres but long-term follow-up results have yet to be published.

Conclusion

RP is a common condition affecting 10% of the female population. Differentiation between primary and secondary RP is important for the correct management strategy. Satisfactory symptomatic relief is possible with a combination of drug therapy and non-pharmacological aids despite the lack of a cure. Surgery may be appropriate in some cases with an obstructive, bony or fibrous cervical rib. Treatment of associated CTD is also important. Occupational RP can sometimes be improved by change of job or a change in work techniques and this should always be considered.

Connective tissue disease

The most common disease associations with RS are the CTDs. Table 12.1 lists these disorders and indicates the relevant incidence of RP. It is found in the majority of patients with systemic sclerosis (SSc) and mixed CTD. RP is a frequent accompanying symptom of CTDs. In some of these the RP is reported as

Table 12.1 • Incidence of Raynaud's phenomenon in connective tissue disorders

Systemic sclerosis	95%
Systemic lupus erythematosus	29–40%
Polymyositis/dermatomyositis	40%
Sjögren's syndrome	33%
Mixed connective tissue disease	85%
Rheumatoid arthritis	10%

merely consisting of a biphasic or triphasic colour change with minimal discomfort. In other conditions RP is the most significant symptom, with the patients complaining of pain, ulcers and even gangrene. The most likely group of patients to be seen by the vascular clinician are those suffering from limited systemic sclerosis because the Raynaud's is often so severe as to require hospital referral. Furthermore, it often predates the other symptoms of CTD by many years. Thus a high index of suspicion for this particular disorder must be held by those seeing patients as a result of their vasospastic symptomatology.

The frequency with which these secondary conditions are recognised varies widely in reported studies and may depend in part on the doctor's referral pattern and the thoroughness with which the screen for a CTD is undertaken. One of the most challenging issues when evaluating patients with RP is the assessment of risk for transition to CTD. Koenig et al. reported that 12.6% of patients referred for assessment of RP progressed to SSc after a median follow-up of 4 years.[52] Ziegler et al.[53] reported a 9% transition in patents presenting with RP alone and 30% from 'possible' secondary RP after a 12.4-year mean follow-up. This study suggests that there is a continuum in transition to CTD and that clinicians should not confidently assure patients with what appears to be isolated primary RP of the benign nature of their symptoms. However, recently more clearly defined abnormalities have been documented in RP that have a strong link with disease progression and could help predict more accurately who will progress to CTD. These include certain clinical features, the presence of abnormal nail-fold vessels as previously described, and abnormal tests of immunology.

The American Rheumatism Association (ARA) criteria for CTDs have high specificity but low sensitivity for the diseases. Thus patients who do not fulfil the ARA criteria for a particular CTD but who have a single feature of the disease, for example sclerodactyly, digital pitting or photosensitivity, are likely with time to develop fully established CTD.[54] Thus isolated features of CTD occurring in association with RP should arouse clinical suspicion. The age of onset of RP may also be important. As stated, RP is common among young women and most of these probably have primary RD. When RP develops in older subjects, the likelihood of an underlying CTD is increased. Kallenberg[55] reports a study in which the median age of onset of vasospastic symptoms in RD was 14 years, and 36 years in patients with definite CTD. About 80% of patients presenting with onset of RP at the age of 60 years or above also have an associated condition,[53] but the incidence of CTD is the same as in the general population. The larger numbers of secondary cases reflect a higher proportion of patients with atherosclerosis (29% vs. 5% in the total Raynaud's population), and to a lesser extent hyperviscosity syndromes secondary to malignancy. Conversely, RP occurring in very young children, though rare, is frequently due to an underlying CTD. It has been estimated in one childhood study that 70% had primary RP and 30% were associated with other diseases.[31] Other suspicious symptoms that should alert the clinician to the likelihood of secondary RS include the presence of digital ulceration. Digital ulceration does not occur in RD. The recurrence of chilblains in adults may also raise suspicions, as should the occurrence of severe attacks persisting throughout the summer.[56] Furthermore, asymmetrical colour change with fewer digits affected suggests RS rather than RD.[57]

There have been a number recent advances in the use of nail-fold capilleroscopy and antibodies. Koenig et al. found the presence of positive ANAs and positive SSc autoantibodies (anti-CENP-B, anti-CENP, anti-Th/To, anti-RNAP III) along with characteristic findings on nail-fold capillary microscopy at initial assessment of RP to be strong independent predictors of progression to definite SSc in patients presenting with RP.[52] Of patients with all these abnormalities 79.5% progressed to SSc, whereas of those with none of these features only 1.3% progressed to SSc. This suggests a potentially useful role of such a comprehensive assessment at initial assessment to identify those at high risk of progression to CTD. Ingegnoli et al. have developed an algorithm using a combination of NCM findings and autoantibody results to predict the risk of transition to SSc.[58]

Vasculitis

Vasculitis is the term used to describe the group of conditions characterised by inflammation within the blood vessel wall and possibly damage to vessel integrity. The vasculitic process may involve only one or many blood vessels and therefore organ systems. In general, the clinical features result in ischaemia of the tissues supplied by the damaged vessel. These symptoms are often accompanied by the constitutional symptoms of fever, weight loss and anorexia that result from widespread inflammation. The vasculitic conditions may have a range of vessel involvement, from a mild obliterative disorder to necrotising vasculitis. Table 12.2 shows some of the common vasculitides, stratified by the size of the vessel most commonly involved. The classification of vasculitis is confusing as there is considerable clinical overlap between the different vasculitic syndromes and often the cause is unknown. Because the diagnosis of vasculitis still requires histological confirmation in most cases, the classification based on the size

Table 12.2 • Relationship between vasculitis classification and vessel size

Type of vasculitis	Aorta and branches	Large and medium-sized arteries	Medium-sized muscular arteries	Small muscular arteries	Arterioles, capillaries and venules
Takayasu's arteritis	✓				
Buerger's disease (thromboangiitis obliterans)	✓	✓			
Giant cell arteritis (temporal arteritis)	✓	✓			
Polyarteritis nodosa		✓	✓		
Wegener's granulomatosis			✓	✓	
Connective tissue disorders				✓	✓
Rheumatoid vasculitis				✓	✓
Cutaneous vasculitis (leucocytoclastic/allergic)					✓

of the predominant vessel involved and the type of inflammatory change is most frequently used. Non-invasive imaging using whole-body contrast-enhanced magnetic resonance angiography (CE-MRA) and multislice computed tomography have made signiticant inroads into conventional angiography in assessing the distribution of many vasculitic conditions. Increasingly, [18F]fluorodeoxyglucose positron emission tomography/computed tomography can be used to demonstrate the presence, distribution and activity of vasculitis as well as to monitor its response to treatment.

Takayasu's arteritis

This is an inflammatory and obliterative arteritis that primarily affects the large elastic arteries. It affects all levels of the aorta, its branches and the pulmonary arteries. The disorder has a striking female predominance, affecting women five to nine times more frequently than men. It usually presents between 10 and 30 years of age, although case reports of older patients have been published. The disease symptomatology can be divided into two phases: the acute systemic phase (pre-pulseless) and the chronic obliterative (pulseless) phase. The acute symptoms are often non-specific and are those one would expect to see with a generalised inflammatory process, including fatigue and malaise, weight loss and fever. Arthralgia and myalgia are common. The symptoms of the chronic phase are the result of the obliterative arterial lesion and depend on which vessels are affected. Possible findings include diminished or absent arterial pulses, vascular bruits, hypertension, inequality of blood pressure between arms and legs, and abnormalities on auscultation of the heart. Upper limb claudication can occur in association with the reduced or absent upper limb pulses.

Laboratory studies in Takayasu's arteritis reflect the inflammatory nature of the disorder. The ESR is elevated in the majority of patients during active disease. CE-MRA plays an important role in the diagnosis of this disease, with findings of vessel occlusions, stenoses (**Fig. 12.5**), aneurysm formation and the development of collaterals around occlusions. All levels of the aorta as well as its major branches may be involved and should be visualised. Pulmonary artery involvement has been seen in up to half of patients with this disorder. Of six diagnostic clinical and imaging criteria issued by the American College of Rheumatology, three are required to reach the diagnosis of Takayasu's arteritis.[59] Biopsy during the early phase shows granulomatous inflammation with patchy involvement of the vessel wall. Later, the changes are characterised by intimal

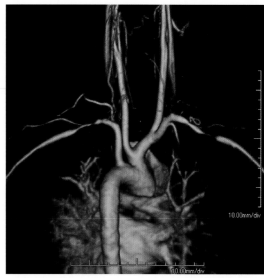

Figure 12.5 • Posterior view of a three-dimensional volume-rendered thoracic aorta magnetic resonance angiogram showing severe bilateral subclavian artery stenoses in a 35-year-old woman who presented with chest pain. In addition there were severe stenoses and occlusions of visceral and lower limb arteries. Image courtesy of Dr John Bottomley, Sheffield Vascular Institute, UK.

> ✓ During the acute inflammatory phase immunosuppression with corticosteroids and/or cyclophosphamide has been found to be effective in halting the angiographic progression.[59]

proliferation and band fibrosis of the adventitia and media.

Other immunosuppressive agents such as methotrexate, mycophenalate mofetil and azathioprine added to corticosteroids can help induce remission.[60] Symptomatic management of the patient is also important and symptoms such as hypertension should be treated aggressively. Therapeutic response is best assessed by improvement in symptoms, a fall in ESR and improvement in serial angiographic studies. Surgery or angioplasty may be required to treat stenosed or occluded segments of vessels. Conventional bypass grafts produce the best long-term results but percutaneous transluminal angioplasty gives good results for shorter lesions.[60]

Buerger's disease (thromboangiitis obliterans)

Buerger's disease is the clinical syndrome characterised by segmental thrombotic occlusions of the small and medium-sized arteries usually of the distal lower limb but occasionally also involving the upper extremities. Buerger's disease usually occurs in young smokers and is frequently associated with both RP and superficial migratory thrombophlebitis. Although previously mainly described in young men, the increased incidence of smoking in women has caused an increase in Buerger's disease in this sex.[61] In a recent review the changing pattern of this disease was recorded, confirming the increased prevalence of Buerger's disease in women.[62] It also documented that older patients (>40 years of age) are being more frequently diagnosed.

In the acute lesion, the internal elastic lamina of the arteries is almost always intact. Thrombus fills the vessel lumen and is hypercellular with an infiltration of lymphocytes, fibroblasts and later giant cells. There is no vessel wall necrosis or vascular wall calcification, and atheromatous plaques and aneurysms are both absent. The consistent presence of an acute hypercellular occlusive thrombus is the hallmark of this disease.

Altered haemorheological parameters have been detected in thromboangiitis obliterans, opening up some new therapeutic avenues.[63]

The symptoms of Buerger's disease are usually related to lower extremity ischaemia and include rest pain and tissue loss. Claudication is a rare symptom, but when present is usually confined to the foot. Femoral or popliteal pulses are usually present but the pedal pulses are absent.[64] The diagnosis of Buerger's disease depends to a great extent on the exclusion of other conditions, particularly early-onset atherosclerosis and immune disorders.

Investigation of the lower limb ischaemia reveals angiographically normal vessels proximal to the

---

☑ Tobacco abstinence is the cornerstone of management for Buerger's disease. In patients who do manage to stop smoking the appearance of new lesions and gangrene requiring amputation is unusual.[64]

---

popliteal. The tibial and peroneal vessels are frequently normal to a point of sudden occlusion.

However, persistent smoking leads to continued progression of the disease. Upper limb RP, finger ulceration and gangrene are treated as described earlier. There have been a large number of medical treatments proposed for the treatment of Buerger's disease affecting the lower limb, and the variety of the treatments proposed testifies to the fact that none are completely satisfactory and nearly all lack documentary efficacy. Corticosteroids, antiplatelet therapy and iloprost infusions are just a few of the treatments that have been used. The evidence for corticosteroid therapy is tenuous, whilst that for the use of iloprost[65] and aspirin-like compounds is

more convincing. Current research is looking at the possibility of using gene transfer to target vascular endothelial growth factor, which has been implicated in disease pathophysiology.[66] Further research is required into the benefits of the various medical treatment regimens currently available.

Giant cell arteritis

Giant cell arteritis, or temporal arteritis, is a systemic granulomatous vasculitis that predominantly affects large and medium-sized blood vessels. It usually involves the cranial branches of the aorta. It is most often seen in patients over 50 years of age and is an important preventable cause of blindness. However, it is recognised that temporal arteritis is a disease with many different manifestations and extracranial presentations are not uncommon. Among the vasculitic disorders, temporal arteritis is one of the more commonly occurring disorders, though it is still relatively rare. The estimated overall incidence rate in persons older than 50 years of age is approximately 17 per 100 000 annually.[67] There is a three to five times higher incidence in women than in men. The risk of this disease occurring is increased in smokers and patients with already established atherosclerotic disease.[68]

Temporal arteritis may present acutely or insidiously. Although headaches and sudden blindness are the classical symptoms, constitutional symptoms such as fever, weight loss and fatigue may be the earliest manifestations. Headaches are the usual complaint and these may be localised to the area overlying the superficial temporal arteries or may be generalised, resembling tension headaches. Scalp tenderness can also be a prominent feature and this can produce difficulty for the patients when combing their hair or sleeping at night on a pillow. This symptom is secondary to the involvement of the superficial temporal and occipital arteries. Jaw claudication occurs in approximately half of patients with this disease. This results from facial and maxillary artery involvement. Tongue claudication and dysphagia have also been reported and rarely glossitis and tongue necrosis are seen.[69] Sudden visual loss is a consequence of disease in the ophthalmic or posterior ciliary artery. Once blindness is established it is irreversible, but amaurosis fugax, a warning sign of impending blindness, is responsive to steroids. Pulmonary, renal and neurological symptomatology have also been reported, as has synovitis, but cutaneous or limb vessel manifestations are rare. This disease is therefore unlikely to present to the vascular clinician.

The diagnosis of temporal arteritis is made by finding an elevated acute-phase response such as the ESR. However, it should be noted that the ESR is not necessarily always elevated in patients with this disorder. The diagnostic hallmark of temporal arteritis

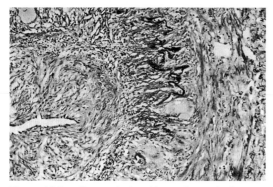

Figure 12.6 • Temporal artery biopsy demonstrating granulomatous inflammation and disruption of the internal elastic lamina.

is a biopsy that shows granulomatous inflammation (**Fig. 12.6**). Because of the intermittent or skip pattern of the lesions, biopsy can be negative in 50% of cases. Thus a negative biopsy in the setting of a high suspicion for the disease does not rule out the disease and should not preclude steroid therapy.

✔ On occasions a trial of steroid therapy can in itself be used to make the diagnosis. Corticosteroids are the mainstay of treatment. This therapy is efficacious in preventing but not reversing blindness.[70]

In studies of cytotoxic agents, methotrexate has been used as a corticosteroid-sparing drug in patients with polymyalgia rheumatica and giant cell arteritis with conflicting results,[71,72] although a meta-analysis of three trials suggests that methotrexate allows a small reduction in steroid dose and a higher probability of steroid discontinuation.[73] This drug may be tried in patients who are taking high doses of corticosteroids to control active disease and who have serious adverse effects from the steroids. Subjects with a raised platelet count are at higher risk of visual loss and should be treated effectively.[74] ESR/plasma viscosity and C-reactive protein (CRP) are generally used to monitor disease activity, but anticardiolipin antibodies, if present, may also be of benefit if there is confounding pathology that will increase ESR/CRP (e.g. infection).[75] Levels of interleukin (IL)-6 may be a sensitive indicator of active disease in polymyalgia rheumatica;[76] however, in giant cell arteritis, subjects with a raised titre of IL-6 may in fact be at lower risk of ischaemic events.[77] Calcium and vitamin D supplementation should be given with corticosteroid therapy in all patients. In patients with reduced bone mineral density, bisphosphonates are recommended.[78] A small open label trial of anti-tumour necrosis factor biologicals has shown potential benefit[79] but further controlled trials are needed before they are used routinely in clinical practice.

Polyarteritis nodosa

Polyarteritis nodosa (PAN) is a unique process characterised by a systemic necrotising vasculitis involving the small and medium-sized muscular arteries. The prevalence of PAN ranges between 5 and 77 per million population, with the higher incidence being reported in hepatitis B hyperendemic populations.[80] PAN is twice as common in men as in women and the average age of diagnosis is between 40 and 60 years, although PAN has been seen in both children and the elderly.

The symptoms reported depend on the vessels affected. The presenting symptoms are often constitutional, such as malaise, abdominal pain, weight loss, fever and myalgia. Organ involvement can occur at the same time or may develop later in the disease process. Renal disease with proteinuria and progressive renal failure occurs in about 70% of patients. Hypertension is a frequent finding. Gastrointestinal involvement is common and manifests as abdominal pain, nausea and vomiting. Acute events such as infarction of the bowel, perforation and haemorrhage are rare but produce the high mortality associated with this condition. Skin manifestations include nail-fold infarcts, digital infarcts (**Fig. 12.7**), palpable purpura and livedo reticularis (**Fig. 12.8**). Damage to the blood vessel wall can result in aneurysm formation. Mononeuritis multiplex is common and other important sites of involvement

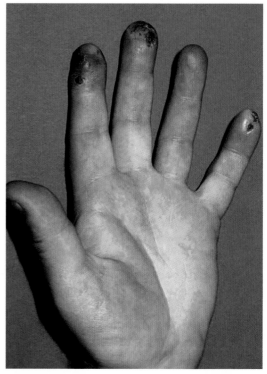

Figure 12.7 • Digital infarct in polyarteritis nodosa.

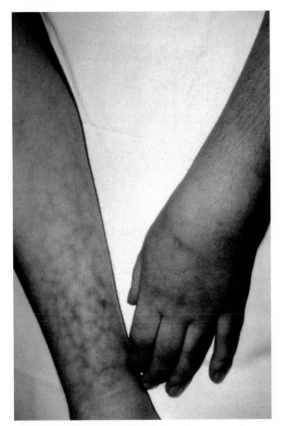

Figure 12.8 • Livedo reticularis in polyarteritis nodosa.

include the retina and testes. Laboratory findings can be non-specific, making the diagnosis difficult, but include anaemia, elevated ESR and a positive test for antineutrophil cytoplasmic antibody (ANCA). Hepatitis B surface antigen and antibodies should be measured in all patients with PAN. Angiography may be diagnostic, showing the characteristic findings of saccular or fusiform aneurysms and arterial narrowing.[81] The diagnosis of PAN must be based on the demonstration of vasculitis by angiography or biopsy.

> ✔ Corticosteroids are the cornerstone of treatment and cyclophosphamide can be added if the disease proves difficult to control.

Wegener's granulomatosis

Wegener's granulomatosis is a form of vasculitis that involves mainly the medium and small arteries and veins of the upper and lower respiratory tract and kidneys. Although it is a systemic necrotising granulomatous vasculitis, it is classically associated with the triad of upper respiratory tract, lung and kidney involvement. The manifestations and severity of the disease at presentation are variable but cutaneous vascular symptoms tend to be less

frequently seen.[82] These consist of cutaneous ulceration, subcutaneous nodules and palpable purpura.

Laboratory findings show an inflammatory response. Sinus radiographs or computed tomography may show evidence of mucosal thickening, sinus opacification or air–fluid levels. The chest X-ray may show mass lesions. Diagnosis is made through biopsy. The finding of elevated blood c-ANCA levels is strongly associated with Wegener's granulomatosis and these should be measured in cases of clinical suspicion.

Circulating endothelial cells may be a novel marker of active ANCA-associated small-vessel vasculitis. The clinical use of this tool and the pathogenic mechanisms leading to these findings require further investigation.[83] Treatment is with immunosuppressants.

Cutaneous vasculitis/small-vessel vasculitis

The vessels primarily involved in small-vessel vasculitis are the postcapillary venules, although capillaries and arterioles may also be involved. When first described, small-vessel vasculitis was named hypersensitivity angiitis. At one time, small-vessel vasculitis was thought to be identical to the microscopic form of PAN. However, the latter affects mainly small arteries and arterioles rather than venules. Box 12.3 lists the clinical syndromes associated with cutaneous vasculitis.

Idiopathic cutaneous vasculitis

This is the most common form of vasculitis in the skin.[8] It is usually manifest by palpable purpura most commonly occurring in the lower limb, often below the knee. The involvement of the lower limb tends to be symmetrical and is worsened by periods of sitting

Box 12.3 • Clinical syndromes of cutaneous vasculitis

Idiopathic cutaneous vasculitis
Necrotising vasculitis secondary to
Drugs, e.g. antibiotics, diuretics, NSAIDs, anticonvulsants
Infection, e.g. upper respiratory tract virus, *Streptococcus*, hepatitis B, HIV
Immunological disorders, e.g. connective tissue diseases
Cutaneous vasculitis as a manifestation of systemic disease
Connective tissue disease
Mixed cryoglobulinaemia
Allergic granulomatosis (Churg–Strauss syndrome)
Behçet's disease
HIV, human immunodeficiency virus; NSAIDs, non-steroidal anti-inflammatory drugs.

or standing. The lesions occur in crops, initially appearing as macular erythema and then progressing to purpura. Uncommonly, this type of vasculitis can present as urticaria and it can be distinguished from typical urticaria by the fact that the lesions persist for more than 24 hours. Biopsies of the lesion show leucocytoclastic vasculitis with endothelial cell swelling, often necrosis as well as haemorrhage, fibrin deposition and infiltration with polymorphonuclear neutrophils.

Necrotising vasculitis associated with infections, drugs or CTD

The aetiology of this form of vasculitis is presumed to be hypersensitivity to various factors, including infective agents and drugs, or underlying systemic disease. Nevertheless, in approximately half the cases no definitive precipitating agent can be found.[84] Infection is associated with cutaneous necrotising vasculitis in approximately 10% of cases. Most often these are viruses associated with the upper respiratory tract and cause vasculitis such as Henoch–Schönlein purpura, although bacterial organisms have also been found capable of inducing a hypersensitivity vasculitis. The most commonly implicated drugs are antibiotics, particularly penicillin and sulphonamides. Diuretics and non-steroidal anti-inflammatory drugs (NSAIDs) have also been linked to the condition. Leucocytoclastic vasculitis may also be associated with a number of immunological disorders with systemic manifestations; most commonly these are of the CTD type.

Cutaneous vasculitis as a manifestation of systemic disease

Small-vessel vasculitis affecting the skin may be a manifestation of underlying systemic disease. The most common diseases in this category are the CTDs, particularly systemic lupus erythematosus but also mixed cryoglobulinaemia. The clinical and histological appearances of this type of vasculitis are often indistinguishable from those of the lesions of idiopathic cutaneous vasculitis. It is of crucial importance to examine any patient with skin vasculitis in a thorough fashion, focusing on the potential for the presence of CTD.

In Churg–Strauss vasculitis the most common type of skin manifestation appears mainly in the extremities and is maculopapular in appearance. It may be accompanied by vesicles and occasionally by bullae. Behçet's disease, which is characterised by oral and genital ulceration, may also present with a variety of non-specific skin changes including papules, vesicles, pyoderma and erythema nodosum-like lesions. Most patients with small-vessel vasculitis have disease limited to the skin. Investigation of these patients should be aimed at confirming the diagnosis by biopsy and then elucidating potential aetiological agents or underlying systemic disorder.

Most patients with small-vessel vasculitis limited to the skin experience a single episode that is often short-lived and associated with minimal symptomatology. Therapy for these individuals may not be required or may be limited to the use of antihistamines or NSAIDs. However, for individuals with more severe or recurrent episodes, treatment with corticosteroids may have to be considered.

Human immunodeficiency virus (HIV) is becoming a rare but reported cause of vasculitis, and it is important for the clinican to be aware of these emerging data in this regard. A broad spectrum of vasculitis is reported in HIV-infected patients, ranging from involvement of the small vessels, in hypersensitivity vasculitis secondary to drug treatment, to involvement of the aorta and branches. Corticosteroids or other immunosuppressive therapies such as intravenous immunoglobulin and cyclophosphamide are used to treat life-threatening vasculitic complications that involve the lungs, kidneys or central nervous system, in conjunction with effective antiretroviral therapy.

Conclusion

Vasculitis will present to the vascular clinician as skin ischaemia. The predilection of a number of vasculitic disorders for the lower limb may mimic large-vessel disease or emboli. The cornerstone of diagnosis is the finding of an acute-phase response, e.g. elevated ESR, plasma viscosity and CRP levels. Screening for autoantibodies may be helpful, but diagnosis is often only made by analysis of biopsy material and this should be considered in all cases of vasculitis, unless the tissue is too ischaemic to sustain wound healing.

Key points

- Raynaud's phenomenon should be classified appropriately into primary Raynaud's disease and secondary Raynaud's syndrome. Management includes general measures, drugs, sympathectomy and attention to any underlying disease.
- Vasculitis may present to the vascular clinician as skin ischaemia. Constitutional symptoms of fever, weight loss and fatigue are often clues to the diagnosis. Key investigations are ESR/plasma viscosity, CRP, autoantibodies and biopsy. Immunosuppression is the cornerstone of treatment of vasculitis.

References

1. Raynaud MD. De l'asphyxie locale et de la gangrene symetrique des extremites. Paris; 1862. (Trans. Thomas Barlow, London, New Sydenham Society, 1988.).

2. Brotzu G, Falchi S, Mannu B, et al. The importance of presynaptic beta receptors in Raynaud's disease. J Vasc Surg 1989;9:767–71.

3. Baron M, Feiglin D, Hyland R, et al. [67]Gallium lung scans in progressive systemic sclerosis. Arth Rheum 1983;26:969–74.

4. Belch JJ, Land D, Park RH, et al. Decreased oesophageal blood flow in patients with Raynaud's phenomenon. Br J Rheumatol 1988;27:426–30.

5. Kahan A, Devaux JY, Amor B, et al. Nifedipine and thallium-201 myocardial perfusion in progressive systemic sclerosis. N Engl J Med 1986;314:1397–402.

6. De Trafford JC, Lafferty K, Potter CE, et al. An epidemiological survey of Raynaud's phenomenon. Eur J Vasc Surg 1988;2:167–70.

7. Suter LG, Murabito JM, Felson DT, et al. The incidence and natural history of Raynaud's phenomenon in the community. Arth Rheum 2005;52(4):1259–63.

8. Porter JM, Bardana Jr EJ, Baur GM, et al. The clinical significance of Raynaud's syndrome. Surgery 1976;80:756–64.

9. Porter JM, Rivers SP, Anderson CJ, et al. Evaluation and management of patients with Raynaud's syndrome. Am J Surg 1981;142:183–9.

10. Kallenberg CG, Wouda AA, The TH. Systemic involvement and immunologic findings in patients presenting with Raynaud's phenomenon. Am J Med 1980;69:675–80.

11. Allen EV, Brown GE. Raynaud's disease: a critical review of minimal requisites for diagnosis. Am J Med Sci 1932;183:187–200.

12. Palmer KT, Griffin MJ, Bendall H, et al. Prevalence and pattern of occupational exposure to hand transmitted vibration in Great Britain: findings from a national survey. Occup Environ Med 2000;57:218–28.

13. Letz R, Cherniack MG, Gerr F, et al. A cross sectional epidemiological survey of shipyard workers exposed to hand–arm vibration. Br J Ind Med 1992;49:53–62.

14. Mirbod SM, Yoshida H, Nagata C, et al. Hand–arm vibration syndrome and its prevalence in the present status of private forestry enterprises in Japan. Int Arch Occup Environ Health 1992;64:93–9.

15. Koskimies K, Pyykko I, Starck J, et al. Vibration syndrome among Finnish forest workers between 1972 and 1990. Int Arch Occup Environ Health 1992;64:251–6.

16. Hedlund U. Raynaud's phenomenon of fingers and toes of miners exposed to local and whole-body vibration and cold. Int Arch Occup Environ Health 1989;61:457–61.

17. Kennedy G, Khan F, McLaren M, et al. Endothelial activation and response in patients with hand arm vibration syndrome. Eur J Clin Invest 1999;29:577–81.

18. Taylor W, Pelmear PL. The hand–arm vibration syndrome: an update. Br J Ind Med 1990;47:577–9.

19. Department for work and pensions. DB1 – A guide to industrial injuries disablement benefits. 2011.

20. Freedman RR, Sabharal SC, Desai N, et al. Increased alpha-adrenergic responsiveness in idiopathic Raynaud's disease. Arth Rheum 1989;32:61–5.

21. Lau CS, O'Dowd A, Belch JJ. White blood cell activation in Raynaud's phenomenon of systemic sclerosis and vibration induced white finger syndrome. Ann Rheum Dis 1992;51:249–52.

22. Lau CS, Bridges AB, Muir A, et al. Further evidence of increased polymorphonuclear cell activity in patients with Raynaud's phenomenon. Br J Rheumatol 1992;31:375–80.

23. Belch JJ, Drury J, McLaughlin K, et al. Abnormal biochemical and cellular parameters in the blood of patients with Raynaud's phenomenon. Scott Med J 1987;32:12–4.

24. Belch JJ, Zoma AA, Richards IM, et al. Vascular damage and factor-VIII-related antigen in the rheumatic diseases. Rheumatol Int 1987;7:107–11.

25. Belch JJ, McLaren M, Anderson J, et al. Increased prostacyclin metabolites and decreased red cell deformability in patients with systemic sclerosis and Raynaud's syndrome. Prostaglandins Leukot Med 1985;18:401–2.

26. Belch JJ, O'Dowd A, Forbes CD, et al. Platelet sensitivity to a prostacyclin analogue in systemic sclerosis. Br J Rheumatol 1985;24:346–50.

27. Zamora MR, O'Brien RF, Rutherford RB, et al. Serum endothelin-1 concentrations and cold provocation in primary Raynaud's phenomenon. Lancet 1990;336:1144–7.

28. Kahaleh B, Fan PS, Matucci-Cerinic M, et al. Study of endothelial dependent relaxation in scleroderma (abstract). Am Coll Rheum 1993;B233:S180.

29. Khan F, Belch JJ. Skin blood flow in patients with systemic sclerosis and Raynaud's phenomenon: effects of oral l-arginine supplementation. J Rheumatol 1999;26:2389–94.

30. Nakamura H, Matsuzaki I, Hatta K, et al. Blood endothelin-1 and cold-induced vasodilation in patients with primary Raynaud's phenomenon and workers with vibration-induced white finger. Int Angiol 2003;22:243–9.

31. Kahaleh MB. Raynaud phenomenon and the vascular diseases in scleroderma. Curr Opin Rheumatol 2004;16(6):718–22.

32. Konttinen YT, Mackiewicz Z, Ruuttila P, et al. Vascular damage and lack of angiogenesis in systemic sclerosis skin. Clin Rheumatol 2003;22:196–202.

33. Lau CS, O'Dowd A, Belch JJF. White blood cell activation in Raynaud's phenomenon of systemic sclerosis and vibration white finger. Ann Rheum Dis 1992;51:249–52.

34. Lau CS, Bridges AB, Muir A, et al. Further evidence of increased polymorphonuclear cell activity in patients with Raynaud's phenomenon. Br J Rheumatol 1992;31:375–80.

35. Kurozawa Y, Nasu Y. Circulating adhesion molecules in patients with vibration-induced white finger. Angiology 2000;51:1003–6.

36. Lau CS. Haemostatic abnormalities in Raynaud's phenomenon and the potential for treatment with manipulation of the arachidonic acid pathway. MD thesis, University of Dundee; 1993.

37. Worda M, Sgonc R, Dietrich H, et al. In vivo analysis of the apoptosis-inducing effect of anti-endothelial cell antibodies in systemic sclerosis by the chorionallantoic membrane assay. Arth Rheum 2003;48:2605–14.

38. Cherkas LF, Williams FMK, Carter L, et al. Heritability of Raynaud's phenomenon and vascular responsiveness to cold: a study of adult female twins. Arth Care Res 2007;57:524–8.

39. Cutolo M, Sulli A, Pizzorni C, et al. Nailfold videocapillaroscopy assessment of microvascular damage in systemic sclerosis. J Rheumatol 2000;27:155–60.

40. Nagy Z, Czirjak L. Nailfold digital capillaroscopy in 447 patients with connective tissue disease and Raynaud's disease. J Eur Acad Dermatol Venereol 2004;18:62–8.

41. Turner JB, Belch JJF, Khan F. Current concepts in assessment of microvascular function using laser Doppler imaging and iontophoresis. Trends Cardiovasc Med 2008;18(4):109–16.

42. Maricq HR, Jennings JR, Valter I, et al., Raynaud's Treatment Study Investigators. Evaluation of treatment efficacy of Raynaud phenomenon by digital blood pressure response to cooling. Vasc Med 2000;5:135–40.

43. La Civita L, Pitaro N, Rossi M, et al. Amlodipine in the treatment of Raynaud's phenomenon. Br J Rheumatol 1993;32:524–5.

44. Rhedda A, McCans J, Willan AR, et al. A double blind placebo controlled crossover randomized trial of diltiazem in Raynaud's phenomenon. J Rheumatol 1985;12:724–7.

45. Leppert J, Jonasson T, Nilsson H, et al. The effect of isradipine, a new calcium-channel antagonist, in patients with primary Raynaud's phenomenon: a single-blind dose–response study. Cardiovasc Drugs Ther 1989;3:397–401.

46. Pope J, Fenlon D, Thomson A, et al. Iloprost and cisaprost for Raynaud's phenomenon in progressive systemic sclerosis. Cochrane Database Syst Rev 2000;2CD000956.

47. Belch JJ, Capell HA, Cooke ED, et al. Oral iloprost as a treatment for Raynaud's syndrome: a double blind multicentre placebo controlled study. Ann Rheum Dis 1995;54:197–200.

48. Wigley FM, Korn JH, Csuka ME, et al. Oral iloprost treatment in patients with Raynaud's phenomenon secondary to systemic sclerosis: a multicenter, placebo-controlled, double blind study. Arth Rheum 1998;41:670–7.

49. Rosenkranz S, Diet F, Karasch T, et al. Sildenafil improved pulmonary hypertension and peripheral blood flow in a patient with scleroderma-associated lung fibrosis and the Raynaud phenomenon. Ann Intern Med 2003;139:871–3.

50. Muir AH, Robb R, McLaren M, et al. The use of Ginkgo biloba in Raynaud's disease: a double-blind placebo-controlled trial. Vasc Med 2002;7:265–7.

51. Rajagopalan S, Pfenninger D, Somers E, et al. Effects of cilostazol in patients with Raynaud's syndrome. Am J Cardiol 2003;92(11):1310–5.

52. Koenig M, Joyal F, Fritzler MJ, et al. Autoantibodies and microvascular damage are independent predictive factors for the progression of Raynaud's phenomenon to systemic sclerosis: a twenty-year prospective study of 586 patients, with validation of proposed criteria for early systemic sclerosis. Arth Rheum 2008;58:3902–12.

53. Ziegler S, Brunner M, Eigenbauer E, et al. Long-term outcome of primary Raynaud's phenomenon and its conversion to connective tissue disease: a 12-year retrospective patient analysis. Scand J Rheumatol 2003;32:343–7.

54. Belch JJ. Raynaud's phenomenon: its relevance to scleroderma. Ann Rheum Dis 1991;50(Suppl. 4):839–45.

55. Kallenberg CG. Early detection of connective tissue disease in patients with Raynaud's phenomenon. Rheum Dis Clin North Am 1990;16:11–30.

56. Franceschini F, Calzavara-Pinton P, Valsecchi L, et al. Chilblain lupus erythematosus is associated with antibodies to SSA/Ro. Adv Exp Med Biol 1999;455:167–71.

57. Cardelli MB, Kleinsmith DM. Raynaud's phenomenon and disease. Med Clin North Am 1989;73:1127–41.

58. Ingegnoli F, Boracchi P, Gualterotti R, et al. Improving outcome prediction of systemic sclerosis from isolated Raynaud's phenomenon: role of autoantibodies and nail-fold capillaroscopy. Rheumatology (Oxford) 2010;49(4):797–805.

59. Arend WP, Michel BA, Bloch DA, et al. The American College of Rheumatology 1990 criteria for the classification of Takayasu arteritis. Arth Rheum 1990;33:1129–34.

60. Liang P, Hoffman GS. Advances in the medical and surgical management of Takayasu arteritis. Curr Opin Rheumatol 2005;17:16–24.

61. Lie JT. The Canadian Rheumatism Association, 1991 Dunlop–Dottridge Lecture. Vasculitis, 1815 to 1991: classification and diagnostic specificity. J Rheumatol 1992;19:83–9.

62. Stvrtinova V, Ambrozy E, Stvrtina S, et al. 90 years of Buerger's disease: what has changed. Bratisl Lek Listy 1999;100:123–8.

63. Bozkurt AK, Koksal C, Ercan M. The altered hemorheologic parameters in thromboangiitis obliterans: a new insight. Clin Appl Thromb Hemost 2004;10:45–50.

64. Mills JL, Porter JM. Thromboangiitis obliterans (Buerger's disease). In: Churg A, Churg I, editors. Systemic vasculitides. Tokyo: Igaku-Shoin; 1991. p. 229–39.

65. Fiessinger JN, Schafer M. Trial of iloprost versus aspirin treatment for critical limb ischaemia of thromboangiitis obliterans. The TAO Study. Lancet 1990;335:555–7.

66. Isner JM, Baumgartner I, Rauh G, et al. Treatment of thromboangiitis obliterans (Buerger's disease) by intramuscular gene transfer of vascular endothelial growth factor: preliminary clinical results. J Vasc Surg 1998;28:964–73.

67. Rao JK, Allen NB. Polymyalgia rheumatica and giant cell arteritis. In: Belch JJF, Zurier RB, editors. Connective tissue diseases. London: Chapman & Hall Medical; 1995. p. 249–70.

68. Machado EB, Gabriel SE, Beard CM, et al. A population-based case–control study of temporal arteritis: evidence for an association between temporal arteritis and degenerative vascular disease. Int J Epidemiol 1989;18:836–41.

69. Sonnenblick M, Nesher G, Rosin A. Nonclassical organ involvement in temporal arteritis. Semin Arth Rheum 1989;19:183–90.

70. Hayreh SS, Zimmerman B. Visual deterioration in giant cell arteritis patients while on high doses of corticosteroid therapy. Ophthalmology 2003;110:1204–15.

71. Hoffman GS, Cid MC, Hellmann DB, et al. A multicenter, randomized, double-blind, placebo-controlled trial of adjuvant methotrexate treatment for giant cell arteritis. Arth Rheum 2002;46:1309–18.

72. Jover JA, Hernandez-Garcia C, Morado IC, et al. Combined treatment of giant-cell arteritis with methotrexate and prednisone: a randomized, double-blind, placebo-controlled trial. Ann Intern Med 2001;134:106–14.

73. Mahr AD, Jover JA, Spiera RF, et al. Adjunctive methotrexate for treatment of giant cell arteritis: an individual patient data meta-analysis. Arth Rheum 2007;56:2789–97.

74. Liozon E, Herrmann F, Ly K, et al. Risk factors for visual loss in giant cell (temporal) arteritis: a prospective study of 174 patients. Am J Med 2001;111:211–7.

75. Liozon E, Roblot P, Paire D, et al. Anticardiolipin antibody levels predict flares and relapses in patients with giant-cell (temporal) arteritis. A longitudinal study of 58 biopsy-proven cases. Rheumatology (Oxford) 2000;39:1089–94.

76. Weyand CM, Fulbright JW, Evans JM, et al. Corticosteroid requirements in polymyalgia rheumatica. Arch Intern Med 1999;159:577–84.

77. Hernandez-Rodriguez J, Segarra M, Vilardell C, et al. Elevated production of interleukin-6 is associated with a lower incidence of disease-related ischemic events in patients with giant-cell arteritis: angiogenic activity of interleukin-6 as a potential protective mechanism. Circulation 2003;107:2428–34.

78. American College of Rheumatology Ad Hoc Committee on Glucocorticoid-induced Osteoporosis. Recommendations for the prevention and treatment of glucocorticoid-induced osteoporosis: 2001 update. Arth Rheum 2001;44:1496–503.

79. Hoffman GS, Merkel PA, Brasington RD, et al. Anti-tumor necrosis factor therapy in patients with difficult to treat Takayasu's arteritis. Arth Rheum 2004;50:2296–304.

80. McMahon BJ, Heyward WL, Templin DW, et al. Hepatitis B-associated polyarteritis nodosa in Alaskan Eskimos: clinical and epidemiologic features and long-term follow-up. Hepatology 1989;9:97–101.

81. Schirmer M, Duftner C, Seiler R, et al. Abdominal aortic aneurysms: an underestimated type of immune-mediated large vessel arteritis? Cur Opin Rheumatol 2006;18(1):48–53.

82. Langford CA, McCallum RM. Idiopathic vasculitis. In: Belch JJF, Zurier RB, editors. Connective tissue diseases. London: Chapman & Hall Medical; 1995. p. 179–217.

83. Woywodt A, Streiber F, de Groot K, et al. Circulating endothelial cells as markers for ANCA-associated small-vessel vasculitis. Lancet 2003;361:206–10.

84. Sanchez NP, Van Hale HM, Su WP. Clinical and histopathologic spectrum of necrotizing vasculitis. Report of findings in 101 cases. Arch Dermatol 1985;121:220–4.

13

Peripheral and abdominal aortic aneurysms

Michael G. Wyatt
John D. Rose

Definition of an aneurysm

Derived from the Greek word *aneurysma* describing 'a widening', an arterial aneurysm is defined by an increased vessel diameter of 50% or more than that of the non-dilated adjacent vessel.[1]

Prevalence of arterial aneurysms

Population screening studies indicate that the prevalence of abdominal aortic aneurysm (AAA) increases with age,[2,3] occurring in 7–8% of men over 65 years.[3,4] The disease prevalence is six times higher in men than in women,[5] with AAA rupture the seventh most common cause of male death in the UK. Between 1951 and 1995 there was a steady increase in age-standardised deaths from all aortic aneurysms in men, from 2 to 56 per 100 000 population in England and Wales. More recently, data suggest that the incidence of abdominal aortic aneurysm (AAA) may now be declining. Between 1997 and 2009 there has been a reduction in age-adjusted mortality from AAA from 40.4 to 25.7 per 100 000 population for England and Wales and from 30.1 to 20.8 per 100 000 population in Scotland.[6]

There is considerably less information about the prevalence of peripheral aneurysms, although it is recognised that these frequently occur in association with AAA. Approximately 25% of patients with AAA have coexisting femoral or popliteal aneurysms.[7] It is likely therefore that peripheral aneurysms share a common aetiology with AAAs and that changes in their prevalence match those of aortic aneurysms.

Pathogenesis of aortic aneurysms

Metabolic regulation of both elastin and collagen proteins in the aortic wall is under the control of several enzymatic agents. The most important group of these mediators appears to belong to the zinc- and calcium-requiring matrix-degrading metalloproteinases (MMPs), and there is compelling evidence that abnormal local MMP production and regulation is associated with the pathogenesis of aortic aneurysms. The elastolytic subtypes MMP-9 and MMP-2 appear to be the most influential in AAA pathogenesis.[8,9] A chronic inflammatory infiltrate composed of T cells, macrophages, B lymphocytes and plasma cells is a typical histological feature of AAA. Although the antecedent trigger for this cellular migration remains unclear, much of the subsequent vessel wall destruction appears to be mediated by the cytokines and chemokines released by the infiltrate with induction and activation of MMP species.[10]

Although certain phenotypes have been associated with increased frequency of disease progression, as yet no single genetic anomaly or polymorphism has been universally identified within all AAA patients. This approach to pathogenesis may eventually form the basis of genetic testing of specific increased-risk populations, allowing more focused surveillance and early intervention.[8]

In an effort to unify all aspects of this complex process, Ailawadi et al.[9] have proposed a model of aortic aneurysm pathogenesis. They postulate that the initial trigger for AAA may be a combination of factors such as fragmented medial proteins, localised haemodynamic stress or a genetic predisposition that causes inflammatory cells to migrate into the aortic wall. This inflammatory infiltrate is rich in cytokines, chemokines and reactive oxygen species, and attracts further cellular influx with expression and activation of proteases, in particular those of the MMP group. Subsequent unregulated connective tissue turnover results in medial degeneration of the aorta and aneurysmal dilatation. The proteolysis is exacerbated by the inherent increase in wall stress with progressive AAA expansion. If untreated, the sequence cascades, with eventual aortic rupture.[10]

Infrarenal abdominal aortic aneurysms

Most AAAs remain asymptomatic until rupture, with approximately 75% being symptom free at diagnosis. The majority of these cases are detected as an incidental finding during the course of investigation of unrelated cause. Aetiological factors include increasing age, male sex, ethnic origin, family history, smoking, hypercholesterolaemia, hypertension and prior vascular disease. Of these, male sex and smoking are the most important, increasing the chances of AAA development by 4.5 and 5.6 times, respectively.[11]

Symptomatic and ruptured AAAs

Rapid expansion (>1 cm/year) or the development of symptoms such as abdominal pain, tenderness and back pain are usually an indication for prompt surgical intervention, irrespective of size. This is because of a higher rupture rate.[12]

Rupture of an aortic aneurysm is a sudden catastrophic event with severe abdominal and/or back pain and circulatory collapse. Frequently, rupture occurs into the retroperitoneum and bleeding may be arrested by a combination of hypotension and tamponade within this space. Although transient and unstable, this circumstance does provide an opportunity for emergency life-saving surgery. Free rupture into the peritoneal cavity is rapidly fatal. Approximately 75% of patients with ruptured AAAs die before reaching hospital.

Inflammatory abdominal aortic aneurysms (IAAAs)

IAAAs account for 3–10% of all AAAs and were not classified per se until the early 1970s.[13] Classical defining features are the triad of a thickened aneurysmal wall, marked perianeurysmal/retroperitoneal fibrosis and dense neighbouring visceral adhesions. Abdominal or back pain, weight loss and an elevated erythrocyte sedimentation rate in a patient with known aortic aneurysm confer a diagnosis of IAAA until proven otherwise.[14]

Population screening for AAAs

Given that (i) the majority of AAAs are asymptomatic, (ii) 75% of patients with rupture die without reaching hospital and (iii) elective surgical treatment of AAAs is effective, then population screening for AAAs is an attractive proposition.

B-mode ultrasound scanning using portable equipment has been shown to be effective in detecting AAAs and is inexpensive.[15] Furthermore, it has been estimated that a single ultrasound scan in males of 65 years of age would detect 90% of aneurysms at risk of rupture.[16]

The Multicentre Aneurysm Screening Study (MASS) trial has provided good statistical evidence to show that the prevalence of aneurysm-related death is reduced significantly in a screened male population aged 65–74 years, with a 53% reduction in those who attended for screening.[2] Because other causes of death overshadow those due to ruptured AAAs, it has not been possible to demonstrate a statistically significant overall survival advantage for the screened population. Nevertheless, the case for extending population-based screening for AAAs is convincing.

Interestingly, the detection of aneurysms in a screened population does not appear to affect quality of life adversely.

The MASS trial data show that over 4 years the mean incremental cost-effectiveness ratio for screening was £28 400 per life-year gained, equivalent to approximately £36 000 per quality-adjusted life-year. It was estimated that this would fall to approximately £8000 per life-year gained at 10 years.[17]

By offering men ultrasound screening in their 65th year, the rate of premature death from ruptured AAA could be reduced by up to 50%. In March 2009, the NHS Abdominal Aortic Aneurysm Screening Programme (NAASP) was introduced; implementation is being phased and the programme aims to cover the whole of England by March 2013.

✅✅ Analysis of the 10-year Multicentre Aneurysm Screening Study (MASS) data shows that the NHS AAA Screening Programme (NAAASP) will prevent significant numbers of AAA ruptures and AAA deaths.[18] It also proves that the number of lives saved will greatly outweigh the number of post-elective surgery deaths. The following figures use the 10-year MASS data and assume an 80% attendance for screening and a 5% post-elective surgery mortality: 240 men need to be invited (192 scanned) to save one AAA death over 10 years and each 2080 men invited for screening (1660 scanned) result in one extra post-elective surgery death. This means that over 10 years, for every 10 000 men scanned under the NAAASP, 65 AAA ruptures will be prevented, saving 52 lives. However, there will also be six post-elective surgery deaths involving men whose aneurysm is detected under the screening programme.

Compared with existing screening programmes, for example for breast and cervical cancer, screening for AAAs appears to be relatively cost-effective.

Principles of AAA management

The fundamental principle underpinning AAA management strategy is the prevention of rupture. The role of medical therapy is important and includes blood pressure control, cholesterol reduction, antiplatelet therapy and smoking cessation. AAA size is still considered the most important factor in prediction of rupture. From a meta-analysis of 13 studies, Law et al. have quantified this annual risk for differing initial size[19] (Table 13.1).

The UK Small Aneurysm Trial and US Aneurysm Detection and Management (ADAM) trials were designed to provide guidelines as to when to offer elective surgery on the basis of aneurysm size.[12,20]

Table 13.1 • Annual AAA rupture risk in relation to size

AAA size (cm)	Risk of rupture per year (%)
<3.0	0
3–3.9	0.4
4–4.9	1.1
5–5.9	3.3
6–6.9	9.4
7–7.9	24

Adapted from Law MR, Morris J, Wald NJ. Screening for abdominal aortic aneurysms. J Med Screening 1994; 1:110–15.

✅✅ These two trials addressed the difficult dilemma of how to manage patients in whom the risks of surgery and rupture are similar. The Medical Research Council-sponsored UK Small Aneurysm Trial randomised 1090 patients with asymptomatic AAAs of 4.0–5.5 cm diameter to either initial ultrasound surveillance (527 patients) or surgery (563 patients). In the surveillance group, 321 patients eventually underwent surgery due to rapid expansion or growth to above the 5.5-cm threshold. In the early surgery group, the 30-day mortality rate was 5.8%. There was no difference in survival between the groups and the UK SAT concluded that early operative intervention for patients with AAAs of less than 5.5 cm diameter was not indicated. The rupture rate for untreated small aneurysms in this trial was less than 2% per annum. However, the rate was relatively higher in females and this suggests that elective surgery may be indicated for smaller aneurysms in this group of patients. However, at present the data are insufficiently robust to support this conclusion convincingly. The results of the ADAM trial and the conclusions drawn were similar.

Surveillance of patients with small aneurysms

Since the publication of the small aneurysm trials, it has been recommended that patients with AAAs of less than 5.5 cm diameter should be managed conservatively with best medical therapy and regular surveillance by interval ultrasound scanning. The timing of such scans remains controversial, requiring a balance between cost/inconvenience and patient safety. It has recently been shown that an aorta with a diameter of <3 cm in a male aged 65 years or over is associated with minimal risk of eventual rupture, hence there is probably no justification for continued surveillance. For larger aneurysms, there is no robust evidence base upon which to base a surveillance programme. However, it is generally accepted that screening intervals of 1 year for aneurysms of 3.5–4.4 cm and 6 months for those of 4.5–5.4 cm would appear to be appropriate.

AAA repair

Currently available evidence supports elective surgical intervention for the treatment of asymptomatic AAAs of 5.5 cm diameter or greater, subject to evaluation of the patient's general health and fitness for surgery.

Investigation of the patient with known AAA

The aims of evaluation of patients diagnosed with an AAA are threefold:

1. to identify patients in whom the balance of risk favours operative intervention;
2. to reduce perioperative morbidity and mortality by identifying patients who may require further investigation or treatment of comorbidity prior to surgery;
3. to assess the anatomical suitability of the aneurysm for open or endovascular repair.

Accurate clinical assessment is imperative as it is recognised that perioperative mortality is related to the pre-existing physiological status of the patient.[20] The majority of early deaths following AAA repair are related to cardiac events and if pre-existing cardiac abnormalities are detected and treated prior to surgery, a substantial improvement in survival rates can potentially be achieved.[21] Respiratory complications are the most common form of morbidity after major abdominal surgery and occur after 25–50% of all such operations, including aortic aneurysm repair.[22] The risk of perioperative renal failure is increased in those with pre-existing renal disease, diabetes or coexisting cardiac disease, and in those aged over 60 years.

Preprocedural imaging

Ultrasound is useful for the initial detection and outpatient surveillance of an AAA. Preoperatively, virtually all elective patients now undergo more detailed cross-sectional imaging with contrast-enhanced computed tomography (CT). With thin-slice acquisition of data, multidetector row scanners provide excellent three-dimensional images from which to plan endovascular repair. Given the wide availability and high quality of multidetector CT angiography (MD-CTA), catheter angiography is rarely required preoperatively.

Elective open AAA repair

General anaesthesia is preferred, and is frequently combined with epidural anaesthesia for postoperative pain control. Epidural anaesthesia may be employed as the sole method, particularly in those patients with severe respiratory disease. At induction, a broad-spectrum antibiotic should be administered as prophylaxis against graft infection. An intravenous bolus of heparin should be given prior to clamp application.

> ✓ A trial conducted by the Joint Vascular Research Group of Great Britain and Ireland showed that while heparin does not have any influence on the risk of bleeding or thromboembolic complications, the incidence of perioperative myocardial infarction was reduced to 1.4% compared with 5.7% in patients who did not receive heparin.[23]

Although elective operative blood loss is usually minimal, excessive bleeding can occasionally be encountered either from back-bleeding lumbar arteries following opening of the sac or from the anastomotic suture lines. The routine use of a cell saver to preserve the patient's own red cells is a useful adjunct under these circumstances.[24]

The aorta is a longitudinal midline structure and most operations for aortic aneurysm repair involve proximal and distal anastomoses within the abdomen. Therefore, the preferred incision is longitudinal and midline and the approach transperitoneal. Alternatives include a transverse incision with a transperitoneal approach, and an oblique left-sided abdominal incision with an extraperitoneal approach, both of which may be advantageous in selected patients. With a transperitoneal approach, the intestines should be retained within the abdominal cavity, being packed to the right side and held in place with a suitable self-retaining retractor.

The aneurysm is exposed by incising the posterior parietal peritoneum and carefully mobilising the duodenum to the right. The renal vein marks the upper limit of dissection for an infrarenal aneurysm. Inferiorly, both common iliac arteries are dissected in preparation for clamping, care being taken to avoid damage to the hypogastric plexus of nerves in sexually active males. Minimal dissection is required to enable placement of clamps inserted from the front. Fabric grafts constructed from coated polyester (Dacron) or polytetrafluoroethylene may be used. Although ectatic dilatation of the common iliac arteries is commonly found in association with AAAs, true iliac aneurysms are comparatively infrequent. Therefore, 60–70% of AAAs can be repaired using a simple tube graft anastomosed to the infrarenal neck proximally and to the aortic bifurcation distally. In the remaining cases, it is necessary to use a bifurcated graft with anastomoses either to the common iliac bifurcation, or to the common femoral artery in the groin if the external iliac arteries are atheromatous or heavily calcified.

For repair of juxtarenal aneurysms, suprarenal clamping is essential. Under these circumstances, clamping of the supracoeliac aorta exposed through the lesser sac with separation of the fibres of the crura of the diaphragm may be preferable, since this allows more explicit exposure of the orifices of the renal arteries and less risk also of renal athero-embolisation than a clamp placed immediately above the renal arteries. A thoraco-abdominal approach with extraperitoneal exposure of the abdominal aorta is rarely necessary for juxtarenal aneurysms, but should be considered especially for obese patients in whom access is predicted to be problematical.

Minimally invasive open AAA repair

The advent of endovascular techniques has stimulated interest in developing other less invasive alternatives to conventional open surgery. These include shorter (6-cm) incisions and totally laparoscopic techniques.[25] Custom-made retractors and other instrumentation have been developed for these procedures. It is claimed that surgical trauma is reduced significantly, with benefits in terms of lower operative mortality and morbidity rates and more rapid recovery of the patients. However, to date, reliable comparative data are lacking.

Emergency open AAA repair

Successful emergency repair of ruptured AAAs relies on a precarious 'window of opportunity' when active bleeding is temporarily arrested by hypotension and tamponade of the haematoma by the posterior parietal peritoneum. In order to adequately conserve this clinical state, minimal resuscitation with permissive hypotension is desirable.

Survival following AAA rupture is poor in patients who have suffered a cardiac arrest, in the very elderly and in those who remain persistently unconscious. A decision not to offer surgical intervention to such patients is justified. Low or absent urinary output should not of itself be a contraindication to surgery, but its consideration within risk-scoring systems such as the Glasgow Aneurysm Score (see later) may help with appropriate patient selection for surgery.[26]

Outcome following open surgical AAA repair

Elective open surgical repair of AAAs has been shown to be an effective procedure with good graft durability.

✔✔ The Canadian Aneurysm Study demonstrated an in-hospital mortality rate of 4.7%, with a 5-year survival rate of 68%.[19] The UK Small Aneurysm Trial reported a 30-day mortality rate of 5.8% and the recent EVAR-1 trial a 30-day mortality rate of 4.7% in patients fit for surgery.[11,27]

Factors associated with a poorer outcome following open AAA repair include increased patient age, larger aneurysm size and the presence of preoperative renal failure.[28,29] In order to assist in the prediction of patients at high risk of perioperative mortality and morbidity after elective and ruptured AAA repair, the Glasgow Aneurysm Score (GAS) has been described.[26,30] In addition to the patient's age, differentially weighted patient-specific variables including the presence of cardiac, cerebrovascular and/or renal comorbidity with/without hypovolaemic shock are summed to yield a numerical value that can be extrapolated to a risk bracket (i.e. GAS = age ± cardiac disease (7 points) ± renal dysfunction (14 points) ± cerebrovascular disease (10 points) ± shock (17 points)). Naturally, the GAS alone should not dictate clinical practice, but it can serve as a useful adjunct for risk stratification in assessing a patient's suitability for AAA surgery.

✔✔ Another important determinant of patient outcome following AAA repair is the ability and experience of the operating surgeon. A recent meta-analysis demonstrated a significantly lower mortality following AAA repair with higher volume surgeons and suggested a minimum caseload of 13 open AAAs per annum for continued practice.[31] With further analysis, this number is likely to rise and, naturally, this has significant implications for the provision of vascular services and would support the argument for fewer, larger, regional vascular centres linked directly to a nationwide targeted AAA screening programme.

Patients with AAAs have a markedly decreased life expectancy in comparison with age- and sex-matched control populations. The 5-year survival of patients postsurgery varies from 62% to 72% (compared with 83–90% in age- and sex-matched populations), with the majority of deaths due to coronary artery disease.[21,28] Quality-of-life studies have shown an improved perception of general health in the first 2 years after open repair in comparison with patients who are under surveillance.[32]

The UK Small Aneurysm Trial showed that only about 25% of patients with ruptured aneurysms make it to theatre for emergency repair.[12] A subsequent meta-analysis showed that there has been a gradual improvement in survival following surgery for ruptured AAAs over the last 40 years of the order of 3.5% per decade. However, this study also showed that the estimate of operative mortality rate remains high at approximately 41%.[33]

Endovascular AAA repair (EVAR)

Since the first case of EVAR was reported by Parodi et al. in 1991,[34] this minimally invasive technique has become increasingly popular with both physicians and patients alike. The fundamental goal of EVAR is sustained aneurysm exclusion from the systemic circulation by means of a preoperatively sized stent graft, preventing further aneurysm expansion and therefore eliminating rupture risk (**Fig. 13.1**).

Indications and eligibility for EVAR

Originally developed as a treatment option for those where existing comorbidity prohibited open surgical repair, the current indications for EVAR are less clear. The approach may well be preferable in cases of a hostile abdomen (e.g. peritoneal adhesions, intestinal stomas) and also where the risk of iatrogenic injury is significant (e.g. IAAA repair).[35] In the absence of such factors and in fitter patients the role of EVAR remains in dispute.

Contrary to open AAA repair, EVAR suitability depends not only on patient fitness but also aneurysmal morphology. Limitations of contemporary endografts and their delivery platforms continue to preclude EVAR in many patients, with current elective eligibility rates quoted between 55% and 74%.[36,37] Features promoting EVAR suitability include a healthy proximal neck with limited angulation, at least 15 mm in length, no more than 30 mm in diameter and with smooth, parallel, endoluminal surfaces without significant mural thrombus. In addition the iliac arteries should be of sufficient calibre, at least 7 mm for most devices, to facilitate the passage of the delivery apparatus into the abdominal aorta. Short ectatic common iliac arteries represent relatively unfavourable anatomy for EVAR in view of the need for a reliable distal seal.[37,38]

EVAR devices

Four distinct generic schemes are currently available for EVAR of infrarenal AAAs: straight aorto-aortic tube endografts, bifurcated systems, aorto-mono-iliac systems and combined bifurcated and iliac branched stent grafts. All devices form their proximal seal within the infrarenal aortic segment but differences exist in the location of the distal 'landing site'. The pioneering aorto-aortic straight stent graft resides entirely in the abdominal aorta but is only suitable for a very limited number of cases. The published early experience of EVAR showed that where aorto-aortic tube endografts were used for fusiform aortic aneurysms, an unacceptably high incidence of late device failure occurred due to extension of the pathological process into the distal neck and aorto-iliac segments.[39] There is still, however, a place for such tube grafts in localised saccular aneurysms, postoperative pseudoaneurysms and penetrating aortic ulcers.

Bifurcated systems offer the best solution by providing the potential for distal fixation beyond the vascular segments most likely to suffer further aneurysmal expansion in the long term, while maintaining normal anatomical relations. The currently available standard bifurcated devices may be appropriate for use in up to 50% of patients,[40] although this figure is increasing as newer devices become available for the treatment of short and angulated proximal necks. The remainder of EVAR-eligible aneurysms with more challenging anatomy (including those with aorto-iliac aneurysms) require the use of branched stent grafts or the aorto-mono-iliac stent graft.[41] Aorto-mono-iliac endografts require an extra-anatomical (femoro-femoral) crossover graft for maintenance of contralateral lower limb blood supply, following endoluminal plugging of the contralateral common iliac artery. Iliac branched stent grafts are a relatively new and unproven development but provide an additional option for younger patients with bilateral aorto-iliac aneurysms.

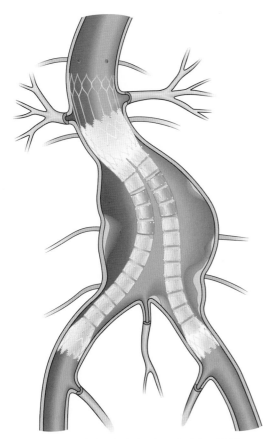

Figure 13.1 • Model depicting the principle of AAA repair using an aortic stent graft.

Patient assessment and EVAR technique

The patient should be formally assessed and prepared for EVAR as if for conventional open surgery. Detailed vascular imaging (preferably MD-CTA) should be obtained to enable calibration of the entire abdominal aorta and iliofemoral segments in order to enable graft sizing and provide information regarding arterial access. Informed consent should include the routine morbidity and also the known EVAR-specific complications, including contrast nephropathy, endoleak (see later) and open surgical conversion. Ideally, the theatre should be designed for combined interventional/operative procedures and equipped with a C-arm or equivalent for intra-operative imaging.

After anaesthetic induction the patient is appropriately positioned, prepped and draped. The procedure usually commences by surgical cut-down to the femoral artery to gain access to the arterial circulation, although some advocate a percutaneous approach[42,43] assisted by the increasing usage of femoral closure devices.[44] After femoral access is achieved, a soft wire and catheter are placed into the suprarenal aorta and a stiff guidewire is introduced through the catheter. Stiff guidewires are not intended to be 'working' wires and it is not sensible to try to negotiate tortuous iliac vessels with them. The stent graft body is introduced over the stiff guidewire and the renal arteries are imaged. The image intensifier should be angled to optimise the view of the renal arteries and this typically requires a small amount of cranio-caudal and oblique tilt.

An imaging catheter is left alongside the graft body as the top stents are released in stages and short angiographic runs should be performed to ensure precise positioning relative to the renal arteries. Modular devices require cannulation in situ of the short leg or 'stump' of the main body of the device prior to introduction of the contralateral limb. This is generally performed by a retrograde approach from the contralateral femoral artery using angled catheters. Confirmation of successful cannulation is needed to avoid the error of inadvertently deploying the contralateral limb alongside rather than within the main graft. The iliac limbs are deployed close to the internal iliac origins, which are defined using oblique projections. Substantial overlap at the modular connections is essential to avoid late disconnections.

Completion angiography is performed to determine whether the aneurysm has been excluded and to ensure that there has been no encroachment by the fabric of the graft on the orifices of the visceral or internal iliac arteries (**Fig. 13.2**). Every effort must be made to resolve all primary type I endoleak before the patient is allowed to leave the operating room.

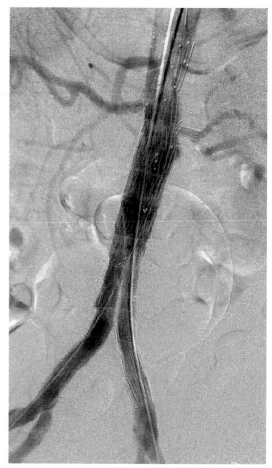

Figure 13.2 • On-table angiogram showing satisfactory fenestrated EVAR placement with good filling of both renal arteries and no evidence of endoleak.

EVAR-related complications and device failure

The physiological advantages of EVAR are reflected by the reduced requirement of postoperative critical care support and incidence of significant cardiac, pulmonary and renal complications. However, in addition to these routine causes of postoperative morbidity following AAA repair, EVAR unfortunately carries with it a distinct spectrum of its own specific complications.

Endoleak

Endoleak is defined as the persistence of blood flow outside the lumen of an endovascular graft but within an aneurysm sac or the adjacent vascular segment being treated by the stent.[45] The leak may be described as primary, originating at the time of EVAR, or secondary, referring to a leak not seen at completion angiography but demonstrated on subsequent imaging. Endoleaks have been classified according to the source of aberrant blood flow, since this characterises

Table 13.2 • Endoleak classification

Endoleak type		Source
I	A: Proximal	Graft attachment site
	B: Distal	
	C: Iliac occluder	
II	A: Simple (single vessel)	Collateral vessel
	B: Complex (>2 vessels)	
III	A: Junctional leak	Graft failure
	B: Mid-graft hole	
	C: Other (e.g. suture hole)	
IV		Graft wall porosity
V	A: Without endoleak	Endotension
	B: With sealed endoleak	
	C: With type I or III leak	
	D: With type II leak	

the endoleak and hence the potential for deleterious sequelae (Table 13.2).[46]

Endoleaks are clinically important since they can be associated with aneurysm enlargement and eventual rupture. This is most often seen in type I (**Fig. 13.3a**) and III (**Fig. 13.3c**) leaks that communicate directly with the aortic lumen, and secondary intervention is almost always necessary in these patients.

> ✅ Of 4291 patients enrolled in the EUROSTAR registry in 2002, analysis of 34 patients with recorded rupture following EVAR showed that type I and III endoleaks and severe modes of structural disintegration of stent grafts with or without migration were the most commonly documented findings at the time of rupture.[47]

Type II (**Fig. 13.3b**) endoleaks denote continued blood flow into the aneurysmal sac from refilling collateral vessels, typically the lumbar and inferior mesenteric arteries. The clinical significance of type II endoleaks is contentious and there is no standard treatment protocol. Many consider these leaks self-limiting and recommend an expectant management course. Others advise early corrective intervention, arguing that any endoleak signifies systemic repressurisation of the aneurysmal sac with reintroduction of rupture risk.[48] Data from the EUROSTAR registry suggested that although they do not warrant

urgent treatment, type II endoleaks are not harmless due to their observed association with aneurysm enlargement and reintervention.[49]

Transwall blood flow through an intact graft within 30 days of EVAR defines the type IV endoleak (**Fig. 13.3d**).[50] These leaks typically seal spontaneously and may be increasingly seen with the thinner and more porous later generation stents of today.

Graft migration and dislocation

Successful EVAR depends on the generation of a fluid-tight seal between stent graft and healthy native vessel for AAA exclusion. Failure at any attachment site renders the endograft insecure and prone to abnormal movement (migration) that is facilitated by systemic arterial blood pressure. Significant device migration at the seal zones predisposes the patient to endoleak (type I), whereas unwanted mobility of modular systems may lead to component dislocation and potential type III endoleak (Fig. 13.3c).

Device migration most likely results from the combined effect of patient and device-related factors with a proximal attachment site failure most often described[51] (**Fig. 13.4**). In view of the significant risk of type I endoleak associated with distal migration of the proximal stent, remedial intervention is almost always indicated. This can usually be achieved with aortic cuff deployment to repair the proximal seal, but occasionally stent revision is required.

Kinking and occlusion

Any distortion ('kinking') of the prosthetic conduit used in EVAR may result in stent stenosis, thrombosis and ultimately device (or limb) occlusion (see **Fig. 13.5**). In a review of 4613 EVAR cases submitted to the EUROSTAR registry over an 8-year period, postoperative graft kinking was described in 3.7% of cases.[52] Patent, symptomatic kinked stents can usually be treated by an endovascular approach (angioplasty or stenting) whereas occluded limbs typically require surgery.

Other EVAR-related complications

Stent manipulation within the aneurysmal sac during positioning and device deployment carries the risk of distal microembolisation of debris with potential for organ infarcts and limb ischaemia.[53–55] Introduction of guidewires, large-bore catheters and the endograft itself risks vessel injury such as rupture or dissection. Delayed presentations of iatrogenic arterial injury may occur with pseudo-aneurysm formation requiring prompt repair.

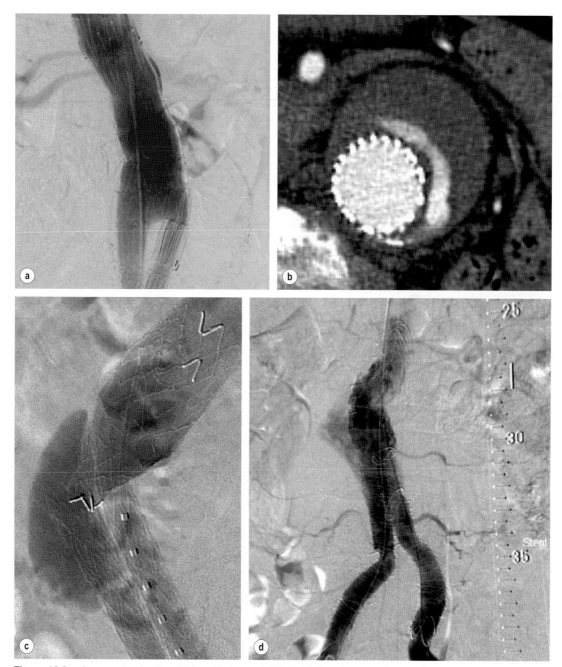

Figure 13.3 • Images showing type I–IV endoleaks post-EVAR. **(a)** Completion angiogram showing a type I endoleak (proximal seal failure). **(b)** Post-EVAR contrast-enhanced CT scan showing a type II endoleak. **(c)** Delayed angiogram showing a type III endoleak (junctional graft failure). **(d)** Completion angiogram showing a type IV endoleak (graft porosity).

Surveillance after EVAR

The modes of failure after endovascular grafting are well documented. It is mandatory that all patients are recruited on to a programme of systematic postoperative surveillance with the aim of detecting causes of late rupture. The principal concerns are graft-related endoleak, aneurysm enlargement and migration of stents at the aortic or iliac landing zones or at the modular connections. Options for the method of surveillance include ultrasound, CT, magnetic resonance imaging (MRI) and plain radiography.

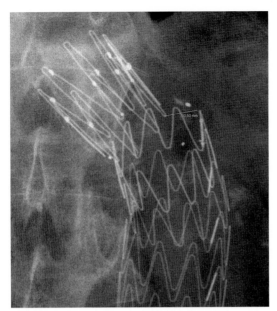

Figure 13.4 • Post-EVAR imaging showing proximal stent graft migration and impending endograft disruption.

It has been shown that ultrasound can be used to detect graft-related (type I) endoleaks reliably.[56] Ultrasound is less effective for the detection of type II endoleaks, but since it is known that type II endoleaks without increased sac diameter are not associated with a significant risk of adverse clinical events, this may be regarded as an acceptable limitation. Plain radiography using a standardised protocol is an effective method for the detection of device migration.[57] Stent fractures and separation of modular components are also relatively easy to identify. It is comparatively inexpensive and usefully complements ultrasound scanning. Used in combination these two methods represent a potentially acceptable alternative to CT for surveillance.

It is generally accepted that surveillance after EVAR should be lifelong. The surveillance intervals vary but typically include baseline imaging with CT and plain radiography at 1 month after EVAR. Most protocols include more frequent surveillance intervals during the first 2 years, with annual surveillance thereafter.

Outcomes after EVAR

Publication of two large multicentre European randomised controlled trials has finally provided some of the level I evidence required to support the continued use of EVAR in the normal AAA population.

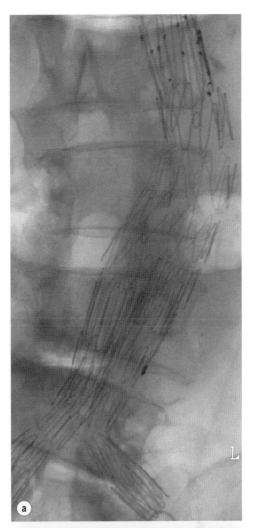

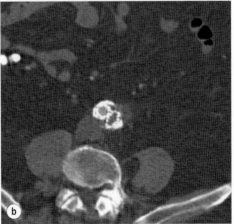

Figure 13.5 • Post-EVAR imaging showing graft kinking and occlusion in the same patient. **(a)** Plain film showing left iliac limb kinking. **(b)** Contrast-enhanced CT scan showing consequent intraluminal occlusion.

✔️✔️ The UK EVAR-1 trial enrolled 1082 patients with suitable aneurysms (mean diameter 65 mm) that were considered fit enough for elective open AAA surgery and randomised them to either EVAR or conventional open repair (OR). Early outcome analysis revealed significantly lower 30-day mortality for the EVAR group (1.7%) compared to open surgical controls (4.7%).[27] Medium-term study follow-up reported EVAR to be as effective as surgery in protecting from late aneurysm-related death, although there was a significantly higher rate of graft-related complications following EVAR (35% vs. 8%).[58] In a smaller but similarly designed study, the Dutch DREAM trial compared outcome following EVAR and OR in 345 fit patients. A significantly lower operative mortality rate post-EVAR was confirmed (1.2% vs. 4.6%) with reduced incidence of early severe postoperative complications.[59] At 2-year follow-up, however, there was no observed survival advantage after EVAR or OR.[60] A recent meta-analysis of 42 trials involving 21 178 patients comparing open AAA repair with EVAR has reinforced these favourable EVAR findings.[61]

Renal failure after EVAR is associated with an increased rate of mortality and its aetiology is probably multifactorial. Implicated factors include radiological contrast-associated nephropathy, renal artery trauma, stent-induced stenosis and aortic neck thromboembolism following vessel instrumentation and manipulation.[62] It is rare for the renal ostia to be inadvertently covered by graft fabric, and careful planning and deployment decrease the risk of this occurring. There was concern that the introduction of suprarenal bare-stent fixation would lead to increased rates of renal failure, especially in patients with pre-existing renal impairment; however, studies have failed to demonstrate this.[62,63]

✔️✔️ The long-term results of the EVAR studies have recently been published.[64] In the EVAR-1 trial, these show that EVAR is not associated with a long-term survival benefit when compared with open repair, with 54% of patients remaining alive in each group after 8 years. Therefore, other long-term outcomes are of great importance to more than half of the patients and, in particular, new endograft-related complications and reinterventions were reported throughout the period of follow-up.

The reporting of new endograft-related complications, in the EVAR group, was highest within the first 6 months of aneurysm repair (48.7 new complications per 100 patient-years of follow-up), reducing to 9.0 new complications per 100 patient-years of follow-up between 6 months and 4 years, and 5.1 new complications per 100 person-years beyond 4 years: these rates are much higher than those reported after open repair, although this is not without complications. In addition, there were 25 secondary ruptures in the EVAR group, compared to 0 in the open group, suggesting that EVAR might not be as durable as open repair in the longer term.

These long-term results question the durability of EVAR and for the moment there is no better evidence. The EVAR trials have now closed and further follow-up data will not be forthcoming.[65] Therefore, the careful long-term follow-up and reporting of patients undergoing EVAR in 2010 and onwards is essential, probably through well-organised registries such as those in Sweden and Finland,[66,67] with some justification for mandatory participation. It is also possible that the uncertainty about the long-term durability of EVAR might swing patient preferences away from endovascular repair; patient preference should now be a key feature in determining the choice of technique for aneurysm repair.

✔️✔️ The UK EVAR-2 trial randomised 338 medically unfit patients who were anatomical candidates for endovascular AAA repair (>55 mm) to either EVAR or best medical therapy. The early mortality in the EVAR limb was 9% and at a mean follow-up of 3.3 years there was no difference in either the all-cause or aneurysm-related mortality between the groups.[68] Many clinicians have adopted these findings as justification not to offer EVAR in the higher-risk population. Caution is advised against this approach to management as closer scrutiny of the EVAR-2 results reveals some complicating issues. Firstly, there appeared to be an unacceptable delay from randomisation to treatment in the EVAR limb, so that nearly half (9 of 20) of the aneurysm-related mortality was explained by rupture prior to planned AAA repair. Operative (EVAR) mortality was surprisingly high (9%) and the rupture rate in the medically treated group (9 per 100 person-years) was significantly lower than expected, raising concern about disparate medical management between the two groups. Clearly, though, EVAR-2 demonstrates the poor long-term prognosis of the unfit AAA patient irrespective of treatment, with only 62–66% alive at 4 years.

The long-term follow-up of the EVAR-2 trial shows that after 8 years EVAR is associated with much improved aneurysm-related survival (86% at 6 years vs. 64% for no intervention), although no clear difference in all-cause survival was observed (30%

at 6 years vs. 26%).[69] The ability of EVAR to reduce aneurysm rupture (and aneurysm-related mortality) but not to improve survival is the sting in the tail for EVAR. However, after 8 years less than 20% of the patients remained alive, so that the long-term outcomes for these patients might carry less weight than for those enrolled in EVAR trial 1.[65]

For the majority of patients EVAR still provides short-term but not long-term benefits but it is clear that long-term surveillance cannot be dispensed with, although this may not need to be through regular CT scans. For the very frail patient with multiple comorbidities, if life expectancy is adequate then EVAR after appropriate medical optimisation may bring some benefits; if life expectancy is short, EVAR is unlikely to bring any benefits. Future work modelling the extent of any benefit in subgroups may help clarify this issue.[65] Clinical decision-making skills clearly remain of crucial importance in the management of patients with large aneurysms.

The future of EVAR

There is little doubt that the principles of EVAR are particularly attractive in the case of AAA rupture, with several groups advocating its role. Avoidance of laparotomy confers a marked physiological advantage over open repair in an already dire situation.[70] However, the urgency associated with ruptured AAA repair results in little or no time being available to gather the required morphological information prior to EVAR. This is of particular importance since these aneurysms tend to have shorter and wider necks and are therefore more challenging for EVAR with current devices.[71] Furthermore, the requirement of a permanently available on-call endovascular team with access to the appropriate facilities for EVAR is a significant obstacle in most centres.[72]

A randomised controlled trial (IMPROVE) is currently recruiting and is designed to determine whether a policy of endovascular repair improves the survival of all patients with ruptured AAA.[73] Recruitment started in October 2009 and 600 patients are required to show a 14% survival benefit at 30 days (primary outcome) for the endovascular first policy. Recruitment will be from the UK and Europe. Secondary outcomes include 24-h, in-hospital and 1-year survival and complications. Until the results of this and similar trials are available, patients with ruptured AAA should only be offered EVAR within the confines of a national registry or clinical trial.

The anatomical requirements for conventional endoluminal grafts exclude many patients from

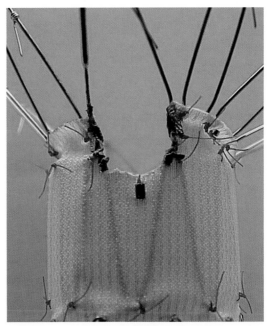

Figure 13.6 • Scalloped stent graft used for the endovascular treatment of AAA with short proximal necks.

elective repair, primarily because of an unsuitable infrarenal aortic neck. The transrenal and juxtarenal aorta can be used to create a neck if holes or fenestrations are custom-manufactured in the graft to precise preoperative plans. The early data on the use of these devices are promising.[74,75] Fenestrations may be one of three types: scalloped, large or small. Scalloped grafts have a U-shaped defect in the leading edge of the endografts for preserved patency of the most proximal visceral arteries (**Fig. 13.6**). Both of the other types of fenestration reside in the body of the device fabric (**Fig. 13.7**). Large fenestrations are traversed by the bare metal scaffold, whereas small fenestrations lie between stent struts and require secondary stenting to achieve a seal and prevent occlusion.[76]

A meta-analysis of fenestrated endovascular aneurysm repair (FEVAR) has recently been published with the aim to highlight current issues around the evidence for the potential benefit of FEVAR.[77] Eleven studies were identified describing a total of 660 procedures. Definitions of aneurysm morphology were variable, and clear inclusion and exclusion criteria were not always documented. Double fenestrations were more common than triple or quadruple fenestrations. Target vessel perfusion rates ranged from 90.5% to 100%. Eleven deaths occurred within 30 days, giving a 30-day proportional mortality rate of 2.0%. Morbidity was poorly reported. The authors conclude that

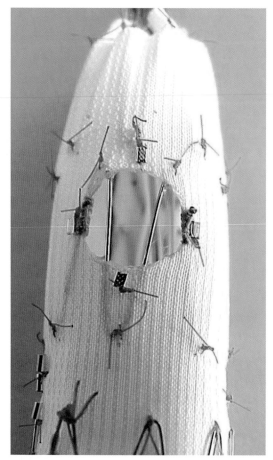

Figure 13.7 • Fenestrated stent graft used for the treatment of perirenal aortic aneurysms. Courtesy of Cook Medical.

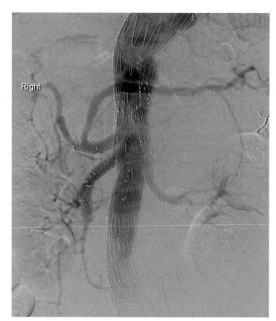

Figure 13.8 • Intraoperative arteriogram showing a completed four-branched stent graft.

FEVAR for repair of suprarenal and juxtarenal aneurysms is a viable alternative to open repair. However, there is no level I evidence for FEVAR, and current evidence is weak, with many unanswered questions.

A similar conclusion must be drawn for branched endografts[78] and snorkel[79] procedures. Although good early results have been published for distal branches used to preserve flow in hypogastric arteries,[78] we await studies to prove the long-term results of these techniques in the treatment of aortic arch and thoraco-abdominal aneurysms (**Fig. 13.8**). Available evidence of efficacy is currently restricted to case reports and a few case series.[80–82] Concerns about these devices include uncertainty regarding the long-term patency of stents in normal branch vessels, the increased number of modular connections and the possibility that the branches may kink if the aneurysm shrinks. Nevertheless, this technology is advancing rapidly and 'off-the-shelf' fenestrated grafts will soon become readily available, and will inevitably result in an increase in numbers of patients treated.[83]

Infected aneurysms

Although much less common than degenerative pathology, infected aneurysms remain an important subgroup of the disease. Since the introduction of antibiotic therapy and concomitant decline of endocarditis, true mycotic aneurysms are now rarely seen. Conversely, with increasingly invasive medical investigation and intravenous drug addiction (IVDA), post-traumatic infected false femoral aneurysms are now a major clinical problem confronting the vascular specialist. These are discussed in more detail in the section on femoral aneurysms.

True mycotic aneurysms

True mycotic aneurysms result when septic emboli of cardiac source (endocarditis) lodge in the vasa vasorum or lumen of an artery. The patients tend to be middle-aged (30–50 years) and may have multiple aneurysms at differing sites. Both normal and abnormal vessels can be affected and although the pathology has a predilection for the aorta, intracranial, visceral and femoral arteries, any vessel can be affected. The usual infecting agents are

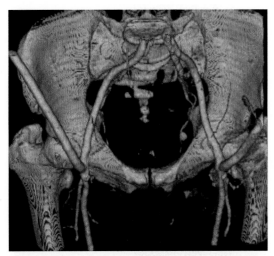

Figure 13.9 • CT reconstruction of a peripheral seeded mycotic aneurysm of the left internal pudendal artery in a patient with an infected aortic stent graft.

Gram-positive cocci, in particular *Streptococcus* spp. and *Staphylococcus aureus*.[84]

Microbial aneurysmal arteritis

With the ageing population and increasing incidence of atherosclerosis, microbial arteritis with aneurysm formation is now more frequently seen than the true mycotic aneurysm. The pathological process involves blood-borne bacteria 'seeding' into diseased arterial intima with subsequent suppuration, localised perforation and pseudo-aneurysm formation (**Fig. 13.9**). Contrary to mycotic aneurysms, healthy native vessels are not affected, atherosclerosis being the prime predisposing factor. Aortic involvement is typical, pathology in this location being three times more common than in the peripheral circulation. The classical infecting micro-organisms are the *Salmonella* spp., but others have been reported, including *Escherichia coli*, *Staphylococcus* spp. and *Klebsiella pneumoniae*.[85]

Clinical features and management principles of infected aneurysms

The clinical presentation of an infected aneurysm depends both on the site of involvement and underlying infective process. Usually, the patient presents with pyrexia of unknown origin and little else; therefore, a high index of suspicion is required. Supporting features include positive blood cultures, leucocytosis, uncalcified aneurysms, vertebral erosion and a first presentation of aneurysm following an episode of bacterial sepsis. Classical radiological appearances on angiography may or may not be present: saccular aneurysm, multilobulated and/or eccentric pathology with a narrow neck.

Following diagnosis, all patients should be commenced on appropriate antibiotic therapy. Unless the patient's general fitness is prohibitive, the definitive management plan is surgical. The principles of surgery for an infected aneurysm are generic, irrespective of site, and include: haemorrhage control, sepsis control (aneurysm resection, wide debridement, irrigation and drainage); confirmation of diagnosis (specimen cultures and sensitivity); and arterial reconstruction with autologous conduit, e.g. superficial femoral vein harvest for aortic disease. Postoperatively, the patient should be prescribed a prolonged course of antibiotics that may be lifelong in some cases.[84] Some authors have advocated using endovascular stents for a definitive treatment of mycotic aneurysms.[86] These can provide good short- and medium-term results, but data regarding long-term efficacy are poor.

Despite recent improvements in diagnosis, surgical techniques and pharmacology, the early outcome for patients with infected aortic aneurysms remains poor, with a mortality rate of 23%. Infected post-traumatic peripheral false aneurysms are associated with better survival (5% mortality), but the lower limb amputation rate can be up to 25–33% if the femoral artery is involved.

Peripheral aneurysms

Iliac aneurysms

Iliac aneurysms usually occur in association with aortic aneurysms. Isolated iliac aneurysms are comparatively unusual, the prevalence having been estimated to be less than 2% of that of aorto-iliac aneurysms. They tend to be large (4–8 cm) and typically involve either the common or internal iliac arteries. Aneurysmal disease of the external iliac artery is extremely rare.

Generally accepted guidance is that elective open or endovascular intervention is indicated for asymptomatic iliac aneurysms greater than 3–4 cm in diameter. Symptomatic and ruptured aneurysms require immediate surgical intervention.

Common femoral aneurysms

Femoral arterial aneurysms can be divided simply into true or false (pseudo) aneurysms. True aneurysms relate to a distinct pathological process involving all three layers of the femoral arterial wall. False aneurysms are so called due to their clinical mimicry of true disease but are, in actual fact, a vessel-associated contained blood collection and typically result from trauma.

Both disease processes may be symptomatic or asymptomatic. Symptomatic femoral aneurysms can present as a pulsatile groin mass that may or may not be painful, leg swelling (due to femoral vein compression and deep vein thrombosis) or features associated with chronic ischaemia attributable to aneurysm thrombosis/embolisation. Rupture can occur but is rare. Asymptomatic pathology is usually discovered incidentally on clinical examination of a patient with an aneurysm elsewhere or with chronic limb ischaemia.

True femoral aneurysms

True femoral aneurysms are the second commonest peripheral aneurysm after the popliteal artery. They occur in between 2% and 3% of patients with aortic aneurysms and tend to be a disease of elderly men (male to female ratio 30:1). The condition is frequently bilateral and a coexistent generalised aneurysmal process may be manifest in other anatomical sites such as the aorto-iliac or popliteal arteries.

Small, asymptomatic true femoral artery aneurysms can be managed expectantly with clinical assessment at intervals. Surgical treatment is indicated for symptoms and probably for most aneurysms of 3 cm or more in size. Usually, a short interposition or inlay tube graft anastomosed proximally at the level of the inguinal ligament and distal to the common femoral bifurcation is required. This is a relatively small operation with durable results.

False femoral aneurysms

Due to its ease of access and the trend for more invasive medical investigation and treatment (e.g. angiography, cardiac catheterisation, EVAR, intra-aortic balloon pumps, etc.), iatrogenic injury leading to false aneurysm is a relatively common occurrence that complicates approximately 1% of transfemoral interventions. The diagnosis should be suspected in any patient with a pulsatile mass at the site of a recent arterial cannulation (**Fig. 13.10**). Initially, a duplex scan should be obtained to both confirm the diagnosis and characterise the false aneurysm. If the pathology is small and associated with minimal symptoms, simple observation with re-scanning may be justified as most of these pseudo-aneurysms will thrombose spontaneously within 2–4 weeks. Other options include compression therapy (direct pressure and/or ultrasound guided) in an effort to seal the feeding arterial jet. Thrombin injection is an effective treatment with a reported success rate of over 95%. If these measures fail or in cases of tense swelling, threatened skin viability or neurology, open surgical repair is indicated. Unlike non-invasive methods, surgery

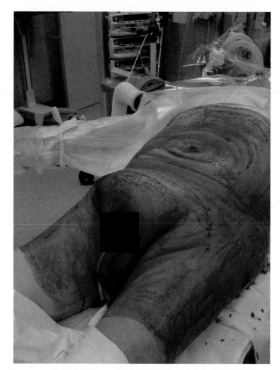

Figure 13.10 • Operative photograph showing a large right false femoral aneurysm.

has the advantage of combining both the arterial repair and field decompression. The former is usually a primary repair of the vessel with a prolene suture, although formal graft reconstruction is sometimes required.[87]

Infected femoral pseudo-aneurysms are now the most common type of infected aneurysm observed in clinical practice, largely explained by increased intravenous drug abuse in recent years. Although the usual micro-organism cultured is a *Staphylococcus* species, the infection may be polymicrobial and close liaison with the microbiology team is required for appropriate antibiotic therapy. The surgical strategy for infected femoral false aneurysms depends largely on its cause. For non-IVDA patients, arterial excision and reconstruction with autologous conduit (e.g. long saphenous vein and obturator bypass) following the operative principles for infected aneurysms outlined earlier is preferred. In the IVDA patient, arterial excision with ligation alone (i.e. no reconstruction) is advised due to the unacceptable risk of subsequent graft infection with continued drug abuse. Ligation of the femoral artery does not necessarily mandate amputation if only one femoral segment is involved. If the femoral bifurcation is excised, however, the risk of limb loss is significant and reconstructive surgery may need to be considered, although this is contentious.[84]

Popliteal artery aneurysms

Popliteal aneurysms are the most commonly encountered peripheral aneurysm, accounting for more than 80% of all peripheral aneurysms. The ratio of popliteal aneurysms to AAAs is approximately 1:15. Half are bilateral, a third asymptomatic and 40% are associated with AAAs.

Although rupture is rare, 50% of cases present with peripheral limb-threatening ischaemia. In common with aneurysms at all other sites, laminated thrombus develops within popliteal aneurysms. The popliteal artery is continually subjected to flexion and extension, greatly increasing the risk of disintegration and embolisation of this thrombus. In many patients, microembolisation of the peripheral circulation occurs silently prior to main vessel occlusion or thrombosis of the popliteal aneurysm itself. For this reason, the viability of the limb may be seriously threatened. Furthermore, compromise of the run-off circulation can impact adversely on the outcome from emergency bypass surgery. The bigger the aneurysm, the more likely there is to be thrombus. The presence of intraluminal thrombus is therefore a more important indication for elective surgical intervention than the size of the aneurysm. Any thrombus detected by ultrasound, CT or MRI constitutes an indication for elective treatment. In the absence of laminated thrombus, it is generally accepted that aneurysms with a diameter of 2 cm or greater warrant consideration for elective surgical repair.

Traditionally, popliteal aneurysms are treated by proximal and distal ligation and bypass using autologous vein undertaken via a medial approach. However, recent studies have identified persistent flow within the popliteal aneurysm in 30% of patients treated in this way.[88] Furthermore, there is a significant risk of continued expansion and even rupture due to pressurisation of the sac resulting from backflow through geniculate branches. Therefore, a posterior approach and insertion of an inlay graft is to be preferred.

An acutely thrombosed popliteal aneurysm is a clinical emergency. Preoperative or on-table thrombolysis has been used to open up the run-off vessels and thereby facilitate bypass surgery. There is some low-level evidence to suggest that this approach may improve the chances of successful limb salvage.[89]

With the evolution of flexible endografts, endovascular repair is now a viable alternative to open surgery for the treatment of some popliteal aneurysms.[90] Long-term follow-up suggests that in selected patients this is a durable technique, capable of achieving excellent patency rates and limb preservation.[91] Further large-scale clinical trials are warranted to help define optimal candidates for this technique.

Aneurysms of the upper limb, carotid and visceral arteries are discussed in their respective chapters.

Key points

- The prevalence of AAAs has increased dramatically over the last four decades, but this trend appears to be reversing.
- The clinical and financial cases for the introduction of a targeted population-based screening for AAAs are convincing.
- The Small Aneurysm Trial did not support a policy of early operative intervention for patients with AAAs of less than 5.5 cm diameter.
- Surgeons working in large-volume hospitals have lower mortality rates.
- The UK EVAR-1 trial reported a significant difference in the 30-day mortality, with 1.7% mortality in the EVAR group compared with 4.7% in those allocated to open repair, but the results are equivalent at 8 years.
- Both the EVAR-1 and DREAM trials confirm EVAR to be at least as effective as open repair in the prevention of aneurysm-related death in the longer term.
- EVAR requires annual surveillance and has an annual reintervention rate of 10%.
- EVAR should be used with caution in patients who are unfit for open surgery as 50% will die within 5 years, mostly from their comorbidity rather than rupture.
- Infected true aneurysms are associated with a poor prognosis but their incidence is declining.
- Post-traumatic false aneurysms are the most common infected aneurysms in clinical practice today and reflect both more invasive medical practice and intravenous drug abuse.

References

1. Johnston KW, Rutherford RB, Tilson MD, et al. Suggested standards for reporting on arterial aneurysms. Subcommittee on Reporting Standards for Arterial Aneurysms, Ad Hoc Committee on Reporting Standards, Society for Vascular Surgery and North American Chapter, International Society for Cardiovascular Surgery. J Vasc Surg 1991;13:452–8.

2. Ashton HA, Buxton MJ, Day NE, et al. The Multicentre Aneurysm Screening Study (MASS) into the effect of abdominal aortic aneurysm screening on mortality in men: a randomised controlled trial. Lancet 2002;360:1531–9.
   A UK multicentre population-based screening study of 67 800 men, aged 65–74 years, who were randomly allocated to be invited to attend for ultrasound assessment or not. The primary outcome measure was aneurysm-related death and there was a 42% risk reduction in the invited group.

3. Lucarotti M, Shaw E, Poskitt K, et al. The Gloucestershire Aneurysm Screening Programme: the first 2 years' experience. Eur J Vasc Surg 1993;7:397–401.

4. Norman PE, Jamrozik K, Lawrence-Brown M, et al. Population based randomised controlled trial on impact of screening on mortality from abdominal aortic aneurysm. Br Med J 2004;329:1259–62.

5. Vardulaki KA, Walker NM, Day NE, et al. Quantifying the risks of hypertension, age, sex and smoking in patients with abdominal aortic aneurysm. Br J Surg 2000;87:195–200.

6. Anjum A, Powell JT. Is the incidence of abdominal aortic aneurysm declining in the 21st century? Mortality and hospital admissions for England & Wales and Scotland. Eur J Vasc Endovasc Surg 2012;43(2):161–6. Epub 2011 Dec 16.

7. Cutler BS, Darling RC. Surgical management of arteriosclerotic femoral aneurysms. Surgery 1973;74:764–73.

8. Wassef M, Baxter T, Chisholm RL, et al. Pathogenesis of abdominal aortic aneurysms: a multidisciplinary research program supported by the National Heart, Lung and Blood Institute. J Vasc Surg 2001;34:730–8.

9. Ailawadi G, Eliason JL, Upchurch GR. Current concepts in the pathogenesis of abdominal aortic aneurysm. J Vasc Surg 2003;38:584–8.

10. Longo GM, Xiong W, Greiner TC, et al. Matrix metalloproteinases 2 and 9 work in concert to produce aortic aneurysms. J Clin Invest 2002;110:625–32.

11. Lederle FA, Johnson GR, Wilson SE, et al. Prevalence and associations of abdominal aortic aneurysm detected through screening. Aneurysm Detection and Management (ADAM) Veterans Affairs Cooperative Study Group. Ann Intern Med 1997;126:441–9.

12. The UK Small Aneurysm Trial Participants. Mortality results for randomised controlled trial of early elective surgery or ultrasound surveillance for small abdominal aortic aneurysms. Lancet 1998;352(9141):1649–55.
    A multicentre randomised controlled trial of 1090 patients with asymptomatic aneurysms of diameter 4.0–5.5 cm were randomly allocated to early elective surgery or ultrasound surveillance. There was no significant survival advantage at 6 years for those undergoing surgical repair.

13. Walker DI, Bloor K, Williams G, et al. Inflammatory aneurysms of the abdominal aorta. Br J Surg 1972;59:609–14.

14. Rasmussen TE, Hallett JW. Inflammatory aortic aneurysms: a clinical review with new perspectives in pathogenesis. Ann Surg 1997;225:155–64.

15. Lindholt JS, Vammen S, Juul S, et al. The validity of ultrasonographic scanning as screening method for abdominal aortic aneurysm. Eur J Vasc Endovasc Surg 1999;17:472–5.

16. Emerton ME, Shaw E, Poskitt K, et al. Screening for abdominal aortic aneurysm: a single scan is enough. Br J Surg 1994;81:1112–3.

17. Multicentre Aneurysm Screening Study Group. Multicentre Aneurysm Screening Study (MASS): cost effectiveness analysis of screening for abdominal aortic aneurysms based on four year results from randomised controlled trial. Br Med J 2002;325:1135.
    See also Ref. 2. Cost-effectiveness analysis at 4 years showed that the cost per quality-adjusted life-year was £36 000. It is projected that this value will fall to £8000 per quality-adjusted life-year at 10 years, which is well below the funding threshold in the UK health service.

18. Thompson SG, Ashton HA, Gao L, et al., Multicentre Aneurysm Screening Study Group. Screening men for abdominal aortic aneurysm: 10 year mortality and cost effectiveness results from the randomised Multicentre Aneurysm Screening Study. Br Med J 2009 Jun 24; 338:b2307. http://dx.doi.org/10.1136/bmj.b2307.

19. Law MR, Morris J, Wald NJ. Screening for abdominal aortic aneurysms. J Med Screen 1994;1:110–5.

20. Katz DJ, Stanley JC, Zelenock GB. Operative mortality rates for intact and ruptured abdominal aortic aneurysms in Michigan: an eleven-year statewide experience. J Vasc Surg 1994;19:804–15.

21. Johnston KW. Non-ruptured abdominal aortic aneurysm: six-year follow-up results from the multicenter prospective Canadian aneurysm study. Canadian Society for Vascular Surgery Aneurysm Study Group. J Vasc Surg 1994;20:163–70.
    A prospective analysis of 680 patients undergoing elective aneurysm surgery showed that cardiac-related death is the major perioperative risk and cardiac and cerebrovascular events are the major causes of death at 6 years.

22. Zibrak JD, O'Donnell CR, Marton K. Indications for pulmonary function testing. Ann Intern Med 1990;112:763–71.

23. Thompson JF, Mullee MA, Bell PR, et al. Intraoperative heparinisation, blood loss and myocardial infarction during aortic aneurysm surgery: a Joint Vascular Research Group study. Eur J Vasc Endovasc Surg 1996;12:86–90.

24. Goodnough LT, Monk TG, Sicard G, et al. Intraoperative salvage in patients undergoing elective abdominal aortic aneurysm repair: an analysis of cost and benefit. J Vasc Surg 1996;24:213–8.

25. Kolvenbach R, Schwierz E, Wasilljew S, et al. Total laparoscopically and robotically assisted aortic aneurysm surgery: a critical evaluation. J Vasc Surg 2004;39:771–6.

26. Samy AK, Murray G, MacBain G. Glasgow Aneurysm Score. Cardiovasc Surg 1994;2:41–4.

27. Greenhalgh RM, Brown LC, Kwong GP, et al. Comparison of endovascular aneurysm repair with open repair in patients with abdominal aortic aneurysm (EVAR trial 1), 30-day operative mortality results: randomised controlled trial. Lancet 2004;364:843–8.
   A multicentre randomised controlled trial comparing open and endovascular repair in patients anatomically suitable for either. The 30-day mortality results show an initial survival advantage for patients treated with EVAR.

28. Batt M, Staccini P, Pittaluga P, et al. Late survival after abdominal aortic aneurysm repair. Eur J Vasc Endovasc Surg 1999;17:338–42.

29. Sahal M, Prusa AM, Wibmer A, et al. Elective abdominal aortic aneurysm repair: does the aneurysm diameter influence long-term survival? Eur J Vasc Endovasc Surg 2008;35:288–94.

30. Korhonen SJ, Ylonen K, Biancari F, et al. Glasgow aneurysm score as a predictor of immediate outcome after surgery for ruptured abdominal aortic aneurysm. Br J Surg 2004;91:1449–52.

31. Young EL, Holt PJE, Poloniecki JD, et al. Meta-analysis and systematic review of the relationship between surgeon annual caseload and mortality for elective open abdominal aortic aneurysm repairs. J Vasc Surg 2007;46:1287–94.
   A meta-analysis involving 115 273 elective open AAA repairs demonstrating significantly lower mortality with higher caseload surgeons. The study suggested a critical case volume threshold of 13 open AAA repairs per annum.

32. Lederle FA, Johnson GR, Wilson SE, et al. Quality of life, impotence, and activity level in a randomized trial of immediate repair versus surveillance of small abdominal aortic aneurysm. J Vasc Surg 2003;38:745–52.

33. Bown MJ, Sutton AJ, Bell PR, et al. A meta-analysis of 50 years of ruptured abdominal aortic aneurysm repair. Br J Surg 2002;89:714–30.

34. Parodi JC, Palmaz JC, Barone HD. Transfemoral intraluminal graft implantation for abdominal aortic aneurysms. Ann Vasc Surg 1991;5:491–9.

35. Hinchliffe RJ, Macierewicz JA, Hopkinson BR. Endovascular repair of inflammatory abdominal aortic aneurysms. J Endovasc Ther 2002;9:277–81.

36. Wolf YG, Fogarty TJ, Olcott CIV, et al. Endovascular repair of abdominal aortic aneurysms: eligibility rate and impact on the rate of open repair. J Vasc Surg 2000;32:519–23.

37. Arko FR, Filis KA, Seidel SA, et al. How many patients with infrarenal aneurysms are candidates for endovascular repair? The Northern California experience. J Endovasc Ther 2004;11:33–40.

38. Dillavou ED, Muluk SC, Rhee RY, et al. Does hostile neck anatomy preclude successful endovascular aortic aneurysm repair? J Vasc Surg 2003;38:657–63.

39. Faries PL, Briggs VL, Rhee JY, et al. Failure of endovascular aortoaortic tube grafts: a plea for preferential use of bifurcated grafts. J Vasc Surg 2002;35:868–73.

40. Simons P, van Overhagen H, Nawijn A, et al. Endovascular aneurysm repair with a bifurcated endovascular graft at a primary referral center: influence of experience, age, gender, and aneurysm size on suitability. J Vasc Surg 2003;38:758–61.

41. Moore WS, Brewster DC, Bernhard VM. Aorto-uni-iliac endograft for complex aortoiliac aneurysms compared with tube/bifurcation endografts: results of the EVT/Guidant trials. J Vasc Surg 2001;33:S11–20.

42. Morasch MD, Kibbe MR, Evans ME, et al. Percutaneous repair of abdominal aortic aneurysm. J Vasc Surg 2004;40:12–6.

43. Perdikides TP, Georgiadis GS, Avgerinos ED, et al. Percutaneous endovascular treatment of aortic aneurysms: Clinical evaluation and literature results. Minim Invasive Ther Allied Technol 2011; Nov 29. Epub ahead of print.

44. Georgiadis GS, Antoniou GA, Papaioakim M, et al. A meta-analysis of outcome after percutaneous endovascular aortic aneurysm repair using different size sheaths or endograft delivery systems. J Endovasc Ther 2011;18(4):445–59.

45. White GH, Yu W, May J. Endoleak: a proposed new terminology to describe incomplete aneurysm exclusion by an endoluminal graft. J Endovasc Surg 1996;3:124–5.

46. Veith FJ, Baum RA, Ohki T, et al. Nature and significance of endoleaks and endotension: summary of opinions expressed at an international conference. J Vasc Surg 2002;35:1029–35.

47. Fransen GA, Vallabhaneni Sr SR, van Marrewijk CJ, et al. Rupture of infra-renal aortic aneurysm after endovascular repair: a series from EUROSTAR registry. Eur J Vasc Endovasc Surg 2003;26:487–93.

48. Choke E, Thompson MM. Endoleak after endovascular aneurysm repair: current concepts. J Cardiovasc Surg (Torino) 2004;45:349–66.

49. van Marrewijk CJ, Fransen G, Laheij RJF, et al. Is a type II endoleak after EVAR a harbinger of risk? Causes and outcome of open conversion and aneurysm rupture during follow-up. Eur J Vasc Endovasc Surg 2004;27:128–37.

50. Chaikof E, Blankensteijn J, Harris P, et al. Reporting standards for endovascular aortic aneurysm repair. J Vasc Surg 2002;35:1048–60.

51. Lee JT, Lee J, Aziz I, et al. Stent-graft migration following endovascular repair of aneurysms with large proximal necks: anatomical risk factors and long-term sequelae. J Endovasc Ther 2002;9:652–64.

52. Fransen GAJ, Desgranges P, Laheij RJF, et al. Frequency, predictive factors, and consequences of stent-graft kink following endovascular AAA repair. J Endovasc Ther 2003;10:913–8.

53. Zhang WW, Kulaylat MN, Anain PM, et al. Embolization as cause of bowel ischemia after endovascular abdominal aortic aneurysm repair. J Vasc Surg 2004;40:867–72.

54. Kramer SC, Seifarth H, Pamler H, et al. Renal infarction following endovascular aortic aneurysm repair: incidence and clinical consequences. J Endovasc Ther 2002;9:98–102.

55. Aljabri B, Obrand DI, Montreuil B, et al. Early vascular complications after endovascular repair of aortoiliac aneurysms. Ann Vasc Surg 2001;15:608–14.

56. McWilliams RG, Martin J, White D, et al. Use of contrast-enhanced ultrasound in follow-up after endovascular aortic aneurysm repair. J Vasc Interv Radiol 1999;10:1107–14.

57. Murphy M, Hodgson R, Harris PI, et al. Plain radiographic surveillance of abdominal aortic stent-grafts: the Liverpool/Perth protocol. J Endovasc Ther 2003;10:911–2.

58. The EVAR Trial Participants. Comparison of endovascular aneurysm repair with open repair in patients with abdominal aortic aneurysm (EVAR trial 1): randomized controlled trial. Lancet 2005;365:2179–86.

59. Prinssen M, Verhoeven EL, Buth J, et al. A randomized trial comparing conventional and endovascular repair of abdominal aortic aneurysms. N Engl J Med 2004;351:1607–18.
A multicentre randomised trial comparing open surgical and endovascular repair in 345 patients with 5 cm or larger AAAs; 30-day mortality was 4.6% in the open repair group and 1.2% in the endovascular group.

60. Blankensteijn JD, De Jong S, Prinssen M, et al. Two year outcomes after conventional or endovascular repair of abdominal aortic aneurysms. N Engl J Med 2005;352:2398–405.

61. Lovegrove RE, Javid M, Magee TR, et al. A meta-analysis of 21178 patients undergoing open or endovascular repair of abdominal aortic aneurysm. Br J Surg 2008;95:677–84.
A meta-analysis of 42 studies comparing outcomes following open and endovascular AAA repair. EVAR was associated with significantly lower early 30-day mortality, postoperative morbidity and late aneurysm-related mortality.

62. Davey P, Peaston R, Rose J, et al. Impact on renal function after endovascular aneurysm repair with uncovered supra-renal fixation (SR-EVR) assessed by serum cystatin C. Eur J Vasc Endovasc Surg 2008;35:439–45.

63. Mehta M, Cayne N, Veith FJ, et al. Relationship of proximal fixation to renal dysfunction in patients undergoing endovascular aneurysm repair. J Cardiovasc Surg (Torino) 2004;45:367–74.

64. The UK EVAR Trial Participants. Endovascular versus open repair of abdominal aortic aneurysm. N Engl J Med 2010;362:1863–71.
In this large, randomised trial, endovascular repair of abdominal aortic aneurysm was associated with a significantly lower operative mortality than open surgical repair. However, no differences were seen in total mortality or aneurysm-related mortality in the long term. Endovascular repair was associated with increased rates of graft-related complications and reinterventions and was more costly.

65. Powell JT, Brown LC. The long-term results of the UK EVAR trials: the sting in the tail. Eur J Vasc Endovasc Surg 2010;40(1):44–6.

66. Troeng T, Malmstedt J, Bjorck M. External validation of the Swedvasc registry: a first-time individual cross-matching with the unique personal identity number. Eur J Vasc Endovasc Surg 2008;36(6):705–12.

67. Kechagias A, Perala J, Ylonen K, et al. Validation of the Finnvasc score in infrainguinal percutaneous transluminal angioplasty for critical lower limb ischemia. Ann Vasc Surg 2008;22(4):547–51.

68. EVAR Trial Participants. Endovascular aneurysm repair and outcome in patients unfit for open repair of abdominal aortic aneurysm (EVAR trial 2): randomized controlled trial. Lancet 2005;365:2187–92.
A multicentre randomised trial comparing EVAR and best medical therapy in 338 unfit patients with morphologically suitable AAAs; 30-day mortality was 9% in the EVAR group and at a mean follow-up of 3.3 years there was no difference in either the all-cause or aneurysm-related mortality between groups.

69. The UK EVAR Trial Participants. Endovascular repair of aortic aneurysm in patients physically ineligible for open repair. N Engl J Med 2010;362:1872.
A randomised trial involving patients who were physically ineligible for open repair. Endovascular repair of abdominal aortic aneurysm was associated with a

significantly lower rate of aneurysm-related mortality than no repair. However, endovascular repair was not associated with a reduction in the rate of death from any cause. The rates of graft-related complications and re-interventions were higher with endovascular repair, and it was more costly.

70. Hinchliffe RJ, Hopkinson BR. Ruptured abdominal aortic aneurysm: time for a new approach. J Cardiovasc Surg (Torino) 2002;43:345–7.

71. Veith FJ, Ohki T. Endovascular approaches to ruptured infrarenal aortoiliac aneurysms. J Cardiovasc Surg (Torino) 2002;43:369–78.

72. Hinchliffe RJ, Yusuf SW, Macierewicz JA, et al. Endovascular repair of ruptured abdominal aortic aneurysm – a challenge to open repair? Results of a single centre experience in 20 patients. Eur J Vasc Endovasc Surg 2001;22:528–34.

73. Powell JT, Thompson SG, Thompson MM, et al. The Immediate Management of the Patient with Rupture: Open Versus Endovascular repair (IMPROVE) aneurysm trial. Acta Chir Belg 2009;109(6):678–80.

74. Greenberg RK, Haulon S, O'Neill S, et al. Primary endovascular repair of juxtarenal aneurysms with fenestrated endovascular grafting. Eur J Vasc Endovasc Surg 2004;27:484–91.

75. Verhoeven EL, Prins TR, Tielliu IF, et al. Treatment of short-necked infrarenal aortic aneurysms with fenestrated stent-grafts: short-term results. Eur J Vasc Endovasc Surg 2004;27:477–83.

76. Parkinson TJ, Rose JD, Wyatt MG. Endovascular aneurysm repair: state of the art 2006. In: Earnshaw JJ, Murie JA, editors. The evidence for vascular surgery. 2nd ed. Shrewsbury: Tfm Publishers; 2007. p. 153–64.

77. Cross J, Gurusamy K, Gadhvi V, et al. Fenestrated endovascular aneurysm repair. Br J Surg 2012;99(2):152–9.
   A search was performed for studies describing FEVAR for juxtarenal abdominal aortic aneurysms. Eleven studies were identified describing a total of 660 procedures. Target vessel perfusion rates ranged from 90.5% to 100%. Eleven deaths occurred within 30 days, giving a 30-day proportional mortality rate of 2.0%. FEVAR for repair of suprarenal and juxtarenal aneurysms is a viable alternative to open repair, although there is no level I evidence.

78. Resch T, Sonesson B, Malina M. Incidence and management of complications after branched and fenestrated endografting. J Cardiovasc Surg (Torino) 2010;51(1):105–13.

79. Lee JT, Greenberg JI, Dalman RL. Early experience with the snorkel technique for juxtarenal aneurysms. J Vasc Surg 2012;55(4):935–46.

80. Abraham CZ, Reilly LM, Schneider DB, et al. A modular multi-branched system for endovascular repair of bilateral common iliac artery aneurysms. J Endovasc Ther 2003;10:203–7.

81. Chuter TA, Gordon RL, Reilly LM, et al. Multi-branched stent-graft for type III thoracoabdominal aortic aneurysm. J Vasc Interv Radiol 2001;12:391–2.

82. Verhoeven EL, Vourliotakis G, Bos WT, et al. Fenestrated stent grafting for short-necked and juxtarenal abdominal aortic aneurysm: an 8-year single-center experience. Eur J Vasc Endovasc Surg 2010;39:529–36.

83. Nordon IM, Hinchliffe RJ, Manning B, et al. Toward an "off-the-shelf" fenestrated endograft for management of short-necked abdominal aortic aneurysms: an analysis of current graft morphological diversity. J Endovasc Ther 2010;17:78–85.

84. Reddy DJ, Weaver MR. Infected aneurysms. In: Rutherford RB, editor. Vascular surgery. 6th ed. Philadelphia: Elsevier Saunders; 2005. p. 1581–96.

85. Reddy DJ, Shepard AD, Evans JR, et al. Management of infected aorto-iliac aneurysms. Arch Surg 1991;126:873.

86. Kritpracha B, Premprabha D, Sungsiri J, et al. Endovascular therapy for infected aortic aneurysms. J Vasc Surg 2011;54(5):1259–65.

87. Knight CG, Healy DA, Thomas RL. Femoral artery pseudoaneurysms: risk factors, prevalence and treatment options. Ann Vasc Surg 2003;17:503–8.

88. Kirkpatrick UJ, McWilliams RG, Martin J, et al. Late complications after ligation and bypass for popliteal aneurysm. Br J Surg 2004;91:174–7.

89. Marty B, Wicky S, Ris HB, et al. Success of thrombolysis as a predictor of outcome in acute thrombosis of popliteal aneurysms. J Vasc Surg 2002;35:487–93.

90. Gerasimidis T, Sfyroeras G, Papazoglou K, et al. Endovascular treatment of popliteal artery aneurysms. Eur J Vasc Endovasc Surg 2003;26:506–11.

91. Jung E, Jim J, Rubin BG, et al. Long-term outcome of endovascular popliteal artery aneurysm repair. Ann Vasc Surg 2010;24(7):871–5.

14

Thoracic and thoraco-abdominal aortic disease

Ian Nordon

Robert Morgan

Matthew Thompson

Introduction

The evolution of endovascular techniques has revolutionised the treatment of thoracic aneurysms and type B aortic dissections. Once the province of cardiologists and cardiothoracic surgeons, these conditions should now be familiar to clinicians dealing with peripheral vascular disease, as they form a potentially important part of vascular practice.

Endovascular repair (EVR) of the thoracic aorta has become an established treatment modality despite a relatively poor evidence base. There are good explanations for the lack of randomised data when the clinical outcomes for pathologies with established indications for treatment are compared between endovascular procedures and open thoracic surgery. Case series and registry data would appear to show that the endovascular procedures offer significantly lower mortality and morbidity rates when compared to open thoracic repair of thoracic aneurysms or acute dissections.[1,2] The lack of randomised trials does, however, pose a problem for endovascular techniques, as much of the evidence base is composed of small retrospective series and registries, which do not offer sufficient detail to facilitate the subgroup analysis that is mandatory to refine indications for treatment.

Despite the change in practice that has encompassed treatment of thoracic aneurysms and dissections, the treatment of thoraco-abdominal aneurysms continues to pose a fundamental clinical challenge, with significant mortality rates attesting to the

pathophysiological derangements that accompany open surgical repair. This chapter reviews the contemporary treatment of thoracic and thoraco-abdominal aortic disease that would be of relevance to the vascular clinician. Readers are referred to more specialised texts for a detailed description of conditions that would still be within the province of cardiothoracic surgery, e.g. ascending aortic aneurysms, type A aortic dissection.

Imaging of the thoracic aorta

The main imaging method used for the assessment of patients with thoracic aortic pathology is computed tomography (CT). Assessment should involve scrutiny of axial and multiplanar images. In general, the axial images are more useful images for assessment of aortic diameters and the multiplanar reconstructions are used for assessment of aortic length. In the present day, endovascular planning should be performed on a workstation that allows three-dimensional reconstruction and centre-line analysis. Magnetic resonance (MR) angiography does not have the required spatial resolution to facilitate the planning of endovascular procedures and there remains concern over the development of nephrogenic fibrosis when certain gadolinium agents[3] are used in patients with renal failure. CT angiography, however, involves the use of ionising radiation and potentially nephrotoxic contrast agents, and as such is largely unsuitable for long-term imaging follow-up of patients with thoracic aortic disease. MR in general is therefore particularly useful for the follow-up of those patients with thoracic aortic disease.

The quality of contemporary CT angiography and the high-level image manipulation available from the workstations means that in the vast majority of patients angiography is only required at the time of intervention.

Transoesophageal echocardiography has a significant role in the classification and diagnosis of thoracic aortic dissection.

Thoracic aortic aneurysms (TAAs)

Classification and aetiology

The descending thoracic aorta is the most common location for aneurysms. Descending thoracic aneurysms are classified on the basis of whether they involve the upper half, the lower half or the entire descending aorta, with the thorax divided at the sixth intercostal space (types A, B and C).[4]

The majority of thoracic aneurysms are non-specific or degenerative, and approximately one-quarter are caused by chronic thoracic aortic dissections. Less frequently, aneurysms are related to Marfan syndrome, Ehler–Danlos syndrome, mycotic aneurysms[5] and connective tissue disorders, e.g. ankylosing spondylitis, rheumatoid arthritis, Reiter's disease and systemic lupus erythematosus. False aneurysms may follow trauma or complication of a previous co-arctation repair. Aneurysms of the descending aorta may extend into the abdomen and are referred to as thoraco-abdominal aortic aneurysms.

The majority of aneurysms are fusiform in morphology. Saccular aneurysms are less common and are usually the result of infection or previous trauma. Thoracic aneurysms have a strong association with coronary artery disease and abdominal aortic aneurysm.

Incidence and clinical presentation

Aneurysms of the descending thoracic aorta are a disease of increasing age and the male to female ratio is 3:1. TAAs are estimated to occur in 10 per 100 000 patient-years.[6] Thoracic aneurysms are most frequently discovered incidentally on routine chest radiography or CT scans. Clinical presentations include substernal, back or shoulder pain, superior vena cava syndrome, dysphagia, dyspnoea, stridor and hoarseness (due to laryngeal nerve compression), and rupture. The survival of patients with untreated TAAs is bleak and is estimated to be 13–39% at 5 years.[7] Eighty per cent of thoracic aneurysms detected at autopsy have ruptured. The risk of rupture increases with the size of the aneurysm, but data regarding estimated annual rupture rates and aortic diameter are sparse and less robust than for the abdominal aorta. Some data suggest that the rupture rate of thoracic aneurysms is 2.7 per 100 000 patient-years as compared to 9.2 per 100 000 patient-years for abdominal aneurysms.

Indications for treatment

The main indications for intervention are symptoms and size. There is controversy regarding the size criteria for treatment of TAAs. Juvonen et al. reported that the 2-year rupture rate for TAAs was 23% in aneurysms less than 7 cm,[8] whereas Elefteriades observed a 30% 5-year rupture rate when the aorta exceeded 6 cm.[9] Practically, most clinicians regard 5.5–6 cm as an indication for possible repair in an asymptomatic patient, the threshold obviously being balanced by the surgical risk. Diameter thresholds should be reduced in patients with defined connective tissue disorders as rupture may occur at smaller aortic diameters.

Technique of surgical repair

The mainstay of traditional surgical repair of TAAs includes a left thoracotomy for access, aortic clamping and inlay grafting, with intercostal reimplantation. The procedures are technically challenging due to the need to maintain visceral and spinal cord perfusion during the procedure. Several surgical adjuncts are available to achieve these aims, including the use of a Gott shunt, left heart bypass and distal aortic perfusion, selective intercostal shunting and routine cerebrospinal fluid (CSF) drainage.

Endovascular repair of thoracic aneurysms

Detailed preoperative imaging is required to assess the proximal and distal landing zones for the endograft and to plan an access route. Ideally, this should be performed using centre-line image reconstruction using vascular-specific software to ensure optimal graft deployment planning.

A segment of normal aorta above and below the lesion to be treated is required (landing zone), so that a seal can be achieved between the endograft and the normal aortic wall. The landing zone length should be at least 15 mm on the lesser curve, although 20 mm is optimal. With respect to the aortic arch, the landing zone length should be measured on the inner curve of the aortic arch and not the outer curve. If the landing zone is considered to be of inadequate length, surgical bypass may be performed to debranch the aortic arch or abdominal aorta so that an effective sealing zone is created. This is often referred to as a hybrid endovascular procedure and examples of surgical bypasses would include ascending aorta to innominate and left common carotid (**Fig. 14.1**), left to right carotid bypass (**Fig. 14.2**) and left carotid–subclavian bypass.

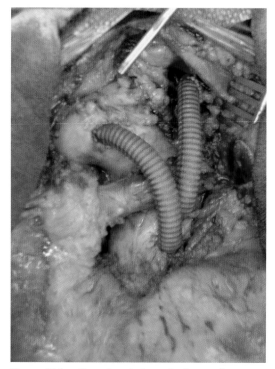

Figure 14.1 • Operative photograph of ascending aorta to innominate and left common carotid. Surgery performed to create an adequate landing zone in a patient with a very proximal thoracic aneurysm.

The diameter thresholds are dictated by the available device sizes. A degree of oversizing is required with respect to the aortic diameter during device selection. In general, for the treatment of aneurysms, devices are oversized by 15–20%. The maximum and minimum diameters of the available stent-grafts are 46 and 22 mm. Therefore, the upper and lower limits of landing zone diameter are 40-42 and 18 mm respectively. If it is necessary to place more than one device because of the long length of aorta to be treated, the operator should also take into account the overlap required between adjacent devices, which is usually around 5 cm. Clearly, as with all endovascular aortic procedures, adequate access is required given the relatively large sizes of the endograft introducer sheaths.

The procedure is usually performed under general or regional anaesthesia, although stents can also be inserted using local anaesthesia alone. A diagnostic angiographic catheter is placed in the ascending aorta via the left brachial artery or the contralateral femoral artery. A femoral arteriotomy is often required (although percutaneous procedures are feasible and gaining in popularity), and an exchange length extra-stiff guidewire (e.g. Lunderquistguidewire, Cook, UK) is advanced so that the tip is placed in the low ascending aorta. The systolic blood pressure should be reduced to below 100 mmHg peak systolic pressure to prevent the windsock effect of the cardiac output displacing the endograft.

The endograft delivery system is advanced over the guidewire to the desired deployment site. Accurate positioning is achieved by serial aortography. When the correct position is achieved, the stent graft is released (Fig. 14.2). Further endografts are placed as necessary with at least 4–5 cm of overlap between endografts.

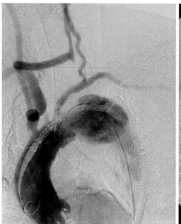 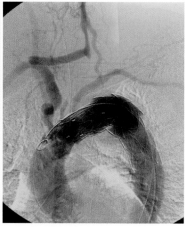

Figure 14.2 • Angiogram demonstrating a large thoracic aneurysm with the landing zone involving the left common carotid artery. To enable endovascular aneurysm repair a right to left common carotid bypass has been performed with ligation of the proximal left carotid artery (arrow).

Management of the spinal cord during endovascular thoracic procedures

One of the most feared complications of thoracic aortic intervention is paraplegia. Placement of an endograft in the thoracic aorta causes coverage of many critical intercostal vessels (T6–L1), with the risk of spinal cord ischaemia (SCI). Some centres advocate prophylactic CSF drainage whilst others adopt an expectant policy. No independent precipitating factor of SCI has been identified, although coexisting infrarenal pathology or previous abdominal aortic repair may reduce the collateral network supplying the spinal cord.[10] Clearly, if there is any sign of SCI the cord perfusion pressure must be increased by reducing CSF pressure (target 10–12 mmHg) through spinal drain insertion, and increasing mean arterial pressure (MAP; target MAP 85–100 mm Hg) with inotropes.[11] This selective approach appears safe for patients developing SCI after thoracic endovascular repair (TEVR), which has an acceptably low permanent neurological deficit, although overall survival of patients experiencing SCI after TEVR is diminished relative to non-SCI patients.[12]

Controversy has surrounded the management of the left subclavian artery during thoracic endografting. Early experience suggested that it was reasonably safe to cover the origin of the subclavian artery with respect to upper limb perfusion. However, more recent evidence has demonstrated that stroke and paraplegia rates are lower when subclavian perfusion is preserved, presumably due to the contribution of the vertebral artery to the anterior spinal artery.[13,14] Routine revascularisation of the left subclavian artery (via left carotid–subclavian bypass) is recommended in the authors' practice for the majority of cases where coverage of the left subclavian origin is planned,[15] and this approach is supported by the recent recommendations from the Society for Vascular Surgery (SVS).

Outcome of treatment

Results of open repair in centres of excellence are good, with 30-day mortality rates for all types of thoracic aneurysm below 12% and paraplegia rates below 4%.[16] Community results that incorporate several centres are more realistic of patient-centred outcomes and demonstrate 30-day mortality rates approaching 20%.[17] Mortality is predicted by renal insufficiency, age and emergency presentation.[18] Outcome data for EVR of thoracic aneurysms are available from several sources. Leurs et al., on behalf of the EUROSTAR collaborators, reported data in 249 patients with 30-day mortality for elective total endovascular repair (TEVR) of 5.3% and paraplegia of 4%.[1] A cohort of patients with TAAs who underwent endografting with the Gore TAG device was compared retrospectively with the results of a cohort of 94 patients who underwent open surgical repair. The perioperative mortality (2.1% vs. 11.7%), paraplegia (3% vs. 14%) and freedom from major adverse event (48% vs. 20%) rates were all better in the endovascular group.[18] Similarly, the European Talent Registry reported technical success of 98%, in-hospital mortality in 5% (4.1% and 7.9% for elective and emergency procedures respectively), paraplegia in 1.7% and stroke in 3.7%.[19] Similar outcomes have been reported for the newest generation of endografts, despite the fact the patients in these later data series had more challenging anatomy compared with earlier series.[13] Endovascular thoracic aneurysm repair has a spectrum of complications unique to the procedure. The most common is endoleak. There seems little doubt that the most common endoleak is an attachment site (or type 1) endoleak. These may occur immediately or during follow-up and should be treated with additional devices. Type 3 leaks (between adjacent devices or through disrupted grafts) may occur and should also be treated with additional devices.

Recommendations for practice

EVR of thoracic aneurysms has changed practice. In the authors' opinion, endovascular procedures should be used as first-line therapy for most thoracic aneurysms. Exclusions to this policy would be patients with unfavourable anatomy, poor long-term durability and patients with documented connective tissue disease, in whom the results of endografting are not well defined, and the results of surgery in experienced centres are excellent.

The management of patients with Marfan syndrome has been the subject of much debate since the introduction of endovascular therapy. Patients with Marfan syndrome develop both thoracic aneurysms and dissections. However, the patients are usually younger and fitter than patients with non-specific aneurysms, have excellent outcomes from conventional surgery[20] and equivocal outcomes from EVR.[21,22] At present, there is no body of evidence to support the routine use of EVR in patients with Marfan syndrome.

Thoraco-abdominal aortic aneurysms (TAAAs)

Thoracic aortic aneurysms that involve the visceral segment of the abdominal aorta are traditionally described as thoraco-abdominal aneurysms and

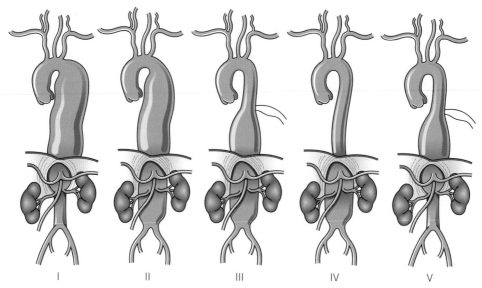

Figure 14.3 • Illustration of the Crawford classification of thoraco-abdominal aneurysms.

are classified according to the extent of the aneurysmal disease (see **Fig. 14.3** for a description of the Crawford classification). The aetiology of thoraco-abdominal aneurysms differs from infrarenal aneurysms, with medial degenerative disease and chronic dissection particularly prevalent.[23] In contrast to infrarenal disease, the majority of patients with thoraco-abdominal aneurysms are symptomatic, the presence of back pain is particularly common, and this symptom may precede aortic rupture or intramural dissection.[24] The rationale for treatment of thoraco-abdominal aneurysms largely derives from a natural history study from Crawford and DeNatale, who reported a series of 94 patients unsuitable for surgery.[25] After 24 months' follow-up, only 24% of these patients were alive, which contrasted with the 59% 5-year survival of a concurrent cohort of patients who underwent operative repair. On the basis of these results, it was concluded that patients with significant thoraco-abdominal aneurysms should have an operative repair unless precluded by coexistent medical conditions.

Surgical management

As with all complex aortic diseases, detailed imaging and careful assessment of comorbid risk factors are essential. Due to the high mortality rates associated with repair of TAAAs, consideration must be given to the balance between predicted surgical risk and aneurysm diameter. Preoperative coronary revascularisation may be appropriate.

A left thoracotomy is usually required, although some type IV aneurysms may utilise an abdominal approach. The abdominal aorta is usually exposed by left medial visceral rotation. The diaphragm is partially divided with a circumferential incision preferred to preserve nerve supply. After the dissection has been completed the aneurysm is clamped at its proximal and distal extents, and an arteriotomy made in the lateral aneurysm wall. It is important that the arteriotomy is sited away from the visceral origins in the abdominal portion of the aneurysm. The proximal anastomosis is performed with a completely transected aorta to prevent aorto-oesophageal fistula. If possible, the proximal anastomosis is fashioned to include adjacent intercostal or visceral arteries, whilst any remaining intercostals are directly reimplanted into the graft or revascularised by separate jump grafts. The visceral arteries are then directly anastomosed into elliptical openings in the graft, utilising an inclusion technique. If possible, the coeliac, superior mesenteric and right renal arteries are taken on one patch; anastomosing the distal graft to the aortic bifurcation or iliac arteries completes the reconstruction (**Figs. 14.4** and **14.5**).

Adjunctive surgical techniques

During thoraco-abdominal aneurysm repair, prolonged visceral ischaemia is the main cause of postoperative renal dysfunction and can also contribute to multiple organ failure. To reduce the severity of organ hypoperfusion, partial left heart bypass with

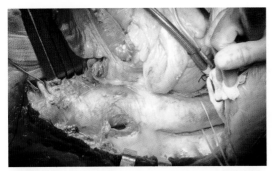

Figure 14.4 • Operative picture demonstrating exposure of a type III TAAA using a left thoracolaparotomy. The diaphragm has been completely divided in this case. The left renal artery is controlled.

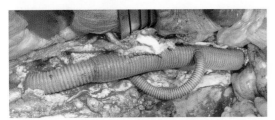

Figure 14.5 • Operative picture of completed reconstruction of a TAAA. The visceral patch has been reinforced with Teflon pledgets. A separate graft has been anastomosed to a large intercostal.

a centrifugal pump may be utilised to drain blood from the left atrium or upper pulmonary vein, and return it via the femoral artery or aorta. This facilitates renal and visceral perfusion whilst the proximal anastomosis is fashioned as long as the distal aortic clamp remains proximal to the visceral vessels.[26] During the abdominal part of the aneurysm repair, the coeliac trunk, superior mesenteric artery and both renal arteries can be selectively perfused with catheters that are connected to the left heart bypass.[27] Paraplegia may complicate thoraco-abdominal aneurysm repair in up to 20% of cases and is increased in more proximal aneurysms, with lengthy clamp time, renal impairment, advanced age and emergency presentations. Paraplegia results from damage to the spinal cord due to a combination of division of spinal cord arteries, prolonged spinal cord ischaemia, reperfusion injury and postoperative hypotension. Maintenance of spinal cord blood supply may be achieved by reimplantation of patent intercostal arteries and by distal aortic perfusion. CSF pressure increases during aortic clamping, and CSF drainage has been advocated to reduce paraplegia.[28,29] A functional approach to the problem of neurological deficit aims at intraoperative monitoring of the spinal cord function. Somatosensory evoked potentials are widely used to detect spinal cord ischaemia during aortic cross-clamping and to identify vessels critical to spinal cord blood supply, which may then be perfused and reimplanted. An alternative approach is to use motor evoked potentials, which have been reported to improve paraplegia rates.[30,31]

Results of surgical repair of thoraco-abdominal aneurysms

The mortality and morbidity rates following conventional repair of TAAAs are still significant, with specialised centres reporting mortality rates of 5–16%, with paraplegia rates of 4–11%.[32–34] However, these excellent results are not representative of outcomes outside of these centres, with national/community mortality rates exceeding 20% at 30 days and 30% at 1 year.[35–37] Identifiable patient risk factors predicting adverse outcomes include emergent presentation, previous aortic replacement, diabetes, smoking history, renal and cardiorespiratory impairment, age beyond 80 years, acute dissection and the extent of TAAA.

Hybrid visceral revascularisation and endovascular repair of thoraco-abdominal aortic aneurysms

The application of combining surgical and endovascular strategies in the management of complex aortic disease has been suggested to reduce the surgical insult, by obviating the need for thoracotomy and aortic cross-clamping whilst also reducing the duration of visceral and renal ischaemia. The exclusion of TAAAs by means of an endoluminal stent graft delivered via a remote arteriotomy or conduit requires sufficient length of proximal and distal landing zones in non-diseased or replaced aorta, and in addition needs to safeguard perfusion of the gut and kidneys. A hybrid repair may be defined as a combined surgical and endovascular approach in which transperitoneal retrograde visceral revascularisation is used to create an adequate distal landing zone for endovascular thoraco-abdominal aneurysm endograft exclusion. The retrograde visceral bypass maintains perfusion to the visceral and renal arteries. This approach may be combined with great vessel transposition or bypass to create an adequate proximal attachment site for the thoraco-abdominal endograft (**Fig. 14.6**).

At present, there are only a few case series reporting the results of this technique (Table 14.1).[38–46] A recent 'collaborative' paper reporting outcomes of 107 consecutive cases across three units described a 15% mortality and 8.4% permanent paraplegia rate in all-comers.[47] Superficially, the results do

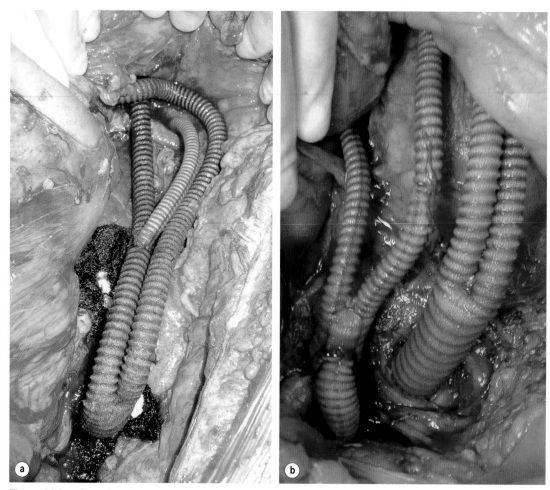

Figure 14.6 • Operative pictures of two patients undergoing retrograde visceral revascularisation. Many different graft configurations are possible with varying numbers of vessels requiring revascularisation.

Table 14.1 • Summary of published independent series of combined surgical and endovascular repair of TAAAs (*n* > 10)

Authors	Institution, year of publication	Number	Type II (%)	Type III (%)	Visceral vessels bypassed	Mortality (%)	Permanent paraplegia (%)
Resch et al.[38]	Cleveland, 2006	13	38.5	15.4	N/A	23.1	30.7
Zhou et al.[39]	Houston, 2006	15	0	53.3	40	6.7	0
Black et al.[40]	St Mary's London, 2006	26	62	26.9	94	23	0
Bockler et al.[41]	Heidelberg, 2007	11	18.2	9.1	N/A	18	0
Chiesa et al.[42]	Milan, 2007	13	15.4	0	32	23.0	7.7
Lee et al.[75]	Gainesville, 2007	17	11.8	47.0	56	24.0	0
Biasi et al.[44]	St George's London, 2008	18	44.4	38.9	48	17.6	5.6
Wolf et al.[45]	Munich, 2010	20	55	35	N/A	10	0
Ham et al.[46]	Los Angeles, 2011	51	0	13	47	3.9	2

not appear to show a significant advantage for the hybrid technique over conventional surgery, but in general patients have more comorbidity, are older, and have a higher proportion of type II and III aneurysms than comparable open series. In the treatment of thoraco-abdominal aortic disease the applicability of any suggested technique must be evaluated – both open surgical replacement and total endovascular solutions may have applicability in approximately 50–60% of patients due to physiological and anatomical considerations, respectively.

Total endovascular repair of thoraco-abdominal aortic aneurysms

Recent technological advances in stent graft design (**Fig. 14.7**) have realised the possibility of deploying customised endografts with fenestrations, allowing target vessel cannulation with additional covered stents to afford antegrade perfusion of the visceral vessels.[48] Similarly, branched endovascular grafts have also been successfully deployed to preserve end-organ perfusion in selected patients, and some TAAAs can now be treated with four-vessel branched grafts.[49,50] The need for accurate measurements and precise manufacturing results in a lag time of several weeks in most, and anatomical constraints with access and vessel tortuosity may not allow all TAAAs to be treated with a total endovascular solution. This evolutionary technology shows significant promise in reducing the mortality and morbidity of TAAA repair, but at present case numbers are extremely small and highly selected. Increased modularity of devices is evolving and will lead to standardised off-the-shelf branched and fenestrated endografts being available, eliminating manufacturing delays and broadening their application.[51] Given the early success of these techniques, which

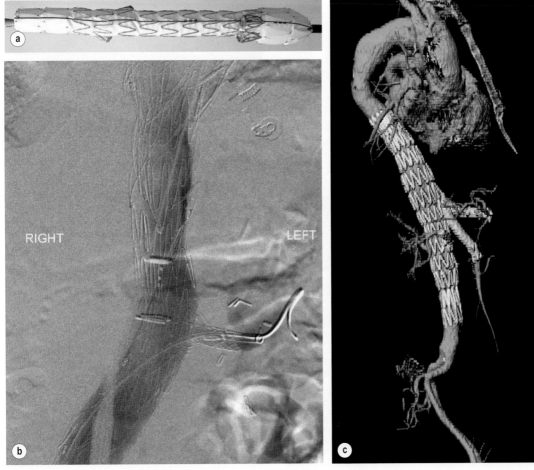

Figure 14.7 • **(a)** Picture of an endograft with four custom-made branches. **(b)** A procedural angiogram demonstrates completed reconstruction of a TAAA with a branched graft to the left renal artery. **(c)** Segmented lateral CT reconstruction of four-vessel branched graft following deployment. Part **(a)** courtesy of Cook, UK.

at present are in their infancy, total endovascular repair is likely to be the future primary treatment modality of thoraco-abdominal aneurysms, with the exception of young patients with defined connective tissue disease.

Recommendations for practice

Endovascular techniques are evolving in this field but the complexities of maintaining visceral and renal perfusion make endovascular solutions technically complex. The hybrid approach is probably best seen as a bridge between traditional surgical techniques and the developing total endovascular solutions. At present, it would seem reasonable to reserve hybrid and endovascular solutions for those patients who have a high predicted mortality for open thoraco-abdominal replacement, whilst acknowledging that as endovascular experience develops, this technique is likely to play a more prominent role in the management of TAAAs.

Thoracic dissection and acute aortic syndrome

Pathology and classification

The acute aortic syndrome may be described as a group of pathological conditions affecting the thoracic aorta that typically cause severe thoracic pain. The syndrome is caused by aortic dissection (**Fig. 14.8**), intramural haematoma (IMH; **Fig. 14.9**) and penetrating aortic ulcers (PAUs;

Fig. 14.10).[52] All three conditions may coexist, and evolution from both IMH and penetrating ulcer to dissection has been described. To a large extent, the management of classic aortic dissection may be applied to both IMH and PAUs.

Aortic dissections result from a tear in the aortic intima that allows blood to penetrate into the aortic wall and propagate a cleavage plane within the media. Two channels of flow result in the formation of true and false lumens. Common causes of dissection include hypertension, trauma and connective tissue disorders. Typically the pressure within the false lumen is higher than the true lumen, leading to compression of the true lumen, which can result in malperfusion or rupture of the false lumen. Malperfusion of the visceral, renal or lower limb arteries may complicate aortic dissection. Such branch vessel malperfusion may be described as dynamic due to true lumen compression or static due to the dissection extending into the branch vessel (**Fig. 14.11**).

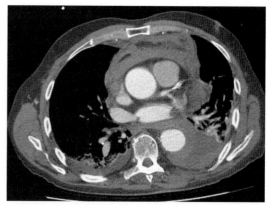

Figure 14.9 • Axial CT appearance of intramural haematoma. There is a relatively high-density crescentic rim of fresh blood in the wall of the aorta.

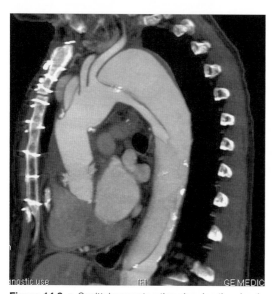

Figure 14.8 • Sagittal reconstruction showing the classic appearance of a type B aortic dissection.

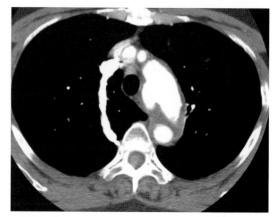

Figure 14.10 • Axial CT appearance of penetrating aortic ulcer.

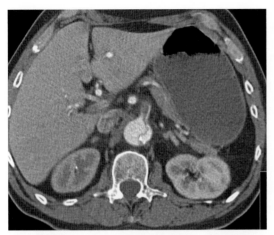

Figure 14.11 • Axial CT demonstrating a patient with visceral ischaemia due to significant true lumen collapse (black arrows) and thrombosis of the false lumen in the superior mesenteric artery.

IMH is defined as a blood clot in the intramural space without an obvious intimal tear. The condition is thought to result from rupture of medial vasa vasora and is often regarded as a precursor to dissection. IMH accounts for up to 20% of acute aortic syndromes and has a prognosis similar to classic aortic dissection.[53]

PAU results from focal ulceration of an atherosclerotic plaque and may be associated with haematoma within the aortic wall. Penetrating ulcers have a poorer prognosis than classical dissection, with higher rates of aortic rupture.[54]

Aortic dissections are classified by site, chronicity and presentation. The most crucial classification involves the site of dissection. Under the commonly used Stanford classification, type A dissections involve the ascending aorta, whereas type B dissection does not. The DeBakey system is also used to classify site. Temporally, dissections are acute when less than 2 weeks after the onset of symptoms, and are termed chronic after this period. In addition, dissections may be termed complicated or uncomplicated. Complications of aortic dissection would include rupture, coronary dissection, aortic valve involvement, malperfusion, impending rupture (persistent pain), refractory hypertension and false aneurysm formation.

Conventional management of acute aortic dissection

Management of aortic dissection involves rapid pharmacological control of blood pressure and dP/dt. Type A dissection has a 1% mortality per hour from aortic rupture, aortic regurgitation, pericardial tamponade or coronary ischaemia and is treated by emergency surgical graft repair of the ascending aorta, with or without aortic valve replacement.[55]

The management of type B dissections is principally medical, with intervention reserved for complications. Overall, medical management of patients with acute aortic dissection has a mortality rate of just over 10%; this includes a mixed group of patients with uncomplicated dissection and some patients with complicated dissection who would be considered unsuitable for surgical intervention. Surgical intervention in patients with complicated dissection has a mortality rate of approximately 30%.[56] Overall, the medical treatment of uncomplicated type B dissection appears appropriate, as in the acute phase uncomplicated type B dissections appear to have a relatively low mortality. In a series of 159 patients presenting with acute type B dissections, 47% of the patients had complicated dissections and had an overall, in-hospital mortality of 18%. In contrast, the 53% of patients with uncomplicated dissection had medical management, with mortality of just 1.2%.[57,58]

Endovascular management of acute type B thoracic dissection

Endovascular therapy has revolutionised the treatment of complicated type B thoracic dissections. The intervention aims to cover the primary entry tear of type B dissections with an endovascular graft. This has the immediate effect of depressurising the false lumen, allowing true lumen expansion. Later thrombosis of the false lumen facilitates aortic remodelling. In the acute phase, covering the primary entry tear will minimise the effects of false lumen aortic rupture by depressurising the false lumen, and treat dynamic branch vessel occlusion by allowing true lumen expansion (**Fig. 14.12**). If there is residual static branch vessel occlusion this is best treated by stent placement.

The technique of EVR is similar to that described above for thoracic aneurysms. The proximal part of the stent graft should be deployed in the proximal non-dissected aorta. Graft oversizing is limited to 10% and proximal bare metal stents are avoided so as not to traumatise the fragile proximal aorta, and balloon dilatation is contraindicated for the same reason. There is controversy as to the length of aorta that requires coverage in acute dissections. A short endograft will allow coverage of the primary tear but will rely on distal aortic remodelling to avoid false lumen perfusion in the lower thoracic aorta. A longer endograft will cause more false lumen thrombosis but will theoretically increase the risk of paraplegia. One recent concept is to use a

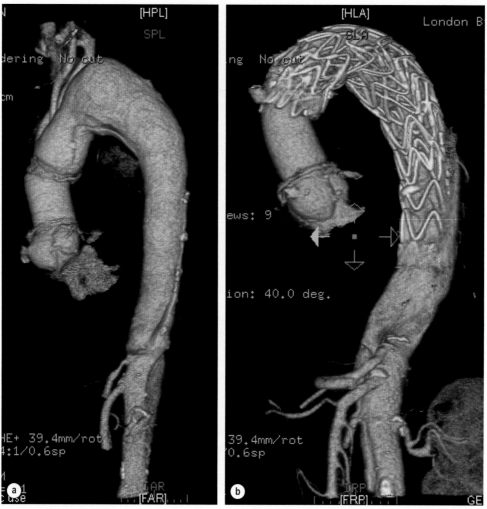

Figure 14.12 • (a) Patient with a residual dissection after a type A repair. **(b)** An endograft has been placed to cover the primary entry tear.

combination of a short covered endograft to cover the primary tear and an uncovered stent to facilitate remodelling.[59] The early results of EVR of complicated type B dissections are vastly better than the open surgical alternative. Most series reported mortality rates of approximately 10%, with paraplegia rates of less than 3%.[1,60,61] These findings stimulated a rapid change in management and most vascular centres would now regard endovascular therapy to be the first-line treatment for complicated type B dissections. EVR of thoracic dissections has its own set of perioperative complications, which include retrograde type A dissection, aortic rupture and continued perfusion of the false lumen.[13] In addition, other endovascular techniques including visceral stenting or percutaneous fenestration[62] may be required to treat malperfusion.

In recent years several authors have suggested that uncomplicated acute type B dissections might benefit from EVR in preventing acute and long-term complications. The rationale for this proposition revolves around the outcome for patients with asymptomatic dissection. Several historical studies have suggested that aortic-related death was high in the group of patients who maintained perfusion of both lumina, and that mortality (from acute complications or late aortic rupture) might be reduced by EVR since this was demonstrated to promote thrombosis of the false lumen. The INSTEAD (INvestigation of STEnt grafts in patients with type B Aortic Dissection) trial explored the difference between optimal medical therapy and TEVR for uncomplicated subacute or chronic type B dissections. TEVR failed to improve 2-year survival and adverse event rates despite favourable aortic remodelling, 2-year cumulative survival rate of 95.6 ± 2.5% with optimal medical therapy versus 88.9 ± 3.7% with TEVR ($P = 0.15$).[63] The clinically important results of the INSTEAD trial will be the mid- and longer-term results to define whether TEVR can reduce the known aortic-related mortality associated with chronic dissection. The European ADSORB (Acute uncomplicated aortic Dissection type B: evaluating Stent-graft placement OR Best medical treatment alone) study started recruitment in 2007 and has yet to report. In contrast to INSTEAD, the ADSORB trial will study patients with acute uncomplicated acute type B dissection and follow patients out to 3 years.[64]

Careful morphological studies and long-term follow-up will be required to define which subgroup of patients may benefit from early TEVR, but some useful data have recently been published that identify a false lumen diameter exceeding 22 mm that predicts rapid aortic expansion.[65]

Endovascular treatment of chronic dissections

Indications for repair of chronic dissections have usually been limited to the onset of complications, and an aortic diameter exceeding 5.5–6.0 cm. The literature surrounding the results of TEVR for chronic dissections is particularly poor. In the series to date the mortality rates have been acceptable but the long-term success in preventing aortic expansion is unclear. There have been anecdotal reports that the false lumen below the stent may continue to expand after treatment and that the rate of repeated intervention is high.[13] This is an area that requires careful documentation to facilitate effective therapy. Again, procedural details require refinement as there is still uncertainty regarding the extent of aorta that should be covered, whether covering the entry tear is sufficient or if all re-entry tears should be treated, and whether aortic remodelling can be predicted by the morphology of the lesion.

Recommendations for practice

EVR should now be considered the gold standard for complicated acute type B thoracic dissections. There appears no justification for unselected repair of uncomplicated non-chronic dissections at present, although this is an evolving field and results from the randomised INSTEAD and ADSORB trials will inform practice. The indications and methodology for the treatment of chronic dissections remain undefined.

Traumatic aortic injury (TAI)

TAI is the second commonest cause of death (after head injury) in patients after blunt injury: 15–30% of deaths from blunt trauma have aortic transaction at post-mortem. TAI is commonly associated with multiple injuries after automobile accidents and falls. The most common site of aortic injury is the isthmus, where the relatively mobile thoracic aorta joins the fixed arch. Aortic ruptures occur at this site in 80% of pathological series and in 90% of the clinical series.[66] There is a spectrum of degree of injury to the aorta ranging from intimal haemorrhage through to complete transaction (grade I: intimal tear; grade II: intramural haematoma; grade III: pseudoaneurysm; grade IV: rupture).[67] The surgical approach to treatment has changed considerably in the last decade. Previously, it was thought that emergency repair was mandatory because of the belief that there was a high risk of early rupture (79% within 24 hours) in immediate survivors, although procedural mortality rates of this approach were in excess of 30%. Recent series suggest that the rupture risk in stable patients is only 10%. Pharmacological lowering of blood pressure and reduction in systolic ejection dynamics facilitate stabilisation of patients and the opportunity for delayed repair. Therefore surgery can be delayed until the immediate threat to life from other injuries is controlled.[68] In the last decade, due to its low complication rate, TEVR has in many centres superseded surgery for TAI. The procedural time is short and the operation confers very little in terms of additional morbidity to these severely ill patients. Due to the focal nature of the injury, only a short length of aorta requires covering with an endograft.

Although TEVR seems to have become the gold standard for TAI, there are relatively limited data on mid- and longer-term outcomes. Data from cohort series involve small numbers of patients. However, the procedural mortality is less than 10% throughout and the reported risk of paraplegia is negligible.[69–71] The largest series to date of TAI patients treated by TEVR ($n = 60$) reported 30-day mortality of 9.1%, and 14.4% at 1 year.[72] The main disadvantage to TEVR for TAI is the relative unsuitability of the devices available for the patients who require TEVR. TAI occurs in a relatively young population with small aortas and more angulated aortic arches than older patients. None of the devices currently available conform very well to angulated arches. There are reports of endografts 'sitting up' in the arch, resulting in endograft collapse and pseudocoarctation.[73] In addition, there is a lack of availability of small-calibre endografts. The smallest endograft is 22 mm, which limits the smallest size of aorta that can be stented to 18–19 mm. This may cause problems in young patients, and in some cases operators may resort to the use of smaller endografts not designed for use in the thoracic aorta, such as abdominal endograft limbs.

Nevertheless, at the very least endografting can act as a temporary measure to prevent rupture until the patient is well enough to undergo definitive surgical repair. In the future, we may expect to see the development of endografts specifically designed to treat aortic trauma.

Recommendations for practice

TEVR should be performed preferentially over open surgical repair for TAI, irrespective of age of the patient, providing anatomical suitability. This should be performed urgently, within the first 24 hours after injury. In the case of minimal grade I injury, intimal tear, expectant management may be followed, with serial imaging and interval review. Following TAI, revascularisation of the left subclavian artery and spinal drainage should be selective and at the discretion of the operating surgeon.[74]

Key points

- There is a lack of randomised data to guide practice in diseases of the thoracic aorta. Most data derive from case series or registries. However, mortality differences, in some diseases, are so disparate between open surgical procedures and the endovascular equivalent that inferences can be drawn.
- Endovascular therapy may now be considered the first-line treatment for thoracic aneurysms, acute complicated type B dissections and traumatic aortic injury.
- There are no data, as yet, to support prophylactic endovascular repair of non-chronic uncomplicated dissections.
- Thoraco-abdominal aneurysms remain a technical challenge with high mortality and morbidity rates from all treatment modalities. Open surgery should still be considered as the first-line therapy for patients with low predicted mortality from open repair. Hybrid and total endovascular approaches might be considered appropriate for patients with high predicted mortality.
- The results of endovascular therapy in patients with Marfan syndrome are equivocal and open surgery should be considered preferable in this patient group.

References

1. Leurs LJ, Bell R, Degrieck Y, et al. Endovascular treatment of thoracic aortic diseases: combined experience from the EUROSTAR and United Kingdom Thoracic Endograft registries. J Vasc Surg 2004;40(4):670–80.

2. Swee W, Dake MD. Endovascular management of thoracic dissections. Circulation 2008;117(11):1460–73.

3. Bellin MF, Van Der Molen AJ. Extracellular gadolinium-based contrast media: an overview. Eur J Radiol 2008;66(2):160–7.

4. Estrera AL, Miller 3rd CC, Porat E, et al. Determinants of early and late outcome for reoperations of the proximal aorta. Ann Thorac Surg 2004;78(3):837–45.

5. Sayed S, Choke E, Helme S, et al. Endovascular stent graft repair of mycotic aneurysms of the thoracic aorta. J Cardiovasc Surg (Torino) 2005;46(2):155–61.

6. Clouse WD, Hallett JW, Schaff HV, et al. Improved prognosis of thoracic aortic aneurysms: a population-based study. JAMA 1998;280(22):1926–9.

7. Perko MJ, Norgaard M, Herzog TM, et al. Unoperated aortic aneurysm: a survey of 170 patients. Ann Thorac Surg 1995;59(5):1204–9.

8. Juvonen T, Ergin MA, Galla JD, et al. Prospective study of the natural history of thoracic aortic aneurysms. Ann Thorac Surg 1997;63(6):1533–45.

9. Elefteriades JA. Natural history of thoracic aortic aneurysms: indications for surgery, and surgical versus non-surgical risks. Ann Thorac Surg 2002;74(5):S1877–80.

10. Clough RE, Modarai B, Topple JA, et al. Predictors of stroke and paraplegia in thoracic aortic endovascular intervention. Eur J Vasc Endovasc Surg 2011;41(3):303–10.

11. Ullery BW, Cheung AT, Fairman RM, et al. Risk factors, outcomes, and clinical manifestations of spinal cord ischemia following thoracic endovascular aortic repair. J Vasc Surg 2011;54(3):677–84.

12. Keith Jr CJ, Passman MA, Carignan MJ, et al. Protocol implementation of selective postoperative lumbar spinal drainage after thoracic aortic endograft. J Vasc Surg 2012;55(1):1–8.

13. Thompson MM, Ivaz S, Cheshire N, et al. Early results of endovascular treatment of the thoracic aorta using the Valiant endograft. Cardiovasc Intervent Radiol 2007;30(6):1130–8.

14. Buth J, Harris PL, Hobo R, et al. Neurologic complications associated with endovascular repair of thoracic aortic pathology: Incidence and risk factors. A study from the European Collaborators on Stent/Graft Techniques for Aortic Aneurysm Repair (EUROSTAR) registry. J Vasc Surg 2007;46(6):1103–11.

15. Holt PJ, Johnson C, Hinchliffe RJ, et al. Outcomes of the endovascular management of aortic arch aneurysm: implications for management of the left subclavian artery. J Vasc Surg 2010;51(6):1329–38.

16. Estrera AL, Miller CC, Azizzadeh A, et al. Thoracic aortic aneurysms. Acta Chir Belg 2006;106(3):307–16.

17. Safi HJ, Estrera AL, Miller CC, et al. Evolution of risk for neurologic deficit after descending and thoracoabdominal aortic repair. Ann Thorac Surg 2005;80(6):2173–9.

18. Bavaria JE, Appoo JJ, Makaroun MS, et al. Endovascular stent grafting versus open surgical repair of descending thoracic aortic aneurysms in low-risk patients: a multicenter comparative trial. J Thorac Cardiovasc Surg 2007;133(2):369–77.

19. Fattori R, Nienaber CA, Rousseau H, et al. Results of endovascular repair of the thoracic aorta with the Talent Thoracic stent graft: the Talent Thoracic Retrospective Registry. J Thorac Cardiovasc Surg 2006;132(2):332–9.

20. Mommertz G, Sigala F, Langer S, et al. Thoracoabdominal aortic aneurysm repair in patients with Marfan syndrome. Eur J Vasc Endovasc Surg 2008;35(2):181–6.

21. Nordon IM, Hinchliffe RJ, Holt PJ, et al. Endovascular management of chronic aortic dissection in patients with Marfan syndrome. J Vasc Surg 2009;50(5):987–91.

22. Ince H, Rehders TC, Petzsch M, et al. Stent-grafts in patients with Marfan syndrome. J Endovasc Ther 2005;12(1):82–8.

23. Svensson LG, Crawford ES, Hess KR, et al. Experience with 1509 patients undergoing thoracoabdominal aortic aneurysms. J Vasc Surg 1993;17(2):357–68.

24. Money SR, Hollier LH. The management of thoracoabdominal aneurysms. Adv Surg 1994;27:285–94.

25. Crawford ES, DeNatale RW. Thoracoabdominal aortic aneurysm: observations regarding the natural course of the disease. J Vasc Surg 1986;3(4):578–82.

26. Safi HJ, Hess KR, Randel M, et al. Cerebrospinal fluid drainage and distal aortic perfusion: reducing neurologic complications in repair of thoracoabdominal aortic aneurysm types I and II. J Vasc Surg 1996;23(2):223–9.

27. Jacobs MJ, de Mol BA, Legemate DA, et al. Retrograde aortic and selective organ perfusion during thoracoabdominal aortic aneurysm repair. Eur J Vasc Endovasc Surg 1997;14(5):360–6.

28. Huynh TT, Miller 3rd CC, Estrera AL, et al. Correlations of cerebrospinal fluid pressure with hemodynamic parameters during thoracoabdominal aortic aneurysm repair. Ann Vasc Surg 2005;19(5):619–24.

29. Estrera AL, Miller 3rd CC, Huynh TT, et al. Preoperative and operative predictors of delayed neurologic deficit following repair of thoracoabdominal aortic aneurysm. J Thorac Cardiovasc Surg 2003;126(5):1288–94.

30. Jacobs MJ, Elenbaas TW, Schurink GW, et al. Assessment of spinal cord integrity during thoracoabdominal aortic aneurysm repair. Ann Thorac Surg 2002;74(5):S1864–8.

31. Shine TS, Harrison BA, De Ruyter ML, et al. Motor and somatosensory evoked potentials: their role in predicting spinal cord ischemia in patients undergoing thoracoabdominal aortic aneurysm repair with regional lumbar epidural cooling. Anesthesiology 2008;108(4):580–7.

32. Coselli JS, Bozinovski J, LeMaire SA. Open surgical repair of 2286 thoracoabdominal aortic aneurysms. Ann Thorac Surg 2007;83(2):S862–4.

33. Conrad MF, Crawford RS, Davison JK, et al. Thoracoabdominal aneurysm repair: a 20-year perspective. Ann Thorac Surg 2007;83(2):S856–61.

34. Estrera AL, Miller 3rd CC, Huynh TT, et al. Neurologic outcome after thoracic and thoracoabdominal aortic aneurysm repair. Ann Thorac Surg 2001;72(4):1225–30.

35. Rigberg DA, McGory ML, Zingmond DS, et al. Thirty-day mortality statistics underestimate the risk of repair of thoracoabdominal aortic aneurysms: a statewide experience. J Vasc Surg 2006;43(2):217–23.

36. Cowan Jr JA, Dimick JB, Wainess RM, et al. Ruptured thoracoabdominal aortic aneurysm treatment in the United States: 1988 to 1998. J Vasc Surg 2003;38(2):319–22.

37. Derrow AE, Seeger JM, Dame DA, et al. The outcome in the United States after thoracoabdominal aortic aneurysm repair, renal artery bypass, and mesenteric revascularization. J Vasc Surg 2001;34(1):54–61.

38. Resch TA, Greenberg RK, Lyden SP, et al. Combined staged procedures for the treatment of thoracoabdominal aneurysms. J Endovasc Ther 2006;13(4):481–9.

39. Zhou W, Reardon M, Peden EK, et al. Hybrid approach to complex thoracic aortic aneurysms in high-risk patients: surgical challenges and clinical outcomes. J Vasc Surg 2006;44(4):688–93.

40. Black SA, Wolfe JH, Clark M, et al. Complex thoracoabdominal aortic aneurysms: endovascular exclusion with visceral revascularization. J Vasc Surg 2006;43(6):1081–9.

41. Bockler D, Schumacher H, Klemm K, et al. Hybrid procedures as a combined endovascular and open approach for pararenal and thoracoabdominal aortic pathologies. Langenbecks Arch Surg 2007;392(6):715–23.

42. Chiesa R, Tshomba Y, Melissano G, et al. Hybrid approach to thoracoabdominal aortic aneurysms in patients with prior aortic surgery. J Vasc Surg 2007;45(6):1128–35.

43. Lee WA, Brown MP, Martin TD, et al. Early results after staged hybrid repair of thoracoabdominal aortic aneurysms. J Am Coll Surg 2007;205(3):420–31.

44. Biasi L, Ali T, Loosemore T, et al. Hybrid repair of complex thoracoabdominal aortic aneurysms using applied endovascular strategies combined with visceral and renal revascularization. J Thorac Cardiovasc Surg 2009;138(6):1331–8.

45. Wolf O, Eckstein H. Combined open and endovascular treatment of thoracoabdominal aneurysms and secondary expanding aortic dissections: early and mid-term results from a single-center series. Ann Vasc Surg 2010;24(2):167–77.

46. Ham SW, Chong T, Moos J, et al. Arch and visceral/renal debranching combined with endovascular repair for thoracic and thoracoabdominal aortic aneurysms. J Vasc Surg 2011;54(1):30–40.

47. Drinkwater SL, Bockler D, Eckstein H, et al. The visceral hybrid repair of thoraco-abdominal aortic aneurysms – a collaborative approach. Eur J Vasc Endovasc Surg 2009;38(5):578–85.

48. Chuter TA. Fenestrated and branched stent-grafts for thoracoabdominal, pararenal and juxtarenal aortic aneurysm repair. Semin Vasc Surg 2007;20(2):90–6.

49. Roselli EE, Greenberg RK, Pfaff K, et al. Endovascular treatment of thoracoabdominal aortic aneurysms. J Thorac Cardiovasc Surg 2007;133(6):1474–82.

50. Anderson JL, Adam DJ, Berce M, et al. Repair of thoracoabdominal aortic aneurysms with fenestrated and branched endovascular stent grafts. J Vasc Surg 2005;42(4):600–7.

51. Chuter TA, Hiramoto JS, Park KH, et al. The transition from custom-made to standardized multibranched thoracoabdominal aortic stent grafts. J Vasc Surg 2011;54(3):660–8.

52. Nordon IM, Hinchliffe RJ, Loftus IM, et al. Management of acute aortic syndrome and chronic aortic dissection. Cardiovasc Intervent Radiol 2011;34(5):890–902.

53. Evangelista A, Mukherjee D, Mehta RH, et al. Acute intramural hematoma of the aorta: a mystery in evolution. Circulation 2005;111(8):1063–70.

54. Coady MA, Rizzo JA, Elefteriades JA. Pathologic variants of thoracic aortic dissections. Penetrating atherosclerotic ulcers and intramural hematomas. Cardiol Clin 1999;17(4):637–57.

55. Mehta RH, Suzuki T, Hagan PG, et al. Predicting death in patients with acute type A aortic dissection. Circulation 2002;105(2):200–6.

56. Hagan PG, Nienaber CA, Isselbacher EM, et al. The International Registry of Acute Aortic Dissection (IRAD): new insights into an old disease. JAMA 2000;283(7):897–903.

57. Estrera AL, Miller CC, Goodrick J, et al. Update on outcomes of acute type B aortic dissection. Ann Thorac Surg 2007;83(2):S842–50.

58. Estrera AL, Miller 3rd CC, Safi HJ, et al. Outcomes of medical management of acute type B aortic dissection. Circulation 2006;114(1, Suppl):I384–1389.

59. Nienaber CA, Kische S, Zeller T, et al. Provisional extension to induce complete attachment after stent-graft placement in type B aortic dissection: the PETTICOAT concept. J Endovasc Ther 2006;13(6):738–46.

60. Eggebrecht H, Nienaber CA, Neuhauser M, et al. Endovascular stent-graft placement in aortic dissection: a meta-analysis. Eur Heart J 2006;27(4):489–98.

61. Bortone AS, De Cillis E, D'Agostino D, et al. Endovascular treatment of thoracic aortic disease: four years of experience. Circulation 2004;110(11, Suppl. 1):II262–7.

62. Beregi JP, Haulon S, Otal P, et al. Endovascular treatment of acute complications associated with aortic dissection: midterm results from a multicenter study. J Endovasc Ther 2003;10(3):486–93.

63. Nienaber CA, Rousseau H, Eggebrecht H, et al. Randomized comparison of strategies for type B aortic dissection: the INvestigation of STEnt grafts in Aortic Dissection (INSTEAD) trial. Circulation 2009;120(25):2519–28.

64. Tang DG, Dake MD. TEVAR for acute uncomplicated aortic dissection: immediate repair versus medical therapy. Semin Vasc Surg 2009;22(3):145–51.

65. Song JM, Kim SD, Kim JH, et al. Long-term predictors of descending aorta aneurysmal change in patients with aortic dissection. J Am Coll Cardiol 2007;50(8):799–804.

66. Shorr RM, Crittenden M, Indeck M, et al. Blunt thoracic trauma. Analysis of 515 patients. Ann Surg 1987;206(2):200–5.

67. Parmley LF, Mattingly TW, Manion WC. Penetrating wounds of the heart and aorta. Circulation 1958;17(5):953–73.

68. Fabian TC, Davis KA, Gavant ML, et al. Prospective study of blunt aortic injury: helical CT is diagnostic and antihypertensive therapy reduces rupture. Ann Surg 1998;227(5):666–77.

69. Melnitchouk S, Pfammatter T, Kadner A, et al. Emergency stent-graft placement for hemorrhage control in acute thoracic aortic rupture. Eur J Cardiothorac Surg 2004;25(6):1032–8.

70. Waldenberger P, Fraedrich G, Mallouhi A, et al. Emergency endovascular treatment of traumatic aortic arch rupture with multiple arch vessel involvement. J Endovasc Ther 2003;10(4):728–32.

71. Fattori R, Napoli G, Lovato L, et al. Descending thoracic aortic diseases: stent-graft repair. Radiology 2003;229(1):176–83.

72. Dake MD, White RA, Diethrich EB, et al. Report on endograft management of traumatic thoracic aortic transections at 30 days and 1 year from a multidisciplinary subcommittee of the Society for Vascular Surgery Outcomes Committee. J Vasc Surg 2011;53(4):1091–6.

73. Hinchliffe RJ, Krasznai A, Schultzekool L, et al. Observations on the failure of stent-grafts in the aortic arch. Eur J Vasc Endovasc Surg 2007;34(4):451–6.

74. Lee WA, Matsumura JS, Mitchell RS, et al. Endovascular repair of traumatic thoracic aortic injury: clinical practice guidelines of the Society for Vascular Surgery. J Vasc Surg 2011;53(1):187–92.

75. Lee YK, Seo JB, Jang YM, et al. Acute and chronic complications of aortic intramural haematoma on follow up computed tomography: incidence and predictor analysis. J Comput Assist Tomogr 2007;31(3):435–40.

15

Renal and intestinal vascular disease

Trevor Cleveland
Jonathan G. Moss
Nicholas J. Cheshire
Robert Kaikini
Mark O. Downes

Renal artery disease

Renal artery stenosis is an anatomical description of a lesion that may represent a variety of pathophysiological disease processes or that may simply be silent throughout life. The pathology in the majority of patients in the Western world is atherosclerosis and the term 'atherosclerotic renovascular disease' has been coined. The remainder are mainly represented by fibromuscular dysplasia, which has little in common with its atherosclerotic counterpart, as well as by manifestations of systemic vasculitis.

Fibromuscular dysplasia (FMD)

FMD is a non-inflammatory, non-atherosclerotic disorder that may be observed in almost any arterial bed and can lead to arterial stenosis. Five different types are recognised and usually affect younger patients, with a female predominance, involving the distal main artery and/or the intrarenal branches. Rarely, FMD may be complicated by an aneurysm. Patients may be asymptomatic but the most usual presentation is hypertension. Hypertension is commonly treated successfully with medication, but renal artery stenosis and renal dysfunction may progress in up to one-third of patients. Occlusion and complete loss of renal function is exceptional. Magnetic resonance angiography (MRA) can detect FMD in the proximal vessels, but is less sensitive for visualising the second- and third-order branches. The diagnosis will usually require conventional digital subtraction angiography and selective views may be necessary to detect subtle branch lesions. When treating FMD, the results of percutaneous angioplasty (PTA) are good, with 10-year cumulative patency rates of 87% and up to 50% of patients cured of their hypertension. The remainder have a reduced drug burden and improved blood pressure control.[1] Stenting is usually reserved for suboptimal PTA.

Arteritis

Involvement of the renal artery is not uncommon in systemic vasculitis. The diagnosis can be difficult and in the absence of other systemic symptoms may require a renal biopsy. Takayasu's arteritis (see also Chapter 12) is a non-specific inflammatory disease that mainly affects large arteries such as the aorta and its main branches including the renal artery, and is the most common cause of renovascular hypertension in India and China. The majority of patients can be managed medically on corticosteroids, with monitoring of disease activity using the erythrocyte sedimentation rate (ESR). In the chronic inactive stage, PTA can produce a reasonable blood pressure response.[2]

Atherosclerotic renal vascular disease

Definition and pathology

Atherosclerotic stenosis is the most common pathological condition of the renal arteries, affecting 1–5% of patients with hypertension.[3] Occlusion of the renal artery is present in up to 50% of patients so the condition is best described as atherosclerotic renovascular disease (ARVD) rather than as renal artery stenosis (RAS). Autopsy data demonstrate that the incidence of ARVD increases with age, affecting 18% of individuals between the ages of 65 and 74 years and >40% of those over 75 years.[4] Medicare data from America indicate that ARVD has an incidence of 3.9 cases per 1000 of the population over 65 years.[5] Usually, ARVD is a manifestation of generalised atherosclerosis involving multiple vessels.

Widespread atheroma is usually present in the aorta and typically compromises the proximal 1–2 cm of one or both renal arteries. If untreated, atherosclerotic stenosis progresses to renal artery occlusion in up to 50% of patients[6] and permanent loss of the renal parenchyma in 15–25% of patients, particularly in the elderly.[7] The exact level of angiographic stenosis that represents significant ARVD is controversial and varies between 50% and 75% in diameter loss. Large-animal experiments have demonstrated a significant pressure gradient across a stenosis of 60%;[8] however, in humans a lesion even less than 50% can be associated with gradients of 15 mmHg.[9]

Pathophysiology

Renal function

ARVD is considered an association, rather than the cause of the majority of cases of chronic and end-stage renal failure.[10] A haemodynamically significant RAS will lead to a reduction in renal artery perfusion pressure and thus an impairment of renal function simply due to a hydraulic effect, in only a minority of patients. Most commonly, renin and angiotensin levels are increased in the poststenotic kidney, constricting the postglomerular efferent arteriole, which in turn helps to support glomerular capillary hydraulic pressure and filtration rate. This might explain why the use of renin–angiotensin–aldosterone system (RAAS) blocking agents such as angiotensin-converting enzyme (ACE) inhibitors is controversial in the management of ARVD. As glomerular perfusion in these patients is critically dependent upon angiotensin II, the risk of developing acute renal failure is significant, especially if the stenosis is bilateral or affects a solitary functioning kidney. Nonetheless, RAAS-blocking drugs are the only agents proven to slow progression to end-stage renal disease, and acute deterioration in renal function is usually immediately reversible on cessation of treatment.

Cholesterol embolisation may cause acute renal failure in renovascular disease. Patients with severe aortic atheroma undergoing arterial surgical or angiographic procedures, thrombolysis or anticoagulation are at a significant risk of developing renal dysfunction secondary to cholesterol emboli. Associated clinical features include livedo reticularis, proteinuria and eosinophilia. Proteinuria appears to be a key marker of renal damage in patients with ARVD and a prospective study has shown that it can be the main predictor of future deterioration in function.[11]

Studies in large cohorts of patients with ARVD have shown that there is often poor correlation between the degree of anatomical atheromatous stenosis, glomerular filtration rate (GFR) and overall renal function.[12,13] Patients with unilateral ARVD can have GFRs that range from normal to stage 5 kidney disease. Nuclear studies in patients with unilateral stenosis reveal that GFR is the same or even lower in the non-stenotic kidney. This lack of correlation between the severity of renal ischaemic injury and kidney function may explain why renal function often fails to improve significantly after revascularisation despite restoration of renal artery patency.

Hypertension

The pathophysiology of hypertension differs in patients with unilateral and bilateral RAS. In both, a drop in renal perfusion pressure distal to the lesion induces an increase in the activity of the RAAS. Vasoconstriction as well as salt and water retention contribute to the initial rise in systemic blood pressure, which tends to increase perfusion pressure of the poststenotic kidney towards normal. In patients with unilateral disease, perfusion pressure also rises in the contralateral, non-stenotic kidney, inducing a pressure natriuresis response. Salt and water excretion increase in the non-stenotic kidney, promoting a return of extracellular volume towards normal. Initially, therefore, patients may experience marked reductions in blood pressure in response to RAAS blockade.

In patients with bilateral RAS, however, the increase in systemic pressure is never transmitted to a kidney, there is no pressure natriuresis, and salt and water retention can persist. Systemic hypertension and volume expansion return renal perfusion pressure toward normal, suppressing activity of the RAAS, and RAAS-blocking drugs may fail to reduce blood pressure effectively in these patients.

Chapter 15

Regardless of whether the disease is unilateral or bilateral, revascularisation may fail to cure hypertension, especially when the stenosis is long-standing.

Diagnosis and presentation

The gold standard for diagnosing RAS is renal arteriography. Non-invasive tests are also used in the diagnosis of RAS, particularly MRA because it does not require either radiation or potentially nephrotoxic iodine-based contrast agents. The use of contrast-enhanced MRA has improved the ability to visualise any accessory renal vessel. It is, however, important to note that for patients with moderate to severe renal disease the administration of some gadolinium contrast agents during MRA has been linked with the development of nephrogenic systemic fibrosis (NSF).

The clinical index of suspicion remains essential in determining an appropriate diagnostic and therapeutic strategy in ARVD. Specific clinical pointers include:

- hypertension;
- renal impairment;
- concomitant cardiovascular disease;
- ACE-induced acute renal impairment;
- 'flash' pulmonary oedema;
- vascular bruits.

ARVD and cardiovascular disease

There is a high incidence of adverse cardiovascular events in patients with ARVD as compared with age-matched subjects with normal renal arteries. ARVD is present in 33–44% of patients with peripheral vascular disease and 38% of those found to have an abdominal aortic aneurysm.[14,15] In an autopsy series of 346 cases of brain infarcts, RAS was found in 10.4% and carotid artery stenosis in 33.6% of subjects.[16]

In a large group of patients in whom renal arteriography was performed at the time of cardiac catheterisation, 15% of patients were found to have significant RAS. Those with RAS had a much higher incidence of adverse cardiovascular events as compared with patients without ARVD.[17] There was also a direct correlation between the degree of stenosis and overall survival. Patients with >95% narrowing had only an approximately 40% 4-year survival as compared with 80% in those with normal arteries. These findings were independent of whether or not the patients subsequently underwent revascularisation.[18]

Sudden-onset left heart failure in patients with no previous cardiac history and well-preserved overall cardiac function ('flash' pulmonary oedema) is a manifestation of ARVD. It affects over 10% of patients, especially those with evidence of bilateral RAS.[19]

The increased risk of adverse cardiovascular events in ARVD may be attributable to concomitant extra burden of atherosclerosis found in other parts of the arterial tree, including the coronary and cerebral circulations.

Management options

Patients with ARVD can be treated with medical therapy and may also be considered for revascularisation by either endovascular or surgical means.

Medical therapy

Optimal medical management should include blood pressure control, antiplatelet therapy, cholesterol management, adequate glycaemic control in diabetics, smoking cessation, diet and exercise (see Chapter 1). It should be noted that the addition of statin therapy to patients with RAS is associated with a reduced likelihood of the progression of the stenosis.[20]

Antihypertensive therapy

Although antihypertensive therapy is proven to be effective in preventing adverse events in patients with essential hypertension, there are no data on its effects on outcomes in patients with ARVD. A target blood pressure of <140/90 mmHg is recommended for individuals without other comorbidities, whereas a lower goal of <130/80 mmHg is recommended for patients with hypertension and diabetes or renal disease with significant proteinuria. Most patients will require combinations of antihypertensive agents to achieve optimal blood pressure control. Surprisingly, RAAS-blocking agents are the first-line antihypertensive choices in patients with ARVD, especially those with evidence of chronic parenchymal disease. Patients should be closely monitored for elevations in serum creatinine and potassium concentrations, particularly in the cases of bilateral RAS or in a solitary kidney.

Endovascular treatment of ARVD

In comparison to surgical techniques, renal stenting is a relatively simple procedure and less hazardous, although careful peri-interventional care is necessary. However, the risk/benefit balance of revascularisation in atherosclerotic RAS is yet to be determined. The recent ASTRAL trial[21] appears to cast doubt on the benefits of an endovascular approach (see below). However, it may be prudent to reserve the procedure for patients in certain subgroups who may be at greatest risk. These include the following indications:

- recurrent flash pulmonary oedema;
- refractory hypertension;
- dialysis-dependent acute renal failure (in such patients with cortical preservation, there is little to be lost and much to be gained by intervention).

Less certain indications include:

- severe stenosis (>70%) in a single functioning kidney with deterioration of renal function;
- severe bilateral stenosis (>70%) with deterioration of renal function;
- ACE inhibitor-related uraemia in patients who require ACE inhibitors for cardiac disease.

Imaging and work-up

Contrast-enhanced MRA had all but replaced other imaging techniques until the association with NSF was recognised. MRA provides the information required prior to renal artery stenting[22] (**Fig. 15.1a**). If a patient has an estimated GFR of <60 mL/min, then computed tomography angiography (CTA) should be considered (**Fig. 15.1b**), which carries the alternative, but perhaps more benign, risk of contrast-induced acute kidney injury. If both MRA and CTA are contraindicated, then CO_2 angiography can be used.

Renal artery anatomy can be determined from the pre-procedural imaging, allowing placement of the stent to cover the lesion and protrude 1–3 mm into the aorta. Kidneys less than 8 cm in length are generally unsuitable for revascularisation. Patients should be adequately hydrated at least 12 hours before and 12 hours following the procedure with intravenous fluids.[23] There is some evidence that administration of N-acetylcysteine reduces the incidence of contrast nephropathy.[24] Patients should receive antiplatelet therapy such as aspirin or clopidogrel for life, and be closely followed up for changes in renal function and blood pressure control.

Procedure (**Fig. 15.1c–e**)

Stenting has effectively replaced angioplasty as the first line in endovascular treatment of atherosclerotic RAS (see later).[25] Typically via a femoral approach, a 5F or 6F shaped sheath is introduced into the abdominal aorta. The renal artery is cannulated and an 0.014–0.018 inch wire is positioned in the renal artery. This allows for usage of low-profile systems for predilatation and stent placement. Vasospasm can be prevented with administration of vasodilators such as glyceryl trinitrate through the sheath. Balloon-expandable stents are now widely used as they are easier to position accurately to achieve full renal ostium coverage.

In patients at risk of contrast-induced nephropathy, alternative contrast agents such as carbon dioxide are available. Cholesterol embolisation may occur at the time of renal artery stenting,[26] and some authors advocate the use of embolic

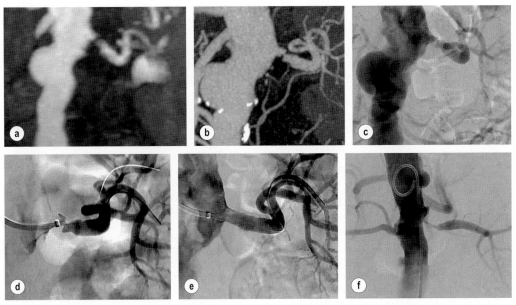

Figure 15.1 • **(a)** Magnetic resonance angiography shows a tight left renal artery stenosis. **(b)** Corresponding CTA. **(c)** Conventional catheter angiogram from a brachial approach at the time of treatment confirms these findings. **(d)** Angiography following cannulation but prior to stent placement. **(e)** Angiography following stent placement. **(f)** Angiography demonstrating in-stent stenosis in a different patient.

protection devices.[27,28] None of the present devices are designed for renal intervention and may add to the complexity of the procedure. Data from treatment of other arterial beds have shown a reduction in complications when statins are used, and administration prior to RAS should be considered.

Complications

For renal PTA/stenting the literature quotes complication rates ranging from 0% to 66%.[29] Major complications include:

- acute deterioration in renal function (usually secondary to contrast acute kidney injury);
- cholesterol embolisation (insidious onset, elevated ESR, eosinophilia, livedo reticularis);
- renal artery perforation (rare) – should this occur, it can usually be treated either by balloon tamponade or a stentgraft.

Most complications can be avoided by the use of low-profile systems, adequate hydration, closure devices, experienced operators and optimisation of patients prior to treatment.

Results of angioplasty and stenting

The treatment of clinically stable patients with high-grade RAS is highly controversial.

✓✓ Van Jaarsveld et al.[30] randomised 106 patients with RAS of greater than 50% and significant hypertension (but only mild to moderate renal impairment; creatinine <200 μmol/L) to angioplasty or medical therapy. No differences were noted in the primary end-point of blood pressure control or in renal function.

Two other trials incorporated a similar design but contained only 49 and 55 patients.[31,32] There are two published meta-analyses of the above trials.[33,34] Both come to the same conclusion, namely that the effect of PTA on hypertension is at best modest and that none of these small trials were powered to detect changes in renal function.

The conclusion of the authors of ASTRAL was that revascularisation conferred substantial risks without significant benefit in patients with atherosclerotic renovascular disease.

✓✓ ASTRAL is the largest randomised trial to date comparing renal artery revascularisation and best medical therapy with best medical therapy alone in 806 patients.[21] Patients were randomised if they had at least one treatable renal artery and clinicians were in equipoise. The clinical status

of the patients was heterogeneous and included hypertension and renal failure. The primary outcome was renal function, as measured by the reciprocal of the serum creatinine level. Secondary outcomes were blood pressure, the time to renal and major cardiovascular events, and mortality. The median follow-up was 34 months.

During a 5-year period, the rate of progression of renal impairment was -0.07×10^{-3} litres per micromole per year in the revascularisation group, as compared with -0.13×10^{-3} litres per micromole per year in the medical therapy group, a difference favouring revascularisation of 0.06×10^{-3} litres per micromole per year (95% confidence interval (CI) -0.002 to 0.13; $P = 0.06$). There was no significant between-group difference in systolic blood pressure. Serious complications associated with revascularisation occurred in 23 patients, including two deaths and three amputations of toes or limbs.

Since its publication, the trial has come under sustained criticism for its methodology. The selection criteria meant that patients were only randomised if there were clinical doubts about the benefit of revascularisation. It is thought that this may have excluded a cohort of patients with severe or unilateral disease who may have benefited from intervention.

Although ASTRAL showed no benefit in revascularisation, recently Kalra et al. have published prospective cohort data suggesting a benefit of stenting among patients with RAS and chronic kidney disease (CKD).[35]

The benefits of revascularisation are controversial and the procedure should be undertaken with caution and only in centres with experience of the procedure. A further large randomised controlled trial, CORAL, is currently under way in the USA.

Stenting versus PTA

✓✓ A recent meta-analysis[25] compared the results of PTA (10 articles, 644 patients) with stenting (14 articles, 678 patients). None were randomised controlled trials. Stent placement had a higher technical success rate and lower re-stenosis rate than PTA and the complication rate was similar for both techniques. The cure rate for hypertension was higher (20% vs. 10%) and the improvement rate for renal function was lower (30% vs. 38%) after stent placement compared with PTA.

A single randomised controlled trial has compared PTA with stenting in 85 patients with ostial lesions.[36] The technical success rate of stents was superior to PTA (88% vs. 55%) and the primary

6-month patency likewise superior (75% vs. 29%). The trial was stopped following an interim analysis of the data.

The clinical outcomes in the two groups were similar, although the study was not powered to detect differences in blood pressure or renal function.

✔ If endovascular treatment of atherosclerotic RAS is undertaken, stenting is preferred to PTA alone.

Re-stenosis and drug-eluting stents

Re-stenosis can be an issue in renal artery stenting as in other vascular territories (**Fig. 15.1f**). If it does occur, it will often be seen in the first 3–6 months after the procedure. Figures vary but a re-stenosis rate of 15% at 6 months is commonly seen.[35] Although bare-metal stenting is superior to PTA alone, drug-eluting stents hold the promise of reducing re-stenosis rates further.

The GREAT trial[37] compared sirolimus-eluting stents with bare-metal stents in a small ($n = 106$) non-randomised trial. Results showed a trend favouring sirolimus-eluting stents but none of the measures reached statistical significance, possibly due to underpowering.

Other trials are currently recruiting and are comparing other drug-eluting stent systems in the treatment of atherosclerotic RAS.

Surgical treatment

There are a range of surgical options available to treat renal artery disease (Box 15.1). Current guidelines recommend surgery in patients with ARVD who have indications for revascularisation and have multiple small renal arteries or require aortic reconstruction near the renal arteries for other indications (e.g. aneurysm, severe aortoiliac occlusive disease). The site of the lesion is also important, and if extra-anatomical bypass is considered, the condition of the donor visceral vessels must be optimal. In patients with renal artery occlusion, renal biopsy (performed either preoperatively or perioperatively) can indicate whether the kidney is viable and functionally salvageable on the basis of collateral vessels. However, this procedure is not without risk of bleeding

Box 15.1 • Surgical revascularisation

Aortic graft and renal bypass
Aortorenal bypass
Aortorenal endarterectomy
Extra-anatomical bypass
Extracorporeal bench surgery

and even the loss of a kidney.[38] Endarterectomy and bypass grafting are the two main surgical options for revascularisation.

Nephrectomy is the oldest surgical procedure used in the treatment of ARVD. In the presence of a normal contralateral kidney, although rarely used, it remains the option if the affected kidney measures less than 8 cm. In this situation measurement of renal vein renin levels is of value, with nephrectomy being indicated when the ratio of renal vein renins is greater than 1.5.

In the presence of aortic aneurysmal disease affecting the renal ostium, aortic graft and renal bypass may be indicated, particularly if the aneurysm is not suited to EVAR. Surgical options include a 6–8 mm limb of Dacron or polytetrafluoroethylene (PTFE) graft sutured onto the aortic graft with an end-to-end renal anastomosis and then bypass on to the affected renal artery in either an end-to-end (usually easiest) or end-to-side manner. Where bilateral RAS is present, an inverted bifurcated Dacron graft is preferred. When the pattern of aneurysm disease dictates that a suprarenal clamp is required for open surgery, transaortic endarterectomy may be performed. The ostial lesion is then carefully endarterectomised and the procedure is completed with patch closure (**Fig. 15.2**). Five-year patencies in large centres can reach 90%.[39]

Extra-anatomical bypass grafting is an attractive option for patients with unilateral RAS in the absence of significant aortic disease. Access is obtained via a subcostal incision, without the need for aortic cross-clamping or extensive dissection, and revascularisation is achieved using inflow from either the hepatic or splenic artery (**Fig. 15.3a**). An interposition saphenous vein graft may be used where there is insufficient arterial calibre and length for an end-to-end anastomosis (**Fig. 15.3b**). The inferior vena cava, the right renal vein and often the left renal vein must be fully mobilised. On the left side, the splenic artery is dissected from its midpoint from the pancreas. Splenectomy can be avoided as there is a rich collateral supply and perfusion via the short gastric arteries. The Cleveland clinic reports 175 extra-anatomical bypass procedures over a 12-year period,[40] with 2.9% operative mortality. Graft patency reached 96%, renal function improved in 40% and hypertension was improved or cured in three-quarters of the series.

Aortorenal bypass can be carried out using the long saphenous vein, PTFE, Dacron or rarely the internal iliac artery. The infrarenal aorta is preferred as an inflow site if it is relatively disease free. If not, then a 'rooftop' incision is necessary in order to expose the aorta above the coeliac

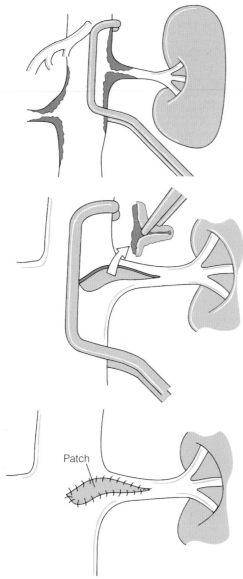

Figure 15.2 • Transaortic renal endarterectomy with patch closure.

Patch

axis. The thoracic aorta can also be used as an in-flow site. Where multiple small anastomoses are required, extracorporeal or bench surgery is performed for patients with disease affecting renal artery branches. Removal of the kidney, cooling and preservation as in renal transplantation surgery will allow multiple microvascular anastomoses to be performed before autotransplantation takes place. The internal iliac artery is commonly used for direct end-to-end anastomosis. The Cleveland clinic

again has the largest reported series of autotrans-plantation, with excellent long-term results.[38]

Surgical revascularisation is considered to be a high-risk option when compared to less invasive treatment methods. Reported results are shown in Table 15.1.[41–47] These morbidity and mortality rates have set the standards against which other treatment modalities can be compared. There have been no large trials to date comparing the outcomes of stenting with surgical revascularisation in ARVD. In young, fit patients surgery may be preferred as it is cost-effective and the long-term re-stenosis rate is reported to be 3–4%. The management of ARVD can be complex and certainly requires a multidisciplinary approach to maximise the therapeutic potential for each individual patient.

> ✔ Stenting should be used as the primary mode of revascularisation as it is minimally invasive, reserving surgery for stent failure or more complex aortic and renal pathology.

Renal artery denervation

Renal artery denervation is a new endovascular procedure for the treatment of resistant hypertension. This condition is thought to involve overactivity of the afferent and efferent sympathetic nerves that run in the adventitia of the renal arteries and is therefore considered here in the discussion of treatment of renal artery disease.

Radical nephrectomy and surgical sympathectomy have been associated with the normalisation of blood pressure in patients with end-stage renal disease (ESRD) and hypertension.[48,49] It has also been established that increased renal sympathetic nerve activity has an important role in the development of essential hypertension.[50]

In 2010, the Symplicity HTN-2 study demonstrated for the first time in humans that endovascular renal denervation is a safe and effective technique to reduce blood pressure in patients with resistant hypertension.[51] Following positioning of a sheath within the renal artery, a probe is positioned with its tip in contact with the inner luminal surface of the vessel. Radiofrequency energy is then applied in order to disrupt the nerve fibres running in the renal artery adventitia. The procedure is repeated at several points in both arteries in order to interrupt the neurogenic signals thought to be involved in the maintenance of sympathetic overactivity and, hence, resistant hypertension. The Symplicity HTN-2 trial randomised 106 patients with uncontrolled blood pressure (systolic >160 mmHg) and taking at least three antihypertensive agents to renal denervation plus best medical therapy or best medical therapy

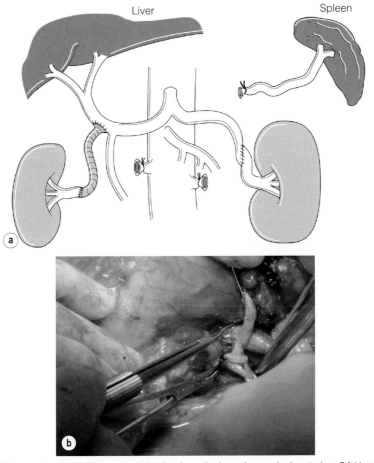

Figure 15.3 • **(a)** Extra-anatomical renal revascularisation from the hepatic or splenic arteries. **(b)** Hepatorenal bypass using the long saphenous vein.

Table 15.1 • Reported results of surgical revascularisation

Benjamin et al. (1996)[41]	Treatment of hypertension (cure or improvement)	63–91%
Dean (1997)[42]		
Benjamin et al. (1996)[41]	Treatment of renal failure (cure or improvement)	33–91%
Reilly et al. (1996)[43]		
Steinbach et al. (1997)[44]	Primary patency rates	93–97%
Darling et al. (1995)[45]		
Novick et al. (1987)[46]		
Darling et al. (1995)[45]	Morbidity	6–43%
Reilly et al. (1996)[43]	Mortality	2–8%
Steinbach et al. (1997)[44]		
Cambria et al. (1996)[47]		

alone. At 6 months the group receiving renal denervation showed a significantly reduced blood pressure measurement of 32/12 mmHg. This is, however, a relatively small study, upon which treatment strategy cannot be based, but a further study is being conducted in the USA (Symplicity HTN-3), which may establish the safety and efficacy of the procedure.

Intestinal vascular disease

Visceral arterial pathology, in common with any arterial disease, falls into two main categories: occlusive and aneurysmal disease. Intestinal ischaemia and visceral aneurysms are uncommon but potentially life-threatening conditions. Despite recent advances in therapeutic techniques and diagnostic tools, their management remains clinically challenging. Significant questions exist with regard to the optimal therapeutic choice and the predictors of clinical outcome. Surgery is the conventional treatment. The endovascular approach is an emerging option and the results have been constantly improving.

Intestinal ischaemia

Mesenteric ischaemia results from hypoperfusion of the gut, most commonly due to occlusion, thrombosis or (vary rarely) vasospasm. The clinical consequences depend upon the number of vessels affected, the adequacy of collateral circulation and the duration of the insult. Early diagnosis and treatment are imperative, otherwise outcomes can be catastrophic.

Acute mesenteric ischaemia (AMI)

Aetiology and incidence

AMI can result from acute occlusion of the superior mesenteric artery (SMA) embolism, thrombosis or iatrogenic, or non-occlusive ischaemia secondary to inadequate mesenteric arterial blood flow and oxygenation. The commonest cause of AMI is embolic occlusion of the SMA (50% of all cases). Such emboli are usually cardiac in origin, but may arise from atherosclerotic plaques or from arterial aneurysms. Acute disruption of the visceral arterial flow can occur during endovascular manipulation as a result of inadvertent plaque dislodgement and embolisation or accidental occlusion of the visceral artery origin with an endograft. Left colon ischaemia can also occur after aortic reconstruction.[52] The majority of emboli progress distally to the tapered segment of the SMA just past the origin of the middle colic artery. In 20% of cases, a pre-existing atherosclerotic lesion at the origin of the vessel will lead to visceral artery thrombosis. Most of these patients are female and have evidence of symptomatic vascular disease at other sites and have often previously undergone vascular interventions. Half of them have symptoms of chronic mesenteric ischaemia. Non-occlusive ischaemia caused during periods of low cardiac output and shock accounts for another 20% of cases.[53] A Swedish population-based study identified 997 cases of intestinal ischaemia using a clinical autopsy database. Fatal heart failure was the leading cause of intestinal hypoperfusion, although stenosis of the SMA and coeliac trunk, atrial fibrillation and recent surgery contributed significantly.[54] Other unusual arteriopathies, such as Takayasu's arteritis, fibromuscular dysplasia and polyarteritis nodosa, may first present with intestinal ischaemia. Isolated dissections of the SMA have also been reported, although more commonly it originates in the thoracic aorta and extends into the SMA.

Pathophysiology

Intrinsic and extrinsic mechanisms are involved in the regulation of mesenteric blood flow. Intrinsic autoregulation of blood flow is most likely to involve direct arteriolar smooth muscle relaxation and metabolic response to adenosine and other metabolites of mucosal ischaemia. Extrinsic control is due to neural and humoral mechanisms. The intestine is able to compensate for a substantial acute reduction of blood flow for up to 12 hours without substantial injury. Extensive collateral circulation opens following occlusion of a major vessel. With prolonged ischaemic time, however, progressive vasoconstriction develops in the obstructed bed, increasing its pressure and reducing collateral flow. This vasoconstriction may persist even after restoration of flow, leading to continuing ischaemia. Ischaemia results in loss of mucosal barrier with translocation of bacteria, endotoxins and cytokines precipitating septicaemia and multiorgan failure. Ischaemic damage can also be caused by reperfusion injury, with the release of free radicals after successful reperfusion causing a pronounced inflammatory response.[55]

Diagnosis and treatment

The classic presentation is with acute severe abdominal pain out of proportion to the physical signs. These patients are usually admitted with an acute abdomen. Left colon ischaemia following aortic reconstruction or aneurysm repair can present with watery diarrhoea (bloody or non-bloody) early in the postoperative period. These patients should all undergo urgent bedside colonoscopy. AMI can lead to sudden decompensation, and therefore a high index of suspicion and experience are required to avoid unnecessary delays in diagnosis and treatment. Mortality rates are high at 70–80%.[54] AMI is a true emergency, and confirmatory angiography should not delay treatment. Initial management includes volume resuscitation, correction of acidosis and intravenous antibiotics. Heparin anticoagulation should be started to prevent further propagation of thrombus. An emergency exploratory laparotomy is usually necessary, although modern computed tomography (CT) scanning may be helpful if this does not result in a delay in surgery.

Whilst reports exist of successful thrombolysis with percutaneous SMA angioplasty,[56] a laparotomy is still strongly advisable to assess bowel viability. The SMA is exposed and there is often a proximal SMA pulse if the cause is embolic. If the bowel is found to be viable, an embolectomy is performed via a transverse arteriotomy using a 3Fr Fogarty catheter. If a longitudinal arteriotomy is performed, it should be closed using a vein patch to prevent stenosis.

If the cause is thrombosis, no pulse is palpable in the SMA and surgical thromboembolectomy is unlikely to be successful or durable. A bypass graft distal to the occlusion is then required to restore arterial blood supply to the gut. This could be antegrade, taking inflow from the supracoeliac aorta, or retrograde from the infrarenal aorta or iliac arteries. Often the latter is chosen because the exposure is familiar and the risks associated with clamping and dissection are less.[57] If there is peritoneal contamination or extensive bowel gangrene, autologous vein as a conduit is preferable to a prosthetic graft. Caution, however, should be taken to avoid graft kinking and subsequent occlusion. Time should be allowed for reperfusion before assessing the bowel for viability. Necrotic bowel needs to be resected. Exteriorisation of the bowel with a planned second-look laparotomy and delayed bowel anastomosis is a safe option. Postoperatively, patients with emboli should be anticoagulated and those with evidence of atherosclerotic disease should receive optimal medical therapy and risk factor management.

Long-term patient outcomes depend on the cardiovascular status, underlying disease and extent of the bowel ischaemia. Mortality rates remain high.

Mesenteric venous thrombosis

This syndrome is rare and accounts for 5–15% of all cases of acute mesenteric ischaemia. It can be primary or secondary, following hypercoagulable states, portal venous stasis, intra-abdominal inflammation, infection, malignancy and oral contraceptive use (4–5% of all cases). Up to 75% of patients with mesenteric venous thrombosis have an inherited thrombotic disorder, the most common being factor V Leiden mutation. Conditions associated with acquired hypercoagulable states that are associated with mesenteric venous thrombosis are paroxysmal nocturnal haemoglobinuria and the myeloproliferative syndromes. Diagnosis is often delayed due to the absence of specific signs, symptoms and laboratory findings. Contrast-enhanced CT can reveal the extent of thrombus, air in the mesenteric vein or portal system and the presence or absence of collateral flow. Unfortunately, the diagnosis is most commonly made at laparotomy or autopsy. Infarcted bowel should be resected and long-term anticoagulation should be established early as recurrence rates are high.

Non-occlusive mesenteric thrombosis

This syndrome develops in severe systemic illness in association with cardiorespiratory shock and multi-organ failure. Typically, this affects patients on the intensive care unit with congestive cardiac failure or severe cardiac dysfunction and the use of inotropic agents may further aggravate the situation. The administration of digoxin and α-adrenergic agonists as well as cocaine have also been implicated. The diagnosis is made with a high index of clinical suspicion and can be confirmed by angiography. This will show intestinal arterial vasospasm and exclude an intrinsic arterial lesion. Treatment depends on optimising cardiac output, treating underlying conditions such as sepsis and, where possible, removing adverse pharmacological agents such as the inotropes. In severe cases, intramesenteric arterial infusion of papaverine at a dose of 30–60 mg/hour is beneficial. Glucagon (2–4 mg/hour) will increase splanchnic blood flow and has the advantage of being given intravenously. However, mortality in this condition remains high at 70–80% despite these therapies.

Chronic mesenteric ischaemia (CMI)

Aetiology and incidence

CMI is the result of progressive atherosclerosis in more than 90% of cases. There is a significant gender difference, with females being affected in 76% of cases.[58] Half of the patients have significant coronary artery disease and/or peripheral arterial occlusive disease. Non-atherosclerotic causes of CMI are unusual and include thrombosis associated with thoraco-abdominal aneurysms, aortic dissection, arteritis, fibromuscular hyperplasia, neurofibromatosis, radiation injury, cocaine abuse, Buerger's disease and extrinsic coeliac artery compression by the median arcuate ligament. Despite the frequency of visceral artery stenosis, symptomatic chronic intestinal ischaemia is rare because of the excellent collateral circulatory network between the main visceral arteries, namely the coeliac trunk, superior mesenteric and the inferior mesenteric arteries, and the systemic circulation (**Fig. 15.4**).

> ✓ At least two of the three intestinal vessels must be stenotic or occluded for symptoms to occur,[58] and patients with single-vessel disease are rarely symptomatic.

Diagnosis

Patients with visceral arterial insufficiency typically suffer from postprandial abdominal pain, which leads to food fear and progressive weight loss. This classical triad is only observed in half of the patients. The clinical picture can be quite non-specific and misdiagnosed for other conditions, such as gastritis, peptic ulcer disease, gastrointestinal malignancy and diverticular disease. Physical examination is also non-specific, although the manifestations of generalised atherosclerotis are very common and in up to 70% of the patients an abdominal bruit can be heard. The natural history is that of malnutrition, and progressive intestinal ischaemia may eventually lead to bowel infarction and death.

Liver

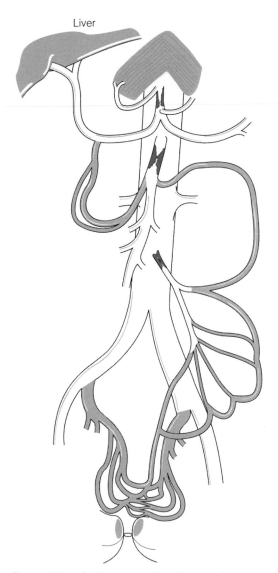

Figure 15.4 • Collateral circulation of the intestine.

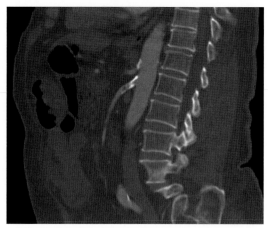

Figure 15.5 • Reconstructed CT angiogram showing a tight superior mesenteric artery stenosis with proximal wall calcification.

Until recently, catheter angiography was the only reliable method of assessing the splanchnic circulation in vivo. Newer techniques such as duplex ultrasound, gastrointestinal tonometry, CTA (**Fig. 15.5**) and magnetic resonance provide non-invasive or minimally invasive examination of the anatomy and function of the splanchnic circulation. As there is no effective medical treatment for CMI, its management is focused on restoration of blood flow.

Surgical intervention

At present no information justifies visceral revascularisation for asymptomatic lesions except for patients with asymptomatic stenosis or occlusion of the SMA who need to undergo aortic surgery.

Postoperative intestinal ischaemia can be prevented by grafting the SMA during the aortic procedure. Reconstruction of the inferior mesenteric artery should be strongly considered for those who have occlusion of all three major visceral trunks.

Patients with symptomatic CMI benefit from surgical intervention but it is associated with a high risk of haemorrhage and death when compared to many other elective vascular procedures. The in-hospital mortality reaches 12.2%, with a postoperative complication rate of 54%, including revascularisation syndrome.[59]

Current surgical techniques usually involve revascularisation of the stenotic or occluded mesenteric vessels using autologous or prosthetic grafts, although the precise configurations remain contraversial. Inflow may be from the supracoeliac aorta or distal thoracic aorta (antegrade reconstruction) or from the infrarenal aorta or the common iliac artery (retrograde reconstruction). Outflow may be either a single-vessel repair to only the coeliac or more commonly to the SMA, or as a multivessel repair. Hollier et al. showed that complete revascularisation in multivessel disease resulted in late recurrence of 11%, while revascularisation of one of the three stenotic vessels resulted in a 50% recurrence rate. They concluded that it is preferable to revascularise as many vessels as possible so that single-vessel thrombosis does not result in bowel infarction.[59] In contrast, Gentile et al. believe that retrograde isolated bypass grafts to the SMA provide comparable long-term prevention of recurrence.[60] Antegrade bypasses have the advantage that the bypass is placed in the direction of the normal blood flow, thus reducing the anastomotic turbulence. This design eliminates the possibility of kinking and thrombosis by compression or traction from the overlying intestinal mesentery that might be observed in retrograde grafts. Early experience with retrograde bypasses with vein as a conduit showed frequent graft kinking and occlusion. This is avoided by using a reinforced prosthetic graft in a lazy loop configuration. Foley et al. reported a 79% primary-assisted patency rate after 9 years. Most of these grafts were done in a retrograde fashion to the SMA only.[61] Taylor et al. prefer to perform a retrograde bypass graft starting from the infrarenal aorta because of its familiar exposure and reduced risks with clamping and dissection. They have a 5-year patency rate of 96% with an operative mortality rate of 7%.[62] Kansal et al. suggest that the retrograde bypass might be preferable to the antegrade bypass in a number of situations, including patients in whom previous surgery might prohibit a safe dissection of the supracoeliac aorta, medically high-risk patients in whom a shorter operative time might be preferable, and the need for simultaneous infrarenal aortic and mesenteric revascularisation.[63]

Since graft occlusion may result in acute mesenteric ischaemia, graft stenoses are of concern. Kazmers found symptomatic assessment of patients insufficient amd therefore recommended graft surveillance using duplex every 4–6 months.[57]

The primary patency of surgical reconstruction has not been matched to date by endovascular techniques.[63–65] Non-randomised comparative studies of surgical revascularisation versus endovascular treatment show better primary and primary-assisted patency rates,[66–68] fewer reinterventions[68] and lower rates of symptom recurrence[69] in favour of surgical bypass. However, the major disadvantage of conventional surgery remains the high perioperative mortality and morbidity.

Endovascular options

The endovascular option for treating this condition is attractive as the open operations are a major undertaking in a group of patients who are almost exclusively elderly and in whom there is significant comorbidity. In addition, the nature of CMI dictates that such patients are chronically undernourished, dehydrated and lacking in metabolic reserves. In such circumstances subjecting these patients to a major surgical procedure, with its associated catabolic consequences, makes little sense.

The technique, although theoretically simple, may be technically challenging because of the difficult angles and heavily calcified, often chronically occluded, lesions. Arterial access is obtained and heparin is routinely administered to ensure anticoagulation during catheter manipulation. The target lesion is identified following a flush aortogram (**Fig. 15.6**). A guidewire is then manipulated across the stenosis and the decision of primary angioplasty

or stenting is made. When stenting has been performed, the literature mostly describes the use of short balloon-mounted stents, allowing as short a stent as possible to cover the lesion (**Fig. 15.7**).

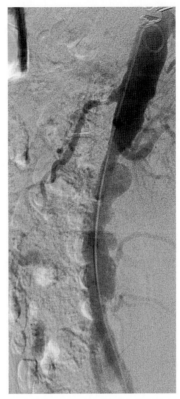

Figure 15.6 • Catheter angiogram showing tandem tight superior mesenteric artery stenoses.

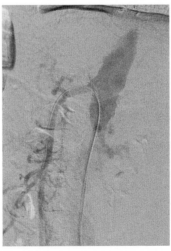

Figure 15.7 • Angiogram showing the same patient as in Fig. 15.6, following placement of a stent.

A series of 27 patients treated endovascularly showed a primary patency of 81% and a secondary patency of 100%.[70] The largest comparative series to date concluded that although the length of stay was reduced with endovascular treatment, stenting was associated with decreased primary patency, primary-assisted patency with an increased need for earlier reintervention.[66] However, the reinterventions are generally of a less invasive nature than open procedures, and carry significantly reduced morbidity. In addition, patients treated endovascularly tend to be those with poorer overall prognosis, in whom long-term patency may be academic.

> ✅ Vascular reconstruction may be more appropriate in younger and fitter patients, while endovascular treatment is preferable for older, less fit, patients.

Coeliac axis compression syndrome

External compression of the coeliac artery by the median arcuate ligament of the diaphragm may result in chronic mesenteric ischaemia and visceral artery aneurysm formation.[71] During inspiration, the aorta and coeliac axis move downward with the abdominal viscera. In expiration, the vessels move upwards and a maximal external compression on the coeliac artery occurs. Reilly et al. developed a group of positive and negative criteria to predict successful relief of symptoms with coeliac axis decompression: female gender, postprandial pain, age 40–60 years, profound weight loss, absence of a psychiatric or drug abuse history, arteriographic findings of coeliac artery decompression with poststenotic dilatation or collateral flow.[72] The diagnosis remains one of exclusion. Surgical division of the arcuate ligament remains the only effective treatment.[73] This procedure can be performed laparoscopically and may be combined with coeliac artery stenting, which is a novel and attractive minimally invasive approach.[74] The debate regarding the clinical importance of this syndrome is compounded by the observation of recurrence after surgical treatment.[75]

Visceral aneurysms

Aetiology and incidence

Visceral artery aneurysms, whilst uncommon, are clinically important since 22% present as clinical emergencies, of which 8.5% result in death.[76] Although more than 3000 cases of visceral artery aneurysms have been documented in the literature, their exact incidence is unknown. The natural history is one of expansion and eventual rupture. In the past, most visceral artery aneurysms were syphilitic or mycotic in origin, but today

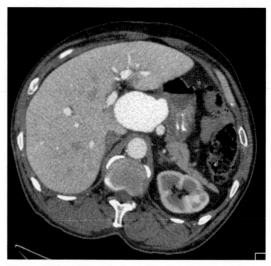

Figure 15.8 • CT angiogram showing a large gastric artery aneurysm.

most true aneurysms are caused by atherosclerosis or medial degeneration, whereas false aneurysms are usually the result of trauma or inflammation (e.g. pancreatitis).[76] The clinical symptoms, natural history and mortality from visceral artery aneurysms vary depending on which vessels are involved.

Vessels affected, in descending order of involvement, include the splenic (60%), hepatic (20%), superior mesenteric (5.5%), coeliac (4%), gastric and gastroepiploic (4%), intestinal (3%), pancreaticoduodenal and pancreatic (2%), gastroduodenal (2%) and rarely inferior mesenteric arteries.[72] An example of a visceral aneurysm is shown in **Fig. 15.8**.

Diagnosis and treatment

Although in the past most visceral artery aneurysms were discovered at the time of rupture or at autopsy, many asymptomatic aneurysms are currently being recognised due to the greater availability of advanced imaging modalities.

Compared to other visceral aneurysms, SMA aneurysms are often symptomatic. This is due to their unique location near the origin of the pancreaticoduodenal and middle colic arteries. If dissection or occlusion of the aneurysm occurs, the distal mesenteric circulation will be isolated. Abdominal discomfort varies from mild to severe pain and in many is suggestive of intestinal angina. SMA dissections may be treated with stents[77] and aneurysms with stent grafts.[78]

> ✅ Modern treatment of splenic, hepatic and postinflammatory pseudoaneurysms is either by endoluminal embolisation or exclusion by placement of a stent graft.[79,80]

Treatment is indicated to prevent catastrophic complications. Operative procedures include aneurysmorrhaphy or simple ligation.[75,81] Bypass reconstruction is seldom required using autologous vein or prosthetic graft.[82] Mortality associated with ruptured visceral artery aneurysms remains high, reaching 50%, whereas mortality from elective surgery is 5%.[82]

Acknowledgements

The authors would like to acknowledge the contributions made to this chapter by Philip Kalra, Michael Dialynas and Celia Riga.

Key points

Renal disease

- Angioplasty (PTA) is the procedure of choice for non-atheromatous lesions.
- The improvement of blood pressure control in non-atheromatous lesions is good to excellent following PTA.
- ARVD usually presents with hypertension, chronic renal failure, acute renal failure or pulmonary oedema. However, it is often asymptomatic and should be considered in patients with extrarenal vascular disease.
- Stents have a higher technical success and patency rate compared with PTA in atheromatous ostial lesions.
- Surgery gives the lowest re-stenosis rates but should be reserved for stent failures or young fit patients.
- Improvement of blood pressure control in atheromatous lesions following stenting is marginal but may reduce the drug burden.
- There is currently no consensus on the role of stenting in ARVD for hypertension or renal insufficiency. Further trials are under way.

Intestinal ischaemia

- Intestinal ischaemia is a rare condition that presents a major diagnostic and management challenge to the vascular specialist.
- Acute intestinal ischaemia remains a surgical emergency that should be treated by laparotomy revascularisation and resection of dead bowel in most cases.
- Chronic intestinal ischaemia may be treated by surgical or endovascular methods. Endovascular techniques should be considered in poor-risk symptomatic patients and merit further objective assessment.

Visceral aneurysms

- Visceral artery aneurysms are uncommon but clinically important since 22% present as clinical emergencies, of which 8.5% result in death. Treatment is indicated to prevent catastrophic complications.

References

1. de Fraissinette B, Garcier JM, Dieu V, et al. Percutaneous transluminal angioplasty of dysplastic stenoses of the renal artery: results on 70 adults. Cardiovasc Intervent Radiol 2003;26(1): 46–51.
2. Tyagi S, Singh B, Kaul UA, et al. Balloon angioplasty for renovascular hypertension in Takayasu's arteritis. Am Heart J 1993;125:1386–93.
3. Rudnick KV, Sackett DL, Hirst S, et al. Hypertension in a family practice. Can Med Assoc J 1997;117(5): 492–7.
4. Schwartz CJ, White TA. Stenosis of renal artery: an unselected necropsy study. Br Med J 1964;2(5422):1415–21.
5. Kalra PA, Guo H, Kausz AT, et al. Atherosclerotic renovascular disease in US medicare recipients aged 67 years or more: risk factors, revascularization and prognosis. Kidney Int 2005;68(1):293–301.
6. Zierler RE, Bergelin RO, Isaacson JA, et al. Natural history of atherosclerotic renal artery stenosis: a prospective study with duplex ultrasonography. J Vasc Surg 1994;19(2):250–8.
7. Herrera AH, Davidson RA. Renovascular disease in older adults. Clin Geriat Med 1998;14(2): 237–54.

8. Haimovici H, Zinicola N. Experimental renal-artery stenosis diagnostic significance of arterial hemodynamics. J Cardiovasc Surg 1962;3:259–62.

9. Wasser MN, Westenberg J, van der Hulst VP, et al. Hemodynamic significance of renal artery stenosis: digital subtraction angiography versus systolically gated three-dimensional phase-contrast MR angiography. Radiology 1997;202(2):333–8.

10. Guo H, Kalra PA, Gilbertson DT, et al. Atherosclerotic renovascular disease in older US patients starting dialysis, 1996 to 2001. Circulation 2007;115(1):50–8.

11. Wright JR, Shurrab AE, Cheung C, et al. A prospective study of the determinants of renal functional outcome and mortality in atherosclerotic renovascular disease. Am J Kidney Dis 2002;39(6):1153–61.

12. Middleton JP. Ischemic disease of the kidney: how and why to consider revascularization. J Nephrol 1998;11(3):123–36.

13. Textor SC. Revascularization in atherosclerotic renal artery disease. Kidney Int 1998;53(3):799–811.

14. Missouris CG, Buckenham T, Cappuccio FP, et al. Renal artery stenosis: a common and important problem in patients with peripheral vascular disease. Am J Med 1994;96(1):10–4.

15. Olin JW, Melia M, Young JR, et al. Prevalence of atherosclerotic renal artery stenosis in patients with atherosclerosis elsewhere. Am J Med 1990;88(1N):46N–51N.

16. Kuroda S, Nishida N, Uzu T, et al. Prevalence of renal artery stenosis in autopsy patients with stroke. Stroke 2000;31(1):61–5.

17. Harding MB, Smith LR, Himmelstein SI, et al. Renal artery stenosis: prevalence and associated risk factors in patients undergoing routine cardiac catheterization. J Am Soc Nephrol 1992;2(11):1608–16.

18. Crowley JJ, Santos RM, Peter RH, et al. Progression of renal artery stenosis in patients undergoing cardiac catheterization. Am Heart J 1998;136(5):913–8.

19. MacDowall P, Kalra PA, O'Donoghue DJ, et al. Risk of morbidity from renovascular disease in elderly patients with congestive cardiac failure. Lancet 1998;352(9121):13–6.

20. Cheung CM, Patel A, Shaheen N, et al. The effects of statins on the progression of atherosclerotic renovascular disease. Nephron Clin Pract 2007;107(2):c35–42.

21. The ASTRAL Investigators. Revascularisation versus medical therapy for renal-artery stenosis. N Engl J Med 2009;361:1953–62.

22. Tan KT, van Beek EJ, Brown PW, et al. Magnetic resonance angiography for the diagnosis of renal artery stenosis: a meta-analysis. Clin Radiol 2002;57(7):617–24.

23. Solomon R, Werner C, Mann D, et al. Effects of saline, mannitol, and furosemide to prevent acute decreases in renal function induced by radiocontrast agents. N Engl J Med 1994;331(21):1416–20.

24. Mainra R, Gallo K, Moist L. Effect of N-acetylcysteine on renal function in patients with chronic kidney disease. Nephrology 2007;12 (5):510–3.

25. Leertouwer TC, Gussenhoven EJ, Bosch JL, et al. Stent placement for renal arterial stenosis: where do we stand? A meta-analysis. Radiology 2000;216:78–85.
   Renal stenting is technically superior and clinically comparable to renal angioplasty alone.

26. Hiramoto J, Hansen KJ, Pan XM, et al. Atheroemboli during renal artery angioplasty: an ex vivo study. J Vasc Surg 2005;41:1026–30.

27. Holden A, Hill A, Jaff MR, et al. Renal artery stent revascularization with embolic protection in patients with ischemic nephropathy. Kidney Int 2006;70:948–55.

28. Hagspiel KD, Stone JR, Leung DA. Renal angioplasty and stent placement with distal protection: preliminary experience with the FilterWire EX. J Vasc Intervent Radiol 2005;16:125–31.

29. Beek FJ, Kaatee R, Beutler JJ, et al. Complications during renal artery stent placement for atherosclerotic ostial stenosis. Cardiovasc Intervent Radiol 1997;20(3):184–90.

30. Van Jaarsveld BC, Krijnen P, Pieterman H, et al. The effects of balloon angioplasty on hypertension in atherosclerotic renal artery stenosis. N Engl J Med 2000;342:1007–14.
   The largest randomised controlled trial (106 patients). In patients with hypertension and atherosclerotic RAS, angioplasty has little advantage over drug therapy alone.

31. Plouin P-F, Chatellier G, Darne B, et al. Blood pressure outcome of angioplasty in atherosclerotic renal artery stenosis. Hypertension 1998;31:823–9.
   In unilateral atherosclerotic RAS, angioplasty is a drug-sparing procedure that involves some morbidity. Previous uncontrolled studies have overestimated its effect on hypertension.

32. Webster J, Marshall F, Abdalla M, et al. Randomised comparison of percutaneous angioplasty vs continued medical therapy for hypertensive patients with atheromatous renal artery stenosis. J Hum Hypertens 1998;12:329–35.
   Angioplasty results in a modest improvement in systolic blood pressure compared with drug therapy alone. This benefit was confined to bilateral disease. No patient was cured and renal function did not improve. Angioplasty was associated with significant morbidity.

33. Ives N, Wheatley K, Stowe RL, et al. Continuing uncertainty about the value of percutaneous revascularisation in atherosclerotic renovascular disease: a meta-analysis of randomised trials. Nephrol Dial Transplant 2003;18:298–304.
   Reported trials are too small to determine reliably the role of angioplasty in ARVD. Trials do exclude a large improvement in hypertension or renal function but are too small to exclude a clinically worthwhile benefit.

34. Nordmann AJ, Woo K, Parkes R, et al. Balloon angioplasty or medical therapy for hypertensive patients with atherosclerotic renal artery stenosis? A meta-analysis of randomised controlled trials. Am J Med 2003;114:44–50.
    Angioplasty has a modest but significant effect on blood pressure and should be considered in poorly controlled hypertension in atherosclerotic patients. There is no evidence to support its use in improving or preserving renal function.

35. Kalra PA, Chrysochou C, Green D, et al. The benefit of renal artery stenting in patients with atheromatous renovascular disease and advanced chronic kidney disease. Cath Cardiovasc Interv 2010;75(1):1–10.

36. Van de Ven PJG, Kaatee R, Beutler JJ, et al. Arterial stenting and balloon angioplasty in ostial atherosclerotic renovascular disease: a randomised trial. Lancet 1999;353:282–6.
    This trial showed convincing superiority of stenting over angioplasty regarding technical success and primary patency.

37. Zahringer M, Sapoval M, Pattynama PM, et al. Sirolimus-eluting versus bare-metal low-profile stent for renal artery treatment (GREAT Trial): angiographic follow-up after 6 months and clinical outcome up to 2 years. J Endovasc Ther 2007;14:460.

38. Novick AC. Extracorporeal microvascular reconstruction and autotransplantation for branch renal artery disease. In: Novick AC, Scoble J, Hamilton G, editors. Renal vascular disease. London: WB Saunders; 1996. p. 497–511.

39. Bergentz SE, Weibull H, Novick AC. Long-term patency after reconstructive surgery and PTA for renal artery stenosis. In: Greenhalgh RM, Hollier L, editors. The maintenance of arterial reconstruction. London: WB Saunders; 1991. p. 384–96.

40. Fergany A, Kolettis P, Novick AC. The contemporary role of extra-anatomical surgical renal revascularization in patients with atherosclerotic renal artery disease. J Urol 1995;153(6):1798–802.

41. Benjamin ME, Hansen KJ, Craven TE, et al. Combined aortic and renal artery surgery. A contemporary experience. Ann Surg 1996;223:555–65.

42. Dean RH. Surgical reconstruction of atherosclerotic renal artery disease. In: Branchereau A, Jacobs M, editors. Long term results of arterial interventions. Armonk, NY: Futura; 1997. p. 205–16.

43. Reilly JM, Rubin BG, Thompson RW, et al. Revascularization of the solitary kidney: a challenging problem in a high risk population. Surgery 1996;120:732–6.

44. Steinbach F, Novick AC, Campbell S, et al. Long-term survival after surgical revascularization for atherosclerotic renal artery disease. J Urol 1997;158:38–41.

45. Darling III RC, Shah DM, Chang BB, et al. Does concomitant aortic bypass and renal artery revascularization using the retroperitoneal approach increase perioperative risk? Cardiovasc Surg 1995;3:421–3.

46. Novick AC, Ziegelbaum M, Vidt DG, et al. Trends in surgical revascularization for renal artery disease. Ten years' experience. JAMA 1987;257:498–501.

47. Cambria RP, Brewster DC, L'Italien G, et al. Renal artery reconstruction for the preservation of renal function. J Vasc Surg 1996;24:371–82.

48. Johal NS, Kraklau D, Cucklow PM. The role of unilateral nephrectomy in the treatment of nephrogenic hypertension in children. BJU Int 2005;95(1):140–2.

49. Medina A, Bell PRF, Briggs JD, et al. Changes of blood pressure, renin and angiotensin after bilateral nephrectomy in patients with chronic renal failure. Br Med J 1972;4:694–6.

50. Schlaich MP, Sobotka PA, Krum H, et al. Renal denervation as a therapeutic approach for hypertension – novel implications for an old concept. Hypertension 2009;54(6):1195–201.

51. Symplicity HTN-2 Investigators. Renal sympathetic denervation in patients with treatment-resistant hypertension (the Symplicity HTN-2 Trial): a randomised controlled trial. Lancet 2010;376:1903–9.

52. Farkas JC, Calvo-Verjat N, Laurian C, et al. Acute colorectal ischemia after aortic surgery: pathophysiology and prognostic criteria. Ann Vasc Surg 1992;6(2):111–8.

53. Stoney RJ, Cunningham CG. Acute mesenteric ischemia. Surgery 1993;114(3):489–90.

54. Acosta S, Ogren M, Sternby NH, et al. Fatal non-occlusive mesenteric ischaemia: population-based incidence and risk factors. J Intern Med 2006;259(3):305–13.

55. Granger DN, Hollwarth ME, Parks DA. Ischemia–reperfusion injury: role of oxygen-derived free radicals. Acta Physiol Scand Suppl 1986;548:47–63.

56. Gartenschlaeger S, Bender S, Maeurer J, et al. Successful percutaneous transluminal angioplasty and stenting in acute mesenteric ischemia. Cardiovasc Intervent Radiol 2008;31(2):398–400.

57. Kazmers A. Operative management of acute mesenteric ischemia. Part 1. Ann Vasc Surg 1998;12(2):187–97.

58. Hansen HJ, Christoffersen JK. Occlusive mesenteric infarction. A retrospective study of 83 cases. Acta Chir Scand Suppl 1976;472:103–8.

59. Hollier LH, Bernatz PE, Pairolero PC, et al. Surgical management of chronic intestinal ischemia: a reappraisal. Surgery 1981;90(6):940–6.

60. Gentile AT, Moneta GL, Taylor Jr. LM, et al. Isolated bypass to the superior mesenteric artery for intestinal ischemia. Arch Surg 1994;129(9):926–32.

61. Foley MI, Moneta GL, Abou-Zamzam Jr. AM, et al. Revascularization of the superior mesenteric artery alone for treatment of intestinal ischemia. J Vasc Surg 2000;32(1):37–47.

62. Taylor L, Moneta G, Porter J. Treatment of chronic visceral ischemia. In: Rutherford RB, editor. Vascular surgery. Philadelphia: WB Saunders; 2000. p. 1532–41.

63. Kansal N, LoGerfo FW, Belfield AK, et al. A comparison of antegrade and retrograde mesenteric bypass. Ann Vasc Surg 2002;16(5):591–6.

64. Park WM, Cherry Jr KJ, Chua HK, et al. Current results of open revascularization for chronic mesenteric ischemia: a standard for comparison. J Vasc Surg 2002;35(5):853–9.

65. Kruger AJ, Walker PJ, Foster WJ, et al. Open surgery for atherosclerotic chronic mesenteric ischemia. J Vasc Surg 2007;46(5):941–5.

66. Atkins MD, Kwolek CJ, LaMuraglia GM, et al. Surgical revascularization versus endovascular therapy for chronic mesenteric ischemia: a comparative experience. J Vasc Surg 2007;45(6):1162–71.

67. Kasirajan K, O'Hara PJ, Gray BH, et al. Chronic mesenteric ischemia: open surgery versus percutaneous angioplasty and stenting. J Vasc Surg 2001;33(1):63–71.

68. Biebl L, Oldenburg W, Paz-Fumagalli R, et al. Surgical and interventional visceral revascularization for the treatment of chronic mesenteric ischemia – when to prefer which? World J Surg 2007;31(3):562–8.

69. Sivamurthy N, Rhodes JM, Lee D, et al. Endovascular versus open mesenteric revascularization: immediate benefits do not equate with short-term functional outcomes. J Am Coll Surg 2006;202(6):859–67.

70. van Wanroij JL, van Petersen AS, Huisman AB, et al. Endovascular treatment of chronic splanchnic syndrome. Eur J Vasc Endovasc Surg 2004;28(2):193–200.

71. Sugiyama K, Takehara Y. Analysis of five cases of splanchnic artery aneurysm associated with coeliac artery stenosis due to compression by the median arcuate ligament. Clin Radiol 2007;62(7):688–93.

72. Reilly LM, Ammar AD, Stoney RJ, et al. Late results following operative repair for celiac artery compression syndrome. J Vasc Surg 1985;2(1):79–91.

73. Gloviczki P, Duncan AA. Treatment of celiac artery compression syndrome: does it really exist? Perspect Vasc Surg Endovasc Ther 2007;19(3):259–63.

74. Carbonell AM, Kercher KW, Heniford BT, et al. Multimedia article. Laparoscopic management of median arcuate ligament syndrome. Surg Endosc 2005;19(5):729.

75. Geelkerken RH, van Bockel JH, de Roos WK, et al. Surgical treatment of intestinal artery aneurysms. Eur J Vasc Surg 1990;4(6):563–7.

76. Graham LM, Stanley JC, Whitehouse Jr WM, et al. Celiac artery aneurysms: historic (1745–1949) versus contemporary (1950–1984) differences in etiology and clinical importance. J Vasc Surg 1985;2(5):757–64.

77. Chu S-Y, Hsu M-Y, Chen C-M, et al. Endovascular repair of spontaneous isolated dissection of the superior mestenteric artery. Clin Radiol 2012;67(1):32–7.

78. Larson SA, Solomon J, Carpenter JP. Stent graft repair of visceral artery aneurysms. J Vasc Surg 2002;36(6):1260–3.

79. Ishii A, Namimoto T, Morishita S, et al. Embolization for ruptured superior mesenteric artery aneurysms. Br J Radiol 1996;820(69):296–300.

80. Lorelli DR, Cambra RA, Seabrook GR, et al. Diagnosis and management of aneurysms involving the superior mesenteric artery and its branches: a report of four cases. Vasc Endovasc Surg 2003;37(1):59–66.

81. Jindal R, Pandey V, Natt R, Jenkins M. Ruptured mycotic aneurysm of a branch of the superior mesenteric artery and pulmonary tuberculosis. Eur J Vasc Endovasc Surg 2005;30(1):107.

82. Huang YK, Hsieh HC, Tsai FC, et al. Visceral artery aneurysm: risk factor analysis and therapeutic opinion. Eur J Vasc Endovasc Surg 2007;33(3):293–301.

16

Central venous and dialysis access

Peter W.G. Brown
David C. Mitchell

Introduction

Access to the venous circulation is an almost universal requirement in hospitalised patients for intravenous fluid administration or blood transfusion. This is most commonly achieved with an indwelling peripheral intravenous cannula but central venous access may be required for pressure monitoring, intravenous nutrition, haemodialysis, haemofiltration or the administration of cytotoxic drugs.

For acute haemodialysis, central venous catheters (CVCs) are the mainstay of access and provide high dialysis flows (>300 mL/min) but have high complication rates and are less suitable for chronic use. For long-term haemodialysis, an arteriovenous fistula (AVF) or graft (AVG) can provide a sufficiently high dialyser flow (>300 mL/min) to allow dialysis via two needles inserted into the efferent vein or the graft itself.

Central venous access

Indications

In addition to central venous pressure monitoring, CVCs can be used to infuse large volumes of irritant solutions, such as antibiotics, blood products, parenteral nutrition and chemotherapeutic agents, particularly if required over long periods. In an emergency, CVCs allow the rapid administration of large volumes of fluid if peripheral access cannot be achieved. Other indications include haemodialysis and plasmapheresis. Implantable injection ports, 'portacaths' (e.g. Bardport, Passport, Infuse-a-Port or MediPort), may be used for chemotherapy or long-term administration of other drugs.[1] One has also been developed for haemodialysis (Lifesite).[2]

Methods

CVCs are generally inserted under local anaesthetic through the internal jugular, subclavian or femoral veins, preferably using ultrasound guidance, by the Seldinger technique.[3] If short-term access is required a multilumen catheter is inserted into the internal jugular vein so that the tip lies in the superior vena cava. For long-term access a catheter with an attached Dacron cuff is placed in a subcutaneous tunnel (e.g. Hickman line) for fixation and to act as a barrier to infection.

Implantable access ports are usually inserted into the subclavian vein in the operating theatre and tunnelled so that the port lies over the anterior chest wall. They contain a diaphragm that may be accessed repeatedly using a special side-hole needle. Central vein access can also be achieved using a peripheral intravenous central catheter inserted in the antecubital or long saphenous vein. These are relatively small but widely used in neonates, as an alternative to umbilical vein catheters.

Complications

Air embolus can be avoided by ensuring a head-down position during insertion.

✔✔ Accurate placement under ultrasound guidance will reduce the incidence of arterial puncture, haematoma, haemothorax and pneumothorax.[4]

The long-term complications of infection and thrombosis are dealt with below.

Temporary dialysis access

Renal replacement therapy may be accomplished by renal transplantation or peritoneal dialysis but most patients require at least a period of haemodialysis. About 75% of patients are known to have deteriorating renal function at least 90 days before dialysis is required so that permanent haemodialysis access can be created in advance. Unfortunately, this opportunity is frequently missed in UK practice, with less than a third of patients starting haemodialysis with definitive access.[5] Dialysis is required for hyperkalaemia or when symptoms of weight loss, nausea, vomiting, anorexia or itching occur, usually at a serum creatinine level of 500–1500 mmol/L.

For patients presenting as an emergency with end-stage renal disease (ESRD) without prior access, haemodialysis can start using a double-lumen CVC whilst awaiting a permanent AVF. However, CVCs have a high risk of infection,[6] cause central venous stenosis or thrombosis[7] compromising further access in the upper limbs, and have a higher mortality than AVFs,[8] so should not be used long term except where other options have been exhausted.

✔ Temporary (non-tunnelled) catheters are used in patients who require short-term dialysis for transient renal failure or who present acutely with ESRD. They are also indicated after failure of a permanent access, whilst awaiting maturation of a new AVF. Tunnelled catheters are preferred if dialysis is required for more than 2 weeks or for permanent access when the creation of an AVF or AVG is contraindicated or technically impossible.

The subcutaneous tunnel may reduce the rate of infection, but this has not been proven in a randomised trial.[9]

Methods

Temporary femoral vein catheters are useful for acute dialysis but have a higher rate of infection than internal jugular CVCs[10] and should be replaced by a tunnelled (preferably jugular) venous catheter at the earliest opportunity. A median survival of 166 days has been reported for tunnelled femoral CVCs.[11]

The right internal jugular vein (IJV) is preferred as this provides the most direct route to the superior vena cava (SVC) and right atrium (RA). The left IJV has a greater complication rate because the catheter has to traverse two 90° bends to reach the RA. The subclavian route is discouraged because of the high incidence of subclavian vein stenosis and thrombosis that compromises future access in the ipsilateral arm. When other routes have been exhausted, tunnelled catheters can be placed in the femoral vein or even the inferior vena cava (IVC) via a transhepatic or translumbar approach.

The catheter tip is usually placed at the SVC/RA junction. Atrial placement minimises recirculation and reduces the risk of migration on standing,[12] but may cause arrhythmias.

✔✔ The preferred site for a CVC is the right IJV. CVCs should be inserted under fluoroscopic or ultrasound guidance, without which there is a malposition rate of 29%.[13]

Complications of CVCs

Insertion
The complications related to catheter insertion are the same as for other CVCs described above and can be reduced by ultrasound guidance and a micropuncture technique.

Catheter dysfunction
Catheter dysfunction occurs when an adequate extracorporeal blood flow of 300 mL/min cannot be achieved. Early dysfunction is usually caused by malposition or kinking and is corrected by repositioning. Later dysfunction is primarily due to thrombosis or fibrin sheath formation. Rarely, tip migration demands repositioning with a snare or exchanging over a wire.

Catheter-locking solutions
Catheter patency can be maintained between dialysis sessions using a catheter-locking solution. The standard procedure has been heparin instillation (1000–10000 u/mL) into the catheter lumen in a volume sufficient to fill to the lumen tip. There is a risk of heparin loss due to diffusion into the blood stream and unintentional systemic anticoagulation. Low-dose heparin (1000–2500 u/mL) seems as effective as high-dose.[14] Trisodium citrate, which also has antibacterial properties, is also an effective catheter lock but there is no randomised trial versus heparin.[15]

A recent randomised study compared 225 patients on haemodialysis who had a central venous catheter using a locking regime of heparin 5000 u/mL or recombinant tissue plasminogen activator (rt-PA)

1 mg in each lumen. The rate of catheter malfunction in the heparin group (34.8%) was significantly worse than in the patients assigned to rt-PA and the risk of bacteraemia was three times higher than in the heparin group.[16]

Catheter lumen thrombosis

Catheter thrombosis is the most common cause of poor long-term function.[17] Prophylactic warfarin can be effective at reducing thrombosis[18] but there are no randomised data comparing international normalised ratio (INR) ranges and controls. There is a risk of bleeding and a need for regular monitoring.

Catheter malfunction due to thrombus can be treated by lytic agents such as rt-PA or urokinase.

rt-PA may be superior to urokinase but this has not been proven in a randomised trial. Urokinase has been withdrawn in the USA due to safety concerns.

Poor flow can be treated by a postdialysis lock or intradialysis lytic infusion. Both are effective but there are no randomised data.

Lytic agents are also used for the treatment of catheter thrombosis. An instillation of rt-PA 1 mg/mL for 30 minutes restored or maintained a flow rate of greater than 300 mL/min without line reversals in 36 of 50 (72%) patients, with a second instillation restoring patency for a further four patients (80%). The majority of patients required further thrombolysis or radiological intervention in the 4-month follow-up period.[19]

The optimal dwell times for lytic agents have yet to be determined. rt-PA infusions are effective even when there is an associated fibrin sheath.[20]

Tenecteplase is a new lytic agent with increased fibrin specificity, greater resistance to plasminogen activator inhibitor 1 and a relatively long half-life. A randomised study showed a 1-hour dwell of 2 mg of tenecteplase more effective than placebo in restoring flow in dysfunctional haemodialysis catheters.[21] An extended dwell improves treatment success.[22]

Central vein thrombosis

Mural thrombus is commonly seen in the SVC and RA with central venous catheters. If it compromises venous return, facial and arm oedema results. Central vein thrombus can be identified by magnetic resonance or conventional venography. Infusion of a fibrinolytic agent is usually successful, although organised thrombus may require angioplasty and stenting.

Fibrin sheaths

Fibrin sheaths cause up to 43% of catheter dysfunction.[23] Contrast injection through the dialysis line may show a filling defect near the catheter tip or retrograde flow along the external surface of the catheter (**Fig. 16.1**). They may be treated by infusing

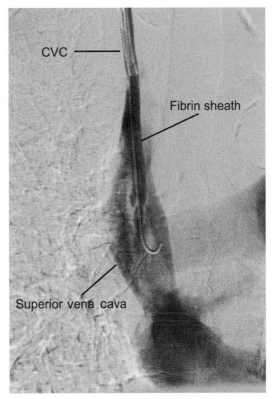

Figure 16.1 • A venogram showing fibrin sheath around a partially withdrawn CVC.

a fibrinolytic agent over 6 hours, mechanical stripping using a snare from the femoral vein, or catheter exchange over a guidewire.

Stripping has a high technical success rate but the fibrin sheath frequently recurs. In a randomised trial there was no significant difference in additional patency between percutaneous stripping or urokinase.[24] In another randomised trial 4-month catheter patency was significantly better after catheter exchange than percutaneous stripping.[25]

If the catheter is exchanged over a guidewire, the sheath must be mechanically disrupted or the new catheter will be reinserted down the existing sheath. There are no controlled trials comparing all three techniques.

Catheter-related infection

Catheter-related infection is a major cause of morbidity and mortality and is related to the duration of placement. Gram-positive bacteria are the usual cause[26] and resistant organisms such as methicillin-resistant *Staphylococcus aureus* (MRSA) are increasing. Catheter-associated sepsis can result in infective endocarditis, osteomyelitis, septic arthritis, epidural abscesses and death. Infection spreads either through the lumen of the catheter or along the outside from the exit site. An associated biofilm reduces the effectiveness of antibiotics.

Infections in non-tunnelled catheters should be treated by catheter removal and systemic antibiotics. In tunnelled catheters 90% of exit-site infections respond to oral antibiotics but intravenous antibiotics and catheter removal may be necessary for more serious tunnel infections. Systemic infections associated with tunnelled catheters can be treated initially with antibiotics but catheter removal is usually required. A new catheter should be inserted at a different site when the systemic sepsis has settled. Catheter exchange over a guidewire is controversial but there is some evidence that infection-free survival is similar to that after removal and delayed replacement.[27]

The cornerstone of prevention is scrupulous asepsis with regular exit-site inspection and dressing changes. Chlorhexidine and alcohol 70% provides superior asepsis to povidone–iodine 10% as an exit-site cleaning solution.[28] Mupirocin ointment is also effective,[29] but may increase colonisation by fungi and multiresistant organisms. Antibiotic-coated catheters reduce line sepsis in intensive care patients[30] and temporary dialysis catheters[31] but there is no evidence of benefit for long-term dialysis as the antibiotic is washed off over time. Bismuth has been demonstrated to have antibiofilm and antibiotic properties. A recent randomised clinical trial of bismuth-coated non-tunnelled dialysis catheters in 77 patients showed a reduction in catheter colonisation compared with non-coated catheters.[32] There is also recent evidence that bacterial growth can be reduced by altering catheter surface irregularities.[33] Antibiotic catheter locks have also been used and are effective at reducing catheter infections but there is a danger of antibiotic resistance. Antibiotic heparin and citrate heparin locks are superior to heparin alone but there are no randomised trials comparing antibiotic and citrate locks.[34]

Permanent dialysis access

✅ An AVF should be constructed 16–24 weeks before the anticipated need for dialysis, when the creatinine clearance falls to 25 mL/min or the serum creatinine level rises above 400 µmol/L (4 mg/dL) to allow time for maturation or redo surgery in the event of failure.[35–37]

Whereas CVCs are usually introduced on the ward or in the radiology department, peripheral arteriovenous (AV) access procedures require an operating theatre. However, most can be performed under local anaesthetic, often as day cases.

✅ Dedicated operating lists organised by a dialysis access nurse are an enormous advantage and one such list is required per week for every 120 patients on dialysis to prevent unacceptable waiting times and prolonged CVC usage.[5,37]

Access planning

✅ In patients with chronic renal failure it is essential that the cephalic and antecubital veins of both arms be reserved for dialysis access. Intravenous cannulae for other purposes should only be inserted into the back of the hand or the small veins on the anterior surface of the wrist, except in emergencies. A CVC, AVF or AVG should only be used for dialysis.[35–37]

An AVF should be created as distally as possible to preserve sites for future access. The non-dominant arm is preferred to allow greater freedom on dialysis or to facilitate self-cannulation for home dialysis patients. When upper limb access sites are exhausted the lower limbs may be used.[35–37] Autogenous AVFs are preferable to prosthetic AVGs as they have higher patency,[38] lower infection rates, require fewer revisions[39] and are associated with a slightly lower mortality, especially in diabetics.[8,40]

Whereas a side-to side radiocephalic AVF was originally described,[41] an end-to side configuration is now preferred as there is less risk of peripheral venous hypertension. Some advocate an end-to-end anastomosis for distal radiocephalic AVFs, provided there is a good ulnar pulse, to reduce the small incidence of steal.[42] Autogenous AVFs require a period of maturation to allow arterialisation of the venous outflow whereas AVGs can be needled directly as soon as the wounds have healed.

Preoperative assessment

✅ In many centres, patients proceed directly to primary AVF formation if there is a satisfactory radial pulse and suitable forearm veins. Opinion is divided on the need for preoperative imaging: the latest US National Kidney Foundation – Dialysis Outcomes Quality Initiative (NKF-KDOQI) clinical guidelines now recommend routine duplex imaging in all patients,[43] whereas the Vascular Access Society recommends a selective approach.[36]

There is an increasing trend for preoperative imaging to reduce primary failure, non-maturation and unnecessary surgery.[35–37,43] This remains untested by clinical trial.

Venography is advisable if central vein stenosis is suspected. In complex cases with unclear venous anatomy, particularly predialysis patients in whom iodinated contrast could exacerbate renal failure, duplex ultrasound or magnetic resonance imaging may be preferable in the first instance. Angiography or arterial duplex is recommended if arterial pulses are diminished.

Duplex ultrasound

Preoperative duplex ultrasound is particularly useful for obese patients with impalpable superficial veins or following previous access failure, but cannot assess central vein patency. In studies from the USA, where AVGs are more frequently used than in Europe, routine preoperative ultrasound significantly increased the prevalence, reduced early failure rate and increased primary patency of autogenous AVFs compared with historical controls.[44–46] Prosthetic AV access reconstruction and access complications also decreased significantly. In another study duplex mapping changed the proposed procedure in a third of patients and almost doubled the proportion of AVFs constructed.[47] However, in a British study, duplex scanning rarely added any useful information except in those patients with poor vessels on clinical examination, when the proposed procedure was altered in 50%. This suggests that patients with good pulses and clinically adequate veins may proceed to surgery safely without preoperative ultrasound mapping.[48]

A radial artery luminal diameter of less than 1.6 mm is associated with early fistula failure[49] and a minimum diameter of 2 mm is now usually advised.[36,37,43] Above this threshold there seems to be no correlation between arterial diameter or flow and fistula success.

Venous diameter is an important determinant of outcome. In prospective studies, mean cephalic vein diameters are significantly smaller in non-functioning AVFs. Minimum venous diameters (with a tourniquet) of 2–2.5 mm have been advised for AVFs and 3.5–4.0 mm for synthetic grafts.[36,37,43]

Venous distensibility is another important predictor of success. Veins were found to dilate 48% with a tourniquet in successful fistulas compared with only 12% in fistulas that subsequently failed.[50]

Venography

✅ For many years, contrast venography was the gold standard and has the advantage of providing a venous map. It is mandatory in patients with prior ipsilateral central vein catheterisation, collateral vein development, oedema or arm swelling, indicating possible central vein obstruction.[36,37] Construction of a peripheral fistula in these patients can cause massive arm swelling. Previous radiotherapy to the shoulder area (e.g. for breast carcinoma) is a further indication for preoperative venography.

Iodinated contrast may precipitate acute renal failure and is relatively contraindicated in predialysis patients. Duplex ultrasound is an alternative but is poor for assessing central vein stenosis. Contrast-enhanced magnetic resonance venography is promising, as the small volume of paramagnetic contrast agent used does not compromise renal function, but there have been concerns about the rare complication of nephrogenic systemic fibrosis. Imaging is likely to improve significantly with new pulse sequences and blood pool contrast agents.

Carbon dioxide venography is not nephrotoxic and is widely used in France but requires a costly injector, causes local pain during injection, overestimation of venous stenoses and occasionally acute right heart failure.

Primary access

The snuffbox AVF is the most distal access possible and gives the longest length of vein for needling. It is possible in about 50% of patients and, in the event of failure, a wrist AVF can still be performed in half of the cases[51] (**Fig. 16.2**).

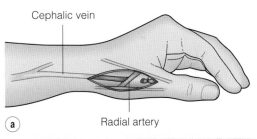

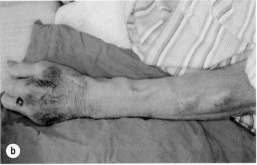

Figure 16.2 • The snuffbox AVF. **(a)** Diagram showing position of anastomosis. **(b)** A mature snuffbox fistula showing the long length of available vein for needling.

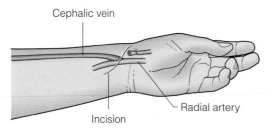

Figure 16.3 • The radiocephalic AVF at the wrist.

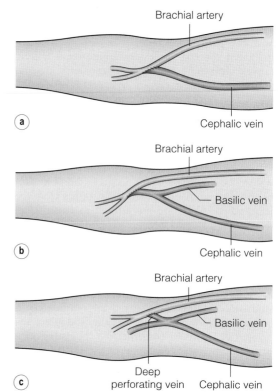

Figure 16.4 • Configurations of the brachiocephalic AVF at the antecubital fossa. **(a)** Direct anastomosis between the cephalic vein and brachial artery. **(b)** Anastomosis including both median basilic and cephalic veins. **(c)** Gracz fistula between the deep perforating vein and the brachial artery.

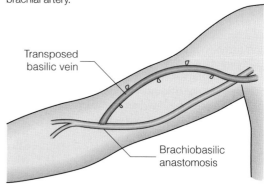

Figure 16.5 • The basilic vein transposition AVF.

The wrist radiocephalic AVF (**Fig. 16.3**) was the first to be described[41] and remains the standard access in most units. It has a low complication rate and gives a good length of available vein. Patencies of 65% at 1 year are usual.[52] If a wrist AVF fails, further forearm radiocephalic fistulas can often be created more proximally. In obese patients the vein may remain difficult to needle so that it may be advisable to excise the subcutaneous fat overlying the vein through one or more transverse incisions.

The brachiocephalic AVF is the next option, which can be performed in a variety of configurations (**Fig. 16.4**), and gives excellent flows at the expense of a greater incidence of steal (see below). To avoid this, some authors advocate anastomosing the cephalic vein to the radial artery 2 cm beyond its origin instead of the brachial artery itself.[53]

The ulnobasilic AVF is often possible after a failed brachial fistula but is more difficult to needle and seems to have a poorer patency than other upper limb AVFs.[54]

When the options are limited by venous thrombosis or arterial disease an ulnocephalic or radiobasilic fistula may be possible in the forearm, but these require more extensive mobilisation and subcutaneous tunnelling of the vein across the forearm.[55]

Secondary and tertiary access

When the cephalic vein is thrombosed, an antecubital brachiobasilic AVF may be possible but this leaves only a short length of vein for needling so the basilic vein is usually mobilised and rerouted superficially over the biceps muscle either in a single procedure or in a second stage after the vein has arterialised (the basilic vein transposition; **Fig. 16.5**).[56]

When an autogenous AVF cannot be performed, a prosthetic graft (AVG) can be used. A variety of graft materials are available, but polytetrafluoroethylene (PTFE) is the most popular. The graft can be used for needling, after 2 weeks, and may be used sooner but this can be associated with perigraft haematoma formation. Grafts have a higher rate of infection compared to AVF. Thrombosis is much more common than in AVF and is usually due to intimal hyperplasia, at or just beyond the venous anastomosis. A wider graft,[57] a vein cuff[58] or an expansion of the venous end of the graft (Venoflo)[59] may reduce this and has better patency. It is widely recognised that revision rates for grafts approach 80% annually compared to about 15% for AVF.

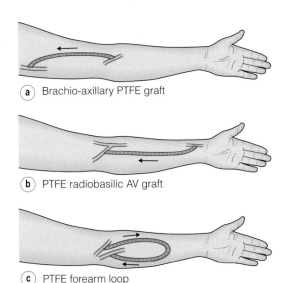

(a) Brachio-axillary PTFE graft

(b) PTFE radiobasilic AV graft

(c) PTFE forearm loop

Figure 16.6 • Popular configurations for upper limb AVGs: straight **(a,b)** and looped **(c)** brachio-axillary forearm grafts.

Biological grafts such as bovine mesenteric vein and bovine ureter are preferred in some units as they have greater resistance to infection, but they are prone to aneurysm formation.[60] A forearm AVG either in a looped or straight configuration allows a basilic vein transposition to be performed if it fails, but has a poorer patency than the latter,[61] so which should be performed first is a matter of dispute. A brachio-axillary AVG is the next option (**Fig. 16.6**).

Lower limb access is less popular but may be the only option when the SVC or both subclavian veins are occluded. An AVF at the ankle between the greater saphenous vein (GSV) and the posterior tibial artery is rarely possible because of underlying arterial disease. The GSV can be anastomosed to the popliteal artery above the knee or used as a subcutaneous loop from the femoral artery in the groin, but these are more difficult to needle. Transposition of the GSV in the thigh is less popular as it is more difficult to needle, but has fewer infective complications than synthetic thigh loop grafts.[62] The superficial femoral vein can be used in the same configurations (or transposed to the forearm) and gives an excellent fistula at the expense of a high incidence of steal.

In desperate cases, a variety of possibilities exist: axillo-femoral, axillo-axillary, ilio-iliac or even aorto-IVC AVGs can be used. Where there are no available veins the RA can be used as an outflow. Alternatively an arterio-arterial graft, usually in the axillary position, is possible but risks distal embolisation to the arm.[63] Occlusion of arterial interposition grafts may precipitate acute limb ischaemia.

Factors affecting access patency

The following factors are known to affect access patency:

- **Vessel size.** Small arteries and veins have higher initial failure rates, more frequent failure to mature and poorer long-term patency.[49]
- **Fistula flow rate.** The flow rate the day after surgery correlates inversely with the risk of thrombosis, although intraoperative flow rates are less reliable.[49] The hyperaemic response of brachial artery blood flow is a strong predictor of access patency and maturation, presumably by detecting proximal arterial stenoses.[64]
- **Mode of presentation.** Patients presenting acutely with renal failure have poorer AVF patency, which may be linked to the need for temporary access via a central venous catheter.[65]
- **Anastomotic method.** Non-penetrating vascular clips, which give an interrupted anastomosis with excellent endothelial apposition and less bleeding, are quicker and have improved patencies compared with sutured anastomoses in randomised trials.[66,67]
- **Access position.** More proximal AVFs have improved patency[67] but leave fewer options for access in the event of failure.
- **Gender.** Patency of AVFs is poorer in women than men.[51,65,68,69]
- **Diabetes.** There is conflicting evidence as to whether diabetes is an adverse factor, with some authors suggesting that AVF patency is poorer[67] whereas others have found no effect.[51,70,71]
- **Age.** In a meta-analysis, access patency was found to be worse in the elderly.[72] Wrist fistulas may perform as well as more proximal AVF.[73]
- **Obesity.** Veins are more difficult to cannulate in obese patients, which may account for poorer patency reported by some authors.[74]
- **Smoking.** Smoking reduces AVF patency.[75]
- **Drugs.** Antiplatelet agents such as aspirin and dipyridamole prolong fistula survival and are used routinely.[76–78] A combination of aspirin and clopidogrel increased haemorrhagic complications without influencing patency in prosthetic AVGs in one study,[79] but clopidogrel alone significantly prolonged graft survival in

another.[80] Warfarin reduces AVF thrombosis in patients with hypercoagulable states,[81] but routine use is best avoided because of the risk of haemorrhage. Surprisingly, warfarin was associated with poorer patency in the Dialysis Outcomes and Practice Patterns Study (DOPPS), but this may reflect its use in patients with a history of fistula thrombosis or known thrombotic disorders.[78] Calcium-channel blockers are associated with improved primary patency.[78] Angiotensin-converting enzyme inhibitors did not affect primary patency in one study[82] but were associated with improved secondary patency in DOPPS.[77] Fish oil reduced AVF thrombosis in one randomised trial.[8,83] Erythropoietin does not reduce and may increase patency, at least in AVGs.[84,85]

- **Thrombotic tendencies and vasculitis.** Increased fibrinogen and vasculitis predispose to access thrombosis.[86]

Access failure

Failure to mature

About 10% of AVFs remain patent but never achieve an adequate flow for dialysis. A duplex scan may reveal a proximal arterial or a venous stenosis, treatable by angioplasty or surgery. Otherwise a more proximal fistula will be required.

Stenosis and thrombosis

Early thrombosis may result from technical error, unrecognised pre-existing arterial stenoses or thrombophlebitis in the outflow vein, usually from previous intravenous cannulation. Late failure can result from hypotension, dehydration and hypercoagulable states, 'blowout' after traumatic needling or inappropriate use for intravenous infusions, but the most common cause is juxta-anastomotic venous intimal hyperplasia in AVG. In AVF failure may result from perianastomotic stenosis, but in long-standing AVF used for dialysis, mid-fistula stenosis between needling sites is also common.

✅ Percutaneous angioplasty of stenoses in AVFs and AVGs preserves veins and may prevent access thrombosis. Stenting is controversial but probably offers little extra advantage. Endovascular thrombolysis or thrombectomy of occluded AV accesses is effective provided that the underlying stenosis is dilated.[35–37]

Prevention of access failure

To prevent damage, careful needling and the avoidance of inappropriate use of AVFs are essential. Attempts to prevent intimal hyperplasia pharmacologically (e.g. with paclitaxel wraps) have yet to lead to routine clinical application.[87,88]

Access surveillance

AVFs and AVGs may suddenly occlude without prior warning, resulting in hospitalisation and the need for a CVC. Most of these will have unrecognised stenoses due to intimal hyperplasia. Detection by routine surveillance and treatment of such stenoses could prevent thrombosis and allow continuous use of the access.

Impending failure may be indicated by the loss of a palpable thrill, needling difficulties or a reduction in dialysis efficiency (e.g. reduced Kt/V (the volume cleared of urea/distribution volume), a reduced urea reduction ratio at each dialysis, a rising predialysis serum potassium or evidence of recirculation through the dialysis machine). Such monitoring is useful but does not identify all failing fistulas.

✅ Access surveillance is controversial but there is increasing evidence that access flow monitoring can identify stenoses in AVFs and AVGs and allow endovascular treatment to prevent access failure.

A variety of surveillance methods using static (with the pump turned off) or dynamic (at a standard pump speed) venous pressure measurements during dialysis have been proposed but are unreliable because the direction of any pressure change depends on whether the venous needle is upstream or downstream of the stenosis. Flow measurements are usually performed by an indicator dilution technique (e.g. ultrasound dilution).[89,90] A low flow (<500 mL/min) is a strong predictor of impending thrombosis in AVGs and is better than dynamic venous pressure.[91-93] The change in graft flow over time is a better predictor than a single value[94] and a 25% drop has been proposed as the trigger for further imaging and intervention.

Detection of stenoses is worthwhile, as intervention-free survival is better for grafts after pre-emptive angioplasty than after thrombectomy and angioplasty,[95] and vascular access flow monitoring reduces access morbidity and costs.[96] Reducing hospitalisation is an important element of providing high-quality care for patients.[97]

Surveillance using flow measurements also reduced thrombosis rates in AVFs in non-randomised[96,98] and randomised studies.[99] Others have failed to show improvement with surveillance but have been criticised on grounds of inadequate sensitivity[100] or inadequate angioplasty of detected stenoses.[101] Duplex

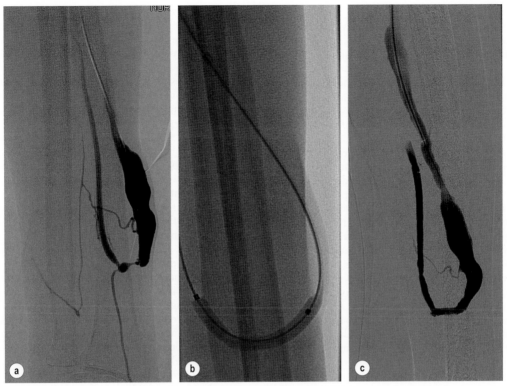

Figure 16.7 • Fistulogram showing a stenosis adjacent to a radiocephalic AVF **(a)** successfully treated by angioplasty **(b,c)**.

surveillance also reduces thrombosis rates,[102] hospitalisation and CVC usage[103] in AVFs and AVGs.

Access salvage

AVF stenosis

In radiocephalic fistulas, most stenoses occur close to the AV anastomosis (**Fig. 16.7**), with the remainder more proximally in the vein. In upper arm AVFs they also occur at the cephalic/subclavian vein junction. Intervention is indicated for stenoses greater than 50% associated with flow reduction, compromised dialysis or arm oedema. Fistulography is usually performed through the draining vein, reserving brachial artery puncture for inflow and anastomotic lesions. The venous run-off and central veins should also be demonstrated.

Primary angioplasty is indicated for upper forearm and upper arm significant stenoses, with technical success rates of over 90% and 1-year primary patency of 51% for forearm and 35% for upper arm fistulas.[104] Secondary patencies of over 80% can be achieved but more frequent interventions are needed in the upper arm. Stents offer no advantage.

Stenoses in the upper arm cephalic vein (cephalic arch) are a common cause of failure in patients with brachiocephalic fistulas. These lesions respond poorly to angioplasty as they are resistant to dilatation, develop early re-stenosis and have high vein rupture rates. Primary patencies at 6 months and 1 year after angioplasty are 42% and 23%, respectively.[105] A small randomised trial of stent grafts versus bare metal stents for the management of cephalic arch stenosis showed a 6-month primary patency of 81.8% for stent grafts and 39.1% for bare metal stents.[106] There have been no randomised studies comparing angioplasty and stent placement. There is a danger of stent migration into the subclavian vein that could jeopardise future access in the whole ipsilateral limb. Surgical revision with cephalic vein transposition to the basilic or axillary veins can be considered if angioplasty fails, although this may be technically difficult in an extensively needled AVF. If recurrent stenoses are angioplastied in patients who have undergone surgical revision, secondary patency rates of 92% at 1 year can be achieved.[107]

If endovascular intervention fails, stenoses can also be repaired surgically using a vein or prosthetic patch. Alternatively, inserting a short PTFE graft segment appears to be as good as an autogenous patch.[108] Stenoses adjacent to a distal AVF are best treated by creating a more proximal fistula, which may have better patency than angioplasty.[109]

AVG stenosis

The most common cause for AVG dysfunction is a stenosis at or near the venous anastomosis. Indications for intervention are similar to those for AVFs, with similar high technical success rates. Re-stenosis is a greater problem and leads to poor primary patency rates of 23–44% at 1 year,[110] but 1-year secondary patencies of 92% can be achieved by repeated angioplasty.[104] Intragraft stenoses from excessive ingrowth of fibrous tissue through cannulation defects can be treated similarly, but may require surgical curettage or segmental replacement.

When angioplasty fails repeatedly, bare metal stents can be considered but their primary patency is generally no better than angioplasty. There is an emerging role for covered stents in the treatment of angioplasty rupture and poor results from simple angioplasty. In one randomised trial, adding a covered stent after AVG angioplasty increased the 6-month patency from 23% to 51%.[111] However, there were similar access assisted and cumulative patency rates at 6 months in both groups, and it remains unclear whether the high cost of stent grafts can justify their routine use.[112] There are no published randomised trials on the use of drug-eluting stents.

Unassisted graft survival after thrombectomy and angioplasty is significantly worse than after elective angioplasty of patent grafts. Graft survival after thrombectomy and angioplasty may also be improved by stent implantation,[113] but there are no prospective controlled data.

There is no evidence favouring surgical revision over endovascular repair, but revisional surgery by segmental replacement or a jump graft to bypass a venous outflow stenosis may be required for recurrent stenoses. A pragmatic approach of reserving surgery for resistant or rapidly recurring stenosis will minimise unnecessary surgical intervention.

AVF and AVG thrombosis

Percutaneous declotting of AVGs is well established and effective, but AVFs are also being increasingly referred for radiological salvage. A thrombosed access should be declotted as soon as possible, preferably within 48 hours, and the underlying stenosis treated by angioplasty (with or without stenting). Available techniques include thrombolysis, thromboaspiration and mechanical thrombectomy. None seems superior but the expertise and experience of the operator are paramount.

Thrombus in an AVF causes phlebitis. Keeping the inflammatory response to a minimum is a key component of successful intervention. Whilst AVG can be declotted up to several weeks after thrombosis, most AVF require intervention within 24–48 hours for success. The amount of thrombus can vary enormously. In some AVFs only a short segment of vein thromboses because a side-branch just proximal to a perianastomotic stenosis maintains patency. These can usually be treated by simple angioplasty. In others the large volume of thrombus in an aneurysmal draining vein has a risk of a significant pulmonary embolus unless it is aggressively aspirated or a mechanical clot-removing device is used.

Technical success is reported as 73–90%, with widely differing 1-year primary and secondary patencies of 9–70% and 44–93%, respectively.[114] Patencies are higher in the forearm than upper arm. There are no randomised trials of percutaneous intervention versus surgery for AVFs. Primary endovascular intervention has the advantage of preserving veins for needling, but surgical revision or a new AVF is often necessary.

AVGs thrombose more frequently than AVFs but are well suited to percutaneous intervention. Radiological declotting is less invasive than surgery and allows accurate treatment of the underlying cause, which is nearly always a venous outflow stenosis. No single device or declotting technique has been shown to be superior, and the success of treatment of the underlying stenosis seems to be the only predictive value for graft patency.[115] Thrombolysis or mechanical thrombectomy have clinical success rates of 74–94% but 6-month primary patencies are only 18–39%.[116] However, with repeated intervention secondary patency rates of up to 83% have been reported.[117] Whilst there has been no prospective randomised multicentre trial, a meta-analysis found surgical intervention to have higher primary patency than endovascular intervention.[118] In many centres endovascular declotting is preferred because of its low morbidity, reserving surgical revision for technical failures or repeated thromboses.[116]

The most common complication of endovascular declotting is distal arterial embolisation, which occurs in 1–9% of cases.[116] Others include vessel rupture (2–4%) and non-puncture site bleeding (2–3%). All methods of declotting, especially mechanical techniques, cause venous embolisation, but this is usually asymptomatic because of the small volume of thrombus displaced.

Surgical thrombectomy is usually easy if the access has failed recently. Any underlying stenosis must be corrected by bypass or patch angioplasty at the same time. If surgery is delayed for 10 days or more it may be best to abandon it and create a new access at another site.

Other access complications

Infection

Infection is the commonest cause of hospital admission and mortality in dialysis patients. It is most

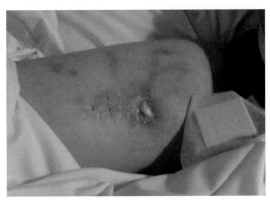

Figure 16.8 • A PTFE thigh loop with an exposed segment.

frequent in patients with CVCs and commoner in patients with AVGs than AVFs. The most frequent organism is *Staphylococcus aureus*. Bacteraemia or septicaemia may lead to endocarditis, mycotic aneurysms and septic arthritis.

Local needle-site infections may be controlled with antibiotics in the early stages but can lead to uncontrollable haemorrhage in autogenous fistulas, requiring emergency ligation or bypass of the infected area. AVGs with chronic needle-site infections or exposed segments (**Fig. 16.8**) may be salvaged by local excision and bypass of the area with appropriate antibiotic cover, but when the whole graft is infected it requires total excision. A further graft may be inserted once the wounds have healed.

Haemorrhage

Traumatic cannulation leads to localised haematomas. Prosthetic grafts can be destroyed by repeated punctures in the same area. This may necessitate local graft replacement.

Steal

An AVF tends to reduce digital arterial pressures[119] by lowering the peripheral resistance and may cause ischaemia (high-flow steal). The presence of a proximal arterial stenosis will amplify the reduction in finger pressures on AVF creation by limiting the increase in inflow (low-flow steal).

> ✓✓ Mild steal symptoms, such as coldness, pain, cramps, diminished sensation or reduced grip strength, are common in patients with AVFs. At least one symptom is present in 80% of brachial AVFs, 50% of those with forearm AV loops and 40% of radiocephalic AVFs,[120] but clinically significant steal with rest pain or tissue loss occurs in only 1–8% of patients.

Table 16.1 • The stages of access steal syndrome

Stage	Clinical features
I	Pale/cyanosed and/or cold hand without pain
II	Pain on exercise and/or dialysis
III	Rest pain
IV	Ulcer/necrosis/gangrene

Four grades of steal are recognised (Table 16.1). Grades 1 and 2 can usually be managed conservatively, but grades 3 and 4 require surgical intervention.

Predisposing factors include proximal AVF, diabetes mellitus, cardiac ischaemia, peripheral vascular disease[121,122] and low preoperative finger pressures.[119] Steal is the most likely cause of unilateral hand or finger ischaemia occurring after AVF creation (**Fig. 16.9**).

The clinical diagnosis can be made by a clear history of steal associated with the finding of an absent radial pulse that returns when the fistula is occluded. If in doubt, the diagnosis is confirmed by a digital pressure of 60 mmHg or less, with a significant increase on AVF occlusion.[123] A digital:brachial pressure index of less than 0.4 is also associated with steal. A duplex scan will demonstrate any proximal stenosis, quantify AVF flow and show reversed flow in the artery distal to the AVF (although this is not diagnostic). Fistulography is rarely required.

Steal syndrome should be treated promptly to avoid permanent neurological sequelae. These rarely recover completely if allowed to persist for any length of time.

AVF ligation cures steal syndrome and may be the sensible course of action in severe cases with rapid onset. Clinicians should only undertake this if they are confident that alternative access can be safely provided. As the majority of patients have similar arterial and venous pathologies in all their limbs,

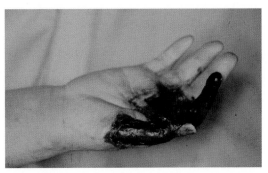

Figure 16.9 • Severe steal with digital gangrene after a brachial AVF.

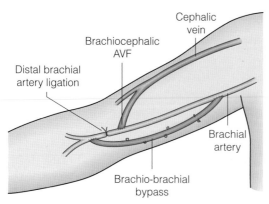

Figure 16.10 • The DRIL procedure.

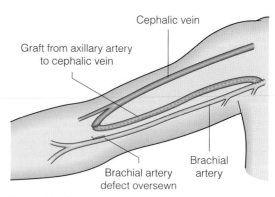

Figure 16.11 • Proximalisation of the arterial inflow.

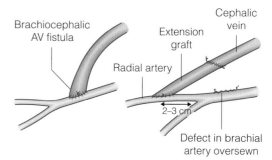

Figure 16.12 • The extension procedure.

attempting new access in the contralateral limb may simply reproduce steal in a new site. Steal syndrome associated with arterial inflow stenosis can usually be corrected by angioplasty or bypass. There are a variety of treatment options for steal with evidence of proximal arterial disease. At the wrist, radial arterial ligation distal to the fistula to prevent reversed flow is usually successful in those AVFs with an intact ulnar artery and palmar arch.

Distal arterial ligation may also be sufficient in brachial AVFs but intraoperative monitoring with finger or needle pressures is essential as in most cases finger pressures rarely improve sufficiently. In these cases a bypass from the proximal brachial (at least 8 cm proximal to the AV fistula anastomosis) or the axillary artery to the brachial artery distal to the ligature increases the distal pressure enough to relieve symptoms in most cases. This is the so-called DRIL (distal revascularisation interval ligation) procedure[124] (**Fig. 16.10**).

Another technique to prevent distal reversed flow is 'proximalisation of the arterial inflow' in which a brachial AVF or AVG is taken down and a prosthetic graft is led from the axillary or proximal brachial artery and anastomosed to the outflow vein or the arterial end of the AVG[125] (**Fig. 16.11**). This preserves fistula flow but transfers the inflow to a larger, high-flow artery capable of adapting to the reduction in peripheral resistance without distal flow reversal. This may be useful in patients where a diseased run-off might compromise the distal revascularisation of a DRIL procedure.

An alternative flow-reduction method is the 'extension procedure',[126] which is also known as the 'revision using distal inflow' (RUDI),[127] in which the cephalic vein or AVG is detached from its origin on the brachial artery and extended onto the radial artery 2–3 cm from its origin using a vein or prosthetic graft. This narrows the inflow and permits hand perfusion through the ulnar artery (**Fig. 16.12**). The choice of procedure depends on experience and personal preference, but the DRIL procedure is currently the most popular.

Fistula flow can be reduced by narrowing the outflow vein ('banding'), but achieving the appropriate degree of stenosis is difficult. It is not uncommon to either narrow the outflow sufficiently to cause thrombosis, or to fail to reduce flow and relieve the steal. However, in a recent report the degree of stenosis was successfully controlled by tightening a polyester band in stages whilst monitoring the flow rate, digital pressures and subclavian venous oxygen saturation.[128] In another report banding was accomplished by a spindle-like suture and a PTFE strip during intraoperative flow monitoring.[129]

Carpal tunnel syndrome

The incidence of carpal tunnel syndrome is increased by the presence of an AVF, possibly due to mild oedema due to venous hypertension.[130]

Cardiac failure

High-output cardiac failure is a rare complication, occurring occasionally with proximal AVFs with fistula flows in excess of 1.5 litres per minute. Bramham's sign (slowing of the heart rate on AVF compression) confirms the diagnosis. Treatment is either by fistula ligation or flow reduction by the extension procedure or controlled banding.[128]

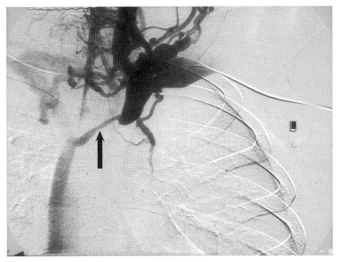

Figure 16.13 • Venogram showing an innominate vein stenosis.

Venous hypertension and central vein obstruction

Venous hypertension with oedema, venous collateral formation, or ulceration and tissue loss can occur with side-to-side AVFs but is more commonly associated with central venous obstruction (**Fig. 16.13**). If venous hypertension occurs with a side-to-side AVF, ligation of the distal vein draining the AVF is easy to perform and usually curative.

An AVF distal to a central obstruction is likely to exacerbate venous hypertension and may precipitate symptoms. Treatment of central vein obstruction by endovascular means or, as a last resort, surgical bypass will preserve the AVF, but sometimes the access must be ligated and created elsewhere, usually in the lower limb.

Subclavian stenosis or thrombosis is usually caused by a previous subclavian CVC. IJV catheters are now preferred but there is still a significant incidence of innominate and SVC stenosis (Fig. 16.13) or thrombosis. Endovascular treatment of these lesions is ideal, but simple angioplasty has a disappointing primary patency rate at 1 year of less than 40% in most studies.[7] Primary assisted or secondary patency rates are more encouraging at 35–97%.[131] Stents have a major role and can either be routinely placed at the initial intervention or reserved for early and frequent re-stenosis. There are no randomised trials versus angioplasty. There is no evidence at present advocating covered stents.

Surgical bypass gave a similar primary patency rate (70–80%) at 1 year to primary angioplasty and stenting in one study,[132] but has significant morbidity and mortality. Isolated subclavian vein occlusions may be repaired surgically by direct patch angioplasty, an axillo-jugular venous bypass or the jugular turndown operation.

SVC obstruction is best treated endovascularly, often requiring stent insertion to achieve patency. The symptomatic relief for the patient is immediate. Surgical bypass is a major undertaking with significant morbidity and should be regarded as a last resort in younger patients. Surgical incisions in an engorged neck can be associated with significant venous bleeding.

Aneurysm

The AVF outflow vein usually hypertrophies but sometimes reaches aneurysmal proportions (**Fig. 16.14**). In general, such aneurysms can be observed, as rupture is rare. Indications for intervention are rapid or persistent enlargement, skin breakdown with or without bleeding and patient request. The psychological effects of large and unsightly access in younger patients should not be

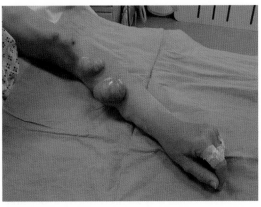

Figure 16.14 • An aneurysmal wrist AVF.

underestimated. Surgical aneurysmorrhaphy can significantly reduce the bulk of AVF whilst excising damaged skin and preserving the AVF for use. In AVF with multiple aneurysms, the author's preference is for sequential aneurysmorrhaphy allowing continued use of the unoperated segment of the AVF while healing occurs.

There is debate as to whether mesh wrapping of the aneurysmorrhaphy is required, but this has not been formally tested.[133,134]

There is interest in the use of covered stents for exclusion of pseudo-aneurysms, but this has not been formally tested in a clinical trial.

Cannulation

Cannulation of AVFs should be performed by adequately trained staff under strict aseptic conditions. A new autologous AVF is usually rested for 6 weeks before needling, to allow the vein wall to thicken, although early cannulation did not appear to be a risk factor in the DOPPS.[135] There may be cultural differences, with a tendency to earlier needling in Japan. An experienced dialysis nurse should always perform the first cannulation. Prosthetic grafts are needled directly and are usable for dialysis after 2 weeks.

There are three major strategies:

- The buttonhole technique, where the same site is needled at each dialysis, which is less painful

and causes less aneurysm formation but is less suitable for grafts because it can cause local graft destruction.
- Area puncture, where the vein or graft is needled over a specific area for each of the withdrawal and reinfusion sites, results in venous dilatation over an area but can also cause stenoses between aneurysmal sections.
- The rope-ladder technique, where needles are inserted for each dialysis by moving along the vein or graft in a sequential pattern. This is probably most suitable for AVGs as the damage of repeated needling is distributed over a larger area and delays the need for revision.

Access in children

The small calibre of the vessels has discouraged many surgeons from constructing AVFs in small children. Alternative methods such as continuous ambulatory peritoneal dialysis (CAPD) are therefore preferred in many units, but when haemodialysis is unavoidable CVCs are commonly used. However, excellent results of radiocephalic or brachial AVFs constructed by microsurgery in small children have been reported from experienced units.[136]

Key points

- The veins of the dorsum of the hand should be the preferred site for intravenous cannulation. The cephalic and antecubital veins should be reserved for dialysis access in patients with renal failure.
- The right IJV is the preferred site for central venous cannulation, which should be performed under ultrasound control.
- The use of CVCs for acute or short-term dialysis should be minimised because of the risks of septic complications, central venous thrombosis and a higher mortality than AVFs.
- Tunnelled CVCs should be used for dialysis if required for longer than 2 weeks but should only be used long term when an AVF or AVG cannot be constructed.
- Permanent vascular access should, wherever possible, be constructed 16–24 weeks before the anticipated need for dialysis.
- For permanent dialysis access an autogenous AVF should be constructed as distally as possible, preferably in the non-dominant arm.
- AVGs should only be used when the construction of an autogenous AVF is not possible.

References

1. Sariego J, Bootorabi B, Matsumoto T, et al. Major long-term complications in 1,422 permanent venous access devices. Am J Surg 1993;165:249–51.

2. Rayan SS, Terramani TT, Weiss VJ, et al. The LifeSite hemodialysis access system in patients with limited access. J Vasc Surg 2003;38:714–8.

3. Seldinger SI. Catheter replacement of the needle in percutaneous arteriography; a new technique. Acta Radiol 1953;39:368–76.

4. Hind D, Calvert N, McWilliams R, et al. Ultrasonic locating devices for central venous cannulation: meta-analysis. Br Med J 2003;327:361–4.

5. Ansell D, Feest T, Williams AJ, et al. editors. UK Renal Registry Report 2005. Bristol: UK Renal Registry, Chapter 6. The National Dialysis Access Survey – preliminary results, p. 87–102. www.renalreg.com.

6. Nasser GM, Ayus JC. Infectious complications of haemodialysis access. Kidney Int 2001;60:1–13.

7. Mickley V. Central vein obstruction in vascular access. Eur J Vasc Endovasc Surg 2006;32:439–44.

8. Dhingra RK, Young EW, Hulbert-Shearon TE, et al. Type of vascular access and mortality in U.S. hemodialysis patients. Kidney Int 2001;60:1443–51.

9. Tokars JI, Miller ER, Stein G. New national surveillance system for hemodialysis-associated infections: initial results. Am J Infect Control 2002;30:288–95.

10. Merrer J, De Jonghe B, Golliot F, et al. Complications of femoral and subclavian venous catheterisation in critically ill patients: a randomised controlled trial. JAMA 2001;286:700–7.

11. Chow KM, Szeto CC, Leung CB, et al. Cuffed tunneled femoral catheters for long-term hemodialysis. Int J Artif Organs 2001;24:443–6.

12. Nazarian GK, Bjarnason H, Dietz CA, et al. Changes in tunnelled catheter tip position when the patient is upright. J Vasc Interv Radiol 1997;8:437–41.

13. Mallory DL, McGee WT, Shawker TH, et al. Ultrasound improves the success rate of internal jugular vein cannulation. A prospective, randomised trial. Chest 1990;98:157–60.
In this prospective randomised trial ultrasound was shown to increase the success rate and reduce the complications of internal jugular cannulation.

14. Brzosko S, Hryszko T, Malyszko J, et al. Femoral localization and higher ultrafiltration rate but not concentration of heparin used for canal locking of hemodialysis catheters are negative predictors of its malfunction. Am J Nephrol 2008;28:298–303.

15. Hemmelgarn BR, Moist LM, Lok CE, et al. Prevention of dialysis catheter malfunction with recombinant tissue plasminogen activator. N Engl J Med 2011;364:303–12.

16. Grudzinski L, Quinan P, Kwok S, et al. Sodium citrate 4% locking solution for central venous dialysis catheters. An effective, more cost-efficient alternative to heparin. Nephrol Dial Transplant 2007;22:471–6.

17. Trerotola SO, Johnson MS, Harris VJ, et al. Outcome of tunneled hemodialysis catheters placed via the right internal jugular vein by interventional radiologists. Radiology 1997;203:489–95.

18. Willms L, Vercaigne LM. Does Warfarin safely prevent clotting of hemodialysis catheters? Semin Dial 2008;21:71–7.

19. Haymond J, Shalansky K, Jastrzebski J. Efficiency of low-dose alteplase for treatment of hemodialysis catheter occlusions. J Vasc Access 2005;6:76–82.

20. Savader SJ, Ehrman KO, Porter DJ, et al. Treatment of hemodialysis catheter-associated fibrin sheaths by rt-PA infusion: critical analysis of 124 procedures. J Vasc Interv Radiol 2001;12:711–5.

21. Tumlin J, Goldman J, Spiegel DM, et al. A phase III, randomised, double-blind, placebo-controlled study of tenecteplase for improvement of hemodialysis catheter function: TROPICS 3. Clin J Am Soc Nephrol 2010;5:631–6.

22. Fishbane S, Milligan SL, Lempert KD, et al. Improvement in hemodialysis catheter function with tenecteplase; a phase III, open label study: TROPICS 4. J Throm Thrombolysis 2011;31:99–106.

23. Suhocki PV, Conlon PJ, Knelson MH, et al. Silastic cuffed catheters for hemodialyss vascular access: thrombotic and mechanical correction of malfunction. Am J Kidney Dis 1996;28:379–86.

24. Gray RJ, Levitin A, Buck D, et al. Percutaneous fibrin sheath stripping versus transcatheter urokinase for malfunctioning well-positioned central venous dialysis catheters: a prospective randomized trial. J Vasc Interv Radiol 2000;11:1121–9.

25. Merport M, Murphy TP, Egglin TK, et al. Fibrin sheath stripping versus catheter exchange for the treatment of failed tunneled hemodialysis catheters: randomised clinical trial. J Vasc Interv Radiol 2000;11:1115–20.

26. Saad TF. Bacteraemia associated with tunnneled, cuffed hemodialysis catheters. Am J Kidney Dis 1999;34:1114–24.

27. Tanriover B, Carlton D, Saddekni S, et al. Bacteraemia associated with tunneled dialysis catheters: comparison of two treatment strategies. Kidney Int 2000;57:2151–5.

28. Onder AM, Chandar J, Billings A, et al. Chlorhexidine-based antiseptic solutions effectively reduce catheter-related bacteremia. Pediatr Nephrol 2009;24:1741–7.

29. Johnson DW, MacGinley R, Kay TD, et al. A randomized, controlled trial of topical exit site mupirocin application in patients with tunnelled, cuffed haemodialysis catheters. Nephrol Dial Transplant 2002;17:1802–7.

30. Kamal GD, Pfaller MA, Rempe LE, et al. Reduced intravascular catheter infection by antibiotic bonding. JAMA 1991;265:2364–8.

31. Chatzinikolaou I, Finkel K, Hanna H, et al. Antibiotic-coated hemodialysis catheters for the prevention of vascular catheter-related infections: a prospective, randomised study. Am J Med 2003;115:352–7.

32. Schindler R, Heemann U, Haug U, et al. Bismuth coating of non-tunelled hemodialysis catheters reduces bacterial colonization: a randomized controlled trial. Nephrol Dial Transplant 2010;25:2651–6.

33. Verbeke F, Haug U, Dhondt A, et al. The role of polymer surface degredation and barium sulphate release in the pathogenesis of catheter-related infection. Nephrol Dial Transplant 2010;25:1207–13.

34. Snaterse M, Ruger W, Scholte OP, et al. Antibiotic-based catheter lock solutions for the prevention of catheter-related bloodstream infections: a systematic review of randomised controlled trials. J Hosp Infect 2010;75:1–11.

35. National Kidney Foundation – Dialysis Outcomes Quality Initiative. NKF-DOQI clinical practice guidelines for vascular access. Am J Kidney Dis 1997;30(4, Suppl. 3):S150–91.

36. Vascular Access Society Guidelines, http://www.vascularaccesssociety.com; [accessed 2.07.12].

37. Winearls CG, Fluck R, Mitchell DC, et al. The organization and delivery of the vascular access service for maintenance haemodialysis patients. Report of a joint working party, 2006. Online. http://www.renal.org/Libraries/Clinical_Service/Report_of_a_Joint_Working_Party_on_Vascular_Access_September_2006.sflb.ashx. [accessed 18.06.12].

38. Huber TS, Carter JW, Carter RL, et al. Patency of autogenous and polytetrafluoroethylene upper extremity arteriovenous hemodialysis accesses: a systematic review. J Vasc Surg 2003;38:1005–11.

A review and meta-analysis comparing 34 non-randomised studies of upper limb AV access showing a significantly better primary patency for autogenous AV fistulas at 6 months (72%) and 18 months (541%) than PTFE AV grafts (58% and 33% respectively).

39. Hodges TC, Fillinger MF, Zwolak RM, et al. Longitudinal comparison of dialysis access methods: factors for failure. J Vasc Surg 1997;26:1009–19.

A large retrospective single-centre study showing similar secondary patency for autogenous and prosthetic access but a much higher revision rate for AV grafts.

40. Astor BC, Eustace JA, Powe NR, et al. Type of vascular access and survival among incident hemodialysis patients: the Choices for Healthy Outcomes in Caring for ESRD (CHOICE) Study. J Am Soc Nephrol 2005;16:1449–55.

A large non-randomised multicentre study on the outcome of different forms of AV access, showing a relative mortality for central venous catheters of 1.5 and prosthetic access 1.2 in comparison with autogenous AV fistulas.

41. Breschia MJ, Cimino JE, Appel K, et al. Chronic hemodialysis using venepuncture and a surgically created arteriovenous fistula. N Engl J Med 1966;275:1089–92.

42. Gelabert HA, Freischlag JA. Haemodialysis access. In: Rutherford RB, editor. Vascular surgery. 5th ed. Philadelphia: Saunders; 2000. p. 1466–77.

43. NKF-DOQI clinical practice guidelines for vascular access. Online, www.kidney.org/professionals/kdoqi/guideline_upHD_PD_VA/index.htm; [accessed 18.06.12].

44. Silva MB, Hobson RW, Pappas PJ, et al. A strategy for increasing use of autogenous hemodialysis access procedures: impact of preoperative non invasive evaluation. J Vasc Surg 1998;27:302–8.

45. Allon M, Lockhart ME, Lilly RZ, et al. Effect of preoperative sonographic mapping on vascular access outcomes in hemodialysis patients. Kidney Int 2001;60:2013–20.

46. Mihmanli I, Besirli K, Kurugoglu S, et al. Cephalic vein and hemodialysis fistula. Surgeon's observation versus color Doppler utrasonographic findings. J Ultrasound Med 2001;20:217–22.

47. Robbin M, Gallichio MH, Deierhoi MH, et al. US vascular mapping before hemodialysis access placement. Radiology 2000;217:83–8.

48. Wells AC, Fernando B, Butler A, et al. Selective use of ultrasonographic vascular mapping in the assessment of patients before haemodialysis access surgery. Br J Surg 2005;92:1439–43.

49. Wong V, Ward R, Taylor J, et al. Factors associated with early failure of arteriovenous fistulae for haemodialysis access. Eur J Vasc Endovasc Surg 1996;12:207–13.

50. Malovrh M. The role of sonography in the planning of arteriovenous fistulae for dialysis. Semin Dial 2003;16:229–303.

51. Wolowczyk L, Williams AJ, Gibbons CP. The snuffbox arteriovenous fistula for vascular access. Eur J Vasc Endovasc Surg 2000;19:70–6.

52. Rooijens PP, Tordoir JH, Stijnen T, et al. Radiocephalic wrist arteriovenous fistula for hemodialysis: meta-analysis indicates a high primary failure rate. Eur J Vasc Endovasc Surg 2004;28:583–9.

53. Ehsan O, Bhattacharya D, Darwish A, et al. 'Extension technique': a modified technique for brachio-cephalic fistula to prevent dialysis access-associated steal syndrome. Eur J Vasc Endovasc Surg 2005;29:324–7.

54. Salgado OJ, Chacon RE, Henriquez C. Ulnar–basilic fistula: indications, surgical aspects, puncture technique, and results. Artif Organs 2004;28:634–8.

55. Tordoir JH, Keuter X, Planken N, et al. Autogenous options in secondary and tertiary access for haemodialysis. Eur J Vasc Endovasc Surg 2006;31:661–6.

56. Dix FP, Khan Y, Al-Khaffaf H. The brachial artery–basilic vein arterio-venous fistula in vascular access for haemodialysis – a review paper. Eur J Vasc Endovasc Surg 2006;31:70–9.

57. Garcia-Pajares R, Polo JR, Flores A, et al. Upper arm polytetrafluoroethylene grafts for dialysis access. Analysis of two different graft sizes: 6 mm and 6–8 mm. Vasc Endovasc Surg 2003;37:335–43.

58. Lemson MS, Tordoir JH, van Det RJ, et al. Effects of a venous cuff at the venous anastomosis of polytetrafluoroethylene grafts for hemodialysis vascular access. J Vasc Surg 2000;32:1155–63.

59. Sorom AJ, Hughes CB, McCarthy JT, et al. Prospective, randomized evaluation of a cuffed expanded polytetrafluoroethylene graft for hemodialysis vascular access. Surgery 2002;132:135–40.

60. Berardinelli L. Grafts and graft materials as vascular substitutes for haemodialysis access construction. Eur J Vasc Endovasc Surg 2006;32:203–11.

61. Keuter XH, De Smet AA, Kessels AG, et al. A randomized multicenter study of the outcome of brachial–basilic arteriovenous fistula and prosthetic brachial–antecubital forearm loop as vascular access for hemodialysis. J Vasc Surg 2008;47(2):395–401.

62. Bhandari Wilkinson A, Sellars L. Saphenous vein forearm grafts and gortex thigh grafts as alternative forms of vascular access. Clin Nephrol 1995;44:325–8.

63. Rudarakanchana N, Davies AH. Complex vascular access. In: Davies AH, Gibbons CP, editors. Vascular access simplified. 2nd ed. Shrewsbury, UK: tfm Publishing; 2007. p. 103–16[chapter 9].

64. Wall LP, Gasparis A, Callahan S, et al. Impaired hyperemic response is predictive of early access failure. Ann Vasc Surg 2004;18:167–71.

65. Rayner HC, Pisoni RL, Gillespie BW, et al. Dialysis Outcomes and Practice Patterns Study. Creation, cannulation and survival of arteriovenous fistulae: data from the Dialysis Outcomes and Practice Patterns Study. Kidney Int 2003;63:323–30.

66. Lin PH, Bush RL, Nelson JC, et al. A prospective evaluation of interrupted nitinol surgical clips in arteriovenous fistula for hemodialysis. Am J Surg 2003;186:625–30.

67. Shenoy S, Miller A, Petersen F, et al. A multicenter study of permanent hemodialysis access patency: beneficial effect of clipped vascular anastomotic technique. J Vasc Surg 2003;38:229–35.

68. Ernandez T, Saudan P, Berney T, et al. Risk factors for early failure of native arteriovenous fistulae. Nephron Clin Pract 2005;101:c39–44.

69. Rodriguez JA, Armadans L, Ferrer E, et al. The function of permanent vascular access. Nephrol Dial Transplant 2000;15:402–8.

70. Murphy GJ, Nicholson ML. Autogeneous elbow fistulae: the effect of diabetes mellitus on maturation, patency, and complication rates. Eur J Vasc Endovasc Surg 2002;23:452–7.

71. Akoh JA, Sinha S, Dutta S, et al. A 5-year audit of haemodialysis access. Int J Clin Pract 2005;59:847–51.

72. Lazarides MK, Georgiadis GS, Antaniou GA, et al. A meta-analysis of dialysis access outcome in elderly patients. J Vasc Surg 2007;45:420–6.

73. Weale AR, Bevis P, Neary WD, et al. Radiocephalic and brachiocephalic arteriovenous fistula outcomes in the elderly. J Vasc Surg 2008;47(1):144–50.

74. Kats M, Hawxby AM, Barker J, et al. Impact of obesity on arteriovenous fistula outcomes in dialysis patients. Kidney Int 2007;71:39–43.

75. Weitzig GA, Gough IR, Furnival CM. One hundred cases of arteriovenous fistula for haemodialysis access: the effect of cigarette smoking on patency. Aust N Z J Surg 1985;55:551–4.

76. Andrassy K, Malluche H, Bornfeld H, et al. Prevention of PO clotting of AV. Cimino fistulae with acetylsalicyl acid: results of a prospective double blind study. Klin Wochenschr 1974;52:348–9.

77. Sreedhara R, Himmelfarb J, Lazarus JM, et al. Antiplatelet therapy in graft thrombosis: results of a prospective randomised double blind study. Kidney Int 1994;45:1477–83.

78. Saran R, Dykstra DM, Wolfe RA, et al. Dialysis Outcomes and Practice Patterns Study. Association between vascular access failure and the use of specific drugs: the Dialysis Outcomes and Practice Patterns Study (DOPPS). Am J Kidney Dis 2002;40:1255–63.

79. Kaufman JS, O'Connor TZ, Zhang JH, et al. Randomized controlled trial of clopidogrel plus aspirin to prevent hemodialysis access graft thrombosis. J Am Soc Nephrol 2003;14:2313–21.

80. Trimarchi H, Young P, Forrester M, et al. Clopidogrel diminishes hemodialysis access graft thrombosis. Nephron Clin Pract 2006;102:c128–32.

81. LeSar CJ, Merrick HW, Smith MR. Thrombotic complications resulting from hypercoagulable states in chronic haemodialysis vascular access. J Am Coll Surg 1999;189:73–9.

82. Heine GH, Ulrich C, Kohler H, et al. Is AV fistula patency associated with angiotensin-converting enzyme (ACE) polymorphism and ACE inhibitor intake? Am J Nephrol 2004;24:461–8.

83. Schmitz PG, McCloud LK, Reikes ST, et al. Prophylaxis of hemodialysis graft thrombosis with fish oil: double-blind, randomized, prospective trial. J Am Soc Nephrol 2002;13:184–90.

84. Fischer-Colbrie W, Clyne N, Jogenstrand T, et al. The effect of erythropoietin treatment on arteriovenous haemodialysis fistula/graft: a prospective study with colour flow Doppler ultrasonography. Eur J Vasc Surg 1994;8:346–50.

85. Martino MA, Vogel KM, O'Brien SP, et al. Erythropoietin therapy improves graft patency with no increased incidence of thrombosis or thrombophlebitis. J Am Coll Surg 1998;187:616–9.

86. Bumann M, Niebel W, Kribben A, et al. Pimary failure of arteriovenous fistulae in auto-immune disease. Kidney Blood Press Res 2003;26:362–7.

87. Kohler TR, Toleikis PM, Gravett DM, et al. Inhibition of neointimal hyperplasia in a sheep model of dialysis access failure with the bioabsorbable Vascular Wrap paclitaxel-eluting mesh. J Vasc Surg 2007;45:1029–37.

88. Kelly B, Melhem M, Zhang J, et al. Perivascular paclitaxel wraps block arteriovenous graft stenosis in a pig model. Nephrol Dial Transplant 2006;21:2425–31.

89. Krivitski NM. Access flow measurement during surveillance and percutaneous transluminal angioplasty intervention. Semin Dial 2003;16:304–8.

90. Bosman PJ, Boereboom FT, Bakker CJ, et al. Access flow measurements in hemodialysis patients: in vivo validation of an ultrasound dilution technique. J Am Soc Nephrol 1996;7:966–9.

91. Bosman PJ, Boereboom FT, Smits HF, et al. Pressure or flow recordings for the surveillance of hemodialysis grafts. Kidney Int 1997;52:1084–8.

92. Bosman PJ, Boereboom FT, Eiklboom BC, et al. Graft flow as a predictor in haemodialysis grafts. Kidney Int 1998;54:1726–30.

93. May RE, Himmelfarb J, Yenicesu M, et al. Predictive measures of vascular access thrombosis: a prospective study. Kidney Int 1997;52:1656–62.

94. Neyra NR, Ikizler TA, May RE, et al. Changes in access blood flow over time predicts vascular access thrombosis. Kidney Int 1998;54:1714–9.

95. Lilly RZ, Carlton D, Barker J, et al. Predictors of arteriovenous graft patency after radiological intervention in hemodialysis patients. Am J Kidney Dis 2001;37:945–53.

96. McCarley P, Wingard RL, Shyr Y, et al. Vascular access blood flow monitoring reduces access morbidity and costs. Kidney Int 2001;60:1164–72.

97. Plantinga LC, Fink NE, Bass EB, et al. Preferences for current health and their association with outcomes in patients with kidney disease. Med Care 2007;45(3):230–7.

98. Schwab SJ, Oliver MJ, Suhocki P, et al. Hemodialysis arteriovenous access: detection of stenosis and response to treatment by vascular access blood flow. Kidney Int 2001;59:358–62.

99. Tessitore N, Lipari G, Poli A, et al. Can blood flow surveillance and pre-emptive repair of subclinical stenosis prolong the useful life of arteriovenous fistulae? A randomized controlled study. Nephrol Dial Transplant 2004;19:2325–33.

100. Ram J, Nassar R, Sharaf R, et al. Thresholds for significant decrease in hemodialysis access blood flow. Semin Dial 2005;18:558–64.

101. Krivitski N. Access flow surveillance – major criteria for success. Proc 5th Int Congress of the Vascular Access Society. Nice; 2007. p. L011.

102. Paulson WD. Access monitoring does not really improve outcomes. Blood Purif 2005;23:50–6.

103. Dossabhoy NR, Ram SJ, Nassar R, et al. Stenosis surveillance of hemodialysis grafts by duplex ultrasound reduces hospitalizations and cost of care. Semin Dial 2005;18:550–7.

104. Turmel-Rodrigues L, Pengloan J, Baudin S, et al. Treatment of stenoses and thrombosis in haemodialysis fistulae and grafts by interventional radiology. Nephrol Dial Transplant 2000;15:2029–36.

105. Rajan DK, Clark TW, Vatel NK, et al. Prevalence and treatment of cephalic arch stenosis in dysfunctional autogenous hemodialysis fistulas. J Vasc Interv Radiol 2003;14:567–73.

106. Shemesh D, Goldin I, Zaghal I, et al. Angioplasty with stent graft versus bare stent for recurrent cephalic arch stenosis in autogenous arteriovenous access for hemodialysis: a prospective randomised clinical trial. J Vasc Surg 2008;48:1524–31.

107. Kian K, Unger SW, Mishler R, et al. Role of surgical intervention for cephalic arch stenosis in the "fistula first" era. Semin Dial 2008;21:93–6.

108. Georgiadis GS, Lazarides MK, Lambidis CD, et al. Use of short PTFE segments (<6 cm) compares favorably with pure autologous repair in failing or thrombosed native arteriovenous fistulae. J Vasc Surg 2005;41:76–81.

109. Turmel-Rodrigues L, Pengloan J, Bourquelot P. Interventional radiology in hemodialysis fistulae and grafts: a multidisciplinary approach. Cardiovasc Intervent Radiol 2002;25:3–16.

110. Gray RJ. AV shunt angioplasty – are patency results good enough? J Vasc Access 2007;8:155–7.

111. Haskal Z, Trerotola S, Dolmatch B, et al. Stent graft versus balloon angioplasty for failing dialysis-access grafts. N Engl J Med 2010;362:494–503.

112. Salman L, Asif A. Stent graft for nephrologists: concerns and consensus. Clin J Am Soc Nephrol 2010;5:1347–52.

113. Maya ID, Allon M. Outcomes of thrombosed arteriovenous grafts: comparison of stents vs angioplasty. Kidney Int 2006;69:934–7.

114. Trerotola SO. AVF declotting: techniques and results. J Vasc Access 2007;8:169–71.

115. Smits HFM, Smits JHM, Wust AF, et al. Percutaneous thrombolysis of thrombosed haemodialysis access grafts: comparison of three mechanical devices. Nephrol Dial Transplant 2002;17:467–73.

116. Aruny JE, Lewis CA, Cardella JF, et al. Quality improvement guidelines for percutaneous management of thrombosed or dysfunctional dialysis access. J Vasc Interv Radiol 2003;14:S247–53.

117. Turmel-Rodrigues L, Pengloan J, Rodrique H, et al. Treatment of failed native arteriovenous fistulae for hemodialysis by interventional radiology. Kidney Int 2000;57:1124–40.

118. Green LD, Lee DS, Kucey DS. A metaanalysis comparing surgical thrombectomy, mechanical thrombectomy, and pharmacomechanical thrombolysis for thrombosed dialysis grafts. J Vasc Surg 2002;36:939–45.

119. Valentine RJ, Bouch CW, Scott DJ, et al. Do preoperative finger pressures predict early arterial steal in hemodialysis access patients? A prospective analysis. J Vasc Surg 2002;36:351–6.

120. Van Hoek F, Scheltinga MR, Kouwenberg I, et al. Steal in hemodialysis patients depends on type of vascular access. Eur J Vasc Endovasc Surg 2006;32:710–7.

121. Yeager RA, Moneta GL, Edwards GL, et al. Relationship of hemodialysis access to finger gangrene in patients with end-stage renal disease. J Vasc Surg 2002;36:245–9.

122. Rocha A, Silva F, Queirós J, et al. Predictors of steal syndrome in hemodialysis patients. Hemodial Int 2012. http://dx.doi.org/10.1111/j.1542-758.2012.00684.x.Epub ahead of print.

123. Schanzer A, Nguyen LL, Owens CD, et al. Use of digital pressure measurements for the diagnosis of AV access-induced hand ischemia. Vasc Med 2006;11(4):227–31.

124. Schanzer H, Schwartz M, Harrington W, et al. Treatment of ischemia due to "steal" by arteriovenous fistula with distal artery ligation and revascularization. J Vasc Surg 1988;7:770–3.

125. Zanow J, Kruger U, Scholz H. Proximalization of the arterial inflow: a new technique to treat access-related ischemia. J Vasc Surg 2006;43:1216–21.

126. Ehsan O, Bhattacharya D, Darwish A, et al. 'Extension technique': a modified technique for brachio-cephalic fistula to prevent dialysis access-associated steal syndrome. Eur J Vasc Endovasc Surg 2006;29:324–7.

127. Minion DJ, Moore E, Endean E. Revision using distal inflow: a novel approach to dialysis-associated steal syndrome. Ann Vasc Surg 2005;19:625–8.

128. Van Hoek F, Scheltinga MR, Lurink M, et al. Access flow, venous saturation, and digital pressures in hemodialysis. J Vasc Surg 2007;45:968–73.

129. Zanow J, Petzold K, Petzold M, et al. Flow reduction in high-flow arteriovenous access using intraoperative flow monitoring. J Vasc Surg 2006;44:1273–8.

130. Gousheh J, Iranpour A. Association between carpel tunnel syndrome and arteriovenous fistula in hemodialysis patients. Plast Reconstr Surg 2005;116:508–13.

131. Peden EK. Central venous obstruction: When to treat? What to do? J Vasc Access 2007;8:161–2.

132. Bhatia DS, Money SR, Ochsner JL, et al. Comparison of surgical bypass and percutaneous balloon dilatation with primary stent placement in the treatment of central venous obstruction in the dialysis patient: one year follow up. Ann Vasc Surg 1996;10:452–5.

133. Balaz P, Rokosny S, Klein D, et al. Aneurysmorrhaphy is an easy technique for arteriovenous fistula salvage. J Vasc Access 2008;9(2):81–4.

134. Berard X, Brizzi V, Mayeux S, et al. Salvage treatment for venous aneurysm complicating vascular access arteriovenous fistula: use of an exoprosthesis to reinforce the vein after aneurysmorrhaphy. Eur J Vasc Endovasc Surg 2010;40(1):100–6.

135. Saran R, Dykstra DM, Pisoni RL, et al. Timing of first cannulation and vascular access failure in haemodialysis: an analysis of practice patterns at dialysis facilities in the DOPPS. Nephrol Dial Transplant 2004;19:2334–40.

136. Bourquelot P. Vascular access in children: the importance of microsurgery for creation of autologous arteriovenous fistulae. Eur J Vasc Endovasc Surg 2006;32:696–700.

17

Varicose veins

Manjit S. Gohel
Alun H. Davies

Introduction

Varicose veins are common, often leading to a significant impact on patient quality of life, and the management of venous disease is a major cause of United Kingdom National Health Service (NHS) expense.[1-4] In view of the wide range of clinical presentations, a variety of clinical teams may be involved in the management of patients with venous disease and associated complications, including vascular surgeons, dermatologists, plastic surgeons and other specialists. Clinicians and researchers have generally underestimated the clinical importance of this condition, but recent advances in treatment have stimulated a spate of research in this field. Optimal patient management involves a detailed assessment and evaluation of the patient expectations from treatment in addition to targeted multimodal therapy to address underlying anatomical abnormalities and reduce venous hypertension.

Pathophysiology

Normal venous function

The venous system returns deoxygenated blood from the capillary beds to the right atrium via low-pressure venous channels. Flow in the direction of the heart is maintained by unidirectional valves throughout the venous system and muscle pumps located in the calf and foot, which contract during ambulation and promote venous flow. Retrograde flow (away from the heart) is termed venous incompetence or reflux and is usually due to damage to the venous valves.

Chronic venous hypertension

The underlying cause of venous disease is chronic venous hypertension. This is usually due to venous reflux secondary to vein valve incompetence, but may also be due to occlusive deep venous disease (usually due to thrombosis) and calf muscle pump failure (usually due to ankle stiffness or poor calf muscle bulk).[5] The clinical consequence of venous reflux depends not only on the severity of reflux, but also the effectiveness of normal measures that reduce venous hypertension (Fig. 17.1), ranging from asymptomatic to ulceration. The belief that venous skin changes and ulceration are only due to deep venous disease has been disproved in recent years; anatomical studies have clearly demonstrated that patients with chronic venous ulceration often have superficial reflux only.[6] Chronic venous hypertension (insufficiency) is dealt with in more detail in the next chapter on chronic leg swelling.

Varicose veins

Varicose veins are usually due to superficial venous reflux affecting the great saphenous vein (GSV) (Fig. 17.2), small saphenous vein (SSV) or non-truncal veins. Whether the valve failure is a primary phenomenon or secondary to vein wall dilatation remains unknown. Two theories have been proposed to explain the development

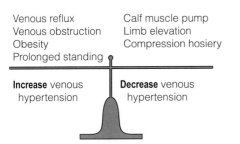

Figure 17.1 • Factors affecting venous hypertension.

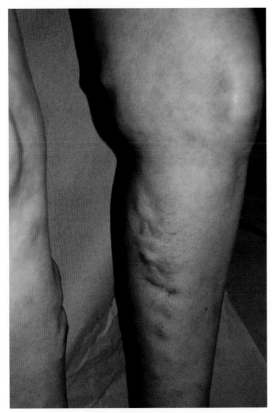

Figure 17.2 • Typical varicose veins in the great saphenous distribution (CEAP C2).

of superficial venous reflux leading to varicose veins. The 'descending theory' was popularised by Trendelenburg in the 19th century and suggests that superficial venous incompetence begins at the saphenous junctions and progresses distally.[7] The 'ascending theory' advocates the proximal progression of distal venous incompetence and is supported by the observation that superficial venous incompetence often occurs with a competent saphenous junction.[8] Although both explanations have merits and proponents, the development of varicose veins is likely to be multifactorial.

Epidemiology and natural history

The incidence of venous disease in the population has been evaluated by large population studies from Edinburgh and Bonn.[9–11] These observational studies have demonstrated that the majority of adults have reticular or thread veins, whereas varicose veins or more severe stages of venous disease (CEAP C2–C6, see Box 17.1) are present in 25–40% of the population. Venous disease is more common in developed rather than developing countries, although the reasons for these differences are poorly understood. Interestingly, deep reflux was more common in men, whereas superficial reflux had a higher incidence in women.[9–11] Overall, the incidence of venous disease was similar in males and females, which is contrary to most clinical studies, where a female preponderance of 3–4:1 is commonly reported. This discrepancy may reflect

Box 17.1 • CEAP classification

Clinical classification
C0: no visible or palpable signs of venous disease
C1: telangiectasies or reticular veins
C2: varicose veins
C3: oedema
C4a: pigmentation or eczema
C4b: lipodermatosclerosis or atrophie blanche
C5: healed venous ulcer
C6: active venous ulcer
S: symptomatic, including ache, pain, tightness, skin irritation, heaviness and muscle cramps, and other complaints attributable to venous dysfunction
A: asymptomatic

Aetiological classification
Ec: congenital
Ep: primary
Es: secondary (post-thrombotic)
En: no venous cause identified

Anatomical classification
As: superficial veins
Ap: perforator veins
Ad: deep veins
An: no venous location identified

Pathophysiological classification
Pr: reflux
Po: obstruction
Pr,o: reflux and obstruction
Pn: no venous pathophysiology identifiable

differences between the sexes in symptoms experienced, or in the threshold to seek medical advice. The prevalence of chronic venous ulceration (CEAP C6) is 0.3–1.0% and venous skin changes (CEAP C4–C5) were present in 5–10%. For all stages of venous disease, the incidence increases with age.

Clinical presentation

Patients with venous disease may seek medical help for a variety of reasons. The Edinburgh Vein Study showed an inconsistent and gender-dependent relationship between a range of lower limb 'venous' symptoms (heaviness/tension, feeling of swelling, aching, restless leg, cramps, itching, tingling) and the presence and severity of thread, reticular or varicose veins. Clinical experience also suggests that there is little concordance between the size and extent of varicose veins and the severity of presenting symptoms. However, venous symptoms correlate with severity of venous reflux on duplex imaging.[12] The CEAP classification was devised in 1994, revised in 2004, and offers a useful and widely used tool to describe a patient using Clinical, aEtiological, Anatomical and Pathophysiological criteria (Box 17.1).[13] The clinical component of the CEAP classification is often used in isolation. Nevertheless, the widespread adoption of this system to characterise venous disease has been a significant advance. Other recognised scoring systems include the venous clinical severity score (VCSS) and venous disability score (VDS).[14,15]

Thread veins and reticular veins (CEAP C1)

These refer to small, superficial veins that may be highly visible and cause cosmetic concern (**Fig. 17.3**). Thread veins (also known as spider veins, telangiectasia, venous flare) are <1 mm, whereas veins of 1–3 mm are termed reticular veins. Superficial, tortuous veins >3 mm are considered varicose veins. Patients with thread or reticular veins may find them unsightly and request treatment. Although not usually funded by state healthcare systems, these veins can be effectively treated using injection sclerotherapy, after underlying truncal reflux has been addressed.

Varicose veins (CEAP C2)

Varicose veins are dilated, tortuous and superficial. They are usually seen below the knee, but are also common in the thigh, with the precise location depending on the anatomical distribution of the

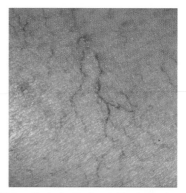

Figure 17.3 • Typical reticular and thread veins.

underlying venous reflux. Most varicose veins are due to an incompetent GSV, although SSV reflux is the cause in around 20% of patients. Some patients may have varicose veins due to an incompetent perforating vein, refluxing pelvic/abdominal or other, unnamed, veins. It should be noted that in thin patients, or those with an athletic physique, superficial veins may be very prominent. However, these veins are usually straight and physiological, rather than abnormal.

Oedema and skin changes (CEAP C3–C4)

Venous oedema is due to an inability of the lymphatic system to adequately drain the excessive interstitial fluid produced as a result of venous hypertension. This usually occurs around the ankle, but may involve the foot and leg. Isolated oedema due to venous disease is unusual, in the absence of other signs of venous disease. Non-venous causes of oedema, including lymphoedema and heart failure, should be considered and may coexist with venous disease.

Chronic venous hypertension is associated with a number of skin changes (**Fig. 17.4**), including:

- **Venous eczema (also known as 'venous stasis dermatitis').** Itchy, dry and scaly skin is a common early skin change due to venous hypertension. As with most venous skin changes, eczema often occurs on the medial aspect of the lower leg (the 'medial gaiter area').
- **Haemosiderinosis and pigmentation.** Chronic venous hypertension may lead to extravasation of red blood cells, resulting in pigmentation due to haemosiderin deposition in the subcutaneous tissues. There is often an associated inflammatory response, which may mimic cellulitis (see 'Lipodermatosclerosis'

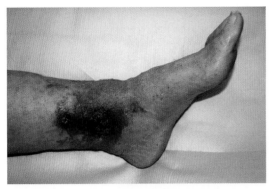

Figure 17.4 • Advanced skin changes secondary to chronic venous hypertension.

below). Once the inflammation has settled, pigmentation is generally considered permanent, despite subsequent treatment.

- **Lipodermatosclerosis.** Chronic venous hypertension and inflammation may result in fibrosis and thickening of the skin and subcutaneous fat in the lower leg, with the classic 'inverted champagne bottle' appearance. Acute inflammation due to venous hypertension may be referred to as 'acute lipodermatosclerosis'. As with haemosiderinosis, chronic skin and subcutaneous changes are generally considered irreversible. The primary aim of venous treatment is usually to reduce symptoms and prevent disease progression.

- **Corona phlebectatica.** Also referred to as 'malleolar flare', this refers to a leash of prominent intradermal veins, located around the medial malleolus. The skin is often fragile and patients may progress to venous ulceration.

- **Atrophie blanche.** Literally translated as 'white atrophy', this refers to a pale, smooth scarring that may occur at the site of previous ulceration.

Chronic venous ulceration (CEAP C5–C6)

Venous ulceration is considered the worst extreme in the spectrum of chronic venous disorders and affects up to 1% of the adult population (increased in patients >65 years[16]). This may be defined as a full-thickness defect of the skin of >4 weeks duration, and commonly occurs on the medial aspect of the lower leg. Other signs of chronic venous hypertension may be present, helping to differentiate chronic venous ulcers from other causes of leg ulceration. Ulcers are usually superficial and although a healthy granulating base is commonly seen, healing times are generally protracted. Microbiological swabs of the ulcer base commonly grow a variety of organisms, but antibiotic therapy is rarely required.

Clinical assessment

History

A detailed history of the presenting symptoms should be elucidated and potential non-vascular causes should be excluded (particularly orthopaedic and arterial disorders). It is important to describe the impact of symptoms on patient quality of life as the decision to treat and the treatment modality will usually be guided by these considerations. Cosmetic appearance is a common concern and should always be a consideration when planning intervention. Other common symptoms include heaviness, aching, itching, cramping or 'tingling'. The correlation between the size of veins and the severity of symptoms reported by the patient is often poor. Those involved in the management of patients with varicose veins should consider that this patient group accounts for a significant proportion of medicolegal claims in surgical specialities.[17] Discontent after treatment is often due to recurrent/residual varicose veins or neurological symptoms.

Specific features that should be elucidated in the history include:

- history of deep vein thrombosis (DVT);
- history of thrombophilia or major risk factors for previous DVT;
- combined oral contraceptive pill use;
- Details of previous venous interventions (open or endovenous).

Patient examination

Patients should be evaluated in the standing position to allow filling of varicosities. Both legs should be examined, in addition to the groins and lower abdomen. The following features should be specifically assessed and documented:

- scars and evidence of previous venous interventions;
- distribution and extent of varicosities (the examiner should specifically document the presence of a saphenovarix and other particularly large or troublesome varicosities);

- presence of skin changes of chronic venous disease (oedema, pigmentation, lipodermatosclerosis, ulceration);
- arterial status (pulses, or ankle brachial pressure index);
- other factors contributing to venous hypertension (immobility, obesity, ankle stiffness, poor calf muscle bulk);
- general patient status (fitness, mobility).

Chronic venous skin changes and ulceration may be present without visible varicose veins. Nevertheless, appropriate venous investigations should be performed to detect those patients with superficial reflux.

Venous investigations

Hand-held Doppler and other bedside tests

The widespread availability and reliability of colour venous duplex scanning has meant that hand-held Doppler assessment of veins should no longer be used to guide venous interventions and has become largely obsolete in many departments. Other bedside tests, such as Trendelenburg's test or the tourniquet test, are well described in clinical textbooks, but rarely utilised in routine practice.

Duplex ultrasound scanning

In recent years, colour duplex ultrasound scanning (DUS) has become established as the 'gold standard' investigation for patients with venous disease.[18] Use of this non-invasive imaging modality can accurately identify the presence of reflux or occlusion in deep and superficial venous systems. Increasing availability and reducing cost of duplex machines has meant that appropriately trained vascular surgeons are able to perform scans in the outpatient clinic and during interventions to improve outcomes. Routine duplex imaging prior to venous intervention should be considered mandatory.[19]

> ✅ All patients being considered for superficial venous intervention should undergo colour venous duplex assessment.

Specific advantages include:

- accurate characterisation of pattern of superficial reflux (including incompetent perforating veins);
- identification of deep venous disease;
- assessment of suitability of superficial veins for endovenous intervention (see 'Treatment' section);
- accurate evaluation of recurrent varicose veins;
- identification of anatomical variants.

There is good justification for the use of DUS post-intervention as a tool for quality control and prognostication. However, economic considerations have meant that routine follow-up with DUS after superficial venous intervention is uncommon in the UK.

Other investigations

In general, DUS is the only venous investigation necessary in the majority of patients. However, other imaging modalities may be useful in specific circumstances:

- **Venography using cross-sectional imaging.** Venous assessment may be performed using computerised tomography (CT) or magnetic resonance imaging (MRI). These investigations may be valuable in visualising iliac veins and the inferior vena cava, as well as identifying sources of pelvis vein incompetence.[20]
- **Invasive venography.** Traditional diagnostic venography (also known as phlebography) for the assessment of superficial veins has virtually no role in modern clinical practice. Venography to assess deep veins may have some value in patients being treated with thrombolysis for DVT and the small group of patients being considered for deep venous reconstruction.
- **Haemodynamic assessments.** A variety of tools are available to assess haemodynamic venous function in the leg. Ambulatory venous pressure (AVP) monitoring is considered the 'gold standard', but is invasive and limited to research use. Potential clinical benefits of digital photoplethysmography and other minimally invasive assessments of venous hypertension have been reported, but these techniques are rarely used in practice.[21]

Treatment

With a range of options now available for the treatment of superficial venous reflux, the clinician should give careful consideration to the optimal management strategy for each individual patient. This may involve using more than one treatment modality and/or more than one treatment episode.

For patients with bilateral varicose veins, opinion varies regarding the optimal approach (one stage or multi-stage intervention). However, there is a growing body of opinion that the treatment of superficial venous disease (particularly bilateral) should be analogous to dental care, with multiple visits and smaller interventions rather than completing treatment in a single sitting.

The CEAP classification is commonly used as a tool for rationing treatment and identifying which patients may get the greatest benefits. However, significant quality-of-life improvements are seen after superficial venous intervention in patients with all classes of venous disease.

Conservative options, drugs and compression therapy

Conservative measures or compression may be the most appropriate therapy in some patients, and are frequently offered prior to surgical or endovenous intervention. Specific groups where conservative therapy or compression may be preferred include:

- pregnant patients;
- elderly patients with significant comorbidity;
- patients with mild symptoms, or symptoms that may not be due to venous disease;
- patients unwilling to accept the risks of surgical or endovenous interventions.

Conservative options

Conservative measures such as weight loss, limb elevation and reduced periods of standing may improve symptoms, but may be difficult to achieve for patients in full-time employment or those with young families.

Pharmacotherapy

A number of venoactive drugs have been studied in patients with venous disease. A large number of studies have evaluated micronised purified flavonoid fraction (Daflon, Servier) and demonstrated that venous symptoms may be reduced, but this is not available in the UK or North America. Small studies have suggested potential benefits with rutins and horse chestnut seed extract, although their use is limited.[22]

Compression stockings

✅ Compression stockings may improve symptoms from varicose veins and reduce oedema.

Compression therapy has been used for the treatment of venous disease for centuries and remains the mainstay of management for patients with venous ulceration.[23] For patients with healed venous ulceration (CEAP C5), the use of elastic compression stockings has been shown to reduce the risk of recurrent ulceration.[24] For patients with CEAP C2–C4 disease, stockings are prescribed frequently, but the evidence for benefit is less clear. Potential benefits include:

- improvement of venous symptoms;
- concealment of visible varicosities;
- prevention of disease progression;
- aiding clinical assessment in patients where there may be uncertainty about the extent to which the symptoms are attributable to venous disease.

Compression stockings may be classified by the sub-bandage pressure applied at the ankle. Using the British standard system for classification, class I stockings apply 14–17 mmHg, class II 18–24 mmHg and class III 25–35 mmHg. In practice, patients are often unable to tolerate stockings greater than class I and many patients find class III stockings virtually impossible to put on or remove. Before commencing compression therapy, arterial disease should be excluded (by clinical assessment±ankle–brachial pressure index measurement). Great care should be taken to fit stockings correctly and to avoid rolling down of the stocking, as this may cause pressure damage to the skin or create a tourniquet effect. Patient compliance remains a major problem with compression stockings, as they may be itchy, hot (particularly in summer months), and difficult to put on and take off, despite the availability of applicator devices. Moreover, any benefit from compression stockings only lasts as long as they are worn and they need to be replaced regularly. Studies have suggested that compliance may be as low as 50% overall and probably much lower with class III stockings.[25]

In a recent systematic review and meta-analysis assessing the efficacy of compression stockings, the paucity of high-quality evidence was highlighted.[26] Although a number of prospective studies were identified, there was significant heterogeneity in patient population, type of compression and outcome measures evaluated. The authors found that wearing compression stockings improved symptom management, although the high number of non-compliant patients, who were excluded, could be a confounding factor. Compression was also found to reduce oedema, but the suggestion that wearing compression can slow the progression or reduce recurrence after intervention was not supported by the published literature.

Principles of surgical and endovenous intervention

The underlying principle of treating patients with symptomatic superficial venous reflux is to remove or obliterate the incompetent venous channel. The treatment of patients with mixed superficial and deep venous reflux presents a challenge. In general, these patients can be safely treated with superficial venous intervention and, in some cases, the refluxing deep veins may even become competent (possibly because the incompetent venous reservoir is removed).[6] However, the level of expected benefit is difficult to predict, as residual deep venous reflux may be a significant cause of venous hypertension. A trial of compression stockings (which generally compress superficial veins only) is a useful test in these circumstances and tourniquet tests using haemodynamic evaluation (digital photoplethysmography) have also been proposed. The treatment of superficial veins in patients with deep venous occlusion is not advisable, as these channels may be contributing to venous drainage, even if incompetent.

Pre-procedure marking

Marking the GSV or SSV

With the routine investigation of patients with DUS prior to intervention and the common use of intraoperative ultrasound during superficial venous interventions, pre-procedure marking of the truncal vein is not generally performed. However, some specialists may prefer to have the GSV or SSV marked on the skin surface, particularly when building experience in endovenous procedures. For those practitioners who prefer the use of local anaesthetic cream prior to office-based procedures, this has the added advantage of indicating where the cream should be applied.

Marking of varicosities

If treatment involves avulsion of visible varicosities, the surgeon should inspect and mark the veins before intervention. The specific technique of marking is a matter of personal preference, but the surgeon should check with the patient (and document) that all symptomatic veins have been marked.

Informed consent

In view of the high number of medicolegal claims following procedures for varicose veins, the process of consent is worthy of specific mention.[27] Patients should be specifically warned of common complications such as bruising and paraesthesia. They should also understand that veins may (and often do) recur and they may suffer DVT or nerve pain. In patients with visible varicosities, they should appreciate that some residual veins may be present and their legs will not be cosmetically perfect. Other complications associated with specific procedures are described below. Information leaflets should be used, specific consent forms may be useful and discussions with the patient should be clearly documented in the medical records. Perhaps most importantly, the patient's expectations from treatment should be clarified before intervention and match those of the treating clinician.

Traditional surgery

Trendelenburg described ligation of the proximal GSV in 1890[28] and modifications of this technique have remained the mainstay of treatment for varicose veins for over a century. With the increasing popularity of minimally invasive, endovenous modalities, the proportion of patients treated with surgical stripping has declined in recent years.[29]

Setting and anaesthesia

With the development of efficient day case units, virtually all varicose vein operations can be performed as day case procedures. Although the majority of procedures are performed using general anaesthesia, regional or local techniques may also be used. Epidural/spinal anaesthesia or femoral nerve blocks can facilitate surgery, but the motor block may persist for several hours, potentially hindering same-day discharge. Surgical stripping may also be performed using dilute local anaesthesia with adrenaline, injected in high volumes around the vein to be stripped ('tumescent' anaesthesia – see below). However, in a generally young and fit patient group, most surgeons (and anaesthetists) favour general anaesthesia for traditional varicose vein surgery. The routine use of prophylactic antibiotics has been shown to reduce the risk of wound complications in one randomised study.[30]

> ✓✓ The routine use of prophylactic co-amoxiclav reduced the risk of wound complications and the need for postoperative antibiotics in one randomised controlled trial.[30]

Great saphenous vein surgery

Saphenofemoral disconnection and GSV stripping is performed with the patient in the supine position, with the legs abducted (using an abduction board). A 'head down' or Trendelenburg position can reduce venous bleeding during the procedure, but may cause head and neck oedema, particularly with prolonged operations. A detailed description of the procedure is beyond the scope of this chapter.

However, some important technical points are listed below:

- The saphenofemoral junction (SFJ) usually lies beneath the skin crease, but may be variable. The use of intraoperative duplex to guide surgical incisions can help ensure technical success.
- No vein should be divided until the SFJ has been clearly identified.
- Divide tributaries as distal as possible (ideally beyond the second branch).
- The deep external pudendal vein (draining to the medial aspect of the common femoral vein, CFV) should be ligated and divided to reduce the risk of recurrence (optional if very small).
- The GSV should be disconnected and transfixed close to the CFV. A number of techniques have been described in an attempt to reduce the incidence of neovascularisation. These include polytetrafluoroethylene (PTFE) patch interposition, closure of the cribiform fascia and formal inverted closure of the CFV after total excision of the GSV. However, none has demonstrated convincing improvements in long-term clinical outcome.
- Although the value of GSV stripping to reduce varicose vein recurrence has been clearly demonstrated, the optimal technique remains a subject of debate. Some believe that using an inversion stripping technique, and stripping from the groin down to the knee (and not the ankle) can reduce the risk of saphenous nerve injury. Irrespective of the technique, intraoperative duplex can help ensure that the entire GSV has been removed. Stripping of the GSV has been clearly shown to reduce the risk of reintervention for recurrent varicose veins.[31]

✓✓ Stripping of the GSV is recommended as part of routine practice during traditional varicose vein surgery, as the risk of reintervention at 11 years was shown to be reduced by 60%.[31]

Small saphenous vein surgery

The patient is usually positioned in the prone position, although some teams prefer the lateral position, as it may be possible to use a laryngeal mask rather than a reinforced endotracheal tube.

- Preoperative marking (or intraoperative verification) of the saphenopopliteal junction (SPJ) should be considered mandatory.[32] The skin incision should be placed slightly below the SPJ to allow for the angle of descent into the popliteal fossa.
- In view of the depth of the junction and risk of nerve damage in the popliteal fossa, a 'flush' SPJ ligation is generally not performed. There is no consensus over whether the gastrocnemius veins (that often join the SSV before the SPJ) should be ligated.
- Stripping of the SSV is an area of great controversy. The traditional view that SSV stripping causes sural nerve injury was challenged by a recent study that demonstrated improved technical results with stripping, with no difference in the incidence of numbness.[33]
- The popliteal fascia should be closed carefully to reduce the risk of muscle herniation, which may be painful and can cause considerable cosmetic distress.

✓ In a prospective study, stripping of the SSV was associated with a lower incidence of recurrent varicosities without greater neurological symptoms.[33]

Redo varicose vein surgery

Redo groin or popliteal fossa dissection in patients with recurrent varicose veins is associated with a rate of significant complications and morbidity that is far greater than the primary procedures. Seroma, infection, bruising and damage to nerves are commonly seen after revision surgery. For these reasons, even for enthusiastic vascular surgeons, endovenous interventions are widely considered the first line in the treatment of patients with recurrent varicose veins, particularly in the popliteal fossa.

Complications

Early and late complications may be seen after any treatment strategy (including conservative management). However, adverse events of specific relevance after traditional superficial venous surgery include:

- **Bruising/bleeding.** Bruising is a very common early complication after surgery, particularly along the track where the truncal vein (GSV or SSV) has been stripped. Bleeding requiring a return to the operating theatre is usually due to persistent venous bleeding in the groin but is rare. Anecdotally, bruising may be reduced by using epinephrine-soaked swabs or local anaesthesia with epinephrine infiltrated in the tract of the stripped vein.[34]

- **Thromboembolic events.** The incidence of DVT after traditional varicose vein surgery ranges from 0.5% to 5.3% in the literature. The risk of pulmonary embolism has been estimated at 1 in 600.[35] Duplex studies have identified that many patients have small, below-knee DVTs of questionable clinical significance. The value of stopping the combined oral contraceptive pill or using DVT prophylaxis is unclear. However, many surgeons take a pragmatic view and do not ask patients to stop the pill, but do prescribe low-molecular-weight heparin at the time of surgery.

- **Nerve damage.** A degree of sensory abnormality may be present in up to 40% of patients after traditional surgery, although this is rarely troublesome. True saphenous nerve injury after GSV stripping (to the knee) is likely to be <10%. The risk of sural nerve injury during SPJ disconnection is unknown, but is likely to be higher. Disabling motor nerve injury may occur, particularly involving the common peroneal nerve at the head of the fibula. This may be injured during stab phlebectomy in this area.

- **Recurrence.** Poor results after traditional varicose vein surgery have often been attributed to poor surgical technique by inexperienced operators. However, it seems clear that even with 'technically' successful surgery, recurrence is common. Reported recurrence rates range from 20% to 80% at 5–20 years, although most patients remain satisfied with surgery.[35]

Endovenous thermal ablation

In an attempt to reduce the early and late risks associated with traditional varicose vein surgery, endovenous thermal ablation techniques have rapidly gained popularity in the last 10 years. Perceived potential advantages of these procedures include:

- avoidance of general anaesthesia;
- ability to perform procedures in modified outpatient or 'office-based' settings (with the associated cost savings);
- improved early morbidity (no groin dissection or stripping) with earlier return to normal activity/work;
- low risk of nerve injury, by avoiding stripping;
- low risk of recurrence, by avoidance of neovascularisation.

Some potential disadvantages of endovenous thermal ablation include:

- expense of the generators, endovenous catheters and consumable items;
- learning curve associated with the new procedure;
- some patients may be unsuitable (tortuous or superficial veins).

In view of the major technical similarities between endovenous laser ablation (EVLA) and radiofrequency ablation (RFA) procedures, both are described in this section.

Setting and anaesthesia

Both EVLA and RFA are ideal for outpatient or 'office-based' therapy as procedures can be performed using only 'tumescent' anaesthesia. This refers to a very dilute mixture of local anaesthesia (0.1% lidocaine) with epinephrine (1:2 000 000), which is injected to surround the truncal vein to be ablated under ultrasound guidance. The use of sodium bicarbonate to neutralise the mixture may reduce the pain during tumescent injections. The anaesthetic allows the ablation to be performed without pain, but also provides a heat buffer to protect surrounding nerves and tissues. Initially, procedures were commonly performed in operating theatres. However, with a growing appreciation of the cost savings that may be possible by taking procedures out of the operating theatre, many centres in the UK now have suitable outpatient treatment rooms.[36]

Summary of technique

Prior to listing the patient for endovenous ablation, the suitability of the vein to be treated should be evaluated using duplex, ideally by the specialist performing the procedure (**Fig. 17.5**). Veins should be straight, >3 mm in diameter and deep enough to be >1 cm from the skin after infiltration of tumescent anaesthesia. The patient should be positioned in the supine position for GSV ablation and prone for SSV procedures. The stages of the procedure are summarised below:

- With the patient in the reverse Trendelenburg position, the vein to be treated is cannulated under ultrasound guidance, using a Seldinger technique. A sheath appropriate to the catheter to be used can then be inserted (**Fig. 17.6**).
- The endovenous ablation catheter is positioned 2 cm from the SFJ or SPJ under ultrasound guidance. The patient position is changed to 'head down'.
- Tumescent anaesthesia is injected around the vein under ultrasound guidance, with the aim of

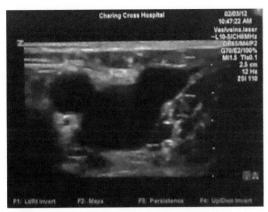

Figure 17.5 • Duplex ultrasound image during endovenous procedure demonstrating the 'Mickey Mouse' appearance of the common femoral artery (left), common femoral vein (middle) and GSV (right).

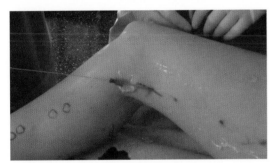

Figure 17.6 • Cannulation of GSV in distal thigh using Seldinger technique under ultrasound guidance.

creating a 'halo' of circumferential infiltration (**Fig. 17.7**). Particular care should be taken to infiltrate between the proximal GSV and CFV and to ensure that the vein is at least 1 cm from the skin. Tumescent injection may be facilitated by using local anaesthetic cream (to reduce the pain of injection) and an injection pump. Volumes of tumescent anaesthesia injected may vary, but are typically around 75–100 mL per 10 cm of vein.

• The technique and speed of ablation will depend on the catheter used. This may be a slow pull-back technique, or segmental ablation.

• After ablation, patency of the deep vein should be verified with duplex and documented.

Endovenous laser ablation (EVLA)

Endovenous ablation using laser was first described in 2001.[37] EVLA procedures must be performed in an appropriate clinical area complying with laser

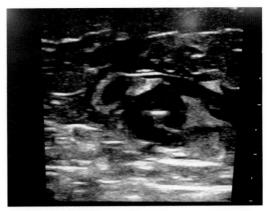

Figure 17.7 • Duplex image demonstrating 'halo' of tumescent anaesthesia around GSV.

safety regulations and protective goggles must be worn during periods of activation. The laser fibre is slowly withdrawn at a steady pace while delivering energy within the vein. The temperatures exceed 1000 °C and although the precise mechanise of action is not fully understood, diffuse thermal damage to the intima has been observed.

Initial fibres were forward firing and utilised laser wavelengths of 810 or 980 nm. Recent advances have included a 1470-nm laser (thought to better target water and therefore the vein wall) and radial firing fibres (better targeting of the vein wall, reducing the risk of vein wall perforations and pain). Using the early laser fibres, a dose of >60 joules/cm is thought to be necessary to ensure vein closure. The dose required may be less for the new radial fibres.

Radiofrequency ablation (RFA)

RFA also involves the delivery of thermal energy to the vein wall, derived from an electrical current.[38] A bipolar catheter is used to generate temperatures of 85–120 °C and an inbuilt feedback mechanism can assess the quality of vein wall contact, which is required for effective energy delivery. Two main types of RFA catheter are currently available. A continuous pull-back device (RFITT) is used in an almost identical way to EVLA catheters, whereas the segmental ablation device (VNUS) treats the vein in 7- or 3-cm segments. Both devices offer a feedback mechanism (either auditory or visual) to confirm energy delivery to the tissues. Histological studies have demonstrated a homogeneous thermal ablation to the vein wall.

Complications

Many of the complications from EVLA and RFA are similar to those seen after traditional surgery.

- **Bleeding/bruising.** In general, the incidence of early complications is significantly lower after endovenous procedures in comparison to traditional surgery. Significant discomfort or bruising is uncommon, but is more likely after EVLA than RFA. Pain using the newer radial laser fibres may be reduced compared to the older fibres.
- **Thromboembolic events.** The incidence of DVT after RFA and EVLA is very low (<1%). However, a tongue of thrombus is sometimes seen at the SFJ or SPJ at the level of or protruding into the deep vein. This phenomenon has been termed endovenous heat-induced thrombosis (EHIT) and four classes have been described:[39,40]
  - Class 1: thrombus to the level of the deep vein, without protrusion.
  - Class 2: protrusion into the deep system, with <50% luminal occlusion.
  - Class 3: protrusion into the deep system, with >50% luminal occlusion.
  - Class 4: protrusion into the deep system, with total deep venous occlusion.
- **Skin burns.** Thermal injury to the skin is a complication almost unique to EVLA and RFA amongst venous interventions. This usually occurs as a result of treating a superficial vein after inadequate tumescent anaesthesia. This may result in an area of pigmentation, although frank ulceration may also occur.
- **Nerve injury.** Although less common than in traditional surgery, an area of abnormal sensation is common after endovenous ablation. This is often an area of paraesthesia over the ablated truncal vein. Thermal injury to saphenous, sural or other nerves may occur, although the generous use of tumescence should reduce this risk. An added advantage of treating the awake patient is that they are likely to feel pain when an EVLA or RFA catheter is in close proximity to a nerve. Most areas of abnormal sensation recover with conservative management.

Ultrasound-guided foam sclerotherapy (UGFS)

The aim of sclerotherapy is to induce chemical ablation and fibrosis by injecting liquid or foam sclerosant into an empty vein.[41,42] Three types of sclerosants are available:

- detergent, e.g. sodium tetradecyl sulphate (STS) and polidocanol;
- osmotic, e.g. hypertonic saline (used in Europe and the USA);
- chemical irritant, e.g. chromated glycerine.

In the UK, STS and polidocanol are in popular use, although the latter is unlicensed. In general, larger veins require a stronger concentration of sclerosant. The conversion of liquid sclerosant into foam by mixing it with air or carbon dioxide (Tessari method) has gained popularity in recent years. This approach has the advantage of increasing the potency and volume of the sclerosant, as well as making it echogenic.

Setting and anaesthesia

UGFS can easily be performed in an outpatient treatment room. Access to a duplex machine and a treatment trolley are the only requirements. As the only injection involves the insertion of small cannulae or butterfly needles into the veins to be treated, the treatment is often possible with minimal or no local anaesthesia.

Technique

Perhaps to a greater extent than other venous treatments, UGFS is associated with a significant learning curve.

- Ultrasound guided cannulation is performed as with other endovenous modalities. However, this may be more challenging with UGFS as multiple cannulae may be required in tortuous varicosities.
- Foam sclerosant is created by combining liquid sclerosant with air in a 1:3 or 1:4 ratio using the 'Tessari' technique (**Fig. 17.8**).
- With the leg elevated (to empty the veins), foam should be injected and movement of the foam should be monitored using ultrasound (**Fig. 17.9**).
- The patient should be encouraged to move the ankle to promote deep venous flow.
- The procedure should be completed by applying eccentric bandaging, with particular compression over the veins treated.

Complications

The safety of UGFS remains the subject of considerable debate, particularly after recent case reports of major neurological complications after treatment.

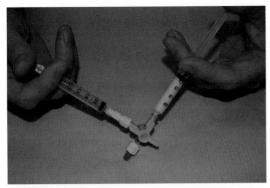

Figure 17.8 • Creation of foam by mixing liquid sclerosant with air (1:4 ratio) using two syringes and a three-way tap (Tessari technique).

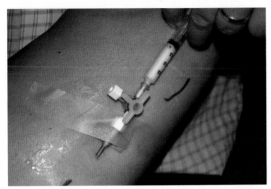

Figure 17.9 • Injection of foam with the leg elevated to empty vein.

There is anecdotal evidence to suggest that adverse events may be more common with larger volumes of foam injection.

> ✔ The incidence of adverse events after UGFS is likely to be related to the volume of foam injected.

The volume injected will depend on the specific case, but most experts would suggest that 10–12 mL (of foam) should be considered a maximum for a single session. Specific risks include:

- **Thrombophlebitis.** Superficial thrombophlebitis is common after UGFS and presents with painful, hard lumpy areas and erythema. Inflammation may respond to topical anti-inflammatory creams, but may require aspiration/expulsion of the thrombus, which usually results in a rapid improvement of symptoms.
- **Thromboembolic events.** Although some foam inevitably enters the deep venous system during treatment, the risk of DVT remains low (approximately 1%). Encouraging ankle dorsiflexion after foam injection (to promote deep venous flow) may reduce the risk of DVT.
- **Skin pigmentation/staining.** May occur (to varying degrees) in a significant proportion of patients. Some experts suggest that aspiration of thrombophlebitis may reduce the severity of pigmentation, which may become a major cosmetic concern.
- **Neurological symptoms/stroke.** A recent review of neurological complications after UGFS demonstrated that transient neurological problems (usually visual disturbances) occur after around 1% of interventions and are more common in patients with a history of migraine.[43] A number of case reports have described post-procedure strokes in patients treated with sclerotherapy, although this is extremely rare. These are thought to be due to paradoxical emboli via a patent foramen ovale. Some experts have suggested that the use of carbon dioxide (rather than air) to produce foam may reduce the risk of neurological events, although robust evidence to support this assertion is lacking.[41]

Treatment of incompetent perforating veins

The optimal management of perforators (veins connecting the deep and superficial systems in the leg) remains an unresolved issue. A number of studies have demonstrated favourable outcomes when incompetent perforators are treated in combination with refluxing superficial veins, but the additional value of perforator treatment is unproven.[44] The sceptical viewpoint is supported by studies that have demonstrated that incompetent perforators may become competent after GSV or SSV treatment. Although each case should be considered individually, many specialists would treat the refluxing truncal vein as an initial intervention and reserve perforator treatment for patients with residual/recurrent disease clearly attributable to an incompetent perforator. Options for perforator treatment include surgical ligation, endovenous ablation or UGFS.

Management of varicosities

As most patients with varicose veins have troublesome varicosities, their management is an important consideration. Traditionally, superficial varicose veins were treated (by stab phlebectomy) at the time of open surgery. However, the use of endovenous interventions in outpatient settings has meant that it may not be possible to treat the varicosities at the time of GSV or SSV intervention. Interestingly, a number of authors have suggested that varicosities often regress after truncal vein ablation and may be unnecessary, particularly if the refluxing superficial vein is ablated to the lowest point of reflux. A benefit for synchronous treatment of varicosities was seen in one randomised study.[45] The strategies for treating varicosities are:

1. Treat at the time of truncal vein intervention.
2. Do not treat varicosities at all.
3. Review the patient after truncal vein treatment and treat varicosities if required.

Once a decision to treat varicosities has been made, options include:

- **Stab phlebectomy.** This is performed via a small incision (made longitudinally) using an Oesch hook. Care should be taken to avoid nerves and other structures,[46] particularly around the lateral knee (common peroneal nerve), the medial malleolus (posterior tibial vessels), and the regions of the saphenous and sural nerves. Although traditionally performed in an operating theatre under general anaesthesia, 'ambulatory phlebectomy' performed in an outpatient setting using tumescent anaesthesia is gaining in popularity.
- **UGFS.** Sclerotherapy may be used to treat varicosities and can be performed in an outpatient setting.
- **Other options.** Although powered phlebectomy has been available for a number of years, evidence demonstrating superiority over stab phlebectomy is lacking.

Other treatment options

Preserving the saphenous vein
Popularised in parts of Europe and contrary to the majority of treatment strategies, the CHIVA technique involves strategic ligation of specific tributaries and/or the saphenofemoral junction without stripping or ablation of the GSV.[47] The aim of such 'saphenous-preserving' approaches is to maintain the venous drainage of GSV and to preserve the option of using the vein as a future vascular conduit. Prospective studies and randomised trials have reported favourable results in comparison to surgical

stripping, but the technique has not been used outside central Europe, mainly due to the excellent results from other, less esoteric treatment options.

Novel endovenous therapies
In addition to EVLA, RFA and UGFS, new varieties of endovenous thermal and chemical ablation therapy are being introduced. The Clarivein system involves mechanical agitation of the venous endothelium using a rapidly rotating catheter whilst simultaneously injecting liquid sclerosant and slowly withdrawing the catheter. Alternative approaches include the use of an intravenous 'glue' or an endovenous thrombogenic plug device at the proximal GSV. In addition to these novel developments, updated versions of laser and radiofrequency catheters and generators are being developed.

Evidence for traditional and endovenous intervention

The development of endovenous treatments has resulted in a diverse and confusing range of interventions for patients with varicose veins.[48] In recent years, a number of randomised clinical trials have been published, comparing various endovenous treatments with traditional surgery and each other.

Traditional surgery
Traditional surgery for varicose veins is associated with a significant improvement in symptoms and patient quality of life. In the REACTIV trial, patients were randomised to surgery or compression stockings.[49] The surgery group experienced greater symptom relief and health-related quality-of-life and satisfaction scores.[50] However, recurrence is common after traditional surgery, with 11-year varicose vein recurrence rates after surgery, (with GSV stripping) reported as 62% in one randomised study.[31,35]

Interestingly, most randomised studies comparing endovenous interventions with traditional surgery have not demonstrated better technical results with the newer treatments. However, poor technical results after surgical stripping have been reported previously by numerous authors, suggesting that intraoperative duplex and other technical refinements may have contributed to improvements in the modern results from surgery. In patients with chronic venous ulceration, the ESCHAR venous ulcer trial clearly demonstrated that superficial venous surgery reduces the risk of recurrent ulceration.[51,52]

✔✔ Traditional surgery is associated with significant symptom relief, quality-of-life improvements and is cost-effective for patients with uncomplicated varicose veins.[49]

Endovenous thermal ablation

A large number of studies have been conducted using EVLA and RFA interventions. As follow-up periods are generally short and rarely longer than 2 years, the long-term effectiveness of EVLA and RFA procedures remains unknown. However, assuming that early outcomes are an accurate surrogate marker for long-term treatment success, it seems likely that endovenous thermal interventions will be deemed superior to traditional surgery. On the basis of recent published studies, the following conclusions can be drawn regarding the effectiveness of endovenous thermal ablation procedures:

- The early post-procedure outcomes (pain, bruising, time to mobilise, return to normal activity) are better after EVLA and RFA in comparison to traditional surgery.[53–57] EVLA procedures performed using forward-firing fibres and lower wavelengths are associated with more early pain than RFA. However, the pain associated with radial fibres using 1470-nm laser energy may be comparable to RFA, though there is no trial evidence to support this.
- GSV occlusion rates of >90% can be expected using RFA and EVLA procedures.

> ☑☑ Early outcomes after RFA, EVLA and UGFS in terms of pain, bruising and return to normal activity are better than traditional surgery.

Ultrasound-guided foam sclerotherapy

UGFS is extremely well tolerated and versatile, although most studies have suggested lower occlusion rates than other treatments.[58] The use of foam sclerosant has been shown to be superior to liquid sclerosant.[59]

> ☑☑ Foam sclerosant is superior to liquid sclerosant in the treatment of truncal veins (such as GSV or SSV).

However, the influence of concentration of sclerosant or adjuvant saphenofemoral junction disconnection as an adjunct to UGFS remains unclear. It seems clear that the technical success after UGFS (as assessed by successful closure of the vein treated) is inferior to other treatments when performed by the majority of venous specialists. However, the unquestionable benefits of sclerotherapy include:

- its versatility to treat almost any vein (recurrent and primary varicose veins);
- it is inexpensive;
- it is quick (in expert hands);
- there is no requirement for specialist equipment or specific safety precautions.

Deciding between treatment modalities

In a recent randomised study of 500 patients comparing EVLA, RFA, UGFS and surgical stripping, 1-year results demonstrated that the highest technical failure rate was seen after UGFS (in keeping with other studies), although longer-term outcomes are awaited.[60] The CLASS trial is a large randomised study comparing EVLA, UGFS and surgical stripping, and it is anticipated that early results will be disseminated in 2013.

A meta-analysis of all endovenous modalities was published in 2009.[58] The authors recognised the enormous heterogeneity in published studies and included randomised trials, prospective and retrospective publications. In view of the variations in follow-up periods reported, the authors performed a meta-regression and presented success rates at different time points up to 5 years. Their analyses suggested that 5-year success rates were greatest after EVLA (95.4%) and lowest after UGFS (73.5%). Numerous other smaller studies are ongoing, but there is significant heterogeneity between studies in terms of intervention performed, operator skill/experience, patients treated and outcomes reported. Interpretation of study results and application into clinical practice is made difficult by these variations. However, it must be recognised that a number of efficacious treatments for varicose veins are now available and have different strengths and weaknesses. Treatment strategies using more than one modality (if necessary) should be adapted to the needs of the patient.

> ☑ Long-term technical success rates are likely to be greatest after EVLA/RFA and lowest after UGFS.

Cost-effectiveness of treatments

Despite the clear clinical benefits of traditional and endovenous treatments for superficial venous disease, state funding for these interventions has been subject to rationing in the UK National Health Service (NHS). State funding has been restricted in many UK regions for all patients other than those with advanced disease (CEAP C4–C6). In general, few studies have scientifically investigated the cost-effectiveness of venous interventions. However, the REACTIV trial clearly demonstrated that saphenous ligation and stripping was cost-effective in comparison to conservative management with an incremental cost-effectiveness ratio of £7175 per quality-adjusted life-year (QALY) at 2 years.[49] A health economic modelling study suggested that endovenous thermal ablation performed in an office setting is highly likely to be cost-effective.[36] It is likely that removing superficial venous procedures from the expensive operating theatre into an outpatient or 'office-based' environment will be the most cost-effective treatment strategy.

✅✅ Traditional surgery and endovenous treatments are likely to be cost-effective in the management of varicose veins.

Atypical varicose veins

Vulval and pelvic varices

In some cases, female patients may have varicose veins as a result of ovarian or internal iliac venous tributary incompetence.[61] Varicose veins of pelvic origin may extend along the medial thigh and join the GSV, which may also be incompetent. Pelvic causes of venous disease should be considered in patients with recurrent varicose veins after GSV intervention. Duplex scanning can often identify an incompetent vein arising from the pelvis that is feeding the visible varicosities. Magnetic resonance venography may identify the typically dilated ovarian vein.

The treatment of choice is endovenous coil embolisation of the incompetent tributary, under fluoroscopic control. Ovarian vein reflux may also be associated with the 'pelvic congestion syndrome', characterised by chronic pelvic pain and menstrual problems.[62]

Congenital causes of varicose veins

A number of researchers have reported that varicose veins may be more common in the families of patients with varicose veins, suggesting a hereditary or genetic contribution to the disease process. In one study, patients with varicose veins were over 20 times more likely to report a positive family history in comparison to controls. However, specific genetic causes of varicose veins have not been identified. Varicose veins may also be seen as part of some inherited disorders, such as Klippel–Trenauney syndrome.[63] Patients may present with a combination of cutaneous capillary malformations (port wine stains), limb hypertrophy/overgrowth and varicose veins. The majority of patients have varicose veins, which are commonly located on the lateral aspect of the leg. Although incompetent superficial veins may be treated, clinicians should be aware that there may be associated deep venous abnormalities, including atresia. Reliable venous mapping with colour duplex is essential before considering intervention, and supplementary investigations may be necessary.

Conclusions

After nearly a century without significant progression, the management of superficial venous reflux has evolved dramatically in the last decade. Endovenous laser, radiofrequency and foam sclerotherapy procedures are rapidly replacing traditional surgery as the 'gold standard'. Despite the lack of long-term evidence for endovenous interventions, the early advantages are becoming more apparent to patients and medical professionals.

Key points

- Varicose veins are part of a spectrum of venous disorders and are associated with significant quality-of-life impairment.
- Interventions for symptomatic varicose veins result in significant clinical and quality-of-life benefits.
- All patients should undergo venous duplex imaging prior to planning intervention.
- Thorough pre-intervention counselling and documented informed consent are essential in view of the risk of medicolegal consequences of adverse outcomes.
- Endovenous treatment modalities including endovenous thermal ablation (using laser or radiofrequency) and ultrasound-guided foam sclerotherapy have become the treatment modalities of choice, ahead of traditional surgery.
- Endovenous modalities are associated with lower early morbidity in comparison to surgical stripping.
- Each of the endovenous treatments has advantages and disadvantages, but the technical success rates are likely to be greatest after EVLA or RFA. Long-term outcomes are awaited.
- Traditional surgical and endovenous treatments are likely to be cost-effective.
- For patients with venous ulceration, superficial venous surgery has been shown to reduce the risk of recurrent ulceration.
- Vascular surgeons and venous specialists should ensure adequate training in duplex ultrasound and endovenous treatments to offer optimal management to patients with venous disease.

References

1. Callam MJ. Epidemiology of varicose veins. Br J Surg 1994;81:167–70.

2. Garratt AM, Macdonald LM, Ruta DA, et al. Towards measurement of outcome for patients with varicose veins. Qual Health Care 1993;2(1):5–10.

3. Sritharan K, Lane TR, Davies AH. The burden of depression in patients with symptomatic varicose veins. Eur J Vasc Endovasc Surg 2012;43(4):480–4.

4. Ratcliffe J, Brazier J, Palfreyman S, et al. A comparison of patient and population values for health states in varicose veins patients. Health Econ 2007;16(4):395–405.

5. Bergan JJ, Pascarella L, Schmid-Schonbein GW. Pathogenesis of primary chronic venous disease: Insights from animal models of venous hypertension. J Vasc Surg 2008;47(1):183–92.

6. Gohel MS, Barwell JR, Earnshaw JJ, et al. Randomized clinical trial of compression plus surgery versus compression alone in chronic venous ulceration (ESCHAR study) – haemodynamic and anatomical changes. Br J Surg 2005;92(3):291–7.

7. Ludbrook J. Valvular defect in primary varicose veins: cause or effect? Lancet 1963;2(7321):1289–92.

8. Labropoulos N, Leon L, Kwon S, et al. Study of the venous reflux progression. J Vasc Surg 2005;41(2):291–5.

9. Evans CJ, Allan PL, Lee AJ, et al. Prevalence of venous reflux in the general population on duplex scanning: the Edinburgh Vein Study. J Vasc Surg 1998;28(5):767–76.

10. Bradbury A, Evans CJ, Allan P, et al. The relationship between lower limb symptoms and superficial and deep venous reflux on duplex ultrasonography: the Edinburgh Vein Study. J Vasc Surg 2000;32(5):921–31.

11. Maurins U, Hoffmann BH, Losch C, et al. Distribution and prevalence of reflux in the superficial and deep venous system in the general population – results from the Bonn Vein Study, Germany. J Vasc Surg 2008;48(3):680–7.

12. Ruckley CV, Evans CJ, Allan PL, et al. Chronic venous insufficiency: clinical and duplex correlations. The Edinburgh Vein Study of venous disorders in the general population. J Vasc Surg 2002;36(3):520–5.

13. Eklof B, Rutherford RB, Bergan JJ, et al. Revision of the CEAP classification for chronic venous disorders: consensus statement. J Vasc Surg 2004;40(6):1248–52.

14. Passman MA, McLafferty RB, Lentz MF, et al. Validation of Venous Clinical Severity Score (VCSS) with other venous severity assessment tools from the American Venous Forum, National Venous Screening Program. J Vasc Surg 2011;54(Suppl. 6):2S–9.

15. Vasquez MA, Rabe E, McLafferty RB, et al. Revision of the venous clinical severity score: venous outcomes consensus statement: special communication of the American Venous Forum Ad Hoc Outcomes Working Group. J Vasc Surg 2010;52(5):1387–96.

16. Margolis DJ, Bilker W, Santanna J, et al. Venous leg ulcer: incidence and prevalence in the elderly. J Am Acad Dermatol 2002;46(3):381–6.

17. Tennant WG, Ruckley CV. Medicolegal action following treatment for varicose veins. Br J Surg 1996;83(3):291–2.

18. De Maeseneer M, Pichot O, Cavezzi A, et al. Duplex ultrasound investigation of the veins of the lower limbs after treatment for varicose veins – UIP consensus document. Eur J Vasc Endovasc Surg 2011;42(1):89–102.

19. Blomgren L, Johansson G, Bergqvist D. Randomized clinical trial of routine preoperative duplex imaging before varicose vein surgery. Br J Surg 2005;92(6):688–94.

20. Arnoldussen CW, Toonder I, Wittens CH. A novel scoring system for lower-extremity venous pathology analysed using magnetic resonance venography and duplex ultrasound. Phlebology 2012;27(Suppl. 1):163–70.

21. Gohel MS, Barwell JR, Heather BP, et al. The predictive value of haemodynamic assessment in chronic venous leg ulceration. Eur J Vasc Endovasc Surg 2007;33(6):742–6.

22. Gohel MS, Davies AH. Pharmacological agents in the treatment of venous disease: an update of the available evidence. Curr Vasc Pharmacol 2009;7(3):303–8.

23. Nelson EA. Venous leg ulcers. (Online) Clin Evid 2011;Dec 21.

24. Gloviczki P, Gloviczki ML. Evidence on efficacy of treatments of venous ulcers and on prevention of ulcer recurrence. Perspect Vasc Surg Endovasc Ther 2009;21(4):259–68.

25. Shingler S, Robertson L, Boghossian S, et al. Compression stockings for the initial treatment of varicose veins in patients without venous ulceration. Cochrane Database Syst Rev 2011;11:CD008819.

26. Palfreyman SJ, Michaels JA. A systematic review of compression hosiery for uncomplicated varicose veins. Phlebology 2009;24(Suppl. 1):13–33.

27. Campbell WB, France F, Goodwin HM. Medicolegal claims in vascular surgery. Ann R Coll Surg Engl 2002;84(3):181–4.

28. Trendelenburg F. Ueber die Unterbindung der Vena Saphena magna bei Unterschenkel Varicen. Beitr Z Klin Chir 1890;7:195–210.

29. Kanwar A, Hansrani M, Lees T, et al. Trends in varicose vein therapy in England: radical changes in the last decade. Ann R Coll Surg Engl 2010;92(4):341–6.

30. Mekako AI, Chetter IC, Coughlin PA, et al. Randomized clinical trial of co-amoxiclav versus no antibiotic prophylaxis in varicose vein surgery. Br J Surg 2010;97(1):29–36.

31. Winterborn RJ, Foy C, Earnshaw JJ. Causes of varicose vein recurrence: late results of a randomized controlled trial of stripping the long saphenous vein. J Vasc Surg 2004;40(4):634–9.

32. Blomgren L, Johansson G, Emanuelsson L, et al. Late follow-up of a randomized trial of routine duplex imaging before varicose vein surgery. Br J Surg 2011;98(8):1112–6.

33. O'Hare JL, Vandenbroeck CP, Whitman B, et al. A prospective evaluation of the outcome after small saphenous varicose vein surgery with one-year follow-up. J Vasc Surg 2008;48(3):669–74.

34. Nisar A, Shabbir J, Tubassam MA, et al. Local anaesthetic flush reduces postoperative pain and haematoma formation after great saphenous vein stripping – a randomised controlled trial. Eur J Vasc Endovasc Surg 2006;31(3):325–31.

35. Perkins JM. Standard varicose vein surgery. Phlebology 2009;24(Suppl. 1):34–41.

36. Gohel MS, Epstein DM, Davies AH. Cost-effectiveness of traditional and endovenous treatments for varicose veins. Br J Surg 2010;97(12):1815–23.

37. Darwood RJ, Gough MJ. Endovenous laser treatment for uncomplicated varicose veins. Phlebology 2009;24(Suppl. 1):50–61.

38. Gohel MS, Davies AH. Radiofrequency ablation for uncomplicated varicose veins. Phlebology 2009;24(Suppl. 1):42–9.

39. Marsh P, Price BA, Holdstock J, et al. Deep vein thrombosis (DVT) after venous thermoablation techniques: rates of endovenous heat-induced thrombosis (EHIT) and classical DVT after radiofrequency and endovenous laser ablation in a single centre. Eur J Vasc Endovasc Surg 2010;40(4):521–7.

40. Mozes G, Kalra M, Carmo M, et al. Extension of saphenous thrombus into the femoral vein: a potential complication of new endovenous ablation techniques. J Vasc Surg 2005;41(1):130–5.

41. Coleridge Smith P. Sclerotherapy and foam sclerotherapy for varicose veins. Phlebology 2009;24(6):260–9.

42. Jia X, Mowatt G, Burr JM, et al. Systematic review of foam sclerotherapy for varicose veins. Br J Surg 2007;94(8):925–36.

43. Sarvananthan T, Shepherd AC, Willenberg T, et al. Neurological complications of sclerotherapy for varicose veins. J Vasc Surg 2012;55(1):243–51.

44. Nelzen O, Fransson I. Early results from a randomized trial of saphenous surgery with or without subfascial endoscopic perforator surgery in patients with a venous ulcer. Br J Surg 2011;98(4):495–500.

45. Carradice D, Mekako AI, Hatfield J, et al. Randomized clinical trial of concomitant or sequential phlebectomy after endovenous laser therapy for varicose veins. Br J Surg 2009;96(4):369–75.

46. Rudstrom H, Bjorck M, Bergqvist D. Iatrogenic vascular injuries in varicose vein surgery: a systematic review. World J Surg 2007;31(1):228–33.

47. Pares JO, Juan J, Tellez R, et al. Varicose vein surgery: stripping versus the CHIVA method: a randomized controlled trial. Ann Surg 2010;251(4):624–31.

48. Gohel MS, Davies AH. Varicose veins: highlighting the confusion over how and where to treat. Eur J Vasc Endovasc Surg 2008;36(1):107–8.

49. Michaels JA, Campbell WB, Brazier JE, et al. Randomised clinical trial, observational study and assessment of cost-effectiveness of the treatment of varicose veins (REACTIV trial). Health Technol Assess 2006;10(13):1–196, iii–iv.

50. Michaels JA, Brazier JE, Campbell WB, et al. Randomized clinical trial comparing surgery with conservative treatment for uncomplicated varicose veins. Br J Surg 2006;93(2):175–81.

51. Gohel MS, Barwell JR, Taylor M, et al. Long term results of compression therapy alone versus compression plus surgery in chronic venous ulceration (ESCHAR): randomised controlled trial. Br Med J 2007;335(7610):83.

52. Barwell JR, Davies CE, Deacon J, et al. Comparison of surgery and compression with compression alone in chronic venous ulceration (ESCHAR study): randomised controlled trial. Lancet 2004;363(9424):1854–9.

53. Nordon IM, Hinchliffe RJ, Brar R, et al. A prospective double-blind randomized controlled trial of radiofrequency versus laser treatment of the great saphenous vein in patients with varicose veins. Ann Surg 2011;254(6):876–81.

54. Carradice D, Mekako AI, Mazari FA, et al. Randomized clinical trial of endovenous laser ablation compared with conventional surgery for great saphenous varicose veins. Br J Surg 2011;98(4):501–10.

55. Shepherd AC, Gohel MS, Brown LC, et al. Randomized clinical trial of VNUS ClosureFAST radiofrequency ablation versus laser for varicose veins. Br J Surg 2010;97(6):810–8.

56. Subramonia S, Lees T. Randomized clinical trial of radiofrequency ablation or conventional high ligation and stripping for great saphenous varicose veins. Br J Surg 2010;97(3):328–36.

57. Darwood RJ, Theivacumar N, Dellagrammaticas D, et al. Randomized clinical trial comparing endovenous laser ablation with surgery for the treatment of primary great saphenous varicose veins. Br J Surg 2008;95(3):294–301.

58. van den Bos R, Arends L, Kockaert M, et al. Endovenous therapies of lower extremity varicosities: a meta-analysis. J Vasc Surg 2009;49(1):230–9.

59. Coleridge Smith P. Foam and liquid sclerotherapy for varicose veins. Phlebology 2009;24(Suppl. 1): 62–72.

60. Rasmussen LH, Lawaetz M, Bjoern L, et al. Randomized clinical trial comparing endovenous laser ablation, radiofrequency ablation, foam sclerotherapy and surgical stripping for great saphenous varicose veins. Br J Surg 2011;98(8): 1079–87.

61. Hobbs JT. Varicose veins arising from the pelvis due to ovarian vein incompetence. Int J Clin Pract 2005;59(10):1195–203.

62. Smith PC. The outcome of treatment for pelvic congestion syndrome. Phlebology 2012;27(Suppl. 1): 74–7.

63. Gloviczki P, Driscoll DJ. Klippel–Trenaunay syndrome: current management. Phlebology 2007; 22(6):291–8.

18

Chronic leg swelling

Timothy A. Lees
Hazel Trender

There are various conditions that can cause chronic lower limb swelling (Box 18.1). The three most common are chronic venous insufficiency, lymphoedema, and dependent oedema, which may be associated with inactivity and obesity. This chapter explores these three conditions further.

Chronic venous insufficiency (CVI)

CVI encompasses disease of the lower limb veins in which venous return is impaired over a number of years, by reflux, obstruction or calf muscle pump failure. This leads to sustained venous hypertension and ultimately clinical complications including oedema, eczema, lipodermatosclerosis and ulceration.

Clinical features

The clinical features of CVI include skin changes, varicose veins, swelling, ulceration and pain.

Swelling

Swelling is due to oedema fluid, which is initially pitting, but as the disease progresses subcutaneous fibrosis and induration occur. If there is any break in the skin, this can lead to copious exudation of fluid.

Skin changes

Varicose eczema presents as dry, scaly and itchy skin. The skin becomes friable and may become infected following scratching. Pigmentation, due to the deposition of haemosiderin in the tissues, produces a brown discoloration characteristic of CVI, which together with fibrosis leads to the clinical picture of lipodermatosclerosis around the ankle (**Fig. 18.1**). There may also be some loss of pigmentation resulting in pale skin changes called atrophie blanche.

Ulceration

Ulceration is often precipitated by minor trauma and venous ulcers occur predominantly on the lower leg, more commonly around the medial aspect of the ankle. There may be surrounding eczema or pigmentation and frequently exudation of fluid that can cause maceration of the surrounding skin. In patients presenting with lower limb ulceration, approximately 80%[1,2] will have evidence of venous disease and 10–25%[3] of limbs will have Doppler-verified arterial disease. Approximately 12% will have coexisting diabetes or rheumatoid arthritis.[4] Immobility is often a contributory cause, and can also cause stasis ulceration in isolation.

Varicose veins

Varicose veins may be present and a history of previous varicose vein treatment should be sought. The absence of visible varicose veins does not exclude the presence of significant superficial reflux. Varicose veins on the lower anterior abdominal wall are a sign of inferior vena cava or iliac vein obstruction and the patient should be examined standing in order to identify these.

Pain

The patient may complain of a general ache and heaviness in the leg after long periods of standing.

Venous disease
Primary varicose veins
Primary deep venous incompetence
Post-thrombotic syndrome
Arteriovenous malformations
Lymphoedema
Primary
Secondary
General disease
Lipidema
Congestive cardiac failure
Pretibial myxoedema
Nephrotic syndrome
Hepatic failure
Tumours
Pelvic tumours causing extrinsic compression
Drugs
Dependency

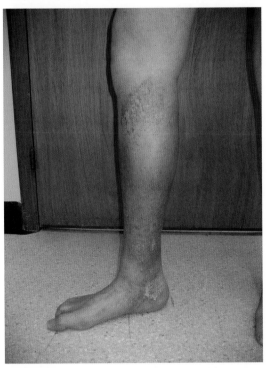

Figure 18.1 • Chronic venous insufficiency with pigmentation and severe lipodermatosclerosis resulting in the typical 'inverted champagne bottle' shape.

This is worse towards the end of the day but improves with elevation or bed rest.

A history of deep vein thrombosis (DVT) should be sought. Venous claudication is an uncommon symptom and is usually due to extensive iliofemoral vein occlusion. The symptoms differ from arterial claudication because the increase in arterial inflow during exercise combined with decreased outflow results in distension of the limb, giving rise to generalised pain and a severe bursting sensation in the leg. The pain often requires elevation for 10–20 minutes for relief after cessation of exercise.

Epidemiology

The prevalence of CVI in the adult population lies between 2% and 9%, and may be higher in males than females.[5,6] The most serious feature of CVI is ulceration, which is a distressing and debilitating condition. Leg ulcers affect approximately 1% of the adult population in developed countries, with 50% of ulcers having been present for more than 12 months, and 72% are recurrent.[7] Within the UK, Australia, Sweden and Italy, overall rates for active ulceration range from 0.15% to 0.5%, and increase with age.[8–12] In the UK, the total cost to the NHS has been estimated to be £230–600 million a year.[13]

Aetiology

To understand CVI, one must consider the changes that occur in both the larger veins (macrocirculation) and the capillary bed (microcirculation).

Macrocirculation

During exercise in the normal individual, effective contraction of the calf muscles combined with vein patency and valvular competence aids venous return and reduces venous pressure in the lower leg from about 90 mmHg to 30 mmHg. Failure of any of these mechanisms may result in postambulatory venous hypertension, which is accepted as the underlying haemodynamic abnormality in CVI. The recognised causes are outlined in Box 18.2.

Deep and superficial reflux

Most venous ulcers were thought to be secondary to previous DVT but duplex scanning has shown us that some patients have primary deep venous reflux. Isolated superficial venous incompetence without deep venous incompetence occurs in between 31%[14] and 57%[15] of patients with venous ulceration.

Perforating vein reflux

The contribution of incompetent perforators to the development of CVI remains controversial. Isolated perforator incompetence occurs in only

Superficial venous reflux
Long saphenous vein reflux
Short saphenous vein reflux
Deep venous reflux and occlusion
Primary (idiopathic)
Secondary to deep venous thrombosis or injury
Perforating vein reflux
Abnormal calf pump
Neurological
Musculoskeletal
Combination of the above

2–4% of limbs with skin changes, and perforator incompetence is usually associated with reflux in the superficial or deep systems. On the other hand, the prevalence of incompetent perforators increases linearly with the clinical severity of CVI.[16] There has been a recent trend towards treatment of incompetent perforating veins with laser and radiofrequency ablation, but the indications for this remain uncertain. In those cases where superficial and perforator reflux coincide, treating only the former results in healing rates of 95%.[17]

Microcirculation

The pathophysiology is still not fully understood but the following two hypotheses exist:

1. **White cell trapping hypothesis.** Increased venous pressures lead to white blood cell plugging of capillaries, adherence of white cells to the endothelium and release of proteolytic enzymes. This leads to increased capillary permeability and tissue damage causing ulceration.[18–21]

2. **Fibrin cuff hypothesis.** A rise in venous pressure causes widening of the pores between the endothelial cells.[22] This results in the passage of fibrinogen out of the intravascular compartment into the tissues, which then polymerises to form fibrin. A defective interstitial fibrinolytic system may also contribute to the build-up of fibrin.[23] This acts as a barrier to oxygen, resulting in local tissue ischaemia and cell death, producing ulceration.[24]

Matrix metalloproteinases help remodel the extracellular matrix by protein degradation, and enhanced matrix metalloproteinase activity has been demonstrated in lipodermatosclerosis.[25] This may also contribute to the development of ulceration.

Classification

CVI involves a variety of anatomical and physiological abnormalities and so a standardised system is required to allow uniformity of reporting.

> ✅✅ A classification was developed in 1994 by an international consensus conference under the auspices of the American Venous Forum and recommendations for change were made in 2004.[26]

This includes clinical signs (C), aetiology (E), anatomical distribution (A) and pathophysiological condition (P), and is therefore known by the acronym CEAP. This system is helpful in comparing limbs for the purposes of research, although it is rather unwieldy for everyday use (Box 18.3).

Investigation

Patients often present with mixed arterial and venous disease and so ankle–brachial pressure indices must be recorded if foot pulses are weak or absent or if compression therapy is being considered. The investigation of the venous disease is discussed below.

Clinical signs (C$_{0–6}$)
Limbs are placed into one of seven clinical classes according to objective signs as follows:
- Class 0: no visible or palpable signs of venous disease
- Class 1: telangiectases, reticular veins, malleolar flare
- Class 2: varicose veins
- Class 3: oedema without skin changes
- Class 4a: pigmentation or eczema class 4b, lipodermatosclerosis or atrophie blanche
- Class 5: skin changes as above with healed ulceration
- Class 6: skin changes as above with active ulceration

Each limb is further classified as asymptomatic (A) or symptomatic (S)

Aetiology (E$_{C,P,S,N}$)
This classification refers to congenital (C), primary (P; unknown cause but not congenital), secondary (S; acquired) and no aetiology identified (N). These groups are mutually exclusive

Anatomical distribution (A$_{S,D,P,N}$)
This refers to superficial (S), deep (D), perforating (P) veins and no venous location identified (N). More than one system may be involved

Pathophysiological condition (P$_{R,O,N}$)
This refers to reflux (R) or obstruction (O), or both may be present. P$_N$ implies no venous pathophysiology identified

Hand-held Doppler

Continuous-wave hand-held Doppler using an 8-MHz probe is a useful outpatient tool in screening for arterial and venous disease. Its limitations are that the exact vein being insonated is unknown, it is operator dependent and the significance of reflux of short duration may be uncertain.

Duplex scanning

Duplex is an important investigation of lower limb venous disease and is now the gold standard. Modern equipment allows easy identification of normal and abnormal venous anatomy, along with the presence of venous reflux. It is also extensively used for the diagnosis of DVT.

> ✔ An international consensus document recommends duplex scanning as an essential investigation for patients with CVI.[27]

Venography

Venography is invasive and to a large extent has been superseded by duplex scanning for the investigation of venous disease. Venography still has a place in the diagnosis of deep venous outflow obstruction, particularly in the iliac veins and inferior vena cava, which are not easily visualised by ultrasound. Such lesions may be amenable to angioplasty or stenting. Magnetic resonance (MR) or computed tomography (CT) venography may be used in place of conventional catheter venography, although the images obtained are not always sufficient to plan treatment.

Functional measurements

Various investigations may be used to examine the function of the venous system in the lower limb.

Ambulatory venous pressure measurement

This provides direct measurement of the superficial venous pressure at the ankle. This is achieved by cannulation of a vein on the dorsum of the foot connected to a pressure transducer, amplifier and a recorder. The pressure changes recorded in the long saphenous vein in the foot during and after 10 tiptoe exercises are shown in **Fig. 18.2**. This investigation is an indicator of overall lower limb venous function including calf muscle pump function.

Plethysmography

There are many different types of plethysmography and these measure either alterations in calf volume directly or other parameters that indirectly reflect volume change. These include photoplethysmography, strain gauge plethysmography and air plethysmography.

Treatment

The management of patients with CVI may be divided into either the prevention or the treatment of clinical complications such as lipodermatosclerosis and ulceration. Correcting the underlying cause will help to stop or reverse these complications. In addition, vigorous treatment of conditions known to lead to CVI, particularly acute DVT, may reduce the incidence of this problem in the long term. Management of patients with ulcers of mixed aetiology will require treatment aimed at each specific cause but this section deals predominantly with the treatment of isolated venous disease.

General measures

These should include elevation of the legs at rest above the level of the heart. This helps to reduce

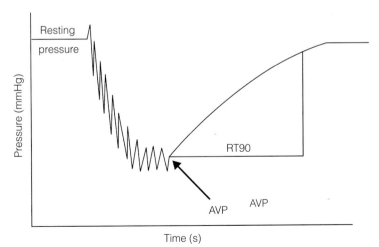

Figure 18.2 • Venous pressure trace recorded from a superficial vein on the dorsum of the foot during 10 tiptoe exercises and return to the resting value after exercise. AVP, ambulatory venous pressure; RT90, time for 90% refilling.

oedema, decrease exudate from ulcers and accelerate regression of skin changes.[4] Immobility, occupation, obesity and coexisting disease may also influence the development of skin complications and should be addressed. Placing the patient in bed reduces the venous pressure at the ankle to about 12–15 mmHg and will therefore usually lead to ulcer healing. However, this is not a treatment enjoyed by most patients and may increase the risk of DVT. It is therefore generally reserved for ulcers that have failed to heal by all other methods.

Graduated elastic compression

Compression therapy remains the primary treatment for CVI. It provides symptomatic relief, promotes ulcer healing and helps in preventing ulcer recurrence. Applying a sustained graduated compressive force that is highest at the ankle and decreases proximally has been shown to reduce venous pressure at the ankle, increase femoral vein blood flow and increase venous refilling time. This improves venous function and can heal up to 93% of venous ulcers.[28] Graduated elastic compression may be applied using either bandages or stockings but this is dependent on factors such as levels of exudate, amount of oedema and leg shape. It is important that these are applied by experienced staff as inexpertly applied compression can cause skin damage. Compression can also be used to treat mixed arterial and venous ulcers but this requires specialist assessment.

✔✔ In the healing of leg ulcers: (i) compression is more effective than no compression; (ii) elastic compression is more effective than non-elastic compression; (iii) multilayered high compression is more effective than single-layer compression; and (iv) there is no significant difference between four-layer bandaging and other high-compression multilayered systems.[29]

In the prevention of ulcer recurrence, there are no randomised trials comparing recurrence rates with and without compression.

✔✔ A review of trials comparing different grades of compression stocking concluded that higher grades of compression are associated with lower recurrence rates, but at a cost of lower patient compliance.[30] Approximately one-third of patients do not comply with the long-term use of compression hosiery.[31]

Stockings are classed according to the pressure they exert at the ankle and are designed to provide a linear graduated decrease in pressure above this, although in practice this may not always be the case.

Table 18.1 • Conventional pressure classes of compression stockings

Class	Pressure at ankle (mmHg)	Indications
I	<25	Mild varicosis, venous thrombosis prophylaxis
II	25–35	Marked varicose veins, oedema, chronic venous insufficiency
III	35–45	Chronic venous insufficiency, lymphoedema, following venous ulceration to prevent recurrence
IV	45–60	Severe lymphoedema and chronic venous insufficiency

Pressures of up to 60 mmHg may be produced by elastic stockings, and conventional pressure classes and indications are given in Table 18.1.

For the majority of patients with CVI or mild lymphoedema, a knee-length compression stocking designed to apply compression of 25–35 mmHg is ideal, but this will be influenced by how well they tolerate the stocking and their ability to apply them. Thigh-length stockings seem to confer little benefit over knee-length ones and as shorter stockings are easier to put on, compliance with these tends to be better. Stocking applicators may also aid patient compliance.

Intermittent pneumatic compression

✔✔ There is some evidence that intermittent pneumatic compression may provide accelerated ulcer healing when used either alone or in combination with elastic compression, although there is a need for further trials in this area.[32]

Laser and electromagnetic therapy

✔✔ A review of low-level laser therapy for venous leg ulcers has not found any benefit in healing rates.[33] Similarly, there is no high-quality evidence that electromagnetic therapy increases the rate of healing of venous leg ulcers.[34]

Pharmacotherapy
Dressings
For those patients with venous ulceration, there are a wide variety of topical dressings available.

The type of dressing applied beneath compression has not been shown to affect ulcer healing, although dressing choice has an impact on pain, frequency of dressing change, maceration and odour. Decisions regarding which dressing to use should be based on local costs and practitioner or patient preference.[35]

Additional factors to consider in choosing a dressing are exudate, odour and patient comfort. Whatever dressing is chosen should be used in conjunction with treatment of the underlying venous insufficiency, usually by adequate graduated elastic compression. Simple non-adherent dressings are all that is required for many ulcers. Vacuum-assisted closure dressing systems are sometimes useful for deep ulceration and can be used under compression. There is recent evidence that they reduce time to healing at a lower cost when compared to conventional dressings.[36] The Vulcan trial suggested that silver dressings made no impact on ulcer healing when compared to any other dressing, although this has been questioned as many of the ulcers treated with silver within the trial would not have had silver applied in clinical practice.[37]

Emollients
These soothe, smooth and hydrate the skin and are indicated for all dry or scaling disorders such as varicose eczema. Their effects are short-lived and frequent application is necessary. Preparations containing an antibacterial should be avoided unless infection is present.

Oxpentifylline (pentoxifylline)

There have been several randomised controlled trials of oxpentifylline compared with placebo, with or without compression, in the healing of venous leg ulcers.[38] These have demonstrated that this drug is more effective than placebo in ulcer healing.

Nutrition
Adequate nutrition is important for ulcer healing; protein, vitamins A and C, zinc and other trace elements are all important. It may be appropriate to consider dietary supplements if these are deficient.

Superficial venous intervention
Superficial venous surgery
Superficial surgery may be of benefit in healing ulcers in situations of isolated superficial venous incompetence or combined superficial and deep venous incompetence. Surgery for isolated superficial venous incompetence may also reduce long-term recurrence rates. With the advent of minimally invasive techniques it may be possible to treat some patients who

previously were not fit for conventional varicose vein surgery. These techniques include radiofrequency ablation (RFA), endovenous laser ablation (EVLA) and foam sclerotherapy, and are discussed in Chapter 17.

A recent randomised controlled trial comparing superficial venous surgery plus elastic compression with compression alone for venous ulceration has demonstrated no difference in initial healing rates but a reduction in recurrence rates at 12 months in the surgical group (12% vs. 28%). The authors concluded that most patients with chronic venous ulceration will benefit from addition of simple venous surgery.[39]

Perforating vein surgery
There has been renewed interest in medial calf-perforating vein incompetence with the advent of subfascial endoscopic perforating vein surgery, and more recently with minimally invasive techniques such as EVLA and RFA. The evidence for the benefit of treatment of incompetent perforating veins by any of these methods is weak and the precise indications and benefit of perforator treatment remain unclear.

Deep venous reconstruction
Worldwide experience of deep venous valvular reconstruction is limited as most patients with CVI can be managed very adequately with superficial venous surgery and the conservative measures described above. Therefore it is usually reserved for those patients with severe symptoms that prove resistant to conservative treatment.

The benefit of deep venous reconstructive surgery is unclear as many of the published series have included ancillary procedures such as high saphenous ligation and stripping, and in the few series where the influence of these procedures has been excluded the numbers involved tend to be small or the follow-up short. A number of different procedures have been described and these are shown in Box 18.4.

A recent Cochrane review has found only one randomised trial of deep venous reconstructive surgery.[40] This trial compared external valvuloplasty plus superficial venous ligation with superficial venous ligation only. There was a moderate improvement in clinical outcome in the valvuloplasty plus ligation group compared with mild clinical improvement in the ligation-only group.

Venous bypass
Following DVT, recanalisation will occur in all affected venous segments in over 50% of limbs by 90 days.[41] Many of these patients, however, will be left with functional outflow obstruction and

Box 18.4 • Procedures for correction of deep venous valvular incompetence

Valvular repair
Valvuloplasty
Valve transposition
Valve transplantation
External support of vein wall
Dacron cuff
Vein wall plication

deep venous reflux. Those that fail to recanalise will also have persistent venous outflow obstruction. If severe, this gives rise to a swollen leg, skin changes and venous claudication. Surgical bypass of an obstructed vein may be possible, but this should be reserved for those patients in whom there is measured evidence of outflow obstruction and in whom there are severe symptoms. As spontaneous improvement may occur due to the development of collaterals up to 4 years after DVT, surgery should not usually be considered before this time. Two principal surgical procedures have been described:

1. The femorofemoral crossover graft for iliac obstruction (Palma operation; **Fig. 18.3**).[42] Only a small number of patients are suitable for this procedure, but in these patients long-term patency and relief of symptoms may be achieved in up to 70% of cases.[43] The long saphenous vein on the unaffected side is used as a crossover graft.
2. Limbs with functional outflow obstruction due to stenosed or occluded deep thigh veins may be suitable for saphenopopliteal bypass, which uses the long saphenous vein as a bypass channel. The theoretical difficulty with this procedure is that the long saphenous vein may already be acting as a collateral channel and to interfere with this may make matters worse should thrombosis occur.

Skin grafting

Large ulcers may be usefully treated with a split-skin graft or pinch grafts which, if successful, will reduce the healing time. Before this is undertaken, it is important that the ulcer bed is clean and free from infection (particularly β-haemolytic streptococci, *Pseudomonas* and *Staphylococcus aureus*). However, unless the underlying venous abnormality is also treated, failure of the graft and subsequent recurrence is inevitable.

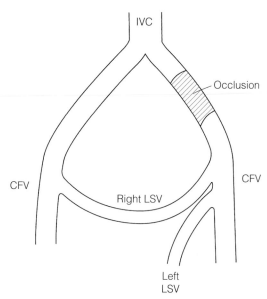

Figure 18.3 • Femorofemoral crossover graft using the long saphenous vein (LSV) to bypass unilateral iliac obstruction. CFV, common femoral vein; IVC, inferior vena cava.

Endovascular management of venous outflow obstruction

With the development of endovascular treatments in recent years it has become clear that iliac venous occlusions and stenoses may be treated by endoluminal stenting, although the long-term results have not been directly compared with surgery. Raju et al.[44] have reported treating a small series of long iliac venous occlusions, with primary and secondary patency rates at 2 years of 49% and 76%, respectively. Further studies have reported patency rates in the region of 90% at 1 year for stenting of iliac venous stenoses (May–Thurner syndrome).[45,46] This refers to the chronic pulsatile compression of the proximal left common iliac vein by the overlying right common iliac artery or aortic bifurcation, resulting in an intraluminal venous spur, web or membrane. This common lesion (20% of the adult population) is an increasingly well-recognised cause of left iliac vein thrombo-occlusive disease, particularly in young patients. The clinical picture is of left leg venous hypertension or DVT and is likely to explain the preponderance of left-sided DVT.

Preventing the post-thrombotic limb

CVI developing secondary to previous DVT is commonly referred to as post-thrombotic syndrome (PTS) or postphlebitic syndrome. The management of DVT has historically been directed at preventing thrombus extension and pulmonary embolus in the acute phase. There has been little focus on long-term treatment in order to prevent the development of PTS. However, 30% or more will develop features of mild or moderate PTS.[47–49] This risk increases with more proximal DVT and recurrent episodes of thrombosis. Even with isolated calf vein thrombosis there is a risk of development of PTS.

✓✓ The risk of developing severe CVI with ulceration following DVT is of the order of 2–10% at 10 years.[47,50]

The causes of PTS related to previous DVT are either valvular incompetence or residual outflow obstruction with eventual calf muscle pump failure. Treatment of the primary DVT should be aimed not only at preventing thrombus propagation and pulmonary embolism, but also at preventing venous damage and preserving or restoring venous function. This may include anticoagulation, limb elevation, elastic compression therapy, and increasingly thrombolysis and catheter thrombectomy are being used in the management of acute iliofemoral DVT. Patients who have had a DVT should be encouraged to wear lifelong elastic compression hosiery, in particular those patients with residual reflux and who are on their feet all day or travel long journeys.[46] They should be encouraged to take regular exercise to stimulate the calf muscle pump and maintain ankle mobility. These simple measures may be required for life but are often all that is needed to prevent a lifetime of debility due to PTS.

Summary

Investigation and treatment must be tailored to the individual patient but a simplified everyday management plan is shown in **Fig. 18.4**.

Dependency and inactivity

Patients who sit for long periods are exposed to a raised venous pressure at the ankle for longer periods of time. Normal daily activity includes activation of the calf muscle pump by walking, thereby decreasing the venous pressure, but without this pressure reduction the effects on the lower limb are similar to those seen in venous reflux due to prolonged venous 'hypertension'. As a result inactive patients, for example those confined to a wheelchair, can develop venous-type leg swelling in the absence of any true venous pathology. Those with a stiff or fused ankle may also be affected. The use of prophylactic compression therapy should

therefore be considered in these patients. Morbid obesity adds to this problem and is becoming a major aetiological factor in lower limb ulceration. The management of obesity is an important component of treatment in these patients and whilst this may be done in primary care in the majority of cases, some may require referral for gastric banding or bypass.

Lymphoedema

Lymphoedema is a progressive, chronic and debilitating swelling that can affect any part of the body, most commonly the limbs, leading to distortion in shape, size, reduction of mobility and impaired function.

Aetiology

Lymphoedema can be caused by intrinsic factors (primary) or extrinsic factors (secondary).

Primary

The traditional classification of primary lymphoedema is shown in Box 18.5. Congenital lymphoedema occurs at or soon after birth and in some rare cases it is autosomally inherited (Milroy's disease). Lymphoedema praecox presents up to the age of 35 years and is more prevalent in females. Typically this is not familial, although lymphoedema–distichiasis syndrome, which develops at puberty, is familial and is linked to the FOXC2 gene mutation.[51] Lymphoedema tarda presents over the age of 35 years. It is likely that these three groups represent different parts of the same spectrum of disease, which has been attributed to aplasia, hypoplasia or hyperplasia of the lymph vessels during development. A fibrotic obstruction in the lymph nodes has also been described.[52]

In addition to this, a functional classification more orientated to the treatment of these conditions may be used. This type of classification was first described by Browse.[53]

- Obliterative (80%): the distal lymphatics undergo progressive obliteration. This occurs predominantly in females and is often bilateral.
- Proximal obstruction (10%): proximal occlusion occurs in the abdominal, pelvic or inguinal lymph nodes. This is predominantly unilateral.
- Lymphatic valvular incompetence and hyperplasia (10%): development of the valve system is incomplete and lymphatic dilatation and hyperplasia occur. This is usually bilateral.

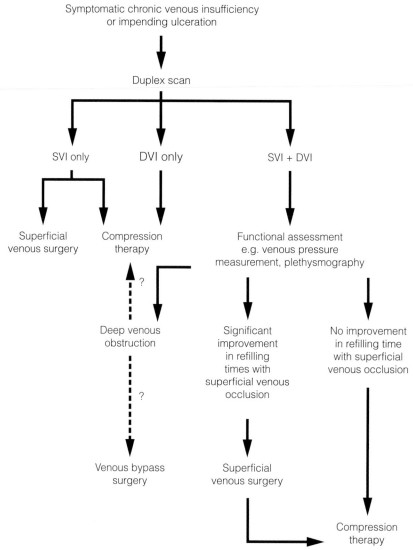

Figure 18.4 • Flow diagram for the management of chronic venous insufficiency. DVI, deep venous incompetence; SVI, superficial venous incompetence.

Secondary

Secondary lymphoedema develops following extrinsic damage to part of the lymphatic system. The lymphatic channels distal to the obstruction become dilated and the valves secondarily incompetent. The commonest cause worldwide is filarial infestation but in Europe the commonest cause is neoplasia and its treatment, for example post-mastectomy lymphoedema. The causes of secondary lymphoedema are also listed in Box 18.5.

Presentation

Initial presentation is with peripheral oedema. History and examination will usually differentiate lymphoedema from other causes of limb swelling and may distinguish between primary and secondary causes.

History

The patient complains of a slowly progressive swelling of the whole or part of the limb, which typically does not reduce overnight with elevation. Limb swelling usually commences distally and may progress during the day, particularly on standing for long periods. The patient may describe the limb as heavy and up to 50% will complain of pain requiring analgesia.[54] There may be a history of recurrent lymphangitis. The age of onset and a history of previous surgery, malignancy or radiotherapy should be sought.

Box 18.5 • Causes of lymphoedema

Primary

Congenital (age <1 year)

- Familial (Milroy's disease)
- Non-familial

Praecox (age <35 years)

- Familial
- Non-familial

Tarda (age >35 years)

Secondary

Malignant disease

Surgery

- Radical mastectomy
- Radical groin dissection

Radiotherapy

Infection

- Parasitic (filariasis)
- Pyogenic (β-haemolytic streptococci, *Staphylococcus aureus*)
- Tuberculosis

Impairment

- Arterial surgery
- Venous disease and venous surgery

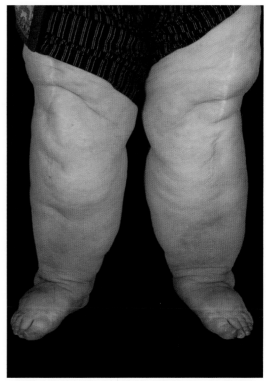

Figure 18.5 • Chronic lymphoedema of the leg with tree-trunk appearance and 'buffalo hump' of the foot.

Lymphoedema can also occur secondary to lipoedema. Lipoedema is abnormal symmetrical swelling due to excess deposit and expansion of fat cells. It is always bilateral, occurs from the waist down and spares the ankles. It cannot be lost through diet and exercise, and often causes pain, particularly surrounding the tibial area. It occurs almost exclusively in women, and can occur in women of all sizes and can be inherited. The expanding fat cells interfere with the lymphatics so many lipoedema patients develop lymphoedema, which is difficult to treat due to the inability to tolerate compression because of pain.

Examination

Examination reveals swelling of the limb, which may be unilateral or bilateral. Initially it will pit like other types of oedema, but with time the swelling becomes non-pitting due to hypertrophy of adipose tissue and increasing subcutaneous fibrosis. The swelling is uniform and as it progresses the leg becomes like a tree-trunk (**Fig. 18.5**). The skin develops a 'peau d'orange' appearance with hyperkeratosis of the toes and skin fissuring with secondary fungal infection. The skin gradually thickens, becoming less elastic until it is not possible to pick up a fold in the lower leg. This inelasticity produces a positive Stemmer sign (the inability to pinch the skin of the dorsum of the second toe between the thumb and

forefinger). The dorsum of the foot is usually involved, producing the characteristic 'buffalo hump' appearance, and chylous vesicles may occur on the pretibial area.

Ankle ulceration is unusual with lymphoedema as the skin remains more elastic than in venous disease, allowing expansion to occur without increased tension.[55] The presence of surgical scars or skin telangiectasia following radiotherapy may indicate a cause of secondary lymphoedema.

Clinical staging

There is no consensus on a universal clinical staging system for all forms of lymphoedema, but the consensus document of the International Society of Lymphology suggests the staging system in Table 18.2.[56,57] Within each stage, severity based on volume difference can be assessed as minimal (<20% increase) in limb volume, moderate (20–40% increase) or severe (>40% increase).

Investigation

The diagnosis of lymphoedema can usually be made clinically. Investigation is needed when the diagnosis

Table 18.2 • Clinical staging of lymphoedema

Stage 0	Latent or subclinical condition where swelling is not evident despite impaired lymph transport
Stage I	Early accumulation of fluid that subsides with limb elevation. Pitting may occur
Stage II	Limb elevation alone rarely reduces tissue swelling and pitting is manifest. Late in stage II, the limb may or may not pit as tissue fibrosis supervenes
Stage III	Lymphostatic elephantiasis where pitting is absent and trophic skin changes such as acanthosis, fat deposits and warty overgrowths develop

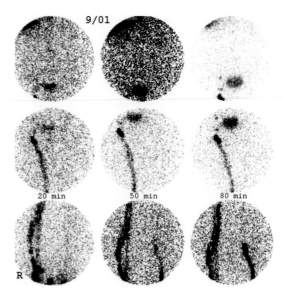

Figure 18.6 • Lymphoscintigram confirming left-sided lymphoedema. On the right, the isotope is travelling up the lymphatics of the leg with concentration in the ilioinguinal nodes (normal). On the left the isotope has remained in the leg.

is uncertain, to exclude sinister underlying causes or, if surgery is being considered, to confirm the diagnosis and plan treatment.

Duplex ultrasonography

This is useful to exclude CVI. The B-mode image will also detect the changes in the dermis and subcutaneous layers and can therefore be used as a means of monitoring the disease.

Lymphangioscintigraphy (isotope lymphography)

This is now one of the most frequently performed investigations as it provides an overall assessment of lymphatic drainage by demonstrating isotope flow up the lymphatics, and in the majority of cases avoids the need for conventional lymphangiography (**Fig. 18.6**). Radiolabelled (usually technetium) colloid is injected into the interdigital space between the second and third toes on both sides and gamma-camera pictures are taken at 5-minute intervals to assess transit through the lymph channels. Scintigraphy has been demonstrated to have a sensitivity of 92% and a specificity of 100% for the diagnosis of lymphoedema.[58] A negative scintigram effectively excludes the diagnosis.[59]

Computed tomography

Computed tomography may show the presence of dilated lymphatic channels, thereby aiding the diagnosis of obstructive lymphoedema and lymphatic valvular incompetence.[60] It will also provide evidence of lymphoedema by the presence of a honeycomb appearance of fluid in the subcutaneous tissues, and has been used to monitor the response to compression therapy by measuring the cross-sectional area of limb compartments. Patients with a previous history of pelvic or abdominal malignancy should be scanned for recurrent disease in order to diagnose enlarged lymph nodes or pelvic masses that may be compressing the lymphatic channels.

Magnetic resonance imaging (MRI)

In patients with chronic lymphoedema, MRI has been shown to demonstrate circumferential subcutaneous oedema, thickening of dermis and a honeycomb pattern of fibrosis between the muscle and subcutis, increased subcutaneous fat and variability in lymph node size and appearance.[61,62]

Interstitial magnetic resonance lymphangiography

Interstitial magnetic resonance lymphography involves intracutaneous injection of a paramagnetic contrast agent for the visualisation of lymphatic vessels.[63] Dilated lymphatic channels are a common finding and collateral vessels along with dermal backflow indicate proximal obstruction.[64,65] Dynamic MR lymphangiography is more sensitive and accurate than lymphoscintigraphy in the detection of anatomical and functional abnormalities in the lymphatic system.[66]

Fluorescence microlymphangiography (FML)

FML involves visualisation of the superficial network of lymphatics with a fluorescence microscope following intracutaneous injection of fluorescein isothiocyanate–dextran. It can confirm the clinical diagnosis of lymphoedema and can distinguish various forms of oedema.[56,67] Emanating from the fluorescent spot, the surrounding network of microvessels is filled and becomes easily visible and is recorded by photography or video. In Milroy's disease, a lack of microlymphatics (aplasia) is typical, while in other primary and secondary lymphoedema the network remains intact but the depicted area is enlarged. In lipoedema, lymphatic microaneurysms are seen.

Contrast lymphangiography

This investigation is now used only rarely in the diagnosis of lymphoedema and has been largely replaced by scintigraphy. It is for patients being considered for microvascular lymphatic reconstruction.

Treatment

The aim of treatment is to reduce limb swelling, reduce the risk of infection and improve function. If management begins early in the disease process when pitting oedema is present, conservative measures should be successful. Once achieved, the improvement must be maintained. Surgical options are available in a few centres for resistant and severely symptomatic cases.

General measures

Once the diagnosis is made, a clear explanation of the condition and its non-life-threatening nature should be given to the patient, along with referral to a specialist service.[51] The treatment is improved by empowering the patient to manage their own condition, and the earlier education and treatment are instituted the better the outcome, hence information leaflets can be helpful. In the early stages elevation of a lymphoedematous limb while resting and at night can reduce oedema by increasing venous return and reducing the production of interstitial fluid. Exercise, such as on an exercise bicycle, encourages movement of lymph along non-contractile vessels and increased contractility of collecting lymph vessels. Managing obesity is also important.

Manual lymphatic drainage

This involves manipulating the leg by squeezing just above the most proximal area of oedema and then working from proximal to distal. This enhances lymphatic flow.

Graduated elastic compression

Compression stockings need to exert a pressure of approximately 50 mmHg or higher. The stockings can be used for maintenance of the limb after oedema reduction but compliance is low in the summer months, and the elderly and frail find them difficult to apply. Multilayer bandaging is an essential stage of the intensive phase of management. Inelastic bandages are applied to the limb, providing a low resting pressure but high exercise pressure. This is used to reduce severe swelling, and improve limb shape and skin condition prior to fitting compression hosiery.

> ✓✓ If graduated elastic compression is used initially followed by a stocking for maintenance, a greater and more sustained limb volume reduction is achieved than if stockings alone are used throughout.[68]

Intermittent pneumatic compression (IPC)

IPC involves placement of the limb in a multicompartmental sleeve. Each compartment consists of air cells that are sequentially inflated to a pressure of about 80 mmHg and deflated from distal to proximal, thus massaging the lymph centrally. Patients use this for 4 hours a day and it can be done at home. If the lymphatic system is obliterated or obstructed more proximally, massaging the lymph centrally can precipitate collections elsewhere, such as the genitals, and high pressures may injure peripheral lymphatics. Reports combining IPC with stockings quote figures of 90% for immediate benefit and long-term maintenance.[69] The poor responders have usually had oedema for more than 10 years. In these chronic patients, compression using the hydrostatic pressure of mercury has had some effect.[70] The leg is placed in a cylinder and is covered by two membranes, which are filled and emptied with mercury in cycles. Pressures of up to 80 mmHg are generated at the foot and this linearly decreases towards normal atmospheric pressure at the surface. This is well tolerated and improvement is even seen in those with fibrosclerotic oedema. Despite its theoretical simplicity, the application and safety precautions are complex.

Thermal treatment

Hyperthermia of the leg is produced by microwave heating or immersion in hot water. There is no change to the flow of lymph but it does reduce the local inflammatory infiltrate and extracellular protein matrix.[71] A reduction in limb volume follows, along with a decrease in the rate of recurrent infections.

Complex decongestive physiotherapy (complex physical therapy)

Complex decongestive physiotherapy generally involves a two-stage treatment programme over 2–4 weeks. The first phase consists of skin care, light manual massage, range of motion exercise and compression, typically applied with multilayered bandage wrapping. Phase 2 aims to conserve and optimise the results obtained in phase 1. It consists of compression by a low-stretch elastic stocking or sleeve, skin care, continued 'remedial' exercise and repeated light massage as needed. With good compliance a 65–67% reduction in limb volume can be achieved, with 90% of the reduction being maintained at 9 months.[72] As an added benefit the incidence of infection almost halves and quality of life is improved.[73]

Prevention of infection

The lymphatic system transports lymphocytes, enabling rapid response to foreign antigens. Stagnation of lymph prevents this and so increases the risk and severity of infection. The common pathogens are β-haemolytic streptococci and *Staphylococcus aureus*. With each attack of cellulitis or erysipelas the organisms further obliterate the lymph channels, making the oedema worse. Well-fitting comfortable shoes prevent small cracks in the skin that may act as a portal of entry. Meticulous skin care is essential and the patient should develop a routine that includes washing followed by thorough drying of the limb, application of an emollient, and monitoring the skin for any problems that develop into cellulitis. Any early signs of infection should be treated aggressively with antibiotics. Recurrent infection can be managed by long-term low-dose prophylactic antibiotics such as amoxicillin, flucloxacillin or a cephalosporin.

> ✅ Current guidelines recommend that antibiotics be taken for at least 14 days after signs of clinical improvement are observed.[74]

Drugs

Benzopyrones are thought to reduce oedema by reducing vascular permeability and thus the amount of fluid forming in the subcutaneous tissues. Advocates for this treatment method believe that the drugs have some beneficial effect on pain and discomfort in the swollen areas. Proponents also claim that these drugs increase macrophage activity, encouraging the lysis of protein, which in turn reduces the formation of fibrotic tissue in the lymphoedematous limb. A Cochrane review in 2009 concluded that it is not possible to draw conclusions about the effectiveness of benzopyrones in the management of lymphoedema from the current available trials.[75] Diuretics are not recommended in the management of lymphoedema as there is no evidence that they improve lymphatic drainage.[51]

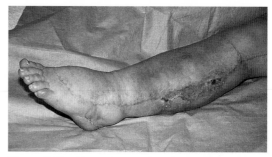

Figure 18.7 • Homan's operation. A long ellipse of skin and subcutaneous tissue has been excised from the lateral side of the leg after a previous procedure on the medial side. Poor wound healing is common.

Surgical treatments

Surgical options are available in some specialist centres. They should be reserved for severely symptomatic patients (e.g. lymphorrhagia or recurrent lymphangitis) in whom all conservative methods have failed. The patient must have realistic expectations of the likely outcome and will need long-term compression therapy after treatment. Surgical procedures can be divided into debulking operations (for obliterative causes) and bypass procedures (for lymphatic obstruction).

Debulking operations

These procedures aim to excise variable amounts of the excess skin and subcutaneous tissue from the affected limb. The techniques range from removal of ellipses of tissue and primary closure (Homan's operation; **Fig. 18.7**) to the radical Charles operation, which excises all the skin and subcutaneous tissues of the calf down to and sometimes including the deep fascia. Primary skin grafting is then required. Good functional results have been obtained with this method but cosmesis is poor and it may be complicated by warts, resistant ulceration, lymph weeping and pantalooning of the thigh. Suction lipectomy, which has good results in the postmastectomy arm,[76] has been advocated in order to overcome these problems but only in the less severe situation because there is a tendency for greater fibrosis in the lower limb. Modern liposuction devices along with the use of tumescent solution and power-assisted cannulae are thought to improve efficacy.[77]

Bypass procedures

These are very rarely performed and are reserved for regional blockage of the lymphatics, due to either primary obstructive or secondary causes. If an iatrogenic secondary cause is suspected, a period of 6 months should elapse to allow any procedural swelling to subside before embarking on a lymphatic bypass. The bypass procedures are listed in Box 18.6.

Box 18.6 • Bypass procedures for lymphoedema

Skin and muscle flaps
Omental bridges
Enteromesenteric bridges
Lymphatico-lymphatic anastomosis
Lymphatico-venous anastomosis

Skin, muscle and omentum have been used to bypass regional obstructions but these tissues tend to have a paucity of lymphatics and as the technique relies on the development of new channels, high levels of success have not been reported. The technique of enteromesenteric bridging was designed to overcome this problem. A 10-cm segment of ileum is resected on its mesentery and opened along its antimesenteric border. The mucosa is dissected off, leaving a submucosal area rich in lymphatics and blood vessels. The uppermost normal nodes are identified and bisected. The submucosal patch is then stitched in place over the top. Investigation has shown the early development of a lymphatic bridge and follow-up for 6 years has demonstrated a maintained improvement in 75% of legs, but the numbers are very small.[78]

Autologous lymphatic vessels harvested from the contralateral normal limb are used to perform lymphatico-lymphatic anastomoses and bypass obstruction. A suitable conduit is identified after the injection of patent blue dye into the interdigital spaces. The anastomoses are technically demanding. Limb volumetry reveals initial improvements in 66% of cases but this falls to about 50% at 1 year. Recent studies show that lower limb bypasses maintain improvement for up to 10 years.[79]

Lymphatico-venous anastomosis is physiological if one considers the termination of the thoracic duct at the subclavian vein. Excellent long-term results have been published, with volume reductions on average of 67% lasting more than 7 years in the 85% of patients followed up, along with an 87% reduction in the incidence of cellulitis.[80]

Key points

- CVI is the commonest cause of chronic leg swelling.
- The risk of mild to moderate chronic venous insufficiency after DVT is 30% at 10 years.
- The risk of severe CVI after DVT is 2–10% at 10 years.
- Superficial venous reflux alone may cause CVI.
- Graduated elastic compression is effective in healing ulcers and preventing recurrence.
- Superficial venous surgery may be of benefit in isolated superficial venous incompetence and combined superficial and deep venous incompetence.
- There is only limited evidence for the benefit of deep venous reconstructive surgery and endovascular therapy.
- Lymphoedema may be classified as primary or secondary.
- A further functional classification of obliterative, proximal obstruction, and valvular incompetence and hyperplasia may be used.
- The commonest cause of lymphoedema worldwide is filariasis but in Europe the commonest cause is malignancy and its treatment.
- Oedema is initially pitting, but becomes non-pitting due to subcutaneous fat deposition and fibrosis.
- Ulceration is rare in lymphoedema.
- Diagnosis is usually confirmed by isotope lymphangioscintigraphy.
- Satisfactory treatment can usually be achieved by conservative measures, including manual drainage, elastic compression, complex decongestive therapy and prevention of infection.

References

1. Ruckley CV, Callam MJ, Dale JJ. Causes of chronic leg ulceration. Lancet 1982;ii:615–6.
2. Cornwall JV, Lewis JD. Leg ulcers: epidemiology and aetiology. Br J Surg 1986;73:693–6.
3. Callam MJ, Harper DR, Dale JJ. Arterial disease in chronic leg ulceration: an underestimated hazard. Lothian and Forth Valley leg ulcer study. Br Med J 1987;294:1389–91.
4. The Alexander House Group. Consensus paper venous leg ulcers. J Dermatol Surg Oncol 1992;18:592–602.

A condensed consensus report summarising the status of various aspects of epidemiology, diagnosis and treatment of venous ulcers. Various investigational and treatment approaches are summarised and recommendations given. Level II evidence.

5. Evans CJ, Fowkes FG, Ruckley CV, et al. Prevalence of varicose veins and chronic venous insufficiency in men and women in the general population: Edinburgh Vein Study. J Epidemiol Community Health 1999;53:149–53.

6. Van den Oever R, Hepp B, Bebbaut B, et al. Socio-economic impact of chronic venous insufficiency. An underestimated public health problem. Int Angiol 1998;17:161–7.

7. Nelzen O, Bergqvist D, Lindhagen A. Venous and non-venous leg ulcers: clinical history and appearance in a population study. Br J Surg 1994;81:182–7.

8. Callam MJ, Ruckley CV, Harper DR, et al. Chronic ulceration of the leg: extent of the problem and provision of care. Br Med J 1985;290:1855–6.

9. Cornwall JV, Dore CJ, Lewis JD. Leg ulcers: epidemiology and aetiology. Br J Surg 1986;73:693–9.

10. Baker SR, Stacey MC, Jopp-McKay AG, et al. Epidemiology of chronic venous ulcers. Br J Surg 1991;78:864–7.

11. Lees TA, Lambert D. Prevalence of lower limb ulceration in an urban health district. Br J Surg 1992;79:1032–4.

12. Cesarone MR, Belcaro G, Nicolaides AN, et al. 'Real' epidemiology of varicose veins and chronic venous disease: the San Valentino Vascular Screening Project. Angiology 2002;53:119–30.

13. Bosanquet N. Costs of venous ulcers: from maintenance therapy to investment programmes. Phlebology 1992;7:44–6.

14. Ruckley CV, Evans CJ, Allan PL, et al. Chronic venous insufficiency: clinical and duplex correlations. The Edinburgh Vein Study of venous disorders in the general population. J Vasc Surg 2002;36:520–5.

15. Lees TA, Lambert D. Patterns of venous reflux in limbs with skin changes associated with chronic venous insufficiency. Br J Surg 1993;80:725–8.

16. Delis KT, Ibegbuna V, Nicolaides AN, et al. Prevalence and distribution of incompetent perforating veins in chronic venous insufficiency. J Vasc Surg 1998;28:815–25.

17. Darke SG, Penfold C. Venous ulceration and saphenous ligation. Eur J Vasc Surg 1992;6:4–9.

18. Lawrence MB, McIntire LV, Eskin SG. Effect of flow on polymorphonuclear leukocyte/endothelial cell adhesion. Blood 1987;70:1284–90.

19. Sahary M, Shields DA, Georgiannos SN, et al. Endothelial activation in patients with chronic venous disease. Eur J Vasc Endovasc Surg 1998;15:342–9.

20. Shoab SS, Scurr JH, Coleridge Smith PD. Increased plasma vascular endothelial growth factor among patients with chronic venous disease. J Vasc Surg 1998;28:535–40.

21. Coleridge Smith PD, Thomas P, Scurr JH, et al. Causes of venous ulceration: a new hypothesis. Br Med J 1988;296:1726–7.

22. Wenner A, Leu HJ, Spycher M, et al. Ultrastructural changes of capillaries in chronic venous insufficiency. Exp Cell Biol 1980;48:1–14.

23. Gajraj H, Browse NL. Fibrinolytic activity of the arms and legs of patients with lower limb venous disease. Br J Surg 1991;78:853–6.

24. Browse NL, Burnand KG. The cause of venous ulceration. Lancet 1982;ii:243–5.

25. Herouy Y, Nockowski P, Schopf E, et al. Lipodermatosclerosis and the significance of proteolytic remodeling in the pathogenesis of venous ulceration. Int J Mol Med 1999;3:511–5.

26. Eklof B, Rutherford RB, Bergan JJ, et al. Revision of CEAP classification for chronic venous disorders: consensus statement. J Vasc Surg 2004;40:1248–52.
This is an international consensus document produced under the auspice of the American Venous Forum that provides a classification for CVI.

27. Coleridge-Smith P, Labropoulos N, Partsch H, et al. Duplex ultrasound investigation of the veins in chronic venous disease of the lower limbs – UIP consensus document, part I. Basic principles. Eur J Vasc Endovasc Surg 2006;31:83–92.

28. Mayberry JC, Moneta GL, Taylor Jr LM, et al. Fifteen year results of ambulatory compression therapy for chronic venous ulcers. Surgery 1991;109:575–81.

29. O'Meara S, Cullum NA, Nelson EA. Compression for venous leg ulcers. Cochrane Database Syst Rev 2009;1: CD000265.
This is a meta-analysis of 39 randomised controlled trials reporting 47 comparisons of compression versus no compression or versus other types of compression in the healing of venous leg ulcers.

30. Nelson EA, Bell-Syer SEM, Cullum NA, et al. Compression for preventing recurrence of venous ulcers. Cochrane Database Syst Rev 2000;4: CD002303.
This is a review of two randomised controlled trials, one of which compared class III stockings with class II stockings and the other compared two different makes of class II stocking in the prevention of ulcer recurrence. Higher grades of compression are associated with lower recurrence rates. Also, not wearing stockings is strongly associated with ulcer recurrence.

31. Ruckley CV. Treatment of venous ulceration: compression therapy. Phlebology 1992;1(Suppl.): 22–6.

32. Nelson EA, Mani R, Thomas K, et al. Intermittent pneumatic compression for treating venous leg ulcers. Cochrane Database Syst Rev 2011;2: CD001899.

This is a review of seven randomised controlled trials; four compared IPC plus compression with compression alone. One of these found increased ulcer healing with IPC, while three found no evidence of benefit. One trial compared IPC without additional compression with compression alone and found no difference, and in one trial more ulcers healed with IPC than with dressings. One trial found that rapid IPC healed more ulcers than slow IPC.

33. Flemming K, Cullum NA. Laser therapy for venous leg ulcers. Cochrane Database Syst Rev 1999;1: CD001182.
Four trials were available, two randomised controlled trials compared laser therapy with sham, one with ultraviolet light and one with red light. Neither of the two randomised controlled trials found a difference in healing rates and there was no significant benefit for laser when the trials were pooled.

34. Aziz Z, Cullum NA, Flemming K. Electromagnetic therapy for treating venous leg ulcers. Cochrane Database Syst Rev 2011;3: CD002933.
This is a review of 3 randomised controlled trials comparing electromagnetic therapy (EMT) with sham treatment. One small trial of 44 patients reported significantly more ulcers healed in the EMT group, one reported no difference and one reported a greater reduction in ulcer size in the EMT group.

35. Palfreyman SSJ, Nelson EA, Lochiel R, et al. Dressings for healing venous leg ulcers. Cochrane Database Syst Rev 2006;3: CD001103.
This is a meta-analysis of 42 randomised controlled trials evaluating various types of dressings in the treatment of venous leg ulcers. In none of the comparisons was there evidence that any one type of dressing was better than others in terms of the numbers of ulcers healed.

36. Vuerstaek JDD, Vainas T, Wuite J, et al. State-of-the-art treatment of chronic leg ulcers: a randomized controlled trial comparing vacuum-assisted closure (V.A.C.) with modern wound dressings. J Vasc Surg 2006;44:1029–37.

37. Michaels JA, Campbell B, King B, et al. Randomized controlled trial and cost-effectiveness analysis of silver-donating antimicrobial dressings for venous leg ulcers (VULCAN trial). Br J Surg 2009;96(10):1147–56.

38. Jull AB, Arroll B, Parag V, et al. Pentoxifylline for treating venous leg ulcers. Cochrane Database Syst Rev 2007;3: CD001733.
This is a meta-analysis of 12 trials, 11 of which compared pentoxifylline (oxpentifylline) with placebo or no treatment. Pentoxifylline is more effective than placebo in terms of complete ulcer healing or significant improvement. The relative risk of ulcer healing with oxpentifylline compared with placebo is 1.70.

39. Barwell J, Davies C, Deacon J, et al. Comparison of surgery and compression with compression alone in chronic venous ulceration (ESCHAR study): randomized controlled trial. Lancet 2004;363:1854.
This is a randomised controlled trial of 500 consecutive patients with chronic venous ulcers randomly assigned to compression alone or in combination with surgery to assess the role of superficial venous surgery in the healing and prevention of recurrence of leg ulcers. There was no difference in initial healing rates but a reduction in recurrence at 12 months in the surgical group (12% vs. 28%).

40. Hardy SC, Riding G, Abidia A. Surgery for deep venous incompetence. Cochrane Database Syst Rev 2004;3: CD001097.
This is a review of randomised trials of surgical treatment of patients with deep venous incompetence. Only one trial was found comparing superficial venous ligation and limited deep anterior valve plication with superficial ligation alone, with moderate improvement in clinical outcome in the former group compared with mild improvement in the latter group.

41. Killewich LA, Bedford GR, Beach KW, et al. Spontaneous lysis of deep venous thrombi: rate and outcome. J Vasc Surg 1989;9:89–97.

42. Palma EC, Esperon R. Vein transplants and grafts in the surgical treatment of the postphlebitic syndrome. J Cardiovasc Surg (Torino) 1960;1:94–107.

43. Halliday P, Harris J, May J. Femoro-femoral cross-over grafts (Palma operation), a long term follow up study. In: Bergan JF, Yao JST, editors. Surgery of the veins. New York: Grune & Stratton; 1985. p. 241.

44. Raju S, McAllister S, Neglen P. Recanalisation of totally occluded iliac and adjacent venous segments. J Vasc Surg 2002;36:903–11.

45. O'Sullivan GJ, Semba CP, Bittner CA, et al. Endovascular management of iliac vein compression (May–Thurner syndrome). J Vasc Interv Radiol 2000;11:823–36.

46. Raju S, Owen Jr S, Neglen P. The clinical impact of iliac venous stents in the management of chronic venous insufficiency. J Vasc Surg 2002;35:8–15.

47. Janssen MC, Haenen JH, van Asten WN, et al. Clinical and haemodynamic sequelae of deep venous thrombosis: retrospective evaluation after 7–13 years. Clin Sci 1997;93:7–12.
In this study, 81 patients with venographically confirmed lower-extremity DVT were clinically and haemodynamically re-examined 7–13 years after DVT (mean 10 years) to assess PTS; 7–13 years after DVT 31% of the patients had moderate and 2% had severe clinical PTS, while 57% of the patients had abnormal haemodynamic findings. Level II evidence.

48. Franzeck UK, Schalch I, Bollinger A. On the relationship between changes in the deep veins evaluated by duplex sonography and the post-thrombotic syndrome 12 years after deep venous thrombosis. Thromb Haemost 1997;77:1109–12.

49. Johnson BF, Manzo RA, Bergelin RO, et al. Relationship between changes in the deep venous system and the development of the postthrombotic syndrome after an acute episode of lower limb deep

vein thrombosis: a one- to six-year follow up. J Vasc Surg 1995;21:307–12.

50. McCollum C. Avoiding the consequences of deep venous thrombosis. Br Med J 1998;517:696.

51. Lymphoedema Framework. Best practice for the management of lymphoedema. International consensus. London: MEP Ltd; 2006.

52. Kinmonth JB, Wolfe JH. Fibrosis in the lymph nodes in primary lymphoedema. Histological and clinical studies in 74 patients with lower limb oedema. Ann R Coll Surg Engl 1980;62:344–54.

53. Browse NL. The diagnosis and management of primary lymphoedema. J Vasc Surg 1986;3:181–4.

54. Moffatt CJ, Franks PJ, Doherty DC, et al. Lymphoedema: an underestimated health problem. QJM 2003;96(10):731–8.

55. Chant ADB. Hypothesis: why venous oedema causes ulcers and lymphoedema does not. Eur J Vasc Surg 1992;6:427–9.

56. The diagnosis and treatment of peripheral lymphedema: consensus document of the International Society of Lymphology. Lymphology 2003;36:84–91.

57. International guidelines on lymphedema and lymphatic disorders. The diagnosis and treatment of peripheral oedema. Consensus Document of the International Society of Lymphology 2009. www.eurolymphology.org.

58. Gloviczki P, Calcagno D, Schirger A, et al. Noninvasive evaluation of the swollen extremity: experiences with 190 lymphoscintigraphic examinations. J Vasc Surg 1989;9:683–98.

59. Szuba A, Shin WS, Strauss HW, et al. The third circulation: radionuclide lymphoscintigraphy in the evaluation of lymphedema. J Nucl Med 2003;44(1):43–57.

60. Monnin-Delhom ED, Gallix BP, Achard C, et al. High resolution unenhanced computed tomography in patients with swollen legs. Lymphology 2002;35(3):121–8.

61. Haaverstad R, Nilsen G, Myhre HO, et al. The use of MRI in the investigation of leg oedema. Eur J Vasc Surg 1992;6:124–9.

62. Case TC, Witte MH, Unger EC, et al. Magnetic resonance imaging in human lymphoedema: comparison with lymphangioscintigraphy. Magn Reson Imaging 1992;10:549–58.

63. Ruehm SG, Shroeder T, Debatin JF. Interstitial MR lymphangiography with gadoterate meglumine: experience in humans. Radiology 2001;220:816–21.

64. Lohrmann C, Foeldi E, Speck O, et al. High resolution MR lymphangiography in patients with primary and secondary lymphedema. Am J Radiol 2006;187:556–61.

65. Lohrmann C, Foeldi E, Bartholoma JP, et al. MR imaging of the lymphatic system: distribution and contrast enhancement of gadodiamide after intradermal injection. Lymphology 2006;39:156–63.

66. Liu NF, Lu Q, Liu PA, et al. Comparison of radionuclide lymphoscintigraphy and dynamic magnetic resonance lymphangiography for investigating extremity lymphedema. Br J Surg 2010;97(3):359–65.

67. Bollinger A, Amann-Vesti BR. Fluorescence microlymphography: diagnostic potential in lymphedema and basis for the measurement of lymphatic pressure and flow velocity. Lymphology 2007;40:52–62.

68. Badger CM, Peacock JL, Mortimer PS. A randomised, controlled, parallel-group trial comparing multilayer bandaging followed by hosiery versus hosiery alone in the treatment of patients with lymphedema of the limb. Cancer 2000;88:2832–7.
This is a randomised, controlled, parallel-group trial in which 90 women with unilateral lymphoedema (of the upper or lower limbs) underwent 18 days of multilayer bandaging followed by elastic hosiery or hosiery alone, each for a total period of 24 weeks. The reduction in limb volume due to multilayer bandaging followed by hosiery was approximately double that from hosiery alone and was sustained over the 24-week period. The mean overall percentage reduction at 24 weeks was 31% (n=32) for multilayer bandaging versus 15.8% (n=46) for hosiery alone, with a mean difference of 15.2% (95% CI 6.2–24.2, P=0.001). Level I evidence.

69. Pappas CJ, O'Donnell TF. Long-term results of compression treatment for lymphedema. J Vasc Surg 1992;16:555–64.

70. Palmer A, Macchiaverna J, Braun A, et al. Compression therapy of limb oedema using hydrostatic pressure of mercury. Angiology 1991;42:533–42.

71. Liu NF, Olszewski W. The influence of local hyperthermia on lymphedematous skin of the human leg. Lymphology 1993;26:28–37.

72. Cheville AL, McGarvey CL, Petrek JA, et al. Lymphedema management. Semin Radiat Oncol 2003;13:290–301.

73. Weiss JM, Spray BJ. The effect of complete decongestive therapy on the quality of life of patients with peripheral lymphedema. Lymphology 2002;35:46–58.

74. Consensus document on the management of cellulitis in lymphoedema. British Lymphology Society. www.thebls.com/consensus.php.

75. Badger C, Preston N, Seers K, et al. Benzo-pyrones for reducing and controlling lymphoedema of the limbs. Cochrane Database Syst Rev 2003;4:CD003140.

76. Brorson H, Svenson H. Liposuction combined with controlled compression therapy reduces arm lymphedema more effectively than controlled compression therapy alone. Plast Reconstr Surg 1998;102:1058–67.

77. Greene AK, Slavin SA, Borud L. Treatment of lower extremity lymphedema with suction-assisted lipectomy. Plast Reconstr Surg 2006;118:118–21.

78. Hurst PAE, Stewart G, Kinmonth JB, et al. Long-term results of the enteromesenteric bridge operation in the treatment of primary lymphoedema. Br J Surg 1985;72:272–4.

79. Baumeister RG, Frick A. The microsurgical lymph vessel transplantation. Handchir Mikrochir Plast Chir 2003;35:202–9.

80. Campisi C, Eretta C, Pertile D, et al. Microsurgery for the treatment of peripheral lymphedema: long term outcome and future perspectives. Microsurgery 2007;27:333–8.

19

The acutely swollen leg

Cees H.A. Wittens
Rob H.W. Strijkers

Introduction

The acutely swollen leg is a common presenting complaint in the emergency room. It may represent a sudden presentation of an underlying chronic disease or it may be the manifestation of a new acute problem, in particular deep vein thrombosis (DVT). A number of diseases can be associated with swelling of the lower extremity. It is important to identify the cause of the swelling, as treatment differs greatly depending on the underlying pathology. The underlying diagnosis may be life threatening and make immediate action necessary, and will also influence long-term prognosis and follow-up.

This chapter will help in the evaluation of the acutely swollen leg and will present up to date information on the treatment of DVT.

Pathophysiology of oedema

Acute swelling of the leg is caused by tissue oedema. Oedema formation is caused by excess water accumulation in the interstitial space of the tissue. Reasons for accumulation of water in the interstitial space are increased hydrostatic pressure, decreased colloid osmotic pressure, increased capillary permeability and lymphatic obstruction. These factors cause rapid fluid shifts in the body. There are also chronic states that cause oedema, but these are beyond the scope of this chapter. The mechanisms causing the shift in fluids are described below.

Increased hydrostatic pressure forces fluid out of the intravascular space. This is usually seen with any process that increases venous pressure. Central causes for increase of hydrostatic pressure include congestive heart failure, right heart failure and tricuspid insufficiency. Focal or unilateral oedema is often the result of DVT causing venous outflow obstruction.

Decreased colloid osmotic pressure allows passive transfer of intravascular fluid to the interstitial compartment. This is generally the result of reduction of intravascular protein content (i.e. hypoalbuminaemia). This mechanism causes generalised oedema and is rarely acute.

Increased capillary permeability removes the barrier to water moving from the intravascular space to the interstitial space. This is observed with focal trauma, burns, infection, ischaemia and immunological injury. This can cause rapid oedema forming in a single leg or it can present as a generalised oedema.

Lymphatic obstruction (lymphoedema) may be the result of hereditary hypoplasia, acute infection, or a consequence of lymphatic ablation following surgery, trauma or radiation. The trigger is usually identifiable and presentation is rarely acute.

Medical history

A good medical history from the patient will often raise suspicion regarding the underlying pathology. A previous history of operations on the leg, trauma or a history of DVT may be useful, along with an overview of the patient's general health. There are often several differential diagnoses despite an accurate history. The correct diagnosis, or exclusion of DVT, is essential to prevent potentially life-threatening complications. Consequently, several decision tools have been developed, including the Wells score.[1] It is important to ascertain the precise time point when symptoms began, as this can influence both treatment and prognosis.

Physical examination

Upon examination of the leg specific features should be identified. The swollen leg may be accompanied by redness, tenderness in the calf and increased temperature. An entry point may be found in cases of erysipelas. Swelling around a specific muscle or muscle compartment may increase suspicion of muscle rupture. Despite a good medical history and thorough physical examination, additional investigations are usually required to confirm a diagnosis. If DVT is suspected, additional imaging may be necessary. Severe pain and loss of sensory and motor function may point towards a compartment syndrome. Skin changes, varicose veins and ulceration of the leg may point towards a chronic venous insufficiency.

Differential diagnosis

There are a few differential diagnoses for the acutely swollen leg. The most frequent cause is a DVT. If DVT is suspected it should be ruled out before any other diagnosis is considered. Other possible causes for acute leg swelling include a ruptured Baker's cyst, erysipelas, cellulitis, fasciitis, muscle rupture or lymphoedema. These causes are mostly limited to one leg. If the patient has swelling of both legs, then alternative causes should be considered, in particular systemic causes such as chronic heart failure, renal failure or sepsis.

Musculotendinous rupture

Sudden intense pain of the calf usually suggests a musculoskeletal aetiology. If associated with sudden dorsiflexion of the foot, rupture of the musculotendinous portion of the medial head of the gastrocnemius muscle or the plantaris muscle (tendon) should be suspected. Localised pain in the medial or mid calf area and swelling at the ankle level is common. Ecchymotic discoloration at the ankle level often follows 2–5 days later due to blood tracking down the fascial planes when the leg is dependent. Excluding DVT with a venous duplex examination is appropriate.

Treatment consists of symptomatic and supportive care until symptoms resolve. Leg elevation, ice early followed by heat, analgesics and reduced weight bearing may be necessary until symptoms resolve, usually within a month.

Baker's cyst

Patients presenting with sudden, instantaneously severe calf pain and swelling of the leg may suffer from a ruptured Baker's cyst. A Baker's cyst forms as a result of overproduction of synovial fluid secondary to an underlying cause such as degenerative arthritis, meniscal tears, gout or rheumatoid arthritis. It is common among adults, but can occur in children.[2] A Baker's cyst is usually located on the dorsolateral side of the knee. If the cyst bursts, immediate pain occurs, with swelling of the leg and redness, often mimicking a DVT.[3] The Baker's cyst is usually easily identified with duplex ultrasound.[4] Treatment consists of anti-inflammatory medication, leg elevation and application of cold packs.[5]

Cellulitis and erysipelas

Sudden swelling of the leg, combined with redness, pain and increased warmth, is seen in patients with erysipelas or cellulitis. Accompanying complaints can be nausea vomiting, headaches and fever. The terms erysipelas and cellulitis are both used. There is however a small distinction between the two diagnosis. They differ in that erysipelas involves the upper dermis and superficial lymphatics, whereas cellulitis involves the deeper dermis and subcutaneous fat. This manifest in a different presentation in erysipelas where there is a clear line of demarcation of the redness and the skin involved. In cellulitis there is no clear demarcation visible. Upon physical examination it is important to look for a break in the skin as a portal for entry of bacteria. Common skin barrier breaks are abrasions, insect bites, or tinea pedis. Any fluid coming from the wound should be cultured. The most likely causative bacteria are *Staphylococcus aureus* and Group A streptococci.[6] Treatment comprises antibiotics targeted towards Gram-positive bacteria, rest and elevation. Duplex ultrasound should be considered to exclude DVT. Patients treated for erysipelas or cellulitis should experience symptom improvement with in 24 to 48 hours.

Necrotising fasciitis

Fasciitis is a very serious condition with a high morbidity and mortality. While this may present as excruciating pain,[7] other clinical signs may be absent. Possible clinical signs include erythema, crepitations due to gas formed by subcutaneous bacteria, fever, nausea, vomiting, local oedema, blisters, and necrosis of the skin and underlying structures. The underlying mechanism is a bacterial colonisation of *Staphylococcus aureus* or Group A streptococci. The micro-organisms produce endotoxins, which cause a severe inflammatory reaction, with destruction of the deep fascia and surrounding structures. Patients with a compromised immune system are more susceptible to infection with opportunistic bacteria. If this situation is left untreated the destruction of the fascia will spread and eventually lead to the death of the patient. Treatment of necrotising fasciitis consists of aggressive surgical debridement of the infected tissues. Broad-spectrum antibiotics should be given to include coverage for Gram-positive, Gram-negative and anaerobic organisms.[8] Additional intensive care support is vital to improve the chance of survival. Even with optimal treatment, the mortality rate is over 30%.[9]

Lymphoedema

Although lymphoedema usually presents as a chronically swollen leg, it can occasionally present acutely. Lymphoedema is the result of impaired lymphatic drainage due to obstruction or destruction of lymphatic tissue. The major causes of lymphoedema can be classified as primary (hereditary) or secondary (acquired). Causes of primary lymphoedema are congenital lymphoedema, lymphoedema praecox and lymphoedema tarda. These causes manifest themselves in childhood (congenital lymphoedema), puberty (lymphoedema praecox) or early adulthood (lymphoedema tarda). Secondary lymphoedema can be caused by malignancy, surgery with lymph dissection, radiation therapy, infection of lymph nodes, recurrent cellulitis or a connective tissue disease. The management of lymphoedema is discussed in Chapter 18.

Bilateral swelling

Swelling of both legs is usually a sign of a systemic problem, such as heart failure, renal failure, liver failure, sepsis, pulmonary hypertension or drugs (non-steroidal anti-inflammatory drugs (NSAIDs) and calcium blockers), but it is essential to rule out bilateral DVT or vena caval obstruction. History and examination will usually guide further investigation.[10] If the patient has a bilateral swelling caused by a systemic disease, treatment should focus on the primary cause. If the patient uses calcium blockers or NSAIDs, alternatives for these medications can be considered.

Deep venous thrombosis

DVT is very common in the western world, with an incidence of 1.6 per 1000 persons per year.[11] The incidence of DVT increases exponentially over the age of 70. In people under 18 years of age, DVT is very uncommon, with an incidence of 0.07 per 10000 per year.[12] In the 19th century, Virchow postulated the mechanisms for clot formation. The three main mechanisms are stasis of blood, vessel wall damage and hypercoagulability. Once the clot has formed it has the tendency to extend. Thrombosis in calf veins does not usually elicit much in the way of symptoms. Once the clot has propagated in the popliteal vein symptoms

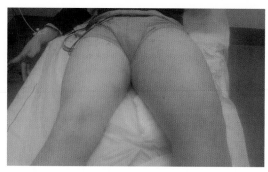

Figure 19.1 • Leg with phlegmasia cerulea dolens.

may become more apparent. If the clot further propagates to the femoral vein and common femoral vein, obstructing venous outflow from the leg, more severe symptoms are likely. At the most severe end of the spectrum is phlegmasia cerulea alba or phlegmasia cerulea dolens (see **Fig. 19.1**). These conditions require immediate attention from the physician, because of possible limb ischaemia and loss of the leg.

Pathophysiology of DVT

DVT should be viewed as a dynamic condition, and often results from a combination of risk factors that shift the balance of coagulation to a hypercoagulable state. A number of risk factors have been identified, which can be categorised relating to Virchow's triad (Table 19.1).[13] Thrombus usually forms around valves on the endothelium. In 80% of cases one or more risk factors can be determined in the patient.

Clinical decision rules

Because clinical signs are not very specific for DVT, clinical decision tools have been developed to aid patient management. The Wells score is the most widely used and validated clinical decision tool.[14,15] The patient's risk for having a DVT is assessed by the criteria shown in Table 19.2. The patient is then categorised into either a high- or low-risk group. A Wells score of 2 or more indicates that the patient has a high risk of DVT.[1] A Wells score of 0 or 1 puts the patient in the low-risk group. The Wells score combined with a D-dimer test can guide the clinician with regard to the need for a duplex scan. A patient with either a Wells score of 2 or more and/or positive D-dimer test will need a duplex scan to look for a possible DVT. Conversely, a Wells score of 0 or 1 with a negative D-dimer almost entirely rules out DVT and the patient does not require a duplex scan. Studies show the negative predictive value for this combination of findings to be 99% for excluding DVT.[16] The clinical decision flow chart is shown in **Fig. 19.2**.

✓✓ If the patient has a low Wells score combined with a negative D-dimer, DVT can be safely ruled out without the need for a duplex scan.

Table 19.1 • Risk factors for DVT

Risk factor	Hypercoagulability	Stasis	Venous injury
Age	X	X	
Immobilisation		X	
Surgery	X	X	
Trauma	X	X	X
Malignancy	X		
Primary hypercoagulable states	X		
History of DVT	X		
Family history	X		
Oral contraceptives	X		
Oestrogen replacement	X		
Pregnancy and puerperium	X	X	
Entiphospholipid and anticardiolipin antibody	X		
Central venous catheters			X
Inflammatory bowel disease	X		
Obesity		X	
Myocardial infarction/ congestive heart failure		X	
Varicose veins		X	

Table 19.2 • Wells score for DVT

Score	Clinical factor
1 point	Active cancer <6 months or palliation
1 point	Paralysis, paresis or recent plaster immobilisation of the lower extremities
1 point	Recently bedridden for more than 3 days or major surgery, within 4 weeks
1 point	Entire leg swollen
1 point	Calf swelling by more than 3 cm when compared with the asymptomatic leg
1 point	Pitting oedema
1 point	Collateral superficial veins (non-varicose)
1 point	Previously documented DVT
−2 points	Alternative diagnosis more likely or greater than that of deep vein thrombosis
Total score	
<2	Low risk of DVT
≥2	High risk of DVT

Imaging techniques

The current standard for diagnosing a DVT is a two-point duplex scan.[17] The non-invasive two-point ultrasound examination looks at the popliteal vein and the common femoral vein. The physician will compress the vein at these two points. If the vein is non-compressible, the presence of thrombus is proven. Thrombus may also be visible on sonography and venous flow may be absent. Alternative diagnoses, such as a Baker's cyst, may also be identified on ultrasound. If the duplex scan is inconclusive, but the suspicion of DVT is still high, a conventional venogram or other imaging may be considered. Conventional venography is still the gold standard, but duplex ultrasound is much more accessible, less invasive and easier to perform. In cases of recurrent DVT it may prove difficult to differentiate between newly formed thrombus and old residual thrombus. Standardised documentation of the previous thrombus location may be helpful. The size of the vein and the identification of scarring may help guide the clinician, with small scarred veins most likely to represent chronic changes. In experienced hands it is also possible to estimate thrombus age based on homogeneity. A thrombus with a homogenous aspect is more likely to be fresh. It should also be recognised that fresh thrombus may form within a recanalised area of old thrombus. **Figure 19.3** shows a duplex scan of the common femoral vein with intraluminal thrombus.

New techniques are becoming more readily available for imaging of the venous system, including computed tomography and magnetic resonance venography. These techniques can be used to identify DVT but are especially useful in determining the precise extent of the thrombus and any underlying stenosis. In particular, the iliac vein segment and the inferior vena cava

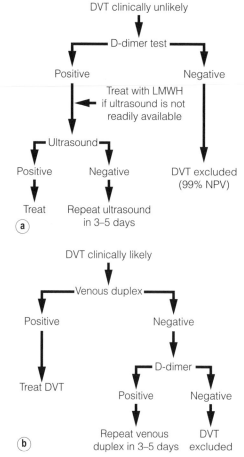

DVT clinically unlikely

D-dimer test

Positive   Negative

Treat with LMWH
if ultrasound is not
readily available

Ultrasound

Positive   Negative   DVT excluded
(99% NPV)

Treat   Repeat ultrasound
in 3–5 days

(a)

DVT clinically likely

Venous duplex

Positive   Negative

Treat DVT   D-dimer

Positive   Negative

Repeat venous   DVT
duplex in 3–5 days   excluded

(b)

Figure 19.2 • Clinical decision flow chart.

can be assessed in a simpler manner than with duplex ultrasound.[18,19] These techniques will become very important in identifying patients suitable for more aggressive intervention than standard anticoagulation

therapy. New reporting standards have been developed to standardise the scoring of venous disease with different imaging techniques (LOVE score). With these standardised reports it is possible to identify and report DVT systematically and stratify patients into different treatment groups (LET score).[20,21] This will become more important as treatment options advance further. **Figure 19.4** shows a magnetic resonance venograph with a DVT present in the popliteal vein and femoral vein of the left leg.

Treatment of DVT

DVT needs to be treated immediately to prevent potentially lethal pulmonary emboli and to stop thrombus propagation. Standard treatment of DVT as formulated by the American College of Chest Physicians (ACCP) guidelines consists of three aspects, namely oral anticoagulation, compression therapy and mobilisation.

Anticoagulation treatment prevents extension of thrombus and pulmonary embolism. Treatment should be started as soon as the diagnosis has been confirmed or in a patient with a Wells score of 2 or more and/or a positive D-dimer test while awaiting duplex scan confirmation. Anticoagulation is achieved by immediate subcutaneous administration of therapeutic levels of low-molecular-weight heparins (LMWHs). Oral anticoagulation with vitamin K antagonists can be started simultaneously. Treatment with the LMWHs can be stopped after the international normalised ratio (INR) has reached the therapeutic range for two consecutive days. The range for a first-time DVT should be between 2 and 3.[22] Anticoagulation should be given for at least 3 months. Depending on the balance of risk of bleeding and further DVT, the physician can choose to prolong the anticoagulation to 6 or 12 months.[23] Patients with malignancy should be treated with

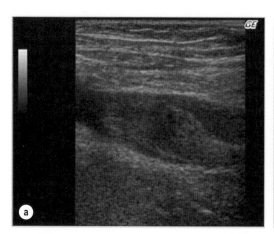
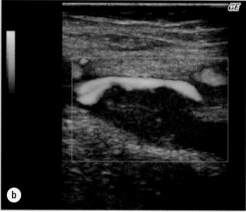

Figure 19.3 • Duplex scan of the common femoral vein with intraluminal thrombus.

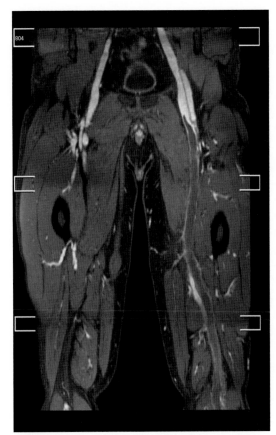

Figure 19.4 • Magnetic resonance venography with a DVT present in the popliteal vein and femoral vein of the left leg.

LMWHs for 3–6 months. Patients with a recurrent episode of DVT should be treated with lifelong anticoagulation. Hospitalisation for anticoagulation therapy is not necessary and treatment can be performed safely in the community.[24] Anticoagulation has no effect on the existing thrombus, resolution of which depends on the patient's own lytic system.[22,23]

> ✔✔ Patients with DVT should be treated with anticoagulation therapy for at least 3 months.

Compression therapy should be started as soon as possible. In the acute phase with leg oedema, compression therapy can be achieved with short stretch bandages. Once this has reduced the acute swelling, the patient can be switched to therapeutic elastic compressive stockings. The stockings should be to the knee, and effect a minimum pressure of between 30 and 40 mmHg. If worn for 2 years, there is a 50% reduction in post-thrombotic morbidity.[25] However, despite encouragement, patient compliance for compression hosiery is low.

> ✔✔ Patients should wear compressive stockings for 2 years in order to reduce post-thrombotic syndrome by up to 50%.

Finally, immediate mobilisation is proven to be safe and does not increase the risk of pulmonary embolism.[26,27]

Thromboprophylaxis is discussed in Chapter 14 of *Core Topics in General and Emergency Surgery*, part of this series.

Prognosis

If patients are treated according to the ACCP guidelines, the risk of recurrent DVT is 30% within 5 years of the initial DVT.[28] More worrisome is the high incidence of post-thrombotic syndrome (PTS), affecting between 20% and 50% of patients with DVT within 2 years,[29,30] because the variability in reported incidence relates to the use of different scales to assess PTS.[31] Patients with iliofemoral DVT have a twofold increased risk of developing PTS than patients with a below-knee DVT.[32] The CaVenT study recently showed that 56% of patients after iliofemoral DVT develop PTS within 2 years.[33]

Iliofemoral deep vein thrombosis

In iliofemoral DVT the thrombus is located proximally, having extended from the common femoral vein segment or commenced within the iliac veins or inferior vena cava. Thrombus in the common femoral vein obstructs outflow of the superficial and deep femoral vein, usually resulting in marked leg swelling and pain. Severe venous obstruction can result in phlegmasia cerulea dolens. This is a dangerous condition, where the circulation is compromised and may lead to amputation. Current ACCP guidelines suggest that immediate clot removal may be considered in specific patients with low bleeding risks. In all other cases of iliofemoral DVT, anticoagulation is still considered the gold standard,[22] though recent studies have challenged this.[34]

Post-thrombotic syndrome

PTS is a chronic disease following DVT, with significant impacts on patient quality of life and healthcare burden.[3] PTS incorporates a range of patient complaints and physical signs of venous disease. The severity of PTS can be recorded using the validated Villalta–Prandoni scale[35] (Table 19.3). The precise aetiology is unknown, though there are identified risk factors that increase the risk of

Table 19.3 • Villalta scale for post-thrombotic syndrome (also incorporates the presence or absence of venous ulceration)

Symptoms and clinical signs	None	Mild	Moderate	Severe
Symptoms				
Pain	0	1	2	3
Cramps	0	1	2	3
Heaviness	0	1	2	3
Paraesthesia	0	1	2	3
Pruritis	0	1	2	3
Clinical signs				
Pretibial oedema	0	1	2	3
Skin induration	0	1	2	3
Hyperpigmentation	0	1	2	3
Redness	0	1	2	3
Venous ectasia	0	1	2	3
Pain on calf compression	0	1	2	3
Venous ulcer	Absent	Present		
Total score	<5	5–9	10–14	≥15 or venous ulcer
PTS classification	No PTS	Mild PTS	Moderate PTS	Severe PTS

developing PTS. Obstruction of the venous outflow tract together with insufficiency, residual thrombus and recurrent DVT are significant risk factors correlating with the development of PTS.[30,36] In particular, poor recanalisation of iliofemoral DVT causes outflow obstruction and a state of venous hypertension, which in turn causes inflammation and vein wall damage.[37–39] The recanalisation process and inflammation also cause valves to be destroyed, resulting in venous insufficiency. Successful early thrombus removal or lysis should avoid these complications and thus lower postthrombotic morbidity.[40] The concept of lysis is not new. Reports and case series from the 1980s stimulated interest in systemic thrombolytic therapy. While results of clinical trials showed that systemic thrombolysis slightly improved complete clot lysis, the high incidence of major bleeding complications has rendered the technique obsolete.[41,42]

✓✓ Systemic thrombolysis should not be given to patients with DVT, because of high major bleeding risk.

However, the severity and chronicity of symptoms is still well recognised,[43] stimulating interest in lysis delivered locally. Catheter-directed lysis has been shown to improve patient quality of life without the high rate of bleeding complications associated with systemic treatment.[44]

Catheter-directed thrombolysis

Catheter-directed thrombolysis (CDT) involves the placement of a catheter directly into the thrombus and local administration of the thrombolytic agent. The drug activates tissue plasminogen, which is converted into plasmin, which in turn can dissolve the fibrin strands of the clot.[45] Local administration in the thrombus enhances the thrombolytic effects but reduces the bleeding complications, because of the lower dosages needed. Retrospective studies have shown that successful lysis directly correlated with improved health-related quality of life.[46] Recently the randomised controlled CaVenT study showed that patients with iliofemoral DVT treated with catheter-directed thrombolysis had an absolute risk reduction of 14% in developing PTS compared to patients treated with standard therapy after 2 years. There was a 3% incidence of major haemorrhage. This is the first randomised controlled trial showing the benefits of early clot removal in iliofemoral DVT with an acceptable bleeding risk.[33] Two other similar trials, ATTRACT and CAVA, are ongoing.[47,48]

The Society for Vascular Surgery (SVS) and American Venous Forum have developed guidelines for the use of CDT and other clot removal techniques (see below). They recommend early thrombus removal in ambulatory patients with good functional capacity and a first episode of iliofemoral DVT of <14 days duration (Grade 2c evidence). They strongly

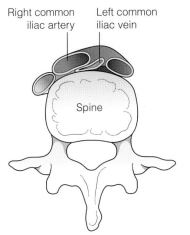

Figure 19.5 • Schematic overview of the May–Thurner syndrome.

recommend such a strategy in patients with limb-threatening ischaemia secondary to iliofemoral DVT (Grade 1a). The guidelines suggest a role for pharmacomechanical strategies over CDT alone if resources are available, and that surgical thrombectomy be considered only if CDT is contraindicated (Grade 2c).[49]

A meta-analysis has suggested that the evidence for surgical thrombectomy is of low quality, reinforcing the recommendation of the SVS. It does, however, confirm the reduced incidence of PTS and venous obstruction follwing CDT.[50]

A number of CDT studies have demonstrated underlying iliac vein stenosis as a potential contributing factor for further DVT.[51,52] May–Thurner syndrome is the most prevalent of the stenotic lesions in the left common iliac vein. This syndrome is a condition where the left common iliac vein is compressed by the overlying right iliac artery, as demonstrated in **Fig. 19.5**.[53] Treatment of the underlying stenosis with balloon venoplasty, stenting, or both, can be performed to relieve venous outflow obstruction, though the role of these interventions remains ill-defined.[54,55] As more data become available regarding CDT for iliofemoral DVT, we will obtain greater understanding of the role and appropriate management of underlying iliac vein stenoses.

> ✔ Patients with iliofemoral DVT should be considered for catheter-directed thrombolysis to reduce the incidence of post-thrombotic syndrome.

New treatment modalities

Although the results of lysis in the CaVenT study are good, the mean treatment time of 2.4 days is considered long. Future techniques will focus on shortening the treatment time, lowering bleeding risk and avoiding the need for expensive intensive care hospitalisation. Therefore the addition of a mechanical component has been suggested to speed up clot removal. This technique is called pharmacomechanical thrombolysis (PMT). At the time of writing, there are three different commercially available devices.

EKOS endowave

The EKOS endowave catheter combines the standard catheter-directed thrombolysis with ultrasound elements. These elements emit high-frequency,

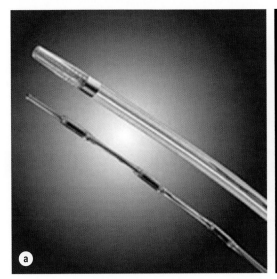
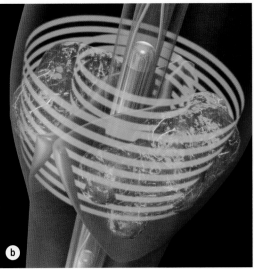

Figure 19.6 • EKOS device.

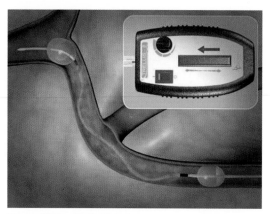

Figure 19.7 • Trellis-8 device.

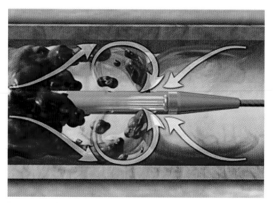

Figure 19.8 • Angiojet device.

low-energy ultrasound waves that enhance the penetration of the thrombolytic drug into the thrombus, enhancing the lytic effect. In vitro studies have shown better permeability of the agent in the thrombus and reduced treatment time. Retrospective case series have shown that thrombolysis with the EKOS catheter is feasible and safe. The ongoing randomised controlled Dutch CAVA trial is further investigating the role of the EKOS endowave system in patients with iliofemoral DVT (**Fig. 19.6**).[48]

Trellis-8

The Trellis-8 device uses balloon containment of thrombus with chemical and mechanical thrombolysis. The thrombus is isolated after placing the catheter by inflating proximal and distal balloons. The drug is then infused through the multiple side holes in the catheter between the balloons. This is followed by removal of the guidewire and placement of a stiff sinusoidal wire between the balloons. A battery-powered motor then turns the wire at 3000 rpm; thus, mechanical dissolution of the thrombus is combined with the actions of the thrombolytic drug (**Fig. 19.7**). Retrospective case series have shown the safety and feasibility of the Trellis-8 device but there are currently no randomised controlled trial data to support routine use in clinical practice.[56]

Angiojet

The Angiojet Power Pulse system uses a complex mixture of rapid fluid streaming and hydrodynamic forces to fracture the thrombus, allowing extraction at the catheter tip as a result of negative pressure (the Bernoulli effect). The catheter infuses normal saline through an infusion port while simultaneously suctioning through the effluent port. If the effluent port is clamped, the infusion port acts as a mechanical 'pulse spray' that delivers the preloaded thrombolytic drug to the thrombus. This is the only device that can be solely used as a mechanical thrombectomy device. Safety and feasibility of the Angiojet (see **Fig. 19.8**) have been demonstrated in retrospective case series only.[57]

The future

A more aggressive approach to the treatment of iliofemoral DVT will reveal underlying venous anomalies in approximately 50% of patients. Additional treatment of the underlying stenosis may enhance patency and improve the prevention of PTS. The ongoing randomised controlled trials ATTRACT and CAVA will provide us with more data on this subject. Dedicated thrombus removal devices and venous stents may further enhance clot lysis and long-term patency, but randomised clinical trials are essential to define their precise role in clinical practice.

Key points

- Acute leg swelling can indicate a number of diseases. The most important differential diagnosis is DVT, which needs to be treated immediately to prevent potentially lethal pulmonary emboli.
- A low Wells score combined with low D-dimer levels is safe for ruling out DVT.
- Duplex sonography is the standard modality to confirm DVT.
- Standard treatment for DVT is oral anticoagulation, compressive stockings and mobilisation.
- Patients with iliofemoral DVT are associated with severe post-thrombotic morbidity and should be considered for additional CDT therapy.

References

1. Engelberger RP, Aujesky D, Calanca L, et al. Comparison of the diagnostic performance of the original and modified Wells score in inpatients and outpatients with suspected deep vein thrombosis. Thromb Res 2011;127(6):535–9.

2. Fritschy D, Fasel J, Imbert J-C, et al. The popliteal cyst. Knee Surg Sports Traumatol Arthrosc 2006;14(7):623–8.

3. Vela P, Pascual E, Ronan J, et al. Cutaneous manifestation of ruptured popliteal cyst. Clin Rheumatol 1991;10(3):340–1.

4. Tarhan S, Unlu Z. Magnetic resonance imaging and ultrasonographic evaluation of the patients with knee osteoarthritis: a comparative study. Clin Rheumatol 2003;22(3):181–8.

5. Acebes JC, Sánchez-Pernaute O, Díaz-Oca A, et al. Ultrasonographic assessment of Baker's cysts after intra-articular corticosteroid injection in knee osteoarthritis. J Clin Ultrasound 2006;34(3):113–7.

6. Eriksson B, Jorup-Rönström C, Karkkonen K, et al. Erysipelas: clinical and bacteriologic spectrum and serological aspects. Clin Infect Dis 1996;23(5):1091–8.

7. Stevens DL. Streptococcal toxic-shock syndrome: spectrum of disease, pathogenesis, and new concepts in treatment. Emerg Infect Dis 1995;1(3):69–78.

8. Anaya DA, Dellinger EP. Necrotizing soft-tissue infection: diagnosis and management. Clin Infect Dis 2007;44(5):705–10.

9. McHenry CR, Piotrowski JJ, Petrinic D, et al. Determinants of mortality for necrotizing soft-tissue infections. Ann Surg 1995;221(5):558–65.

10. Ely JW, Osheroff JA, Chambliss ML, et al. Approach to leg edema of unclear etiology. J Am Board Fam Med 2006;19(2):148–60.

11. Nordström M, Lindblad B, Bergqvist D, et al. A prospective study of the incidence of deep-vein thrombosis within a defined urban population. J Intern Med 1992;232(2):155–60.

12. Andrew M, David M, Adams M, et al. Venous thromboembolic complications (VTE) in children: first analyses of the Canadian Registry of VTE. Blood 1994;83(5):1251–7.

13. Bulger C. Epidemiology of acute deep vein thrombosis. Tech Vasc Interv Radiol 2004;7(2):50–4.

14. Bahia A, Albert RK. The modified wells score accurately excludes pulmonary embolus in hospitalized patients receiving heparin prophylaxis. J Hosp Med 2011;6(4):190–4.

15. Wells PS, Owen C, Doucette S, et al. Does this patient have deep vein thrombosis? JAMA 2006; 295(2):199.

16. Wells PS, Anderson DR, Rodger M, et al. Evaluation of D-dimer in the diagnosis of suspected deep-vein thrombosis. N Engl J Med 2003;349(13):1227–35.
This randomised controlled trial evaluates the value of D-dimer testing in combination with the Wells score in evaluating the chance of the patient having DVT and the ability to safely exclude DVT.

17. Miller N, Satin R, Tousignant L, et al. A prospective study comparing duplex scan and venography for diagnosis of lower-extremity deep vein thrombosis. Cardiovasc Surg 1996;4(4):505–8.

18. van Langevelde K, Tan M, Šrámek A, et al. Magnetic resonance imaging and computed tomography developments in imaging of venous thromboembolism. J Magn Reson Imaging 2010;32(6):1302–12.

19. Baldt MM, Zontsich T, Stümpflen A, et al. Deep venous thrombosis of the lower extremity: efficacy of spiral CT venography compared with conventional venography in diagnosis. Radiology 1996;200(2):423–8.

20. Arnoldussen CWKP, Toonder I, Wittens CHA. A novel scoring system for lower-extremity venous pathology analysed using magnetic resonance venography and duplex ultrasound. Phlebology 2012;27(Suppl. 1):163–70.

21. Arnoldussen CWKP, Wittens CHA. An imaging approach to deep vein thrombosis and the lower extremity thrombosis classification. Phlebology 2012;27(Suppl. 1):143–8.

22. Kearon C, Kahn SR, Agnelli G, et al. Antithrombotic therapy for venous thromboembolic disease: American College of Chest Physicians evidence-based clinical practice guidelines (8th edition). Chest 2008;133(Suppl. 6):454S–5.
These guidelines extend a level 1A recommendation for treating DVT with anticoagulation for at least 3 months. These guidelines are composed after an exhaustive search of multiple studies carefully selected by authorities in the field.

23. Büller HR, Agnelli G, Hull RD, et al. Antithrombotic therapy for venous thromboembolic disease; the seventh ACCP Conference on Antithrombotic and Thrombolytic Therapy. Chest 2004;126(Suppl. 3): 401S–28S.

24. Othieno R, Affan MA, Okpo E. Home versus in-patient treatment for deep vein thrombosis. Cochrane Database Syst Rev 2001;2:CD003076.

25. Prandoni P, Lensing AWA, Prins MH, et al. Below-knee elastic compression stockings to prevent the post-thrombotic syndrome: a randomized, controlled trial. Ann Intern Med 2004;141(4):249–56.
This randomised controlled trial compares treatment of DVT with and without compression therapy and the impact on incidence of PTS on both groups.

26. Partsch H, Blättler W. Compression and walking versus bed rest in the treatment of proximal deep venous thrombosis with low molecular weight heparin. J Vasc Surg 2000;32(5):861–9.

27. Partsch H, Kechavarz B, Köhn H, et al. The effect of mobilisation of patients during treatment of thromboembolic disorders with low-molecular-weight heparin. Int Angiol 1997;16(3):189–92.

28. Prandoni P, Noventa F, Ghirarduzzi A, et al. The risk of recurrent venous thromboembolism after discontinuing anticoagulation in patients with acute proximal deep vein thrombosis or pulmonary embolism. A prospective cohort study in 1,626 patients. Haematologica 2007;92(2):199–205.

29. Prandoni P, Kahn SR. Post-thrombotic syndrome: prevalence, prognostication and need for progress. Br J Haematol 2009;145(3):286–95.

30. Kahn SR, Kearon C, Julian JA, et al. Predictors of the post-thrombotic syndrome during long-term treatment of proximal deep vein thrombosis. J Thromb Haemost 2005;3(4):718–23.

31. Kolbach DN, Neumann HAM, Prins MH. Definition of the post-thrombotic syndrome, differences between existing classifications. Eur J Vasc Endovasc Surg 2005;30(4):404–14.

32. Kahn SR, Shrier I, Julian JA, et al. Determinants and time course of the postthrombotic syndrome after acute deep venous thrombosis. Ann Intern Med 2008;149(10):698–707.

33. Enden T, Haig Y, Kløw N-E, et al. Long-term outcome after additional catheter-directed thrombolysis versus standard treatment for acute iliofemoral deep vein thrombosis (the CaVenT study): a randomised controlled trial. Lancet 2012;379(9810):31–8.

The first randomised controlled trial to study the effects of additional CDT on the incidence of PTS in patients with acute iliofemoral DVT.

34. Comerota AJ. Catheter-directed thrombolysis is the appropriate treatment for iliofemoral deep venous thrombosis. Dis Mon 2010;56(11):637–41.

35. Villalta S, Bagatella P, Piccioli A, et al. Assessment of validity and reproducibility of a clinical scale for the post-thrombotic syndrome. Haemostasis 1994;24:158a.

36. Young L, Ockelford P, Milne D, et al. Post-treatment residual thrombus increases the risk of recurrent deep vein thrombosis and mortality. J Thromb Haemost 2006;4(9):1919–24.

37. Comerota AJ, Grewal N, Martinez JT, et al. Postthrombotic morbidity correlates with residual thrombus following catheter-directed thrombolysis for iliofemoral deep vein thrombosis. J Vasc Surg 2012;55(3):768–73.

38. Delis KT, Bountouroglou D, Mansfield AO. Venous claudication in iliofemoral thrombosis. Ann Surg 2004;239(1):118–26.

39. Akesson H, Brudin L, Dahlström JA, et al. Venous function assessed during a 5 year period after acute ilio-femoral venous thrombosis treated with anticoagulation. Eur J Vasc Surg 1990;4(1):43–8.

40. Meissner MH, Manzo RA, Bergelin RO, et al. Deep venous insufficiency: the relationship between lysis and subsequent reflux. YMVA 1993;18(4):596–608.

41. Watson LI, Armon MP. Thrombolysis for acute deep vein thrombosis. Cochrane Database Syst Rev 2004;4: CD002783.

Systematic review reporting on the effects of systemic thrombolysis for acute DVT. The results show an increase in clot lysis and a decrease in PTS incidence, and also a high rate of major bleeding. Systemic thrombolysis is therefor considered obsolete.

42. Alesh I, Kayali F, Stein PD. Catheter-directed thrombolysis (intrathrombus injection) in treatment of deep venous thrombosis: a systematic review. Cathet Cardiovasc Interv 2007;70(1):145–50.

43. Kahn SR, Hirsch A, Shrier I. Effect of postthrombotic syndrome on health-related quality of life after deep venous thrombosis. Arch Intern Med 2002;162(10):1144–8.

44. Grewal NK, Martinez JT, Andrews L, et al. Quantity of clot lysed after catheter-directed thrombolysis for iliofemoral deep venous thrombosis correlates with postthrombotic morbidity. YMVA 2010;51(5):1209–14.

45. Comerota AJ, Throm RC, Mathias SD, et al. Catheter-directed thrombolysis for iliofemoral deep venous thrombosis improves health-related quality of life. YMVA 2000;32(1):130–7.

46. Mewissen MW. Catheter-directed thrombolysis for lower extremity deep vein thrombosis. Tech Vasc Interv Radiol 2001;4(2):111–4.

47. Comerota AJ. The ATTRACT Trial: rationale for early intervention for iliofemoral DVT. Perspect Vasc Surg Endovasc Ther 2009;21(4):221–5.

48. Grommes J, Strijkers RHW, Greiner A, et al. Safety and feasibility of ultrasound-accelerated catheter-directed thrombolysis in deep vein thrombosis. Eur J Vasc Endovasc Surg 2011;41(4):526–32.

49. Meisner MH, Gloviczki P, Comerota AJ, et al. Early thrombus removal strategies for acute deep vein thrombosis: Clinical Practice Guidelines of the Soiety for Vascular Surgery and the American Venous Forum. J Vasc Surg 2012;55(5):1449–62.

50. Casey ET, Murad MH, Zumaeta-Garcia M, et al. Treatment of acute iliofemoral DVT. J Vasc Surg 2012;55(5):1463–73.

51. Mewissen MW, Seabrook GR, Meissner MH, et al. Catheter-directed thrombolysis for lower extremity deep venous thrombosis: report of a national multicenter registry. Radiology 1999;211(1):39–49.

52. Baeligkgaard N, Broholm R, Just S, et al. Long-term results using catheter-directed thrombolysis in 103 lower limbs with acute iliofemoral venous thrombosis. Eur J Vasc Endovasc Surg 2010;39(1):112–7.

53. Heniford BT, Senler SO, Olsofka JM, et al. May–Thurner syndrome: management by endovascular surgical techniques. Ann Vasc Surg 1998;12(5):482–6.

54. O'Sullivan GJ, Semba CP, Bittner CA, et al. Endovascular management of iliac vein compression (May–Thurner) syndrome. J Vasc Interv Radiol 2000;11(7):823–36.

55. Enden T, Kløw NE, Sandvik L, et al. Catheter-directed thrombolysis vs. anticoagulant therapy

alone in deep vein thrombosis: results of an open randomized, controlled trial reporting on short-term patency. J Thromb Haemost 2009;7(8):1268–75.

56. O'Sullivan GJ, Lohan DG, Gough N, et al. Pharmacomechanical thrombectomy of acute deep vein thrombosis with the Trellis-8 isolated thrombolysis catheter. J Vasc Interv Radiol 2007;18(6):715–24.

57. Kasirajan K, Gray B, Ouriel K. Percutaneous AngioJet thrombectomy in the management of extensive deep venous thrombosis. J Vasc Interv Radiol 2001;12(2):179–85.

20

Vascular anomalies

James E. Jackson

Introduction

Vascular anomalies are common in infants and children, but their classification is frequently a source of great confusion and, as a result, they are often poorly managed. This is despite the fact that, as long ago as 1982, Mulliken and Glowacki proposed a new way of classifying vascular anomalies[1] that is now the most widely recognised system in use. It is based upon differences in the cellular kinetics and natural history of these lesions and describes two separate groups: vascular tumours and vascular malformations, which will be discussed in turn. Vascular tumours include the common infantile haemangiomata as well as rarer congenital haemangiomata and other vascular tumours, many of which are high flow. Vascular malformations comprise low-flow venous and lymphatic malformations and high-flow arteriovenous malformations. An acquired arteriovenous fistula following trauma is a separate entity that may occasionally be misdiagnosed as a vascular malformation.

Vascular tumours

Haemangioma of infancy

The haemangioma of infancy is the most common soft-tissue tumour of childhood, occurring in up to 12% of Caucasian infants by the age of 1 year with a female:male ratio of 3:1. Congenital haemangiomata share some of the characteristics of the common infantile lesions but have very different natural histories. Other tumours in this arm

of the classification system include the pyogenic granuloma, tufted angiomas and kaposiform haemangioendotheliomas. All are rare.

Infantile haemangioma

Typically, this lesion is not present on the day of birth but becomes visible within the first 2 months of life. An initial stage of rapid proliferation first brings the lesion to attention, although the clinical appearance of the haemangioma at this time will depend upon its depth of involvement of the skin. Those involving the superficial dermis produce lobulated, bright red lesions that are commonly referred to as 'strawberry birthmarks' (**Fig. 20.1**). A haemangioma involving the deep dermis and subcutis, however, will produce a swelling with either no discoloration or a blueness of the overlying normal skin. The term 'cavernous haemangioma' is often used to describe such lesions, but it is important to recognise that their appearance is due solely to their depth of involvement of the skin and not to any variation in their histology.

The proliferative phase of a haemangioma varies in its duration, but rapid growth will usually occur during the first 6 months of life. Growth will often continue at a slower rate after this until about 1 year of age, following which the haemangioma will gradually involute completely in 50% of individuals by 5 years, in 70% by 7 years and 90% by 9 years. Residual skin changes following complete involution are common but in the majority are mild and inconspicuous, and include mild hypopigmentation, focal telangiectases and cutaneous atrophy.

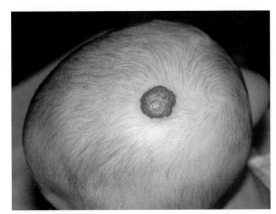

Figure 20.1 • Typical infantile haemangioma of the scalp with a 'strawberry-like' appearance.

As mentioned above, many haemangiomata are focal nodular lesions but others have a plaque-like configuration involving a larger area of skin and these 'segmental' haemangiomata involving the face are important to recognise, as they may be associated with other abnormalities, as outlined below.

Subglottic haemangiomata

Infants with large segmental haemangiomata of the neck and 'beard area' require careful follow-up during the first 12–16 weeks of life as they have a 60% risk of associated airway haemangiomata. These tumours may be life threatening and if symptoms of airway obstruction are present prompt surgical or medical treatment is mandatory.

Parotid gland haemangiomata

A segmental haemangioma involving the pre-auricular region may be accompanied by a haemangioma within the underlying parotid gland.

PHACE syndrome[2]

PHACE (an acronym for: Posterior fossa; Haemangioma; Arterial anomalies; Coarctation of the aorta and other cardiac defects; Eye abnormalities) syndrome describes the association between large segmental facial haemangiomata and several structural abnormalities. Affected individuals are nearly always female and the majority will have one or two of the described structural anomalies rather than all of them. The haemangioma most commonly involves the upper face and forehead, but this is not invariable. A child with such a lesion should be carefully examined for signs and symptoms of the syndrome and appropriate investigations should be performed to exclude anomalies of the heart and aorta, including coarctation. Neurological symptoms will prompt magnetic resonance scanning of the brain with or without catheter angiography.

Diagnosis and imaging

The diagnosis of a haemangioma of infancy is usually straightforward based upon the clinical history and findings on clinical examination; imaging is often unnecessary unless there is a concern about associated underlying structural anomalies (see above). It may occasionally be difficult, however, to differentiate between a deep-seated haemangioma and other vascular anomalies or tumours, and in such instances further investigation, and rarely biopsy, may be necessary.

The imaging features during the proliferative phase are usually characteristic: ultrasound demonstrates a well-defined, echogenic lesion that is highly vascular, with large central feeding arteries and draining veins. Magnetic resonance imaging (MRI) will demonstrate a well-defined lobulated tumour that is isointense or hypointense when compared with normal muscle on T1-weighted images and hyperintense on T2-weighted images. If contrast medium is given the tumour will enhance homogeneously and dilated feeding arteries and draining veins will be visualised.

Biopsy may be required in the rare instance that doubt remains as to the diagnosis. Infantile haemangiomata express glucose transporter-1 (GLUT-1), a simple diagnostic marker that may be very helpful in the differentiation between this entity and other vascular tumours. Core needle biopsy is usually straightforward under ultrasound guidance as lesions are typically superficial.

Management of haemangiomata of infancy

The majority of haemangiomata can be managed conservatively but intervention is indicated when a lesion causes significant mass effect or disfigurement, when it involves the airway and when it obstructs the visual axis. Pharmacological management is now the mainstay of treatment in this group, with beta-blockers the preferred first-line therapy.[3] Rarely, high output cardiac failure occurs in children with very large infantile haemangiomata, particularly when there is hepatic involvement, and this requires urgent intervention. Management consists of a combination of optimal medical therapy and particle embolisation of the capillary bed, with the aim of reducing the vascularity of the lesion and stabilising the child's cardiovascular status until the natural history of the lesion causes involution.

The surgical management of haemangiomata can be divided into those procedures performed during the proliferative phase of development and those performed later when partial or complete involution has occurred but a persistent cosmetic deformity remains. Early surgery is generally reserved for lesions obstructing the visual axis when more conservative measures have failed. Later surgery, between the ages of 3 and 5 years, may be considered when a large haemangioma persists that is slowly involuting and which is thought to be having a detrimental effect on the child's social development because of its appearance. The surgical scar that is likely to result from such an operation should, however, be weighed against the likely outcome if the haemangioma were allowed to involute completely.

Congenital haemangioma[4]

These haemangiomata differ in their natural history and prognosis when compared with infantile haemangiomata. Unlike the infantile subgroup, classical haemangiomata are fully formed at birth and have subtle differences in colour and contour on clinical examination. They form two distinct clinical subgroups defined by their natural history: the first involute very rapidly in the first few months of life and are termed rapidly involuting congenital haemangiomata (RICH) and the second never involute (non-involuting congenital haemangiomata, NICH). Both types are histologically and immunophenotypically distinct from infantile haemangiomata and neither of them expresses GLUT-1.

Other vascular tumours

Infantile and congenital haemangiomata make up the vast majority of the lesions in the vascular tumour arm of the Mulliken and Glowacki classification of vascular anomalies, but it is important to recognise other much less common lesions. These include the pyogenic granuloma, the tufted angioma and the kaposiform haemangioendothelioma.

The lobular capillary haemangioma, or pyogenic granuloma, is the second most common vascular tumour of childhood after the haemangioma of infancy, although it can occur at any age. It most often involves the head and neck and presents as a rapidly growing, bright red papule varying in size from a few millimetres to about 2 cm, which frequently ulcerates and may bleed profusely. Most can be removed surgically.

The tufted angioma (TA) presents initially as a small red or purple patch involving the skin of the neck or upper trunk, which grows slowly and may reach a large size. Its natural history is unpredictable, however, and some lesions will resolve spontaneously. The kaposiform haemangioendothelioma (KHE) most frequently occurs in the skin

of the trunk, shoulder and thigh. Seventy-five per cent of these tumours occur in early infancy and are manifest as a deep reddish-purple discoloration of the skin that may appear tense, shiny and bruised. Recognition of these two vascular tumours (TA and KHE) is important as they are sometimes associated with the Kasabach–Merritt phenomenon (KMP). Both are GLUT-1 negative on biopsy and have characteristic histology, so biopsy is often useful.

KMP describes a pattern of variable but often severe coagulopathy and thrombocytopenia seen in association with a variety of soft-tissue lesions, most commonly KHE, and is associated with a high mortality. It is not a complication of the common haemangioma of infancy[5] and should not be confused with the coagulopathy that may be associated with large venous malformations in which there is consumption of clotting factors with elevated D-dimers but a much less profound reduction in platelet and fibrinogen levels. The management of this condition lies outside the scope of this chapter but evolving pharmacological approaches to other vascular tumours may have a role to play in the management of these lesions and embolisation may be helpful in some cases.

Vascular malformations

Classification

Vascular malformations are inborn errors of vasculogenesis of unknown aetiology. All are believed to be present at birth but they may not become evident clinically for many years. They persist for life, will never spontaneously regress and may undergo periods when they increase in size, most commonly during puberty or pregnancy, or following trauma or spontaneous thrombosis, although a triggering event is not always recognised. They are most conveniently divided into low- and high-flow lesions, a differentiation that is usually obvious on clinical examination. Low-flow malformations are further subdivided into capillary, venous and lymphatic types. Lesions in the high-flow group are termed arteriovenous malformations.

Low-flow malformations

Capillary malformations
Capillary malformations come in a variety of forms.

Salmon patch (naevus simplex; erythema nuchae)
A salmon patch is a red macule present at birth, which most commonly involves the skin of the nape of the neck, the upper eyelids or glabella. It is usually central, does not follow a dermatomal distribution

and will usually fade by 2 years of age, especially if it involves the skin of the face; the nuchal lesion is more likely to persist into adult life.

Port-wine stains (naevus flameus)

Port-wine stains are well-demarcated vascular stains that are present at birth and increase in size commensurately with the child's growth. They are relatively uncommon and have an equal sex distribution. They tend to follow a dermatomal distribution and are usually unilateral, although they may occasionally cross the midline. Those involving the face are usually flat in early childhood but have a tendency to become thickened and nodular over time and may be associated with bony and soft-tissue hypertrophy, particularly when they involve the cutaneous distribution of the second branch of the trigeminal nerve. Most of these facial lesions occur as an isolated abnormality but some are part of a syndrome complex, the most relevant of which is Sturge–Weber syndrome,[6] which describes the triad of a facial port-wine stain in a V1 distribution, an ipsilateral leptomeningeal vascular malformation and a choroidal vascular malformation of the eye that can cause glaucoma. MRI is helpful to document an intracranial abnormality, although only 10% of children with a port-wine stain in the V1 distribution will have the syndrome.

Venous malformations

These lesions consist of dilated venous spaces of varying size, within which blood flow is sluggish. They vary considerably in size from small lesions localised to the skin or superficial fat to very large abnormalities involving skin, muscle and bone. The most common symptoms of pain and swelling are highly variable and are not directly related to the extent of the malformation, but rather to its site and the size of the vessels of which it is composed. Thus, for example, a relatively small venous malformation involving the superficial soft tissue of the sole of the foot is often the cause of more disability than an extensive intramuscular malformation involving quadriceps femoris, but a quadriceps malformation made up of large venous sacs that become engorged during exercise is likely to be more symptomatic than one at the same site consisting of numerous much smaller veins. Pain and swelling may also be caused by spontaneous episodes of in-situ thrombosis, which are relatively common.

On clinical examination a non-pulsatile soft-tissue swelling is often apparent (**Fig. 20.2a**), often with a bluish discoloration of the overlying skin, which may be tender when compressed. Firm, mobile, pea-sized phleboliths, which have developed as a result of episodes of spontaneous thrombosis, are commonly palpable.

It is very important to recognise that a chronic intravascular coagulopathy is common in patients with very large, bulky malformations causing low fibrinogen and elevated D-dimers, which may result in severe bleeding during surgery.

Most venous malformations are single but they may rarely be multiple, involving the skin and gastrointestinal tract (and other organs including the liver, lung, renal tract and brain) as part of the Blue rubber bleb naevus or Bean syndrome. Most of these cases are sporadic, although some are inherited in an autosomal dominant fashion.

Imaging

A vascular malformation may be likened to an 'iceberg' as its visible, superficial portion often belies its involvement of the deeper tissues and it is imperative that this is appreciated prior to therapy. The full extent of venous malformations will be exquisitely delineated with MRI and this is often the only pretreatment imaging that is required; fat suppressed sequences will show these lesions as areas of high signal intensity. If there

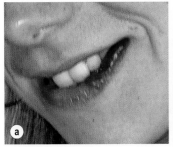 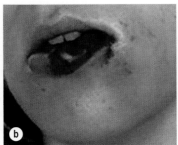 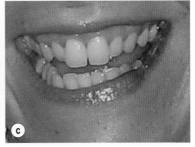

Figure 20.2 • (a) Venous malformation of the lower lip treated by percutaneous sclerotherapy. **(b)** Clinical photograph demonstrating lobulated blue swelling involving the left lower lip. On clinical examination this lesion rapidly increased in size when the patient leant forward. Following percutaneous sclerotherapy performed with a total of 3 mL of 3% sodium tetradecyl sulphate injected at two separated sites, there is tense swelling of the malformation and adjacent bruising. **(c)** Three months later the appearance is considerably improved.

is any concern that there is direct involvement of underlying bone by the malformation, or that there is secondary osseous hypertrophy or atrophy, this is best visualised by computed tomography (CT). It is important, however, that this is only performed if the documentation of the bony abnormality is likely to affect treatment, in order to avoid unnecessary radiation exposure. Arteriography is not required.

Management of venous malformations

The treatment of a venous malformation will depend on a number of factors, including its size, location, depth of soft-tissue involvement and the presence or absence of associated bony deformity. The aim of therapy should clearly be to improve symptoms and the cosmetic appearances, and the two modalities used to try and achieve this are percutaneous sclerotherapy and surgery, sometimes in combination. Patients should be clear from the outset that a 'cure' is not possible, although there are obviously some lesions that do respond very well to therapy with no symptomatic recurrence on long-term follow-up.

Percutaneous sclerotherapy (Fig. 20.2) involves the direct puncture and injection of a liquid sclerosant such as sodium tetradecyl sulphate or absolute alcohol under fluoroscopic control into the abnormal venous sacs within the malformation.[7] The former agent is often 'foamed' by the addition of air or carbon dioxide before injection and this may improve the results. Malformations consisting of large compressible venous spaces are likely to respond especially well to this form of therapy. Multiple treatment sessions performed at intervals of several weeks or months may be necessary for extensive malformations but satisfactory control of such lesions may be achieved; subsequent re-expansion is likely to occur, however, that will necessitate further sclerotherapy at a later date. Low-flow malformations that are relatively firm, poorly compressible and that show little increase in size when held dependent – signs that usually indicate that they contain numerous small venous sacs – tend to respond less well to this form of treatment.

Surgical techniques that are most commonly used for venous malformations include staged excisions and Popescu sutural compartmentalisation, which may be usefully combined with percutaneous sclerotherapy.[8]

Lymphatic malformations

Lymphatic malformations are best subclassified into macrocystic and microcystic lesions. Most are evident at birth but some may not become apparent until early childhood. MRI is the best imaging modality as it will beautifully demonstrate the full extent of the abnormality on fat-suppressed images. Ultrasound is helpful to differentiate between macro- and microcystic varieties and to guide percutaneous therapy.

Management[9]

Percutaneous sclerotherapy is generally considered a first-line treatment option for the macrocystic subtype of lymphatic malformation. A large number of sclerosing agents have been reported as producing satisfactory long-term cyst decompression, including OK-432, bleomycin, ethanol, sodium tetradecyl sulphate, doxycycline and cyclophosphamide.

Microcystic and mixed micro- and macrocystic lymphatic malformations are commoner than the macrocystic variety and are much more difficult to treat successfully. Multiple modalities may be required, including percutaneous sclerotherapy of larger cysts and surgical debulking.

High-flow malformations

Although present at birth, many arteriovenous malformations (AVMs) do not become apparent until puberty or even adult life. Progression of high-flow malformations may also occur in response to pregnancy or trauma, which may be accidental or iatrogenic – for example, proximal surgical ligation or embolisation of feeding arteries, and subtotal resection.

A pulsatile soft-tissue swelling is usually evident on clinical examination, with prominence of draining veins, and the high-flow nature of a malformation is often apparent on simple palpation. A deeper-seated lesion may be less obviously pulsatile, however, and in such cases the detection of an arteriovenous signal using a simple hand-held Doppler probe in the outpatient clinic will allow its high-flow nature to be appreciated. The differential diagnosis of a vascular soft-tissue tumour should be considered, although a history of a long-standing, pre-existing swelling or the clinical finding of an associated overlying cutaneous stain will help make the diagnosis; there is rarely a need for a biopsy, although this should be performed if there is doubt as to its true nature. Recognised complications of AVMs include thinning of the overlying skin, frank ulceration, infection and bleeding, and these should obviously be documented at the time of clinical examination.

An acquired post-traumatic arteriovenous fistula (AVF) may have an identical appearance on clinical examination to that of a high-flow AVM. There should be a history of previous trauma but some patients will not volunteer this information and indeed may have forgotten an antecedent injury, which may have occurred many years previously. The development of an AVF usually requires penetrating trauma but this is not always the case and may follow a significant blunt injury. A single fistulous communication is usually present and this will sometimes be the first indication of this diagnosis, which is an important one to make as a cure is likely if treated appropriately.

Imaging

Other than Doppler ultrasound, which may be very helpful during initial clinical assessment of a vascular malformation, other cross-sectional imaging of high-flow malformations, although often performed, is rarely essential as the decision regarding the requirement for treatment is based upon clinical findings and symptoms. Many patients require no more than reassurance about the diagnosis and a frank discussion about its nature and natural history. If treatment is felt to be necessary then MRI is the non-invasive modality of first choice to demonstrate the extent of the AVM. Magnetic resonance angiography may be helpful to document its angiographic anatomy but this is often better visualised by catheter angiography. Bone involvement is best demonstrated on CT. Contrast-enhanced CT is rarely helpful and should be avoided if possible in order to avoid unnecessary radiation exposure. Even when MRI is contraindicated, CT is unlikely to give any more information than catheter angiography, which will be necessary if the decision has been made that treatment is required.

Management

AVMs that are quiescent, not associated with significant symptoms and that cause little in the way of cosmetic deformity are usually best left alone. Patients should be informed that a change in the malformation may warrant re-evaluation.

Patients with symptomatic AVMs who require treatment are often best managed by embolisation, although surgical excision or debulking, often combined with embolisation, may be necessary in some individuals.

Embolisation

The anatomy of the vascular communications within a high-flow AVM directly influences the method of vascular occlusion and the final result, and it is important to be fully aware of the various forms that may be present. Houdart et al.[10] classified intracranial arteriovenous malformations into three main types based upon the anatomy of the arteriovenous communications. This classification is equally appropriate for peripheral malformations (**Fig. 20.3**):

- Type I: arteriovenous. These AVMs have a first identifiable venous component that is supplied by three or fewer arterial pedicles.
- Type II: arteriolovenous. Here the first identifiable venous component is supplied by more than three (often very many) arterial pedicles.
- Type III: arteriolovenulous. Here the arteriovenous communications are so small and numerous that they cannot be separately identified and the first obviously venous component is often at some distance from them.

These anatomical variations can coexist within the same malformation. In particular, AVMs with a dominant type III anatomy may also contain type II communications.

The general principle of embolisation is that occlusion is performed at the site of the abnormal arteriovenous shunts and not in the vessel proximal to this point. If embolisation is directed at the arteriovenous communications themselves – from the arterial side, by a direct percutaneous puncture or via a retrograde venous approach[11,12] – and these are totally obliterated using a liquid embolic agent such as sodium tetradecyl sulphate or absolute alcohol, then a long-term

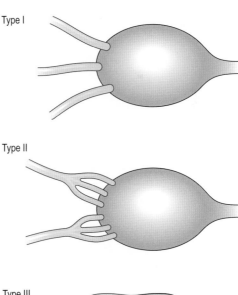

Type I

Type II

Type III

Figure 20.3 • Classification of arteriovenous malformations based upon the anatomy of the arteriovenous communications.

improvement in symptoms can be achieved. Type I and type II lesions are particularly suited to this form of treatment (**Fig. 20.4**).

There has been much written about the importance of occluding the 'nidus' but this term is unhelpful; it is better to think of high-flow vascular malformations as 'venous sumps' as it is the low-pressure first venous component, at the site of abnormal arteriovenous communication, that drives the AVM. If this is left untouched and only the feeding vessels are occluded, the low-pressure 'sump' continues to draw in blood from adjacent collaterals. If the venous component is occluded from the start, however, the low-pressure 'drive' disappears and arteriovenous shunting is obliterated.

AVMs with a largely intraosseous component are especially well suited to treatment by this method of embolisation because they usually have a type II (arteriolovenous) anatomy and are usually best approached by a direct, transosseous, puncture of the dilated venous component of the malformation.

Embolisation and surgery

If surgery is to be performed the aim should be to excise the AVM totally, if at all possible. Preoperative embolisation may be very helpful but it is very important to understand that this is performed in order to make surgery easier by reducing the vascularity of the AVM rather than to reduce the extent of resection. The technique of preoperative embolisation differs from that which has been described above. The aim is clearly to make the malformation avascular so as to give the surgeon as near bloodless a field as possible and is usually best achieved with a particulate embolic material such as polyvinyl alcohol. A particle size should be chosen that will allow deep penetration into the malformation without passing through the arteriovenous communications.

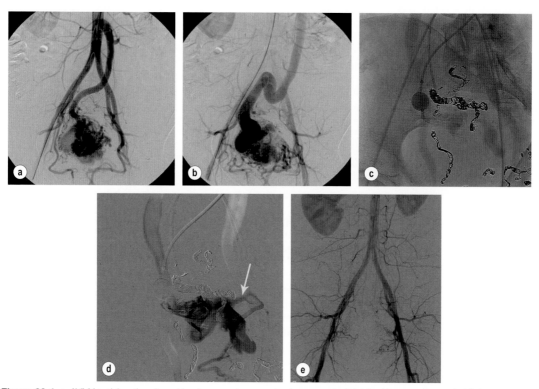

Figure 20.4 • AVM involving the sigmoid colon causing massive lower gastrointestinal haemorrhage. **(a,b)** Arterial and venous images from an abdominal aortogram demonstrate rapid arteriovenous shunting through an AVM in the pelvis supplied by a massively hypertrophied inferior mesenteric artery and haemorrhoidal branches of both internal iliac arteries. Venous drainage is via an enlarged inferior mesenteric vein. Coil embolisation of many of the arterial feeding vessels was performed at the referring hospital, which temporarily stopped active bleeding. **(c,d)** Via a transhepatic puncture of the portal vein, the inferior mesenteric vein has been retrogradely catheterised into the pelvic and an occlusion balloon has been inflated to control venous outflow. There is stasis of contrast medium in the venous sac. The arrow shows filling of a haemorrhoidal artery that was catheterised with a coaxial catheter via the lumen of the occlusion balloon and embolised with coils before the sac was sclerosed with 3% sodium tetradecyl sulphate. **(e)** Aortogram performed 6 months later documents obliteration of arteriovenous shunting through the AVM.

Larger communications may require embolisation with other agents such as 'glue' introduced via a co-axial arterial catheter or via a direct puncture route. Coil occlusion alone of feeding arteries is useless as the malformation will remain very vascular via collaterals. Indeed, it is important not to embolise feeding vessels with coils or plugs even when distal embolisation has been performed with particles, as this will only hamper future angiographic assessment or treatment if the malformation recurs.

As regards surgical technique, tissue expansion and muscular flap transfer techniques may be necessary when a large cutaneous defect is likely to result from excision.

Results

The best results are undoubtedly achieved in specialist centres that are able to provide multidisciplinary input. When treatment is necessary, long-term symptomatic improvement is achieved in the majority of individuals and there is no doubt that radiological and clinical obliteration of more malformations has come with a better understanding of their radiological anatomy and the use of agents that are directed at the arteriovenous shunts themselves rather than at the proximal feeding vessels.

Conclusions

Vascular anomalies are simply classified into vascular tumours and vascular malformations. The common haemangioma of infancy makes up the vast majority of the former group and most of these will involute spontaneously without the need for active intervention.

Vascular malformations are difficult to treat successfully and a cure is unlikely. Patients with these anomalies are best treated in specialised units providing multidisciplinary expertise, including diagnostic and interventional radiology and surgery.

Key points

- Vascular anomalies are classified into vascular tumours and vascular malformations.
- The commonest vascular tumour is the haemangioma of infancy.
- The majority of haemangiomata of infancy require no treatment.
- Vascular malformations are inborn errors of vasculogenesis and persist throughout life.
- Vascular malformations are most conveniently classified into high- and low-flow lesions.
- Not all vascular malformations require treatment.
- Venous and lymphatic malformations may cause marked disfigurement and their treatment is often difficult, involving percutaneous sclerotherapy and/or surgery.
- A chronic intravascular coagulopathy is common in patients with very large, bulky venous malformations causing a low fibrinogen and elevated D-dimers, which may result in severe bleeding during surgery.
- High-flow malformations are equally difficult to manage and may require multimodality treatment, including embolisation and surgery.
- An understanding of the angioarchitecture of a high-flow malformation is essential as this influences the approach to treatment and predicts the likely response to embolisation.

References

1. Mulliken JB, Glowacki J. Hemangiomas and vascular malformations in infants and children: a classification based on endothelial characteristics. Plast Reconstr Surg 1982;69:412–22.

2. Metry D, Heyer G, Hess C, et al. PHACE Syndrome Research Conference. Consensus statement on diagnostic criteria for PHACE syndrome. Pediatrics 2009;124(5):1447–56.

3. Itinteang T, Withers A, Leadbitter P, et al. Pharmacologic therapies for infantile hemangioma: is there a rational basis? Plast Reconstr Surg 2011;128:499–507.

4. Mulliken JB, Enjolras O. Congenital hemangiomas and infantile hemangioma: missing links. J Am Acad Dermatol 2004;50:875–82.

5. Sarkar M, Mulliken JB, Kozakewich HP, et al. Thrombocytopenic coagulopathy (Kasabach–Merritt phenomenon) is associated with kaposiform hemangioendothelioma and not with

common infantile hemangioma. Plast Reconstr Surg 1997;100:1377–86.

6. Baselga E. Sturge–Weber syndrome. Semin Cutan Med Surg 2004;23:87–98.

7. Stimpson P, Hewitt R, Barnacle A, et al. Sodium tetradecyl sulphate sclerotherapy for treating venous malformations of the oral and pharyngeal regions in children. Int J Pediatr Otorhinolaryngol 2012;76(4):569–73.

8. James CA, Braswell LE, Wright LB, et al. Preoperative sclerotherapy of facial venous malformations: impact on surgical parameters and long-term follow-up. J Vasc Interv Radiol 2011;22(7):953–60.

9. Perkins JA, Manning SC, Tempero RM, et al. Lymphatic malformations: review of current treatment. Otolaryngol Head Neck Surg 2010;142(6):795–803.803.e1

10. Houdart E, Gobin YP, Casasco A, et al. A proposed angiographic classification of intracranial arteriovenous fistulae and malformations. Neuroradiology 1993;35:381–5.

11. Jackson JE, Mansfield AO, Allison DJ. Treatment of high-flow vascular malformations by venous embolization aided by flow occlusion techniques. Cardiovasc Intervent Radiol 1996;19:323–8.

12. Cho SK, Do YS, Kim DI, et al. Peripheral arteriovenous malformations with a dominant outflow vein: results of ethanol embolization. Korean J Radiol 2008;9(3):258–67.

21

Future developments

Alan G. Dawson
Julie Brittenden

Introduction

Secondary prevention is the first-line management of all patients with peripheral arterial disease (PAD). The first section of this chapter will discuss new advances and emerging pharmacotherapy in secondary prevention therapy, specifically with regard to cholesterol-lowering and antiplatelet agents. A significant proportion of patients with PAD are unsuitable for surgical or endovascular revascularisation and refractory to pharmacotherapy. In these patients, recent interest has focused on strategies to improve neovascularisation. The next two sections will discuss the role of gene therapy and cell-based therapy as a potential treatment option for patients with PAD in terms of therapeutic angiogenesis and vasculogenesis. The final section will discuss the role of gene therapy in the prevention of neointimal hyperplasia within vein grafts and stents.

Cholesterol-lowering and antiplatelet therapy

Novel cholesterol-lowering secondary prevention therapies

Increasing high-density lipoprotein (HDL)

Multiple large-scale epidemiological studies have consistently shown an inverse relationship between HDL cholesterol levels and cardiovascular risk. Studies have shown that for every 0.03 mmol/L increase in HDL there is an associated 2–3% reduction in cardiovascular risk.[1] HDL mediates its cardioprotective role through several mechanisms. One of these is the ability of HDL to remove macrophage cholesterol through its involvement in reverse cholesterol transport (**Fig. 21.1**). It transports excess cholesterol from the arterial macrophages to the liver, where it can be excreted in the bile. HDL also has direct anti-inflammatory and antithrombotic effects that have been attributed to the action of apolipoprotein A-I, a protein derived from HDL that will be discussed below (**Fig. 21.2**).

It should be noted that HDL particles and apolipoproteins which are dysfunctional and exhibit pro-inflammatory properties have been identified in some patient cohorts.[4] Thus the functionality as well as the quantity of HDL cholesterol that is present is important.

Cholesterol ester transfer protein inhibitors

Various pharmacotherapies have aimed to increase HDL levels. Recent interest has focused on the use of inhibitors of cholesterol ester transfer protein (CETP). In a randomised double-blind study of 15 000 patients with a history of cardiovascular disease, including PAD, the CETP inhibitor torcetrapib was associated with increased risk of cardiovascular events and mortality.[5] Torcetrapib when used in patients already on atorvastatin resulted in a 72% increase in HDL cholesterol and a 25% reduction in low-density lipoprotein (LDL) cholesterol. However, the increased HDL generated by torcetrapib was shown to be less effective with regard to reverse cholesterol transport. Torcetrapib reduced serum potassium and increased bicarbonate levels,

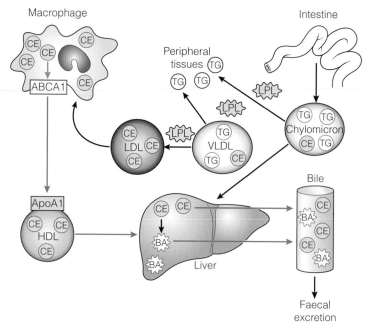

Figure 21.1 • Overview of lipid transport and metabolism. Dietary lipids in the form of triglycerides (TG) and cholesterol esters (CE) are absorbed through the intestinal wall and packaged as chylomicrons. These triglyceride-rich particles are rapidly metabolised by lipoprotein lipase (LPL), which hydrolyses triglycerides into free fatty acids and glycerol that are subsequently taken up by peripheral tissues. Chylomicron remnants are removed from circulation by the liver. The liver synthesises triglyceride-rich very-low-density lipoprotein (VLDL) particles as a means of transport for de novo cholesterol and triglycerides. VLDL particles can also be converted to low-density lipoproteins (LDL) through the actions of LPL and function to deliver cholesterol to peripheral tissues such as macrophages. Small phospholipid-rich high-density lipoprotein (HDL) can be made by the liver or from pinched-off VLDL or chylomicron remnants. HDL functions in a process known as reverse cholesterol transport (RCT; red arrows). RCT involves HDL-mediated removal of excess cholesterol from peripheral tissues through the interactions of apolipoprotein A-I (ApoAI) on the surface of HDL and ABCAI on the surface of peripheral cells. This cholesterol is transported to the liver in the form of HDL, where it is converted to bile acids (BA) or secreted directly into the bile. Both bile acids and cholesterol present in the bile can be removed from the body through excretion in the faeces.[2] Reproduced from Hanniman EA, Sinal CJ. Nuclear receptors: novel therapeutic targets for the treatment and prevention of atherosclerosis. Drug Discovery Today: Therapeutic Strategies 2004; 1:155–61. With permission from Elsevier.

aldosterone levels and blood pressure. These effects were not related to CETP inhibition and further work led to the development of the more specific CETP inhibitors: anacetrapib, dalcetrapib and evacetrapib, which have been evaluated in phase I trials.[6]

The safety and efficacy of anacetrapib in increasing HDL cholesterol has been assessed in a randomised placebo-controlled double-blind study involving 1623 patients with cardiac disease or high risk of cardiac disease.[7] In the Randomised Evaluation of the Effects of Anacetrapib through Lipid Modification study (REVEAL), patients at high risk of vascular events, which includes patients with PAD, are currently being recruited into a large multicentre trial with the aim of determining if anacetrapib prevents vascular events.[8] The patients will undergo optimisation of LDL cholesterol via atorvastatin therapy prior to entering the study and will be randomised to receive anacetrapib 100 mg daily or placebo for 5 years.

Niacin

Niacin is known to increase HDL cholesterol levels, but the ability to reduce cardiovascular events in patients on statin therapy is unknown. One large randomised trial of niacin monotherapy was performed before the introduction of statin therapy.[9] Niacin causes flushing, which may be reduced by laropiprant (formerly MK-0524), a selective prostaglandin D receptor antagonist. In the Treatment of HDL to Reduce the Incidence of Vascular Events (HPS2-THRIVE) randomised placebo-controlled study, 25 000 patients with atherosclerotic vascular disease including PAD have been randomised to niacin (1 g)/laropiprant in addition to pre-existing simvastatin or combination simvastain/ezetimibe therapy for 4 years.[10] Prior to entry into the study the patients' LDL cholesterol level was below 2 mmol/L. The aim is to determine if increasing HDL cholesterol levels through niacin therapy reduces the primary outcome of myocardial infarction, stroke or revascularisation.

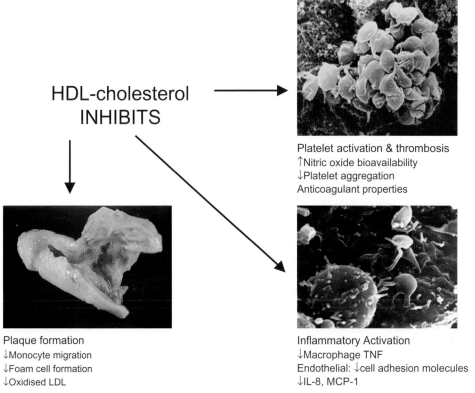

HDL-cholesterol INHIBITS

Platelet activation & thrombosis
↑Nitric oxide bioavailability
↓Platelet aggregation
Anticoagulant properties

Plaque formation
↓Monocyte migration
↓Foam cell formation
↓Oxidised LDL

Inflammatory Activation
↓Macrophage TNF
Endothelial: ↓cell adhesion molecules
↓IL-8, MCP-1

Figure 21.2 • Anti-inflammatory properties of HDL. IL, interleukin; MCP-1, monocyte chemoattractant protein 1; TNF, tumour necrosis factor.[3]

In the study of niacin in patients with low HDL cholesterol levels receiving intensive statin therapy (AIM-HIGH), 3414 patients with atherosclerosis were randomised to extended-release niacin (1.5–2 g daily) or matching placebo.[11] All patients had an LDL cholesterol level of 1.03–2.07 mmol/L and were on simvastatin plus ezetimibe if required. The primary end-point was the first event of a composite, myocardial infarction, stroke, hospitalisation for an acute coronary syndrome, revascularisation or death from coronary heart disease. The study was stopped after a mean follow-up period of 3 years since due to a lack of efficacy, as despite significant increases in HDL-cholesterol there was no observed increase in clinical benefit.

Apolipoprotein A-I and mimetic peptides

Apolipoprotein A-I is a gatekeeper in reverse cholesterol transport and binds to the ABCA1 receptor on macrophages (Fig. 21.1). Apolipoprotein A-I has been shown in several preclinical studies to reduce the development and progression of atherosclerosis through its lipid-binding properties. It is, however, a large protein that has to be administered intravenously. Thus, D-4F peptide has been developed, which appears to mimic the lipid-binding actions

of apolipoprotein A-I and can be administered orally.[12] Preclinical trials have shown that D-4F has anti-inflammatory and anti-atherogenic effects. In a small phase I clinical trial, D-4F had low bioavailability but a single dose appeared safe and well tolerated.[13] Further studies are awaited.

Summary: therapy to increase levels of HDL cholesterol

While there is robust epidemiological evidence that low levels of HDL cholesterol are associated with increased risk of cardiac events, to date there is no evidence that therapy which aims to increase HDL cholesterol levels reduces this risk. In the era of aggressive statin therapy, which can achieve very low LDL cholesterol levels, the clinical benefit of improving HDL cholesterol levels remains to be proven.

Lipoprotein metabolism and inflammatory response

The role of lipids in the pathogenesis of atherosclerosis has been discussed in Chapter 1.

Secretory phospholipase A_2 and lipoprotein-associated phospholipase A_2 are two inflammatory biomarkers that have been shown to predict cardiovascular events in population-based studies of healthy volunteers and in patients with known coronary heart disease.[14] They have not been studied in patients with PAD.

Secretory phospholipase A$_2$ causes hydrolysis of phospholipids on lipoproteins and cell membranes, and the generation of pro-inflammatory lipids (non-esterified fatty acids, lysophospholipids and eicosanoids). Lipoprotein-associated phospholipase A$_2$ generates pro-inflammatory lipids from oxidised LDL (oxidised non-esterified fatty acids and lysophosphatidylcholine).[15]

Secretory phospholipase A2 inhibitors

The secretory phospholipase A2 inhibitor, varespladib methyl, has been shown in two large phase II studies to significantly reduce the levels of LDL cholesterol, non-HDL cholesterol and ApoB.[16,17] A phase III study involving 6500 patients with acute coronary syndrome is currently underway.[18]

Lipoprotein-associated phospholipase A$_2$ inhibitors

The lipoprotein-associated phospholipase A$_2$ inhibitor darapladib has been evaluated in two phase II studies.[19,20] Darapladib reduced lipoprotein phospholipase activity and concentrations both within the blood and in carotid plaques. The concentrations of other inflammatory mediators were also reduced but there was no change in lipid profiles. Currently, there are two phase III studies underway that aim to determine the effect of darapladib on clinical outcome in patients with a recent cardiovascular event and patients with stable disease.[21,22] The ability of these drugs in combination with statin therapy to improve clinical outcome needs to be determined.

Novel antiplatelet agents

The value of antiplatelet therapy in patients with PAD has been discussed in Chapter 1. The three major pathways involved in platelet activation are triggered by thromboxane, adenosine diphosphate and thrombin (**Fig. 21.3**).

We are currently able to block the synthesis of the enzyme cyclo-oxygenase by aspirin and thus prevent the synthesis of thromboxane A$_2$ which normally causes platelet aggregation. Thienopyridines (such as clopidogrel and prasugrel) and non-thienopyridine derivatives (such as ticagrelor, cangrelor) inhibit the binding of adenosine diphosphate (ADP) to the P2Y(12) receptor which in turn prevents the activation of the glycoprotein IIb/IIIa complex by fibrinogen. However, thrombin is the most potent platelet activator. It acts mainly through the protease-activated receptor (PAR-1) and this pathway is not affected by current anti-platelet agents. Thrombin receptor antagonists such as vorapaxar and E-555 are a new class of anti-platelet agents that block thrombin-mediated platelet activation via a PAR-1 inhibition.

While antiplatelet therapy has been effective at reducing thrombotic risk in patients with atherosclerosis, patients continue to experience thrombotic events. Many of these events occur because patients may be non-responsive to current antiplatelet therapy. For instance, the thienopyridine clopidogrel needs to be activated by cytochrome

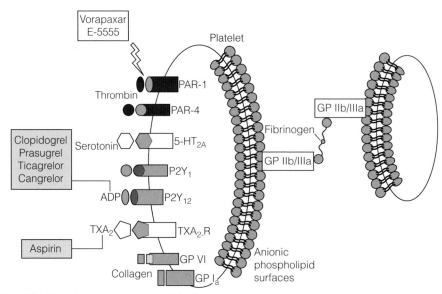

Figure 21.3 • Platelet activation and current antiplatelet agents.

P450 metabolism, and recent studies have shown that clopidogrel is inactive in patients who lack a functional allele of CYP2C19.[23] A newer generation of P2Y$_{12}$ receptor antagonists and novel agents such as thrombin receptor antagonists have recently been developed and are discussed below.

Thrombin receptor antagonists: protease-activated receptor 1 (PAR-1)

Platelet thrombin receptor antagonists, also known as protease-activated receptor 1 (PAR-1) antagonists, are a novel class of antiplatelet agents.[24] In phase II clinical trials, two oral PAR-1 antagonists, vorapaxar (SCH 530348, Merck/Schering-Plough) and atopaxar (E-5555, Eisai Co), have been evaluated in combination with standard antiplatelet therapy. In the thrombin receptor antagonist trial of patients undergoing percutaneous coronary angioplasty (TRA-PCI), vorapaxar was found to be safe and effectively inhibited platelet function in a thousand patients.[25] Results of the phase II trials involving atopaxar are awaited.[26]

Vorapaxar: phase III trials

In the phase III TRACER study (Thrombin Receptor Antagonist for Clinical Event Reduction in Acute Coronary Syndrome), 12 944 patients with acute coronary syndrome without ST-elevation were entered into a double-blind randomised controlled trial of vorapaxar. The primary end-point was a composite of myocardial infarction, stroke, and death from cardiovascular causes, recurrent ischaemia or urgent coronary revascularisation. The study was terminated early after 6473 patients were randomised, due to the increased risk of major bleeding in patients randomised to vorapaxar, which included intracranial haemorrhage. The study failed to show any difference in its composite end-points.[27]

However, in the phase III TRA-2P (Thrombin Receptor Antagonist in Secondary Prevention of atherothrombotic ischaemic events) study, 26 449 patients with a prior history of myocardial infarction, ischaemic stroke or symptomatic PAD were randomised to vorapaxar or placebo in addition to standard care.[28] Patients randomised to vorapaxar had a significantly reduced risk of sustaining the primary end-point, which was a composite of cardiovascular death, myocardial infarction, stroke or urgent coronary revascularisation (hazard ratio 0.88; 95% confidence interval (CI) 0.82–0.95; $P = 0.001$). This, however, was associated with an increased risk or moderate and severe bleeding complications. In particular, as in the TRACER study, a significantly increased risk of bleeding, including intracranial haemorrhage (ICH), was observed in patients randomised to vorapaxar.

P2Y12 receptor antagonists

Prasugrel is a third-generation thienopyridine, which is more potent, has a faster onset of action and, unlike clopidogrel, its bioconversion is not affected by CYP genetic polymorphisms.[29] In a phase III trial, 3534 patients with ST-elevation myocardial infarction who were due to undergo percutaneous coronary intervention were randomised into a placebo-controlled double-blind trial (TRITON-TIMI38).[30] Prasugrel was more effective than clopidogrel in reducing the primary end-point of cardiovascular death, non-fatal myocardial infarction or stroke. The major bleeding rates were similar apart from increased bleeding after coronary artery bypass graft (CABG) surgery.

Ticagrelor is the first oral reversible P2Y$_{12}$ antagonist, it is a cyclopentyltriazoloprimidine which does not require metabolic activation and may be of value in patients who require to undergo surgery. In the PLatelet Inhibition and Patient Outcomes (PLATO) trial, ticagrelor reduced the incidence of death as a result of cardiovascular causes with no increase in overall major bleeding or bleeding related to CABG compared with clopidogrel. However, it was associated with increased non-CABG major bleeding and non-procedural-related major bleeding after 30 days on study treatment.[31] Ticagrelor was also associated with increased side-effects such as dyspnoea, hypotension and arrhythmias (ventricular pauses). Cangrelor is an intravenous P2Y$_{12}$ antagonist with a very fast onset and short half-life. It may have benefit in patients undergoing cardiac surgery.[32] Further studies are awaited.

EP3 receptor antagonists

Production of prostaglandin E$_2$ by an inflamed plaque potentiates atherothrombosis. Similar to the P2Y$_{12}$ receptor, the platelet EP3 receptor for prostaglandin E$_2$ also inhibits cyclic AMP synthesis, thus resulting in platelet activation. EP3 receptor antagonists such as DG-041 may have the potential to selectively reduce atherothrombosis without increasing the risk of bleeding and are currently being evaluated in clinical trials.[33,34]

Summary: novel antiplatelet agents

At this stage it is unclear if these novel antiplatelet agents will have a role in the treatment of high-risk patients with PAD. It is apparent that they are generally associated with an increased risk of moderate or severe bleeding complications such as intracranial haemorrhage. With the exception of vorapaxar they have not yet been studied in patients with PAD. While the results from the TRA-2P study appear promising, the full cost–benefit analysis is awaited.

Angiogenesis

Therapeutic angiogenesis aims to stimulate the development of new vessels from the pre-existing vasculature in order to bypass occluded segments.[35,36] Angiogenesis is a complex process involving many growth factors interacting to produce the end-result of neovascularisation and reversal of ischaemia. The natural trigger for angiogenesis is hypoxia. Hypoxia induces expression of a variety of growth factors, including vascular endothelial growth factor (VEGF) and angiopoietin-2 (Ang-2). These act on cells located within the basement membrane of capillaries known as pericytes, which play an important role in endothelial cell proliferation, migration and stabilisation. A number of phases are involved in the angiogenesis process (**Fig. 21.4**). In the initiation phase, pericytes detach from the capillaries, basement membrane is degraded by matrix metalloproteinases (MMPs) and plasma proteins extravasate to form a protein-rich matrix in the interstitial space. In the neovascular phase, growth factors up-regulated by hypoxia and released from the extracellular matrix induce proliferation and migration of endothelial cells and pericytes. In the adaptation phase, excessive neovessel network is then trimmed to respond to the metabolic needs of the tissue and vessels that receive insufficient blood flow regress. In the maturation phase, vessels with sufficient flow mature, achieve pericyte coverage and deposit a basement membrane.[37] VEGF is the most potent angiogenic factor and is the most studied gene in trials to date.[38] Other pertinent factors and genes that have been studied are fibroblast growth factor (FGF), hypoxia-inducible factor-1 alpha (HIF-1α), hepatocyte growth factor (HGF) and developmental endothelial locus-1 (Del-1).

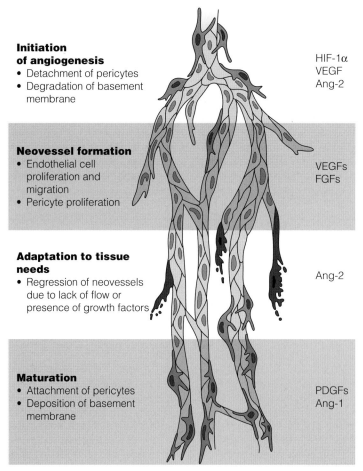

Initiation of angiogenesis
- Detachment of pericytes
- Degradation of basement membrane

HIF-1α
VEGF
Ang-2

Neovessel formation
- Endothelial cell proliferation and migration
- Pericyte proliferation

VEGFs
FGFs

Adaptation to tissue needs
- Regression of neovessels due to lack of flow or presence of growth factors

Ang-2

Maturation
- Attachment of pericytes
- Deposition of basement membrane

PDGFs
Ang-1

Figure 21.4 • Angiogenic growth factors and their effect on the angiogenesis pathway. Ang-1, angiopoietin-1; Ang-2, angiopoietin-2; FGF, fibroblast growth factor; HIF-1α, hypoxia-inducible factor-1 alpha; PDGF, platelet-derived growth factor; VEGF, vascular endothelial growth factor. Reproduced from Markkanen JE, Rissanen TT, Kivela A et al. Growth factor-induced therapeutic angiogenesis and arteriogenesis in the heart–gene therapy. Cardiovasc Res 2005; 65:656–64. With permission from Oxford University Press.

Target genes in use for gene therapy in peripheral arterial disease

A highly specific mitogen for endothelial cells, VEGF is a potent initiator of angiogenesis. Its signal transduction results in endothelial cell proliferation, migration and ultimately new vessel formation.[38] These pro-angiogenic cytokines are a multigene family, of which VEGF-A is the most commonly studied, particularly VEGF-A$_{121}$ and VEGF-A$_{165}$, as these are associated strongly with new vessel formation.[39] Similarly, FGF is a family of heparin-binding polypeptide proteins that are powerful stimulators of angiogenesis. They control the proliferation of endothelial cells, smooth muscle cells and fibroblasts, and the most widely studied FGF, FGF-1, has been shown to play a key role in neoangiogenesis in preclinical trials in vivo.[40,41] A regulator of angiogenesis, HIF-1α, plays a vital role in the cellular response to hypoxia. In the presence of low oxygen tensions, this factor is released and stimulates the production of several pro-angiogenic growth factors, including VEGF-A.[42] Hepatocyte growth factor is a pro-angiogenic growth factor that has a predilection for the stimulation and proliferation of epithelial and endothelial cells.[43] Del-1 is expressed widely during vascular development in the embryonic period. It has the role of encouraging endothelial cell adhesion and preclinical studies have proven its presence in ischaemic tissue, suggesting it has a role as an intermediary of neoangiogenesis[44,45] (Fig. 21.4).

Gene therapy vectors

The identification of the above genes was a major development in the field of gene therapy and the next biggest challenge facing gene therapists is the choice of vector. Vectors allow the carriage of genetic material from an exogenous source to the target cell. The two major limitations are the rates of transfection and the potential to induce an immune response. The vectors in use in clinical trials can be divided into non-viral and viral vectors.

Non-viral methods

Non-viral methods for stimulating angiogenesis make use of naked plasmid DNA. Several advantages are associated with the use of plasmids: ease of production, high yields and, owing to its low immunogenic potential, its safety profile.[46] Despite these advantages, large randomised trials have shown that gene transfer efficiency is low, limiting its overall effect.[47] This has led to a greater focus in developing viral vectors as the method of choice.

Viral methods

Viruses, as part of their replication cycle, will enter the cell and integrate their genetic information with the DNA of the native cell, with subsequent expression of the desired effects. However, they initiate an immune response and older viral types were unable to integrate with cells in the quiescent phase of the cell cycle, which are found abundantly in vascular tissues.[48] The best known and most widely used viral vectors studied come from the family of adenoviruses.[49] These vectors have the associated advantages of: low mutagenesis (as they do not integrate with the host genome); high titres; broad tissue tropism; and ability to induce cells in the quiescent phase.[50] Stimulation of the immune response is, however, unavoidable and this acts to decrease their effectiveness, especially after repeated administrations, accounting for the short-term improvements with poorer longer-term outcomes.[51]

Delivery methods of vectors

The delivery of viral vectors can be directly into the circulation at the time of surgery or endovascular techniques, or by the intra-arterial route, or by the intramuscular route in those patients not suitable for any form of endovascular or surgical approach. Direct intra-arterial administration is limited by its transient response as it is distributed to a wide area, while intramuscular injection has the advantage of local penetration to the area of ischaemia with a longer-lasting response.[52]

Non-viral methods use physical or chemical forces, which are intended to induce cell membrane defects to allow the DNA (in plasmid form) to diffuse and create its effect intracellularly. The physical methods include microinjection, ultrasound and hydrodynamic administration, while chemical approaches use natural or synthetic substances to bind cellular receptors to gain entry into the cell and then interact with the DNA to exert their response. This non-viral method is associated with low transfection rates and transient gene expression. However, its advantages are its ease of use and low immunogenic potential.[37]

Therapeutic angiogenesis has been used in in vitro models, animal models and clinical trials.[53,54] This section will outline the clinical trials that have been conducted and summarise the current issues in the field of gene therapy for PAD (Table 21.1).

Vascular endothelial growth factor (VEGF)

Phase I clinical trials

The first clinical study using vascular endothelial growth factor (VEGF) was conducted in 1996 by Isner and yielded positive results: digital substraction angiography at 4 weeks post-treatment confirmed

Table 21.1 • Methodology employed by the trials assessing gene therapy for peripheral arterial disease

Reference	Year	Administration	Vector	No. of patients	Outcomes
Phase I trials					
VEGF					
Isner et al.[55]	1996	Intra-arterial	Plasmid	1	Collateral vessels, distal flow
Baumgartner et al.[57]	1998	Intramuscular	Plasmid	9	ABPI, collateral vessels, ulcer, healing, distal flow
Rajagopalan et al.[59]	2002	Intramuscular	Virus	18	ABPI, peak walking time
Shyu et al.[56]	2003	Intramuscular	Plasmid	21	ABPI, distal flow, ulcer healing, rest pain
Kim et al.[58]	2004	Intramuscular	Plasmid	9	ABPI, collateral vessels, ulcer, healing, rest pain
FGF					
Comerota et al.[63]	2002	Intramuscular	Plasmid	51	ABPI, ulcer healing, rest pain, transcutaneous oxygen pressure
HGF					
Morishita et al.[66]	2004	Intramuscular	Plasmid	6	ABPI, rest pain, ulcer healing, transcutaneous oxygen pressure
HIF-1α					
Rajagopalan et al.[69]	2007	Intramuscular	Virus	34	Rest pain, ulcer healing
Phase II trials					
VEGF					
Mäkinen et al.[60]	2002	Intra-arterial	Virus/plasmid	54	Distal vascularity
Rajagopalan et al.[61]	2003	Intramuscular	Virus	105	No differences from placebo
Kusumanto et al.[62]	2006	Intramuscular	Plasmid	54	ABPI, ulcer healing
Del-1					
Grossman et al.[71]	2007	Intramuscular	Plasmid	105	ABPI, peak walking time and quality of life
FGF					
Nikol et al.[64]	2008	Intramuscular	Plasmid	125	Amputation rates
HGF					
Powell et al.[67]	2008	Intramuscular	Plasmid	104	Transcutaneous oxygen pressure
Shigematsu et al.[68]	2010	Intramuscular	Plasmid	40	Rest pain, ulcer healing, quality of life
HIF-1α					
Creager et al.[70]	2011	Intramuscular	Virus	289	No differences from placebo
Phase III trials					
Belch et al.[65]	2011	Intramuscular	Plasmid	525	No differences from placebo

increased vessel collateralisation in the ischaemic leg at the knee, mid-tibial and ankle levels, and this was maintained at 3 months; arterial flow was found to be 82% greater and maximum flow was found to be 72% greater than that measured prior to therapy.[55] Magnetic resonance angiography (MRA) performed at 4 and 12 weeks confirmed improvement in distal flow to the pre-existing occlusion to the peroneal and tibial arteries. However, despite the improved blood flow and demonstrable neovascularisation, an amputation of the ischaemic leg was required 5 months post-gene therapy.

In 2003, Shyu et al. published the largest phase I clinical trial to date, involving 21 patients (24 limbs) with severe limb ischaemia.[56] A plasmid vector containing phVEGF$_{165}$ was administered via two intramuscular injections 4 weeks apart. Five different doses were studied. A statistically significant increase in ankle–brachial pressure index (ABPI) was found from pre-therapy values (0.58 ± 0.24 to 0.72 ± 0.28; $P<0.001$). MRA was performed, which showed qualitative evidence of improved distal flow with a mean MRA score of 0.37 ± 0.10 pre-treatment to 0.47 ± 0.11 post-treatment ($P<0.01$). Regression of rest pain was evident in 83% of limbs and improved ulcer healing was reported in 75% of limbs. The optimum dose was found to be 1.6 mg.

Two further trials with VEGF showed significant improvements in ABPI values post-therapy,[57,58] while Rajagopalan et al. noted improved but non-significant increases in ABPI.[59] Significant improvements in rest pain or pain-free walking distance and in distal flow as evidenced by angiography or MRA are supported by other studies that have assessed VEGF.[57,58]

Phase II clinical trials

Three phase II clinical trials using VEGF as the study gene were continued from the positive results obtained from the phase I clinical trials.[60–62] The Regional Angiogenesis with Vascular Endothelial Growth Factor (RAVE) study was the largest phase II randomised, double-blind, placebo-controlled study, consisting of 105 patients with intermittent claudication and critical limb ischaemia (CLI).[61] An adenovirus containing $VEGF_{121}$ was injected intramuscularly into patients. Patients were randomised to receive placebo, 4×10^9 particle units (low dose) or 4×10^{10} particle units (high dose). The study showed no differences in walking distances, quality of life or ABPI.

Kusumanto et al. reported the GRONINGEN trial of 54 patients, which concluded similar findings in that there were no significant differences in ABPI values or rates of ulcer healing, although both did clinically improve.[62] Furthermore, this study also demonstrated that there was no significant difference in amputation rates at 100 days.[60] While the VEGF-PVD trial was able to demonstrate a statistically significant increase in peripheral vascularity downstream from the injection site of the VEGF vector in 54 patients ($P=0.02$), but no statistically significant differences in ABPI, amputation rates or re-stenosis rates. In keeping with the above studies, this study supported the lack of association between VEGF and major amputation rates, ulcer healing, resolution of rest pain or ABPI measurements.

Fibroblast growth factor (FGF)

Phase I clinical trials

Up until 2002, VEGF had dominated the field of gene therapy for PAD. Comerota et al. published the first series of 51 patients treated with CLI undergoing treatment with FGF-type I.[63] Naked DNA encoding for FGF was delivered by intramuscular injections and the dose ranged from 0.5 to 16 mg;

follow-up was for 24 weeks. Statistically significant reductions were obtained in pain scores at 8, 12 and 24 weeks' follow-up ($P=0.001$). Transcutaneous oxygen measurement, a surrogate marker for tissue healing, improved over the 3-month period with significant increases at week 8 ($P=0.035$) and at week 12 ($P=0.0012$), but no final measurement was made at the end of the follow-up at week 24. No significant ABPI difference was noted between groups and no patients had complete healing of their ulcer.

Phase II clinical trials

In the Therapeutic Angiogenesis Leg Ischaemia Study for the Management of Arteriopathy and Non-healing Ulcer (TALISMAN),[64] 125 patients were randomised to receive naked DNA encoding (16 mg, i.m.) or placebo. The risk of all amputations (hazard ratio (HR)=0.498, $P=0.015$) and major amputations (HR=0.371, $P=0.015$) was significantly reduced in patients randomised to FGF. Similar rates of ulcer healing were noted between both groups (19.6% vs. 14.3%, FGF vs. placebo, $P=0.514$). There were no differences noted in ABPI values or pain levels between the treatment and placebo groups.

Phase III clinical trials

In 2011, the first, and only, phase III clinical trial, entitled Therapeutic Angiogenesis for the Management of Arteriopathy in a Randomised International Study (TAMARIS), reported its findings.[65] This randomised, placebo-controlled clinical trial of 525 patients assessed the effect of naked DNA encoding for FGF (16 mg i.m., over four treatment sessions separated by 2-week intervals) on amputation-free survival. At 36 months there was no significant difference between the groups in terms of major amputation and/or death.

Hepatocyte growth factor (HGF)

Phase I clinical trials

In 2004, Morishita et al. were the first to study the effect of HGF as a potential therapy in six patients with CLI.[66] HGF was delivered by an intramuscular injection of a plasmid vector at a dose of 2 mg, which was repeated after 4 weeks. ABPI values increased significantly from baseline (0.426 ± 0.046) to 0.626 ± 0.071 at 4 weeks after the second injection and then to 0.596 ± 0.046 at 8 weeks following the second injection ($P=0.036$). The transcutaneous oxygen levels increased significantly at 12 weeks (21.7 ± 4.5 to 31.2 ± 6.4); of the 11 ulcers present, two healed completely and eight improved, supporting the increase in transcutaneous oxygen levels. Resting pain levels were also noted to have reduced in response to HGF.

Phase II clinical trials

In 2008, Powell et al., in a double-blind, placebo-controlled study (HGF-STAT), randomised 104 patients with CLI to receive: placebo, 0.4 mg of HGF at 0, 14 and 28 days (low dose); 4 mg at 0 and 28 days (middle dose); or 4 mg at 0, 14 and 28 days (high dose) via the i.m. route.[67] Follow-up was for 12 months. At 6 months, the transcutaneous oxygen levels increased significantly in the high-dose subgroup, but there were no improvements in ABPI, pain, ulcer healing or reductions in major amputations.

A multicentre, randomised, double-blind, placebo-controlled clinical trial (HGF-CLI) used HGF to assess the improvement of rest pain in those patients without ulcers and the reduction of ulcer size in patients with ulcers.[68] The results of 40 patients showed that 70.4% in the HGF-treated group versus 30.8% in the placebo group had significant improvement in pain at rest ($P=0.014$) and also a significant improvement in ulcer size with 100% versus 40% (HGF vs. placebo, respectively, $P=0.018$). An improvement in quality of life was observed, but no difference was found between both groups in terms of ABPI values or rates of amputation.

Hypoxia-inducible factor-1α

Phase I clinical trials

In 2007, Rajagopalan et al. were the first to publish phase I trial results on the use of HIF-1α.[69] This was tested in patients with end-stage CLI and was an adenovirus transfected intramuscularly to 34 patients. This study failed to demonstrate any differences in ABPI or blood flow post-treatment using MRA at 6 and 12 months. Clinically significant but statistically insignificant results were observed for the reduction in pain (occurring in 12 of 32 patients at 6 months, increasing to 14 of 32 patients at 12 months) and for ulcer healing (3 of 18 patients at 6 months and 5 of 18 patients at 12 months).

Phase II clinical trials

The only phase II trial assessing HIF-1α (the WALK trial) was published in 2011 and assessed the safety and efficacy of this gene in patients with intermittent claudication.[70] Randomisation of 289 patients to one of three doses of HIF-1α (2×10^9, 2×10^{10}, 2×10^{11} viral particles) or placebo took place by 20 i.m. injections to each leg. Follow-up was for a total of 1 year. The primary end-point of peak walking time increased by 0.82 minutes in the placebo group and by 0.82, 0.28 and 0.78 minutes in the HIF-1α 2×10^9, 2×10^{10}, 2×10^{11} viral particles groups respectively, which failed to achieve statistical significance. There were also no significant differences in claudication onset time, ABPI or quality-of-life assessment between both groups.

Developmental endothelial locus-1 (Del-1)

No phase I studies have been conducted assessing the safety or efficacy of the Del-1 gene.

Phase II clinical trials

This study was the first study to assess the Del-1 gene in the treatment of patients with moderate-to-severe peripheral arterial disease (DELTA-1).[71] Patients ($n=105$) received either placebo or 42 mg of Del-1 administered by an intramuscular injection. This study showed clinically significant benefits in peak walking time, ABPI and quality of life in the Del-1-treated group, but no statistically significant differences were noted from the placebo group.

Summary

The phase II trials and the one phase III trial of gene therapy for peripheral vascular disease have generally, with the exception of FGF, yielded disappointing results. The end-points between the phase I and phase II trials differed due to the fact that some phase II trials included patients with intermittent claudication while the phase I studies tended to involve patients with more severe limb ischaemia. The various gene therapies, methods of delivery and different clinical outcomes make it difficult to compare trials. However, in a meta-analysis of gene therapy in PAD in 2008, Ghosh et al. pooled data from five studies.[72] No differences were found in the following outcomes: peak walking time, claudication onset at 90 and 180 days post-treatment, and change in ABPI at 90 days. It was thought that the placebo response, which is well documented in trials involving patients with claudication may have masked any positive effects of gene therapy.

The complications associated with the stimulation of angiogenesis are currently theoretical and include tumorigenesis, retinal neovascularisation (particularly in diabetic patients), risk of haemorrhage, inflammatory responses and oedema.[49] The safety profile analysis of all the genes used in the phase I to phase III trials has shown the commonest side-effect to be peripheral oedema, which can be managed optimally with medical therapy. There have been no associations as evidenced in the safety analyses of the above trials of increased tumorigenesis, neovascularisation of any non-target sites including the retina, or haemorrhage, but current follow-up has only been to 3 years.

It is likely that future studies will look at combinations of gene and cell-based therapy.

Cell-based therapy

Vasculogenesis refers to the formation of blood vessels from circulating endothelial progenitor cells (EPCs) and vascular progenitor cells. Human blood has been shown to contain EPCs, which can develop into functioning endothelial cells in sites of tissue ischaemia.

The major site of origin of EPCs is the bone marrow. Recent studies on cell-based therapies have used both autologous bone marrow and peripheral blood mononuclear cells. Preclinical studies have shown that implantation of bone marrow-derived mononuclear cells into ischaemic limbs leads to collateral vessel formation and increased concentrations of angiogenic growth factors.

Clinical

The Therapeutic Angiogenesis using Cell Transplantation (TACT) study was the first to assess the possible role of bone marrow-derived mononuclear cells obtained from the iliac crest.[73] In a pilot study, 25 patients with unilateral limb ischaemia were injected with bone marrow cells into the gastrocnemius muscle in one limb and saline into the contralateral limb. At 4 and 24 weeks there was a significant increase in the ABPI, transcutaneous oxygen pressure, rest pain and collateral formation. The same group then randomised 20 patients to receive either bone marrow or peripheral mononuclear cells. Overall, those who received the bone marrow mononuclear cells had significant increases in the ABPI, pain-free walking time, rest pain, transcutaneous oxygen pressure and collateral formation at 4 and 24 weeks. However, it was noted that one-third of patients failed to respond.

Granulocyte macrophage colony-stimulating factor pre-treatment

Granulocyte colony-stimulating factor (G-CSF) can mobilise stem cells from the bone marrow to the circulation. Preclinical models showed beneficial effects of G-CSF on collateral artery growth in the peripheral circulation. G-CSF has also been shown to increase collateral flow index in patients with coronary artery disease. In a randomised trial involving 39 patients with PAD, GM-CSF was associated with improvement in symptoms, ABPI and transcutaneous oxygen pressure.[74] In the STimulation of ARTeriogenesis trial (START), GM-CSF was injected subcutaneously in 40 patients with intermittent claudication in a randomised placebo-controlled manner.[75] Both the placebo group and the treatment group showed a significant increase in walking distance at day 14, but the change in walking time did not differ between groups. In 2007, Huang et al. assessed the safety, efficacy and feasibility of the use of autologous transplantation of peripheral blood mononuclear cells (PBMNCs) in 28 patients with CLI who had received G-CSF.[76] Patients randomised to the active group received subcutaneous injections of recombinant human G-CSF for 5 days to mobilise progenitor cells, and then their PBMNCs were collected and injected intramuscularly into the ischaemic limb. At 3-months patients who received G-CSF PBMNC experienced reduced lower limb pain, improvement in ulcer healing, Doppler blood perfusion of lower limbs ($P<0.001$) and ABPI ($P<0.001$) were significantly improved in the G-CSF PBMNC group. Further work is required to determine if, as suggested from this pilot study, treatment of autologous bone marrow mononuclear cells with G-CSF is of value.

Summary

In 2009, De Haro et al. pooled the data from six studies including cell-based and gene therapies.[77] A meta-analysis of a total of 543 patients found that clinical improvement (defined as peak walking time, resolution of rest pain, ulcer healing and limb salvage) was significantly higher in the treatment group compared with placebo (odds ratio (OR)=1.437, 95% CI 1.03–2.00, $P=0.033$). Stratifying patients into those with claudication and those with CLI, it was seen that clinical benefit could not be demonstrated with significance for claudicants ($P=0.16$), but significant associations were deduced in patients with CLI (OR=2.20, 95% CI 1.01–4.79, $P=0.046$; **Fig. 21.5**). Thus, it was concluded that patients with CLI have symptomatic benefit when treated with gene or cell-based therapy.

Preventing neointimal hyperplasia

The medium- and long-term benefit of surgical or endovascular revascularisation is limited by the development of neointimal hyperplasia. Twenty per cent of vein grafts will occlude within 1–18 months after surgery, primarily as a result of intimal hyperplasia.[78] This is also an issue following angioplasty were the primary patency rates are 90% for iliac lesions and 53% for the superficial femoral artery at 4 years.[79]

Intimal hyperplasia represents an abnormal response to injury, with endothelial damage leading to tissue factor release, platelet and monocyte activation, adhesion and an ongoing inflammatory response that includes increased matrix metalloproteinase activation.[80] Vascular smooth muscle cells (VSMCs), which are the predominant

	Statistics for each study					Odds ratio and 95% CI
	Odds ratio	Lower limit	Upper limit	Z-Value	p-Value	
MAKINEN K	1,103	0,243	5,017	0,127	0,899	
TACT	2,821	0,143	6,961	2,250	0,024	
	2,205	0,015	4,790	1,998	0,048	

0,01 0,1 1 10 100

Favour placebo   Favour TA

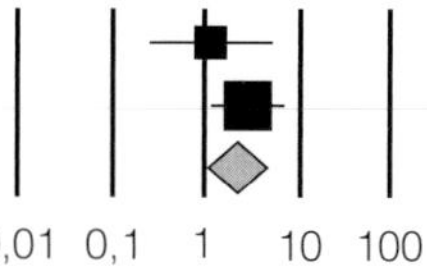

Figure 21.5 • Meta-analysis of patients with CLI and the benefit of gene and cell therapy. Reproduced from De Haro J, Acin F, Lopez-Quintana A et al. Meta-analysis of randomised, controlled clinical trials in angiogenesis: gene and cell therapy in peripheral arterial disease. Heart Vessels 2009; 24:321–8. With permission from Springer.

cell type in neointimal hyperplasia, proliferate and migrate from the media to the intima.[80] In order to migrate, VSMCs alter their phenotype from contractile to proliferative.[81,82] Mitogen-activated protein kinases play an essential role in this process and, in particular, extracellular regulated kinase (ERK) 1/2 is involved in the final step of the mitogen-activated protein kinase cascade. This is essential for signalling the stimulus to VSMC proliferation and is activated by mitogens such as platelet-derived growth factor (PDGF).[83]

Gene therapy may have a role in inhibiting this process through targeting smooth muscle migration, proliferation or apotosis. Potential therapeutic genes may be applied ex vivo to the vein graft, as will be discussed below. Likewise, delivery of gene therapy from stents has been achieved in a number of studies using antibody binding of the gene vector or through the development of various stent surface formulations to which the vectors are bound and then released.

Vein grafts

The studies involving gene therapy to date have all involved preclinical studies involving human vein in vitro studies or animal models. Tissue inhibitors of matrix metalloproteinases have been shown to reduce neointimal formation,[84] as have studies involving adenoviral gene transfer of nitric oxide synthase[85] or P53.[86]

To date, there are no clinical studies aimed at increasing gene expression within vein grafts but there have been a series of phase I–III trials using a synthetic oligonucleotide gene inhibitor, which is discussed below. EF-2 is a transcription factor that leads to up-regulation of a number of cell cycle genes. Inhibition via the E2F decoy oligodeoxynucleotide edifoligide has led to significantly reduced neointimal hyperplasia formation in a rabbit model.

Edifoligide and the PREVENT (Project of Ex Vivo Vein Graft Engineering via Transfection) trials

Gene inhibition strategies have a number of potential benefits in that small, synthetic oligonucleotides can be delivered easily without the need for specific vectors.

In the phase I PREVENT study, 41 patients undergoing lower limb bypass were randomised to E2F decoy oligodeoxynucleotide or saline.[87] E2F decoy was delivered by an ex vivo pressure-mediated transfection that did not involve distending the veins. The treatment was found to be feasible and safe. Mean transfection efficiency was high (89%) and accompanied by inhibition of cell cycle gene expression and DNA replication. Although clinical outcome was not an end-point, patients in the E2F decoy-treated group had fewer graft occlusions, revisions or critical stenosis.

In the phase II PREVENT study, 200 patients undergoing CABG were randomised to receive ex vivo E2F decoy or saline.[88] There were no adverse events or complications, and a significant 30% reduction in critical stenosis was observed in the E2F group.

In the phase III PREVENT study, 1404 patients with CLI were randomised in a multicentre, double-blind, placebo-controlled trial of ex vivo E2F decoy.[89] The primary outcome was graft failure at 1 year. There was no difference observed in the primary or secondary end-points of primary graft patency or limb salvage. A significant but non-clinical improvement was observed in secondary graft patency rates.

The PREVENT IV trial randomised 3014 patients undergoing CABG surgery to ex vivo E2F decoy.[90] No difference was found in the primary outcome or critical stenosis at 1 year.

Gene-eluting stents

In animal models a number of genes have been shown to reduce in-stent stenosis. These include

VEGF, inducible nitric oxide synthetase and tissue inhibitors of matrix metalloproteinases.

Clinical trials

Stent-based gene therapy has the potential to prevent neointimal hyperplasia and yet preserve the integrity of the endothelium. However, to date there have only been two phase I studies involving VEGF transfer via an infusion–perfusion catheter. There have been no studies involving gene-eluting stents in either coronary or peripheral arterial disease patients.[91]

Overall summary

While several novel therapeutic cholesterol-lowering and antiplatelet agents are currently under investi-gation, many of these have not yet been specifically studied in patients with PAD. We await the outcome of ongoing trials to determine if these novel therapies will have a future role in the treatment of high-risk patients.

It is encouraging that there are ongoing new strat-egies and therapies for treating patients with CLI. However, in the new fields of gene therapy or pro-genitor cell therapy it is clear that there are still many issues that need to be addressed, such as the optimal dose, mode of delivery, single or combina-tion therapy. It may also be possible to use gene or progenitor cell therapy in patients who are suitable for revascularisation in order to improve durability and patency rates. Further studies are required to determine if gene and cell-based therapy are viable therapeutic options for the treatment of PAD.

Key points

- Low levels of HDL cholesterol are associated with increased risk of cardiac events. Trials are currently underway to determine if improving HDL cholesterol in patients already on effective statin therapy levels will lead to clinical benefit.
- The novel antiplatelet therapies may have a role in reducing cardiac and thrombotic events in the treatment of high-risk PAD patients. However, with the exception of vorapaxar they have not been evaluated in patients with PAD.
- Further studies in the area of gene and progenitor cell therapy are required to address outstanding issues before these treatments can be considered as viable options in the treatment of PAD.
- Further studies are required to determine if gene therapy has a role in inhibiting the development of neointimal hyperplasia.

References

1. Gordon DJ, Probstfield JL, Garrison RJ, et al. High-density lipoprotein cholesterol and cardiovas-cular disease: four prospective American studies. Circulation 1989;79:8–15.

2. Hanniman EA, Sinal CJ. Nuclear receptors: novel therapeutic targets for the treatment and preven-tion of atherosclerosis. Drug Discovery Today: Therapeutic Strategies 2004;1:155–61.

3. Navab M, Reddy ST, Van Lenten BJ, et al. HDL and cardiovascular disease: atherogenic and atheroprotec-tive mechanisms. Nat Rev Cardiol 2011;8:222–32.

4. Onat A, Hergenc G. Low-grade inflammation, and dysfunction of high-density lipoprotein and its apolipoproteins as a major driver of cardiometabolic risk. Metab Clin Exp 2011;60:499–512.

5. Barter PJ, Caulfield M, Eriksson M, et al. Effects of Torcetrapib in patients at high risk for coronary events. N Engl J Med 2007;357:2109–22.

6. Niesor EJ. Different effects of compounds decreasing cholesteryl ester transfer protein activity on lipopro-tein metabolism. Curr Opin Lipidol 2011;22:288–95.

7. Cannon CP, Shah S, Dansky HM, et al. Safety of Anacetrapib in patients with or at high risk for coro-nary heart disease. N Engl J Med 2010;363:2406–15.

8. Clinical Trial Service Unit (Oxford University). Randomised evaluation of the effects of anacetrapib through lipid modification (REVEAL). Available at http://www.ctsu.ox.ac.uk/reveal/index.htm; [ac-cessed 26.02.12].

9. Canner PL, Berge KG, Wenger NK, et al. Fifteen year mortality in Coronary Drug Project patients: long-term benefit with niacin. J Am Coll Cardiol 1986;8:1245–55.

10. University of Oxford Clinical Trial Service Unit. Treatment of HDL to Reduce the Incidence of Vascular Events (HPS2 THRIVE). Available at http://www.thrivestudy.org; [accessed 26.02.12].

11. The AIM-HIGH Investigators. Niacin in patients with low HDL cholesterol levels receiving intensive statin therapy. N Engl J Med 2011;365:2255–67.

12. Sherman CB, Peterson SJ, Frishman WH. Apolipoprotein A-I mimetic peptides: a potential new therapy for the prevention of atherosclerosis. Cardiol Rev 2010;18:141–7.

13. Bloedon LT, Dunbar R, Duffy D. Safety, pharma-cokinetics, and pharmacodynamics of oral apoA-I

mimetic peptide D-4F in high-risk cardiovascular patients. J Lipid Res 2008;49:1344–52.

14. Rosenson RS. Phospholipase A2 inhibition and atherosclerotic vascular disease: prospects for targeting secretory and lipoprotein-associated phospholipase A2 enzymes. Curr Opin Lipidol 2010;21: 473–80.

15. Garcia-Garcia HM, Serruys PW. Phospholipase A2 inhibitors. Curr Opin Lipidol 2009;20:327–32.

16. Rosenson RS, Hislop C, McConnell D, et al. Effects of 1-H-indole-3-glyoxamide (A-002) on concentration of secretory phospholipase A2 (PLASMA study): a phase II double-blind, randomised, placebo controlled trial. Lancet 2009;373:649–58.

17. Rosenson RS, Elliott M, Stasiv Y, et al. Randomized trial of an inhibitor of secretory phospholipase A_2 on atherogenic lipoprotein subclasses in statin-treated patients with coronary heart disease. Eur Heart J 2011;32:999–1005.

18. ClincialTrials.gov. VISTA-16 Trial: evaluation of safety and efficacy of short-term A-002 treatment in subjects with acute coronary syndrome. Available at http://clinicaltrials.gov/ct2/show/NCT01130246; [accessed 26.02.12].

19. Mohler ER, Ballantyne CM, Davidson MH, et al. The effect of Darapladib on plasma lipoprotein-associated phospholipase A2 activity and cardiovascular biomarkers in patients with stable coronary heart disease or coronary heart disease risk equivalent. J Am Coll Cardiol 2008;51:1632–41.

20. Serruys PW, García-García HM, Buszman P, et al. Effects of the direct lipoprotein-associated phospholipase A_2 inhibitor darapladib on human coronary atherosclerotic plaque. Circulation 2008;118:1172–82.

21. ClinicalTrials.gov. The stabilization of atherosclerotic plaque by initiation of Darapladib therapy trial (STABILITY). Available at http://clinical trials.gov/ct2/show/NCT00799903; [accessed 26.02.12].

22. ClinicalTrials.gov. The stabilization of plaques using Darapladib – thrombolysis in myocardial infarction 52 trial (SOLID-TIMI 52). Available at http://clinicaltrials.gov/ct2/show/NCT01000727; [accessed 26.02.12].

23. De Labriolle A, Doazan JP, Lemesle G, et al. Genotypic and phenotypic assessment of platelet function and response to P2Y12 antagonists. Curr Cardiol Rep 2011;13:439–50.

24. Leonardi S, Tricoci P, Becker C. Thrombin receptor antagonists for the treatment of atherothrombosis: therapeutic potential of vorapaxar and E-555 (Review). Drugs 2010;70:1771–83.

25. Becker RC, Moliterno DJ, Jennings LK, et al. Safety and tolerability of SCH 530348 in patients undergoing non-urgent percutaneous coronary intervention: a randomized, double-blind, placebo-controlled phase II study. Lancet 2009;373:919–28.

26. Goto S, Ogawa H, Takeuchi M, et al. Double-blind, placebo-controlled Phase II studies of the protease-activated receptor 1 antagonist E5555 (atopaxar) in Japanese patients with acute coronary syndrome or high-risk coronary artery disease. Eur Heart J 2010;31:2601–13.

27. Tricoci P, Huang Z, Held C, et al. Thrombin receptor antagonist Vorapaxar in acute coronary syndromes. N Engl J Med 2012;366:20–33.

28. Morrow DA, Braunwald E, Bonaca MP, et al. Vorapaxar in the secondary prevention of atherothrombotic events. N Engl J Med 2012;366(15):1404–13.

29. Oliphant CS, Doby JB, Blade CL, et al. Emerging P2Y12 receptor antagonists: role in coronary artery disease. Curr Vasc Pharmacol 2010;8:93–101.

30. Montalescot G, Wiviott SD, Braunwald E, et al. Prasugrel compared with clopidogrel in patients undergoing percutaneous coronary intervention for ST-elevation myocardial infarction (TRITON-TIMI 38): double-blind, randomised controlled trial. Lancet 2009;373:723–31.

31. Becker RC, Bassand JP, Budaj A, et al. Bleeding complications with the P2Y12 receptor antagonists clopidogrel and ticagrelor in the PLATelet inhibition and patient Outcomes (PLATO) trial. Eur Heart J 2011;32:2933–44.

32. Angiolillo DJ, Firstenberg MS, Price MJ, et al. Bridging antiplatelet therapy with cangrelor in patients undergoing cardiac surgery. A randomized controlled trial. JAMA 2012;307:265–74.

33. Fabre JE, Gurney ME. Limitations of current therapies to prevent thrombosis: a need for novel strategies. Mol Biosyst 2010;6:305–15.

34. Singh J, Zellert W, Zhou N, et al. Antagonists of the EP3 receptor for prostaglandin E2 are novel antiplatelet agents that do not prolong bleeding. ACS Chem Biol 2009;4:115–26.

35. Carmeliet P. Angiogenesis in health and disease. Nat Med 2003;9:653–60.

36. Helisch A, Schaper W. Angiogenesis and arteriogenesis – not yet for prescription. Z Kardiol 2000;89:239–44.

37. Dvorak HF, Brown LF, Detmar M, et al. Vascular permeability factor/vascular endothelial growth factor, microvascular hyperpermeability, and angiogenesis. Am J Pathol 1995;146:1029–39.

38. Markkanen JE, Rissanen TT, Kivela A, et al. Growth factor-induced therapeutic angiogenesis and arteriogenesis in the heart – gene therapy. Cardiovasc Res 2005;65:656–64.

39. Latham AM, Molina-Paris C, Homer-Vanniasinkam S, et al. An integrative model for vascular endothelial growth factor A as a tumour biomarker. Integr Biol 2010;2:397–407.

40. Murakami M, Simons M. Fibroblast growth factor regulation of neovascularisation. Curr Opin Hematol 2008;15:215–20.

41. Baffour R, Berman J, Garb JL, et al. Enhanced angiogenesis and growth of collaterals by in vivo administration of recombinant basic fibroblast growth factor in a rabbit model of acute lower limb ischaemia: dose–response effect of basic fibroblast growth factor. J Vasc Surg 1992;16:181–91.

42. Hirota K, Semenza GL. Regulation of angiogenesis by hypoxia-inducible factor 1. Crit Rev Oncol Hematol 2006;59:15–26.

43. Galimi F, Brizzi MF, Comoglio PM. The hepatocyte growth factor and its receptor. Stem Cells 1993;11:22–30.

44. Penta K, Varner JA, Liaw L, et al. Del1 induces integrin signaling and angiogenesis by ligation of alphaVbeta3. J Biol Chem 1999;274:11101–9.

45. Ho HK, Jang JJ, Kaji S, et al. Developmental endothelial locus 1 (Del-1), a novel angiogenic protein: its role in ischemia. Circulation 2004;109:1314–9.

46. Rissanen TT, Ylä-Herttuala S. Current status of cardiovascular gene therapy. Mol Ther 2007;15:1233–47.

47. Kastrup J, Jorgensen E, Ruck A, et al. Direct intramyocardial plasmid vascular endothelial growth factor-A165 gene therapy in patients with stable sever angina pectoris. A randomised double-blind placebo-controlled study: the Euroinject One trial. J Am Coll Cardiol 2005;45:982–8.

48. Gaffney MM, Hynes SO, Barry F, et al. Cardiovascular gene therapy: current status and therapeutic potential. Br J Pharmacol 2007;152:175–88.

49. Yla-Herttuala S, Alitalo K. Gene transfer as a tool to induce therapeutic vascular growth. Nat Med 2003;9:694–701.

50. Varenne O, Pislaru S, Gillijns H, et al. Local adenovirus-mediated transfer of human endothelial nitric oxide synthase reduces luminal narrowing after coronary angioplasty in pigs. Circulation 1998;98:919–26.

51. Mughal NA, Russell DA, Ponnambalam S. Gene therapy in the treatment of peripheral arterial disease. Br J Surg 2012;99:6–15.

52. Mack CA, Magovern CJ, Budenbender KT, et al. Salvage angiogenesis induced by adenovirus-mediated gene transfer of vascular endothelial growth factor protects against ischaemic vascular occlusion. J Vasc Surg 1998;27:699–709.

53. Van-Royen N, Piek JJ, Buschmann I, et al. Stimulation of arteriogenesis: a new concept for the treatment of arterial occlusive disease. Cardiovasc Res 2001;49:543–53.

54. Laitinen M, Zachary I, Breier G, et al. VEGF gene transfer reduces intimal thickening via increased production of nitric oxide in carotid arteries. Hum Gene Ther 1997;8:1737–44.

55. Isner JM, Pieczek A, Schainfeld R, et al. Clinical evidence of angiogenesis after arterial gene transfer of phVEGF165 in patient with ischaemic limb. Lancet 1996;348:370–4.

56. Shyu KG, Chang H, Wang BW, et al. Intramuscular endothelial growth factor gene therapy in patients with chronic critical leg ischemia. Am J Med 2003;114:85–92.

57. Baumgartner I, Pieczek A, Manor O, et al. Constitutive expression of phVEGF165 after intramuscular gene transfer promotes collateral vessel development in patients with critical limb ischaemia. Circulation 1998;97:1114–23.

58. Kim HJ, Jang SY, Park JI, et al. Vascular endothelial growth factor-induced angiogenic gene therapy in patients with peripheral artery disease. Exp Mol Med 2004;36:336–44.

59. Rajagopalan S, Trachtenberg J, Mohler E, et al. Phase I study of direct administration of a replication deficient adenovirus vector containing the vascular endothelial growth factor cDNA (CI-1023) to patients with claudication. Am J Cardiol 2002;90:512–6.

60. Mäkinen K, Manninen H, Hedman M, et al. Increased vascularity detected by digital subtraction angiography after VEGF gene transfer to human lower limb artery: a randomised, placebo-controlled double-blinded phase II study. Mol Ther 2002;6:127–33.

61. Rajagopalan S, Mohler III ER, Lederman RJ, et al. Regional angiogenesis with vascular endothelial growth factor in peripheral arterial disease: a phase II randomised, double-blind, controlled study of adenoviral delivery of vascular endothelial growth factor 121 in patients with disabling intermittent claudication. Circulation 2003;108:1933–8.

62. Kusumanto YH, van Weel V, Mulder NH, et al. Treatment with intramuscular vascular endothelial growth factor gene compared with placebo for patients with diabetes mellitus and critical limb ischaemia: a double-blind randomised trial. Hum Gene Ther 2006;17:683–91.

63. Comerota AJ, Throm RC, Miller KA. Naked plasmid DNA encoding fibroblast growth factor type 1 for the treatment of end-stage unreconstructible lower extremity ischaemia: preliminary results of a phase I trial. J Vasc Surg 2002;35: 930–6.

64. Nikol S, Baumgartner I, Van Belle E, et al. Therapeutic angiogenesis with intramuscular NV1FGF improves amputation-free survival in patients with critical limb ischaemia. Mol Ther 2008;16:972–8.

65. Belch J, Hiatt WR, Baumgartner I, et al. Effect of fibroblast growth factor NV1FGF on amputation and death: a randomised placebo-controlled trial of gene therapy in critical limb ischaemia. Lancet 2011;377:1929–37.

66. Morishita R, Aoki M, Hashiya N, et al. Safety evaluation of clinical gene therapy using hepatocyte growth factor to treat peripheral arterial disease. Hypertension 2004;44:203–9.

67. Powell RJ, Simons M, Mendelsohn FO, et al. Results of a double-blind, placebo-controlled study to assess

the safety of intramuscular injection of hepatocyte growth factor plasmid to improve limb perfusion in patients with critical limb ischaemia. Circulation 2008;118:58–65.

68. Shigematsu H, Yasuda K, Iwai T, et al. Randomised, double-blind, placebo-controlled clinical trial of hepatocyte growth factor plasmid for critical limb ischaemia. Gene Ther 2010;17:1152–61.

69. Rajagopalan S, Olin J, Deitcher S, et al. Use of a consitutively hypoxia-inducible factor-1 alpha transgene as a therapeutic strategy in no-option critical limb ischaemia patients: phase I dose-escalation experience. Circulation 2007;115:1234–43.

70. Creager MA, Olin JW, Belch JJF, et al. Effect of hypoxia-inducible factor 1 alpha gene therapy on walking performance in patients with intermittent claudication. Circulation 2011;124:1765–73.

71. Grossman PM, Mendelsohn F, Henry TD, et al. Results from a phase II multicenter, double-blind placebo-controlled study of Del-1 (VLTS-589) for intermittent claudication in subjects with peripheral arterial disease. Am Heart J 2007;153:874–80.

72. Ghosh R, Walsh SR, Tang TY, et al. Gene therapy as a novel therapeutic option in the treatment of peripheral vascular disease: systematic review and meta-analysis. Int J Clin Pract 2008;62:1383–90.

73. Taiteishi-Yuyama E, Matsubara H, Murohara T, et al. Therapeutic angiogenesis for patients with limb ischaemia by autologous transplantation of bone marrow cells: a pilot study and a randomised controlled trial. Lancet 2002;360:427–435.

74. Arai M, Misao Y, Nagai H, et al. Granulocyte colony stimulating factor: a noninvasive regeneration therapy for treating atherosclerotic peripheral artery disease. Circ J 2006;70:1093–8.

75. Van Royen N, Schirmer SH, Ataserver B, et al. START trial. A pilot study on stimulation of arterogenesis using subcutaneous application of granulocyte macrophage colony stimulating factor as a new treatment for peripheral artery disease. Circulation 2005;112:1040–6.

76. Huang P, Li S, Han M, et al. Autologous transplantation of granulocyte colony stimulating factor-mobilised peripheral blood mononuclear cells improves critical limb ischaemia in diabetes. Diabetes Care 2005;28:2155–60.

77. De Haro J, Acin F, Lopez-Quintana A, et al. Meta-analysis of randomised, controlled clinical trials in angiogenesis: gene and cell therapy in peripheral arterial disease. Heart Vessels 2009;24:321–8.

78. Mills JL. Mechanism of vein graft failure: the location, distribution and characteristics of lesions that predispose to graft failure. Semin Vasc Surg 1993;6:78–91.

79. Balzer JO, Thalhammer A, Khan V, et al. Angioplasty of the pelvic and femoral arteries in PAOD: results and review of the literature. Eur J Radiol 2010;75:48–56.

80. Varty K, Porter K, Bell PR, et al. Vein morphology and bypass graft stenosis. Br J Surg 1996;10:1375–79.

81. Macleod DC, Strauss BH, De Jong M, et al. Proliferation and extracellular matrix synthesis of smooth muscle cells cultured from human coronary atherosclerotic and restenotic lesions. J Am Coll Cardiol 1994;23:59–65.

82. Huang B, Dryer T, Heidt M, et al. Insulin and local growth factor PDGF induce intimal hyperplasia in bypass graft culture models of saphenous vein and internal mammary artery. Eur J Cardiothorac Surg 2002;21:1002–8.

83. Che W, Abe J, Yoshizumi M, et al. p160 Bcr mediates platelet derived growth factor activation of extracellular signal related kinase in vascular smooth muscle cells. Circulation 2001;104:1399–1406.

84. Akowuah EF, Gray C, Lawrie A, et al. Ultrasound-mediated delivery of TIMP-3 plasmid DNA into saphenous vein leads to increased lumen size in a porcine interposition graft model. Gene Ther 2005;12:1154–7.

85. Cooney R, Hynes SO, Sharif F, et al. Effect of gene delivery of NOS isoforms on intimal hyperplasia and endothelial regeneration after balloon injury. Gene Ther 2006;14:396–404.

86. Wan S, George SJ, Nicklin SA, et al. Overexpression of p53 increases lumen size and blocks neointima formation in porcine interposition vein grafts. Mol Ther 2004;9:689–98.

87. Mann MJ, Whitmore AD, Donaldson MC, et al. Ex vivo gene therapy of human bypass grafts with E2F decoy: the PREVENT single-centre, randomised, controlled trial. Lancet 1999;354(9189):1493–8.

88. Grube E, Felderhoff T, Fitzgerald PJ, et al. Genetic manipulation of human coronary artery bypass grafts with E2F decoy (cgt003) reduces clinical graft failure – results of the randomized, controlled PREVENT II trial (abstract). Late Breaking Clinical Trials American Heart Association; 2001.

89. Conte MS, Bandyk DF, Clowes AW, et al., PREVENT III investigators. Results of PREVENT III: a multicentre, randomized controlled trial of edifoligide for the prevention of vein graft failure in lower limb extremity bypass surgery. J Vasc Surg 2006;43:742–51.

90. Alexander JH, Hafley G, Harrington RA, et al. Efficacy and safety of edifoligide, an E2F transcription factor decoy, for prevention of vein graft failure following coronary artery bypass graft surgery – PREVENT IV: a randomized controlled trial. JAMA 2005;294:2446–54.

91. Attanasio S, Snell J. Therapeutic angiogenesis in the management of critical limb ischaemia: current concepts and review. Cardiol Rev 2009;17:115–20.

Index

NB: Page numbers followed by *f* indicate figures, *t* indicate tables and *b* indicate boxes.

B

Index

W

X